Practical Orthopedic Examination Made Easy®

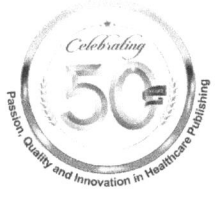

Practical Orthopedic Examination Made Easy®

Third Edition

Manish Kumar Varshney
MS (Ortho) DNB (Ortho Surg) MNAMS MRCS (Glasgow)
Senior Consultant Orthopedic Surgeon
SMVD Narayana Superspeciality Hospital
Reasi, Jammu and Kashmir, India

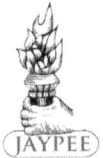

JAYPEE BROTHERS MEDICAL PUBLISHERS
The Health Sciences Publisher
New Delhi | London

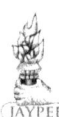
Jaypee Brothers Medical Publishers (P) Ltd.

Headquarters
Jaypee Brothers Medical Publishers (P) Ltd.
4838/24, Ansari Road, Daryaganj
New Delhi 110 002, India
Phone: +91-11-43574357
Fax: +91-11-43574314
Email: jaypee@jaypeebrothers.com

Overseas Office
JP Medical Ltd.
83, Victoria Street, London
SW1H 0HW (UK)
Phone: +44 20 3170 8910
Fax: +44 (0)20 3008 6180
E-mail: info@jpmedpub.com

Website: www.jaypeebrothers.com
Website: www.jaypeedigital.com

© 2020, Jaypee Brothers Medical Publishers

The views and opinions expressed in this book are solely those of the original contributor(s)/author(s) and do not necessarily represent those of editor(s) of the book.

All rights reserved. No part of this publication may be reproduced, stored or transmitted in any form or by any means, electronic, mechanical, photocopying, recording or otherwise, without the prior permission in writing of the publishers.

All brand names and product names used in this book are trade names, service marks, trademarks or registered trademarks of their respective owners. The publisher is not associated with any product or vendor mentioned in this book.

Medical knowledge and practice change constantly. This book is designed to provide accurate, authoritative information about the subject matter in question. However, readers are advised to check the most current information available on procedures included and check information from the manufacturer of each product to be administered, to verify the recommended dose, formula, method and duration of administration, adverse effects and contraindications. It is the responsibility of the practitioner to take all appropriate safety precautions. Neither the publisher nor the author(s)/editor(s) assume any liability for any injury and/or damage to persons or property arising from or related to use of material in this book.

This book is sold on the understanding that the publisher is not engaged in providing professional medical services. If such advice or services are required, the services of a competent medical professional should be sought.

Every effort has been made where necessary to contact holders of copyright to obtain permission to reproduce copyright material. If any have been inadvertently overlooked, the publisher will be pleased to make the necessary arrangements at the first opportunity. The **CD/DVD-ROM** (if any) provided in the sealed envelope with this book is complimentary and free of cost. **Not meant for sale**.

Inquiries for bulk sales may be solicited at: jaypee@jaypeebrothers.com

Practical Orthopedic Examination Made Easy®

First Edition: 2009
Second Edition: 2012
Third Edition: **2020**
ISBN: 978-93-89188-99-8

Dedicated to

*All my students, my teachers from
whom I learned Orthopedics,
both my sons—Siddhant and Mrigank
who taught me how to teach,
and my loving wife—Neeta
who spared me from my homely duties
while being engaged in preparing this book.*

PREFACE TO THE THIRD EDITION

The book *Practical Orthopedic Examination Made Easy* has received tremendous response from the orthopedic students and it provides relevant viva voce reading material for preparation for most of the orthopedic cases given in a standard practical evaluation. With changing times and growing need for better understanding of the concepts, it has been a continuous demand from the students to incorporate figures and include some of the cases. The third edition precisely includes the same and aims to improve the preparation of students for practical examination. A new chapter on reading an X-ray has been added along with the addition of new cases like tuberculosis of knee joint, foot drop, and deltoid contracture. Lots of questions with relevant answers have been added for hip cases. All these are amply supplemented with adequate figures.

I hope the book continues to meet the expectation for orthopedic students in their endeavor to become fantastic clinicians and surgeons.

Manish Kumar Varshney

PREFACE TO THE FIRST EDITION

The first edition of *Practical Orthopedic Examination Made Easy* has emerged after giving immense thought over the imminent need for a text that could serve to guide the postgraduates in the field for preparing through the ultimate acknowledgment of degree. The book specifically serves the stratified group of people preparing for orthopedic practical examinations, but also it does help a beginner in the field; gain theoretical knowledge and grab some basics often not found in modern orthopedic textbooks.

It has been an endeavor to keep the text as simple and directed to maintain interest of the reader. Also preservation of continuity in the text and standardization of information has been specifically dealt with. This gives an advantage for reader rehearse the examination scenario virtually and identify weaknesses to improve upon and strengths to maintain. While providing the most frequently asked questions and the 'expected' answers, consideration has also been given to some uncommon or unique questions with diligent answers. I have tried to provide as non-controversial an answer as possible with direct impact on the next possible questions while simultaneously being adequate. Still, some controversial answers are detailed and are expected to be accepted by prevailing popular choice.

The examination points given at the beginning of every region serve as a quick synopsis along with comments on some uncommon tests that are still uncommonly asked. Figures have deliberately been omitted to make the material less bulky which considering the same are easily found in standard textbooks for orthopedic clinical examination. This work should be perceived in the deserved perspective and is not expected to substitute the standard orthopedic textbooks that have been the masterpieces in the field. When read as contemporary to the standard textbooks, this work helps one understand the meaning of 'reading between lines' that is often the basis of some formidable questions stumbling even some avid book lovers. Organization of the book into regional affections and pertinent cases is more deliberate than accidental considering the relevance of 'regions' to examination cases. Some short cases however, have to be clubbed into miscellaneous section as they are either common to various sections or are full sections by themselves. Named signs, tests, procedures have been kept only to bare minimum necessary level as they are stressed only by an exceptionally uncommon unrealistic examiner unless one heads for a gold medal. No work is impeccable (that's why future editions follow) and readers' comments are delightfully welcome to improve upon the present text.

I personally wish appreciation to the various chapter contributors, colleagues and my seniors and junior residents in bringing this book to fruition in a timely manner. Particularly the constructive criticism and helpful suggestions given by Dr Mohit Singh in formatting the book needs mention. The book is a concise upshot of training and teaching from the expert and experienced teachers at Department of Orthopedics, All India Institute of Medical Sciences to whom I am grateful.

All my sincere dedications and gratitude towards my wife Mrs Neeta Verma, will always fall short of the immense help I received from her in preparing the major part of this work.

Finally, I am highly indebted to the dedicated team of M/s Jaypee Brothers Medical Publishers (P) Ltd, New Delhi, India for giving constant encouragement and sage advice in the preparation of this book.

I wish the readers astounding success in examinations and accomplishments!

Manish Kumar Varshney

CONTENTS

1. **How to Approach Examinations?** 1
   - What is Expected in Examinations? *1*
   - How to Prepare for Examinations? *3*
   - Do's and Don'ts in Examinations *3*
   - How to Read this Book? *4*

2. **The Hip** 6
   - Examination Points for a Hip Case *6*
   - Case I: Tuberculosis of Hip Joint *45*
   - Case II: Nonunion Fractured Neck of Femur (The Unsolved Fracture—Speed) *62*
   - Case III: Osteonecrosis of Femoral Head *77*
   - Case IV: Perthes Disease *89*
   - Case V: Congenital and Developmental Coxa Vara *99*
   - Case VI: Slipped Capital Femoral Epiphysis *102*
   - Case VII: Late Sequelae of Septic Arthritis of Hip Joint *105*
   - Case VIII: Developmental Dysplasia of Hip *111*
   - Case IX: Poliomyelitis Affection of Hip *125*
   - Case X: Old Unreduced Dislocations and Fracture Dislocation *127*
   - Case XI: Malunited/Old Neglected Fracture Intertrochanteric *131*

3. **The Knee** 143
   - Examination Points for a Knee Case *143*
   - Case I: Recurrent Dislocation of Patella *154*
   - Case II: Angular Deformity of Knee (Genu Varum and Genu Valgum) *163*
   - Case III: Quadriceps Contracture *176*
   - Case IV: Exostosis (Osteochondroma ICD 10: C40-C41; ICD-O: 9210/0) *181*
   - Case V: Polio Knee *189*

- Case VI: Injury to Anterior Cruciate Ligament *195*
- Case VII: Injury to Posterior Cruciate Ligament *203*
- Case VIII: Tuberculosis of the Knee Joint *205*

4. Foot and Ankle 212
- Examination Points for Foot and Ankle Cases *212*
- Case I: Congenital Talipes
  (Latin—Talus = Ankle; Pes = Foot) Equinovarus *222*
- Case II: Congenital Vertical Talus *246*
- Case III: Polio Affection of Foot and Ankle *251*
- Case IV: Tendo-Achilles Rupture *266*
- Case V: Foot Drop *274*

5. The Shoulder 279
- Examination Points for a Shoulder Case *279*
- Case I: Tuberculosis of Shoulder Joint *291*
- Case II: The Unstable Shoulder *294*
- Case III: Deltoid Contracture *302*

6. The Elbow Joint 305
- Examination Points for an Elbow Case *305*
- Case I: Tuberculosis of Elbow Joint *313*
- Case II: The Stiff Elbow and Ectopic Ossification *314*
- Case III: The Unstable Elbow *322*
- Case IV: Cubitus Varus *328*
- Case V: Cubitus Valgus *344*
- Case VI: Old Unreduced Monteggia Fracture Dislocation *351*

7. Wrist and Hand 358
- Examination Points for a Wrist and Hand Case *358*
- Case I: Peripheral Nerve Injuries
  (Radial, Median, and Ulnar Nerves) *369*
- Case II: Leprosy Hand *394*
- Case III: Dupuytren Disease *409*
- Case IV: Flexor Tendon Injury *413*
- Case V: Carpal Tunnel Syndrome (Tardy Median Palsy) *425*
- Case VI: Malunited Distal Radius Fracture *433*

Contents

8. **The Spine** **444**
   - Examination of Spine *444*
   - Case I: Spinal Tuberculosis (Pott's Disease) *463*
   - Case II: Lumbar Disk Disease
     (Prolapsed Intervertebral Disk Disease) *481*
   - Case III: Scoliosis *497*

9. **Miscellaneous Short Cases** **520**
   - Case I: Chronic Osteomyelitis *520*
   - Case II: Nonunion of Long Bones *537*
   - Case III: Pseudoarthrosis of Tibia *559*
   - Case IV: Amputation Stump *564*
   - Case V: Examination of Swelling *572*
   - Case VI: Volkmann's Ischemic Contracture and
     Compartment Syndrome *586*
   - Case VII: Torticollis [Tortus (L.): Twisted; Collum (L.): Neck] *594*

10. **Miscellaneous Topics** **598**
    - Gait *598*
    - Prosthetics and Orthotics *608*
    - Wound Infection, Wound Coverage, and Dressings *615*
    - Principles of Fracture Fixation *620*
    - Arthroplasty of Hip, Elbow, and Shoulder *626*
    - Elbow Arthroplasty *635*
    - Shoulder Arthroplasty *636*

11. **How to Read an X-ray and Some Common
    Radiographs as Examples?** **639**

12. **Long and Short Questions for
    Orthopedic Theory Examination** **651**

Index *663*

1
How to Approach Examinations?

WHAT IS EXPECTED IN EXAMINATIONS?

After the immense hard work at orthopedic residency program and practical experience spree, it's difficult to put forward the argument in favor of a one- or two-day assessment of the candidate deciding his fate to procure degree. Everyone has to still undergo the same stereotyped manner of judgment deciding one's "fitness" for the degree. Nevertheless it is a matter of fact that the examiners have also undergone the same course over the years making it easier for a candidate to pass examination if it is taken in its "true perspective", which is often unknown! Candidates often find it an "uphill" task to "please" the examiners in examinations for want of understanding of the main purpose of examinations and the "desired perspective". The following points are projected to give an outline about what exactly is expected from candidate:

- *The way a candidate approaches the patient*: This should ideally be reflected upon as a firm but sober and professional approach to the patient (*always remember to be gentle and kind, be keen, be confident, be smart, be professional—it's not too much an ask!*). Give patient enough time (from your stipulated time, do not be thrift—believe me it helps; sometimes you will find that the patient tells you the diagnosis!). Explain every procedure to the patient and confirm the doubtful points to streamline your "history taking" part. Follow the basic norms such as, to examine the normal side first for comparative assessment, etc. Always pay particular attention to the surroundings, e.g. footwear, assistive appliances, and make a note of them before starting "your probation". This will tell the examiner that you know how to start solving the problem.

- *The way a candidate approaches the given problem*: Perhaps the most difficult part in the absence of practical experience (*good judgment comes from experience and experience from bad judgment*). A hands-on experience in outpatient department which is often time constrained and theory and academic classes give excellent opportunity to present patients to "well-experienced" consultants—who are surely examiners for others and possess immense experience—never flee away from them (Mistakes teach you the most—*The biggest fault of life is to think that you have none*). Ward rounds and patient workup immensely help develop one's skills. Examination anxiety imposes a sense of hurry and uncertainty about cases throws up disarray in approach, which is often striven in the end by a quick fix solution that indeed jumbles up the problem turning on the vicious cycle. Always attempt to develop a unique but well-manageable and adequate approach for most common cases. Regular practice should make one comfortable in examinations.
- *The way a candidate presents the problem and his viewpoint*: After examining the case, which appears to be the "true" encounter whereby you will be assessed regarding to your capability to communicate with the examiner about the case. For this, *you should be a part orator, part clinician, and part politician!* You should be smooth and focused in presentation with tactful representation of the facts leading to diagnosis but not projecting at the same time to the examiner that you are biased by a diagnosis. Keep your mind open to anything and be unprejudiced for criticism.
- *The understanding about the given problem and possible solutions*: Always answer to yourself in the following sequence of the problem and solution (What is the problem? → What can be done? → Why should it be done? → When to do it? → How to do it?; *What, Why, When, and How*). Just making a diagnosis in a long case and particularly in a short case does not surmise the assessment. One is required to know the basic etiopathogenesis and management perspectives of the same. Particularly for some cases, being a specialist in the field you may even be asked of the popular historical perspectives (*so you also need to be a historian!*). The treatment or management options you give require that you know fully about them and that it should

fit the case. Do not beat around the bush, take your time. No one will fail you for being sloppy if your answers are correct, as even the best of clinicians are perplexed sometimes by simple problems in unusual circumstances!
- *Explanation of the most common solutions*: You should be the "boss" of the most common procedures performed. Any question asked right-left or center should be answered with the ease of cutting butter with a "spoon" in summers.

HOW TO PREPARE FOR EXAMINATIONS?

This is the shortest written portion of this book specifically reiterating the fact that it's individual's way of learning, however, there may be some advice of help.
- Refer and follow the standard practice
- Continuously practice and revise the important cases
- Be focused
- Develop communication skills! (Difficult; but of tremendous help, most candidates who fail are just unable to express what they actually mean although they are correct in essence).

DO'S AND DON'TS IN EXAMINATIONS

There are a few things that should be done and more importantly few that should not be done:

DO'S

- Be calm and patient
- Be tactful but considerate
- Be clear in perspective
- Be confident with apt knowledge
- Be frank
- Accept your mistakes if pointed out, be flexible, open-minded
- Finish with a smile to patient and examiner.

DON'TS

- Be in a hurry or anxious or overzealous
- Try to be clever
- Try to jumble up problems or become a researcher with innovative ideas

- Mess up with facts or try guessing work
- Be overconfident and arrogant
- Be dominative
- Argue
- Show disappointment or frustration over disagreement
- Make hasty conclusions!

HOW TO READ THIS BOOK?

A concise yet comprehensive attempt to recreate the questions may make some aspects of the book difficult to grab! It is well accepted that basic concepts regarding the management and diagnostic perspectives differ depending upon the personal and practiced algorithms by various "experts". You too may differ in various respects being amateur in the field (*Information consists of differences that make a difference*). The book definitely does not give a holistic approach to all the cases, but is a willful attempt to introduce the basics for revision with address to some intricacies of the cases that may need further refinement according to the local practice. It is imperative that at the important juncture of examinations one needs support from the internal examiners who are basically "internal experts" and would be able to better explain the "locally practiced" protocols. I would appeal the readers to go through the book as-it-is once and then practice the cases. Mutual/group discussions over particular problems make fundamentals clear and easy to grab. Do not be in an illusion by "illegitimate" concepts that are unacceptable. The book has been prepared after considerate and careful analysis of the various standard texts (more than 21 textbooks) and review papers (more than 650) that are acceptable to most by and large (the acceptability threshold may however, differ!). The concepts given are standard for orthopedic practice, but personally I will prohibit quoting of the texts or concepts or guidelines given herein, one should adhere to standard textbooks or reviewers to this rescue. I feel here to reiterate the fact that what is written in this book is not a hypothesis or personal research work, to give a sense of security to the readers. You will gradually come to know the source for manuscript while reading your textbooks. The read times are calculated approximations depending upon the general practice and exposure of graduates, complexity of topic, importance of topic and compactness of information provided.

How to Approach Examinations?

This, in general holds true but "exceptions are a rule" so one may diverge considering his own knowledge and exposure and the local prevalence of particular topics (e.g. shoulder may be omitted fully while hip may be read twenty times!). General flow of questions in examinations does not necessarily follow the pattern given herein and in a "virtually-realistic" examination it is bound to differ, but one is always questioned of the reasons for giving a particular diagnosis, possible differential diagnoses (with reasons), management protocols, etc. That is primarily stressed upon in this compilation. Some stereotyped questions are oft repeated like "What will you do next", the answer to which is often wrong in an anxious environment! And will hence be found in most of the chapters so that it becomes a habit of the candidate to correctly reply the same as it is the watershed between the diagnosis (considered less important part by the candidate) and management (more stressed part).

Try reading the chapters from beginning unless revising particular concepts as continuity has been specifically dealt with, otherwise some concepts may be overlooked. Teaching notes or text in italics is often ancillary and sometimes includes controversial and unsettled issues needing individual judgment for acceptance. Lastly, where a large amount of knowledge is presented with alternative procedures, the underlined text serves as the standard or most commonly followed method, but is again subjected to individual assessment for want of standardization.

In spite of the best efforts one may not accomplish the desired. The disheartening fate dictates some lapse in fundamental approach which all cannot be laid down in a narration and entails experience—remember hair do not just turn gray in sun (*Experience enables you realize a mistake when you make it again!*). I surely do not mean that one needs to "fail" to understand the cause of failure but it should be emphasized that prevention by a masterly carved approach pays rewards. There is no shortcut to success and exhausting effort with indelible persistence is required to become a specialist. Destiny is not a matter of chance but of choice, and the choice is still yours till you have to face examinations. You can achieve what you want with a good strategy. Strategy building is not just a subject of fighting wars or winning elections—remember those times you devised time to see a movie or attend friend's marriage by quickly shuffling day's work—that is also strategy.

2

The Hip

The hip joint is by far the most popular and common case given to candidates. The candidates are supposed to know all details of the case, especially the examination. Final diagnosis may not matter as much as the approach to it; however, it should not be waywardly different from the expected ones. Being so frequent case and multitude of approaches to the same, a detailed presentation covering some controversial aspects also have been remarked.

Read times: 6–8 times (MS and DNB candidates).

EXAMINATION POINTS FOR A HIP CASE

It is considered immoral to not introduce yourself to the patient and just barge on examination. So, first introduce yourself and take consent (verbal) of examination from patient or guardians, if minor. Note general details and be sure to have a "neutral" female attendant for examining female patient. Before starting examination, always have a look around room to look for assisting devices like crutches/walker/stick and have a look at the footwear for shoe raise, wearing pattern of the sole of shoe, etc.! It has not been repeated everywhere below, but it is imperative to explain all procedures to the patient before performing them and it is better to perform them first on the uninvolved part to reassure him.

HISTORY TAKING

Note the presenting complaints in chronological order and the describe history of presenting illness under following heading details:

The Hip

- *Pain*: Ask to localize pain with fingertip if possible instead of vague description. Onset [acute—traumatic/infective/reactive/muscular; insidious—degenerative, arthritic, osteonecrosis, tuberculosis (TB) (chronic infection)], duration, character (sharp shooting pain of trauma versus dull aching pain of early osteonecrosis and arthritis to throbbing of infection), diurnal variation ("night cries" of tuberculosis, morning stiffness, and pain of ankylosing spondylitis and monoarticular rheumatoid arthritis and rheumatoid arthritis), pain present at first step—arthritis but pain appearing after exertion—uncommonly of hip joint origin except early osteonecrosis, progression over time [undulating course-chronic disease, undulating course with sudden increase—collapse in osteonecrosis or fracture, e.g. bone cyst or slipped capital femoral epiphysis (SCFE)]. Pain localized to groin suggests hip as origin, but patient pointing pain over anterolateral region/back of thigh suggest pain of upper lumbar and lower lumbar origin, respectively. Pain that increasingly involves leg during exertion, "thermometer pain" suggests LCS. If pain is reported to be present laterally above trochanteric region in c-fashion, it suggests femoroacetabular impingement. Note important negative history, pain in multiple joints (arthropathy), pain of spine origin as above, and associated history, e.g. pregnancy. Importantly, unexplained knee pain, especially anterolateral region mandates hip examination. In itself, pain is rarely of help in pointing out hip disorder.
- *Limp*: A very important symptom that quite reliably localizes site of pathology. First symptom to appear in TB of hip (even before pain). Note onset in relation to pain, progression, and assistance in walking. Painless limp is often congenital [developmental dysplasia of the hip (DDH), coxa vara, and dysplastic disorders] or due to healed disease with deformity (healed infection with ankylosis or ankylosing spondylitis) or neuromuscular disorder (poliomyelitis/cerebral palsy).
- *Stiffness (in patients' language, it is better to refer this as to "Limitation of movement")*: It indicates spasm secondary to inflammatory disorder or enthesopathy or cartilage eburnation. It is often seen following treatment of primary disorder

or prolonged immobilization. Morning stiffness is often characteristic of noninfective inflammatory disorder.

- *Deformity and limb length discrepancy:* Often patient will be able to tell shortening but very infrequently you will find a patient telling you flexion/rotational deformities! Ask about when first noticed, association with pain, and progression. Enquire about specific deformities like varus/valgus, equinus, etc. Note the onset, progression-associated symptoms, and any history of trauma/infection/treatment taken for deformity.
- *Swelling:* Small swellings are often masked by bulk of muscle, large progressing swellings like that of TB of hip and acute marked pyogenic infections should be indicated. Other swellings are often superficial and arise due to unrelated disorders (lymphadenopathy, saphena varix, etc.). Old unreduced dislocation is hardly mentioned by patient as swelling in gluteal region unless specifically asked for.
- Describe the event (usually trauma) into mode (road traffic accident, fall from height, fall of heavy object, slip on floor, missing stairs, etc.), site of injury, post-injury mobility, and ability to bear weight, injury to other regions, and treatment received.
- End your history by current disability experienced by patient, mobility status of the patient before event in question, and finally mentioning all negative history:
  - Trauma, fever, history of contacts for TB, affections of other joints, treatment history for TB, and birth disorder. (*Never forget to ask about symptoms in other hip and ipsilateral and contralateral knee, ankle and foot, and mention it*).
  - It is good to mention current functional status of the patient in terms of walking ability (restricted/unrestricted, walking distance, aided or unaided walk, and type of aid used), ability to squat, ability to sit cross-legged, ability to tie shoes or wear socks, and ability to drive vehicle.

Past history: TB and treatment, respiratory, renal, dermatological, cardiac (hypertension, etc.), endocrinological (diabetes mellitus, etc.), and neurological disorders, hematological disorder, connective tissue disorder, organ transplants, liver disorder, trauma and treatment, congenital/developmental disorder and treatment, surgery around hip, diabetes, hypertension, and work tolerance (for treatment planning and anesthesia). In a child, additionally enquire prolonged intravenous (IV) infusion, childhood limping, umbilical sepsis, and episodes of prolonged fever or frequent bleeding.

Personal history: Occupation, diet, smoking, alcohol intake, addiction, menstrual history, sexual history, and recreational activities.

Family history: Dysplasia, inflammatory disorder, and storage disorders.

General Examination

Apart from other routine examination, specifically look for eyes (color of sclera, iritis, uveitis, microphthalmos, and use of unusual glasses for vision), pinna color and low-set pinna, cheeks [Systemic lupus erythematosus (SLE) rash], oral cavity (dental hygiene and dentinogenesis, arch of palate), hair line, neck (webbing and thyroid swelling), shape of chest, clubbing of nails, pitting of nails (psoriasis—psoriatic arthropathy), skin changes (discoloration, café au lait spots, hyperkeratosis, pustules, etc.), lymphadenopathy (external/internal iliac, paraaortic), abdomen for psoas abscess, and rarely tubercular ileitis, hernia sites, hemophilia, dysplasia, and hypermobility syndrome (vide Brighton criteria and Beighton score in chapter on shoulder examination and cases).

Local Examination

(Expose from nipples below and cover private parts to avoid embarrassment).

Inspection

The following order is for comfort of patient—walking and gait (*See* Chapter 10).

Then inspection in standing, sitting, and finally lying down position.

From front: Attitude and Alignment [always start with "A"—hip flexion, knee (patella) pointing out (external rotation) and vice versa and knee flexion, foot pointing out/in, equinus at ankle. Balance (front—flexion at hip is indicates by trunk bent forward, and lateral—

tilt to side). Level of ASISs helps identify pelvic tilt, swelling(s), skin for scar/sinus/loss of creases, dilated veins, and discoloration. Wasting of quadriceps and prominent muscle (e.g. adductor spasm). Hernia sites and perineal widening (post-traumatic/DDH).

From side: Lordosis of spine, pelvic tilt/nutation, trochanteric prominence, flexion at hip, knee and equinus at ankle and skin as above.

From behind: PSIS level (dimple of Venus), midline shift (natal cleft), and curvature of spine, lumbar triangle for fullness, lordosis, gluteal wasting, gluteal folds and symmetry, and skin as above.

Note the skin for (SEADS): Swelling, erythema, atrophy (of appendages), discoloration, and suppuration (scars and sinuses).

Palpation: (before one starts palpation to confirm/refute the findings of inspection, kindly systematically *mark all bony points—both ASIS, greater trochanter, pubic tubercle, PSIS, ischial tuberosities, xiphisternum, center of patella, Gerdy's tubercle, center of hip joint and iliac crest/tubercle; follow your set sequence but keep it constant throughout*). Rotational deformities can be better commented in supine position, so pay attention there. Confirm above findings.

Anteriorly: Note temperature from back of hand, ASIS levels, groin tenderness at base of Scarpa's triangle (hip joint is 2 cm below and lateral to mid inguinal point), femoral pulsations (best palpable just inferolateral to midinguinal point), swelling and abscesses, and palpate femur along length.

From side: Trochanteric upriding, tenderness, broadening, thickening, and levels of iliac crest.

From back: Tenderness over sacroiliac (SI) joint (lies just distal to PSIS), gluteal tenderness (short external rotators underlying gluteus can be a cause of pain), coccygeal tenderness (coccygodynia), tenderness over ischial tuberosity (Weaver's bottom and bursitis), gluteal fold tenderness (gluteus maximus tendinitis), feel for swelling (spherical, smooth, bony hard of head of femur in dislocations), and also feel for soft tissue swellings and abscesses.

Medially: Adductor spasm, Ludloff sign (tenderness over anteromedial aspect of thigh at base of Scarpa's triangle—lesser trochanteric affections).

The Hip

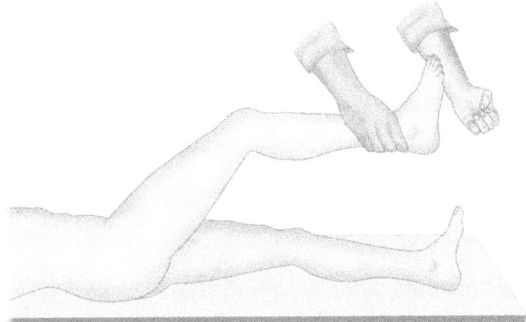

Fig. 1: Anvil sign.

Roll test: This helps in eliciting adductor muscle spasm. Gently roll the patients limb holding at thigh internally and externally like rolling pin to make chapattis. The patient reports pain and there is resistance to rotations if there is adductor spasm, also the spastic muscles may become more prominent.

Percussion: Firm percussion at heel [Anvil sign **(Fig. 1)**—elicits pain at hip in inflammatory conditions].

Deformities:

- *Fixed flexion deformity*: Reveal the deformity by doing Thomas test, then measure using goniometer. For bilateral flexion deformities as in ankylosing spondylosis, one has to use the modification by examining the patient prone at edge of couch supporting both thighs together (*see* further in Thomas test) **(Figs. 2A and B)**.
- *Fixed adduction and abduction deformity*: By squaring the pelvis.
- *Fixed rotational deformities*: There is no indirect way of measuring/estimating it. The deformity has to be measured using goniometer. One can take center of heel to 2nd toe as reference or medial border of foot as reference. Restriction of internal rotation in a child is seen with slipped capital femoral epiphysis/slipped upper femoral epiphysis (SCFE/SUFE) classically while in an adult-restricted internal rotation occurs with osteoarthrosis or degenerative disease of hip.

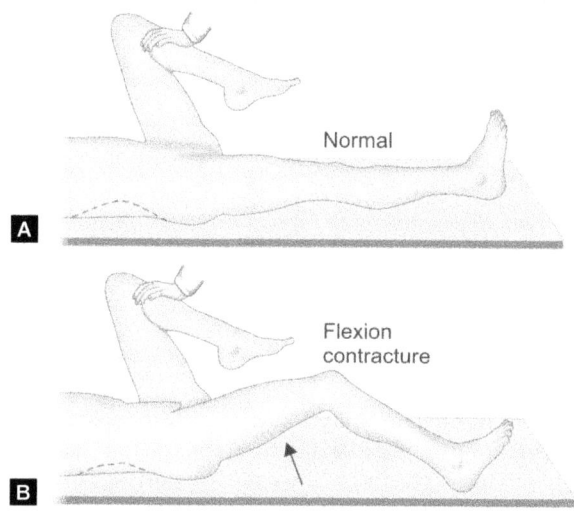

Figs. 2A and B: Thomas test.

Movements (range of common movements is depicted in adjoining figure):

(*For all movements, hold the pelvis firmly with left hand with thumb at the ASIS and fingers embracing trochanter—to detect even the slightest movement of pelvis, hold the affected limb with left hand*).

- *Flexion:* First reveal deformity in affected limb by performing Thomas test, then passively move the limb further and measure the range taking couch as reference **(Figs. 3A and 20)**.
- *Adduction and abduction*: First square the pelvis, then measure the further range of respective movement taking body midline as reference (*If someone speaks 20° of abduction then it usually means 20° abduction beyond deformity, which is more appropriately expressed as range say 20–40° of abduction range of movement*) **(Fig. 3B)**.
- *Rotational movements:* Measure both in extension and 90° flexion at hip (if possible) as above **(Figs. 3C and D)**, in extension; measure further movement possible from deformity in that direction but for opposite movement measure from

The Hip

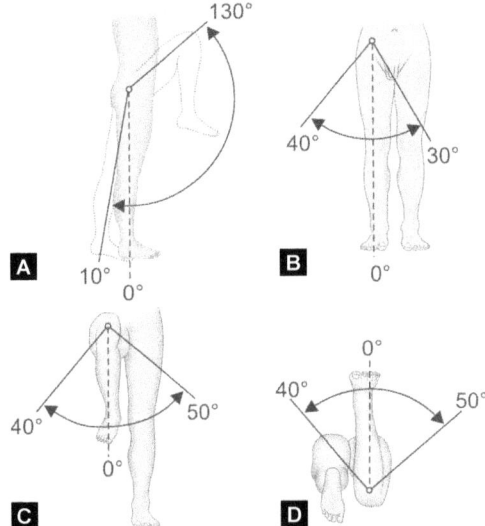

Figs. 3A to D: (A) Flexion-extension; (B) Adduction-abduction; (C) and (D) Internal and external rotations as can be measured in supine and prone positions respectively.

zero position (patella horizontal to ceiling facing directly up). In flexion, measure from zero position only (hip flexed at 90° and leg parallel to midline). *Additional note on assessing rotations of lower extremity at hip in examination.*

There are two main ways to assess rotation:

1. *With the hips extended*: With the patient lying supine (hips and knees extended), hold both lower limbs just above the malleoli, and rotate in reciprocal directions to examine the angle at which the patella faces **(Fig. 4)**. The normal angle of internal rotation is 30°, while the normal angle of external rotation is 45°. If patellar reference is not possible, then one can also use great toe or medial border of foot or heel-center to 2nd toe line on sole of foot (better) as reference to look for rotational inequality.
   - This can also be examined while keeping the patient supine or sitting and letting his legs hang down the edge

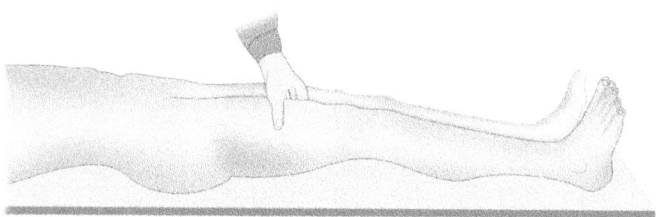

Fig. 4: Measurement of hip rotation in extension.

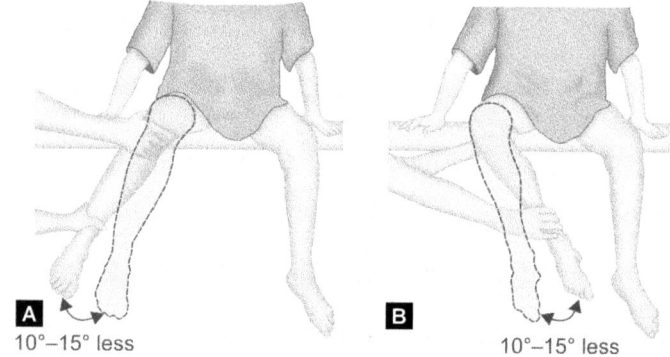

10°–15° less   10°–15° less

Figs. 5A and B: Measuring hip rotations with legs hanging (the patient can be supine or sitting).

of table thus flexing the knees. In this position, the tibia is the pendulum, which measures the angles of internal and external rotation at the hip joints **(Figs. 5A and B)**.

2. *With the hips flexed*: Here the patient is kept supine again but the hips are flexed to 90° and knees also at 90°—"the 90-90 position" for both lower limbs simultaneously or better do sequentially (normal → pathological). Keep the knees touching (in simultaneous method) and move ankles away from midline. Now the rotation is checked from the angle made by tibial shin (look method of using goniometer below) to imaginary midline for internal rotation. For external

The Hip

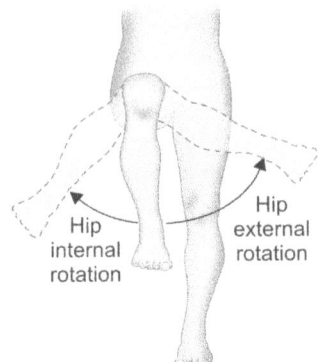

Fig. 6: Measuring hip rotation in flexion.

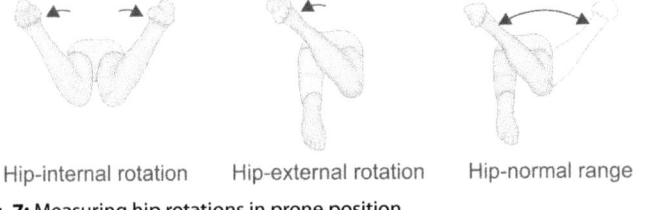

Fig. 7: Measuring hip rotations in prone position.

rotation, cross the sole of foot for the index limb across the midline and repeat measure for other limb. Holding sole of foot together and letting knees fall is not recommended, as this manner actually tests external rotation and abduction together **(Fig. 6)**.

- *Rotations in prone position*: This is a good method to access rotation at hip, provided the hip is not fixed in flexion. Ask patient to lie prone and flex the knees together at knee to 90°. Let the feet then fall apart keeping knees together to check for external rotation. Let the legs cross across midline for checking internal rotation at hip **(Fig. 7)**.

- *Extension:* Measure in prone position. The pelvis and hip are stabilized with one hand on the pelvis while the other hand flexes the knee to relax the hamstrings.

  [*Remember always to speak the movements of affected limb in comparison to other (deemed normal) limb, e.g. flexion of 25–120° as compared to 0–135° in left hip*]

  (***How to use goniometer and where to place it?*** This is a hot and more or less irritating topic for students as hardly ever anyone uses a goniometer later in practice! But examination has to be cleared only by using and showing how to use goniometer).

- *For measuring fixed flexion deformity (FFD) with Thomas test and further flexion range of motion (ROM)*: The axis of femur can be drawn as a straight line from tip of trochanter to lateral epicondyle (better) or Gerdy's tubercle (rough measure). Goniometer should be kept with center at the tip of trochanter and one limb is placed parallel to the couch while other limb is along the axis of femur. Alternate method is to first bring the patient at the edge of couch, place the goniometer center at the point where posterior border of thigh appears to meet couch, and then one limb is placed along the couch for horizontal line while the other limb is placed along the posterior border of thigh to give measure. Both methods are acceptable but first one is more accurate and acceptable; alternative measure is rough and posterior border of thigh is ill defined giving wrong measures often.

- *For measuring adduction/abduction deformity and ROM*: Place the center of goniometer at center of hip joint (1.5 cm below and lateral to mid-inguinal point). The neutral line is taken as straight line passing through center of body (it can be drawn as a line joining xiphisternum and pubic symphysis extended distally). Femoral axis is taken as line from center of hip joint joining center of patella.

- *For rotations*: In supine position, take heel-center as the point of placement of goniometer kept in vertical plane parallel to sole. Vertical line is the reference line while limb rotation is found from angle made by the line joining heel-center to 2nd toe with the vertical reference. For measuring rotations by flexion method (hip and knee flexed), take center of patella as center for goniometer, midline is the reference while line joining center of patella to ankle joint center (midpoint of bimalleolar line) is the measuring line. When measuring the rotation with knees flexed down the couch—keep goniometer again in vertical plane with center at patella and use shin of tibia or line joining patellar center to ankle center as the measuring line.

Measurements

(*Limb length discrepancy*)

- *Apparent length:* Measure in an unsquared pelvis with limbs lying parallel (the comfortable supine position of patient) from *xiphisternum* to tip of medial malleolus **(Fig. 8)**. This is one of the reasons to strip the patient below from level of nipples!
- *True length:* Square the pelvis and put the limbs in mirror image (viz. flexion at hip and knee), and then measure from *ASIS* to medial malleolus **(Figs. 8 and 9)**. More reliably, it is measured by wooden block method.
- *Wasting:* Measure thigh circumference 15 cm from medial knee joint line **(Fig. 10)**.
- Femoral (thigh) and tibial (leg) lengths Galeazzi's sign **(Fig. 11)** and Ally's test.

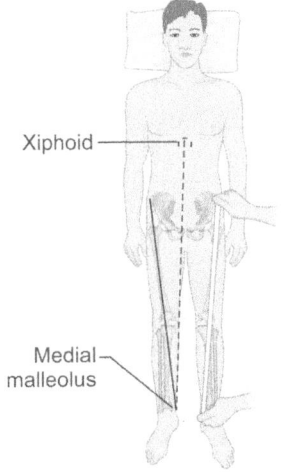

Fig. 8: Apparent length measurement for right lower limb from xiphoid (unsquared pelvis) and true length measurement for left lower limb (limbs in mirrored position).

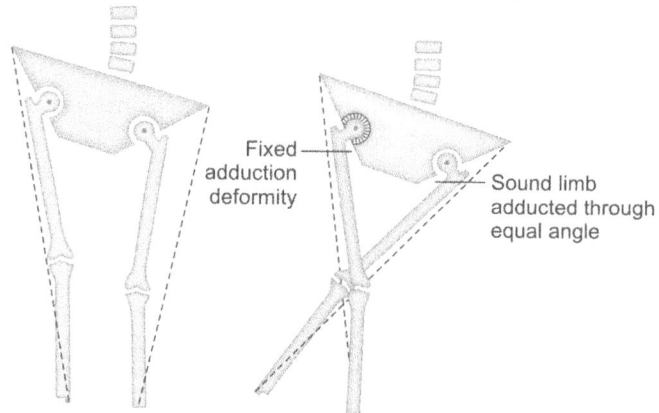

Fig. 9: There is adduction deformity of right hip, lengths of limbs measured in this position from xiphoid will give apparent lengths. To measure true length the left lower limb also should be first placed in mirrored position then true length is measured.

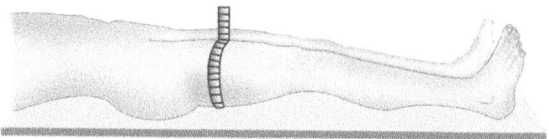

Fig. 10: Measurement of thigh girth.

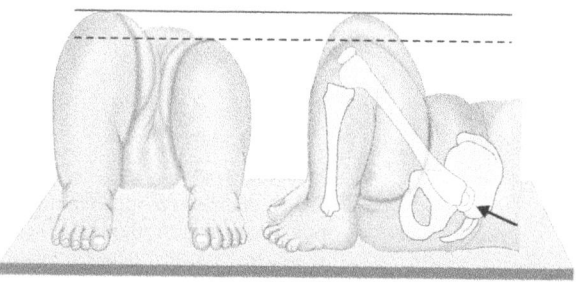

Fig. 11: Galeazzi's sign.

The Hip

- *Bryant's triangle:* First square the pelvis. Draw a line from ASIS laterally horizontal (perpendicular to midline), draw a line joining tip of trochanter to ASIS (hypotenuse); draw a line passing straight up from tip of trochanter to intersect first line (base). Measure all in cm. Some people refer to "digital" Bryant's triangle, which is nothing related to technology! Here approximation of measurements is done by placing fingers as follows. Place the thumb at ASIS, middle finger at tip of greater trochanter and index finger vertically below the ASIS along horizontal plane to make perpendicular. Remember, this is only for quick reference and no accurate measurements can be derived. Square the pelvis before making this and do it simultaneously for both sides so as to have comparison. This implies that whole philosophy of Bryant's triangle is wasteful, if there is bilateral deformity at hip joint.
- Femoral anteversion (Craig's test and Ryder method) **(Fig. 12)**
- *Kothari's parallelogram (ML Kothari):* Unsquared pelvis—join both ASIS and drop perpendicular from each ASIS to midline, measure the angle formed between lines—this gives idea of adduction/abduction in affected hip (*can be used as adjunct to classical method and is easy*).

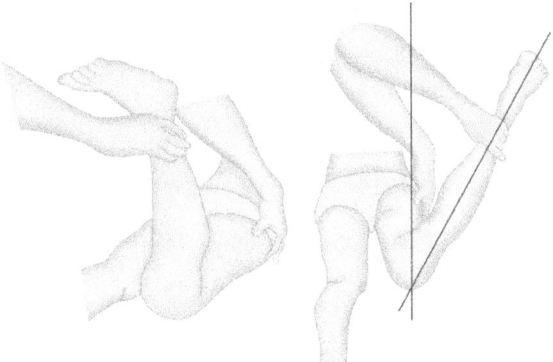

Fig. 12: Measuring femoral anteversion clinically. With patient in prone position, flex the knee to 90° and the internally rotate the hip to feel for trochanter. Stop at the place where greater trochanter is most prominent, measure the angle between shin and vertical.

Special Tests

- *Qualitative assessment of supratrochanteric shortening:*
  - *Nelaton's line:* Turn the patient lateral to *bring affected side up* and flex the hip to 90°. Join ischial tuberosity (often the most distal part is the one most easily palpable) to ASIS. Supratrochanteric shortening is present if tip of greater trochanter crosses this line. As such it is drawn *only on the affected side* **(Fig. 13)**.
  - *Shoemaker line:* In supine position join tip of trochanter to ASIS and extrapolate it to abdomen crossing umbilicus. Draw a similar line from *other side*. Normally the lines cross at or above umbilicus in midline. In unilateral supratrochanteric shortening, the crossing always misses the midline and lies on the opposite side below umbilicus. In bilateral symmetrical deformities, the crossing point is below umbilicus but may be in center (if perfectly symmetrical) **(Fig. 14)**.
  - *Chiene's test:* Horizontal lines joining both ASIS and both tips of trochanter should be parallel—converge on the side of upriding.
  - *Morris bitrochanteric test:* Interpretation as for hypotenuse of Bryant's triangle.

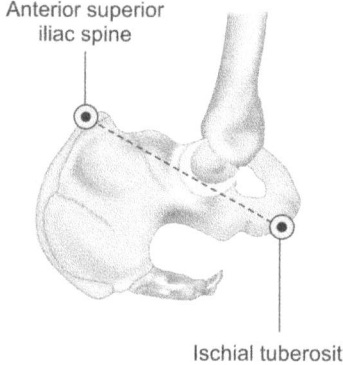

Fig. 13: Nelaton's line.

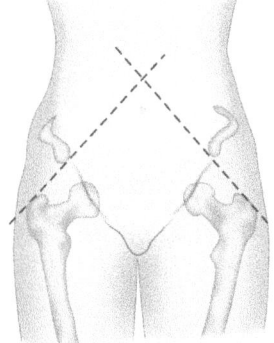

Fig. 14: Shoemaker's lines.

- *Tests for stability:*
    - *Active straight leg raise test (SLRT) (Stinchfield's test)*: If patient is unable to do then it indicates dislocation/fracture of neck or hip joint instability.
    - Trendelenburg test (kindly *see* details below)
    - Telescopy
    - Ortolani's sign and Barlow maneuver (relevant only to pediatric patients).
- Ober's test **(Fig. 15)** to test for iliotibial band (ITB) contracture (*See Chapter 3 also*).
- *Gauvain's sign:* Spasm of abdominal muscles on initiating rotatory movements of hip in active tuberculosis, seen in stage of synovitis.
- *Ely's test (Rectus phenomenon):* Tests rectus tightness in a prone patient, passive flexion of knee leads to flexion at hip joint **(Fig. 16)**. Grading can be done by noting the degree of knee flexion at which hip starts flexing.
- Noble compression test for iliotibial band friction.
- *Yeoman's test:* Active hip extension against resistance to test Gluteus maximus tendinitis.
- *Phelp's test:* To test gracilis tightness—In prone position, abduct the limbs then flex knee to 90° (relaxing gracilis), if further abduction present, it indicates contracture.
- *Tripod sign:* In sitting position, passively extend knee fully if patient leans back and supports himself with both hands and

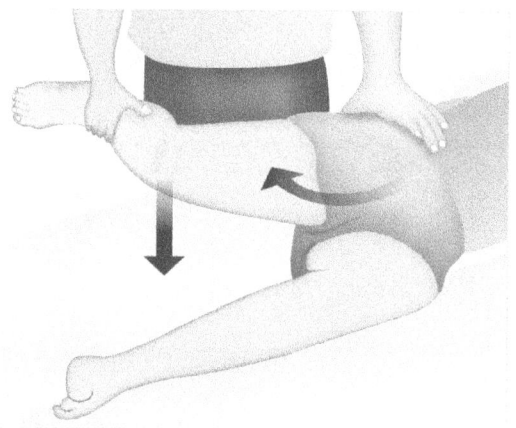

Fig. 15: Ober's test.

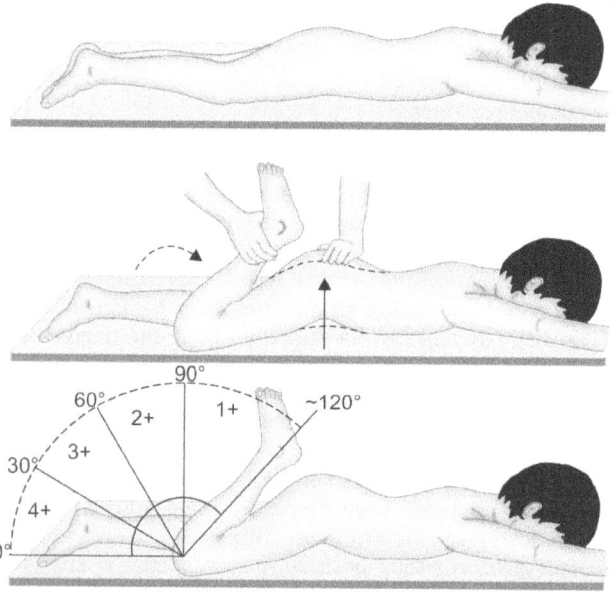

Fig. 16: Ely's test.

The Hip

extension at hip indicates hamstring tightness (remember Lasègue's sign should be negative otherwise tripod sign could very well be positive in sciatica or even Pott's spine).

- *Piriformis test (FADIR):* Flexion, adduction and internal rotation in lateral position stretches piriformis—produces pain in piriformis tendinitis/syndrome. *Same test if produces pain at groin is useful for femoroacetabular impingement (called impingement sign).*
- *Patrick's test [FABER (flexion, abduction, external rotation) test] and Jansen's sign:* Flexion, abduction, and external rotation at index hip is produced by placing lateral malleolus at patella of the other limb (making a figure of "4", where straight line is made by uninvolved limb while involved limb makes the bent portion of the 4)—pain produced at SI joint. *Same test if produces pain at groin is useful for femoroacetabular impingement* **(Fig. 17)**.
- *Erichson's pelvis compression test:* Press iliac crests together—pain over SI joint.
- *Gaenslen's test:* Patient at edge of bed with ipsilateral hip hanging out. Flex both hips together then ask to release ipsilateral limb to extend hip—pain indicates SI joint affection **(Fig. 18)**.
- *Yeoman's test for sacroiliitis:* Passive hyperextension of thigh in a prone patient.
- *Fulcrum test:* To test stress fracture of femur—keep forearm below midthigh and press knee.

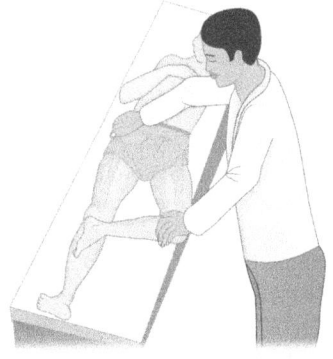

Fig. 17: Patrick's test.

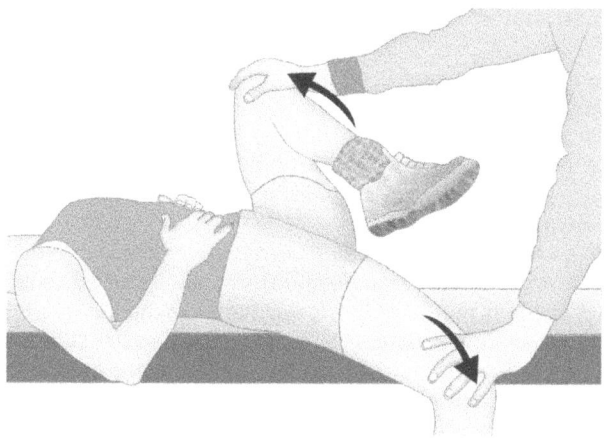

Fig. 18: Gaenslen test.

- *Desault's sign:* On passively rotating femur, the tip of greater trochanter subtends an arc as the pivot is at the head of femur, but if the neck is fractured (nonunion) then tip of trochanter remains stationary and rotates along longitudinal line passing through tip of trochanter itself (long axis of femur).
- *Alli's sign:* Relaxation of the fascia between trochanter and iliac crest (seen in fractures of hip).
- *Gill's sign:* Swollen hip due to effusion feels thicker than other hip felt with thumb at base of Scarpa's triangle and four fingers over buttocks.
- *Ludloff test:* Inability to raise thigh in sitting position especially against resistance (avulsion of lesser trochanter).
- *Sectoral sign:* Seen in osteonecrosis—reduced internal rotation in extension that improves when checked in flexion.
- *Gear-stick sign:* Limitation of abduction in extension but abduction improves with flexion of hip. These are due to replacement of diseased segment by healthy portion of bone so that impingement effect is gone (osteonecrosis and Perthes).
- *Figure of "4" sign:* Click felt on making figure of 4 in osteonecrosis due to collapse of subchondral bone and leftover shell of cartilage.

The Hip

- *Schober's test: See Chapter 8 also.*
- *McFarland's test:* During flexion, hip points to opposite shoulder but in SCFE and osteonecrosis with superolateral collapse the hip points to ipsilateral shoulder.

Per rectal examination: For central fracture dislocation, Otto pelvis (protrusio acetabuli).

Distal neurological and vascular examination: Check for distal motor deficit especially in sciatic nerve distribution, reflexes and sensations. Palpate all peripheral pulses (popliteal, anterior and posterior tibial, dorsalis pedis).

Always conclude with the status of other hip and ipsilateral and contralateral knee and ankle.

Some common classic findings as an example:

- *Posterior dislocation of hip:* FADIR deformity with true (supratrochanteric) and apparent lower limb shortening, upridden trochanter (crosses Nelaton's line), head palpated in gluteal region, limitation of abduction and external rotation, telescopy and Trendelenburg positive, and Gill's sign positive.
- *Developmental dysplasia of the hip*: Upridden trochanter, adduction contracture, absent/reduced femoral pulsations, asymmetric thigh folds, widened perineum (bilateral dislocations), Galeazzi sign shows femoral shortening, higher gluteal fold, restricted abduction, increased internal rotation, limited hip abduction with 90° knee flexion, positive Barlow maneuver and Ortolani's sign. In a young child, "duck-like" or "sailor's gait" is seen (B/L) or a lurching gait (U/L), increased lordosis, true shortening as above, absent/reduced femoral pulses, and positive Trendelenburg's sign.

1. What are the prerequisites of examining hip joint?

Ans. The following points should be observed:
- Patient should be lying supine on a couch or other firm mattress positioned away from wall.
- Expose from below nipples and cover private parts.
- Female attendant should accompany while examining a female patient.
- Make patient comfortable by discussing with him and explaining the procedure before proceeding.

- There should be ample light in the examining room preferably daylight.
- Warm up your hands before palpation.
- Avoid hurting the patient.
- Examine in standing, supine, and sitting positions.

2. What are the causes of asymmetry of gluteal folds?

Ans. DDH, gluteal abscess, gluteal atrophy, fixed pelvic obliquity, gluteus maximus contracture, hematoma/collection/psoas abscess in gluteal region, and tumors.

3. How do you identify various bony points?

Ans. The bony points are marked by a black or blue skin marking pen using the mark ⊗:

Xiphisternum (Xiphoid process): First identify the clavicles and sternoclavicular joints medially. Then along a line centrally between SC joints, slide the metal end of tape that will encounter first the manubrium → the angle of sternum → body of sternum and finally will suddenly dip in epigastrium. The lower edge of bone from where the metal end of tape slid is the tip of xiphoid or ensiform cartilage. One can also follow the lower edge of rib cages from both side and the point where they meet is the xiphoid process but it may be difficult in obese patients and females would be embarrassed.

ASIS: Slide metal end of tape (or thumb) gently along the inguinal ligament superolaterally in the groin fold and the first bony prominence encountered is ASIS.

Iliac tubercle: This is felt as a bony prominence on the outer wall of the iliac crest when palpating posteriorly along the iliac crest from ASIS. It lies some 5 cm behind ASIS.

Pubic tubercle: Lies about 2–2.5 cm lateral to pubic symphysis (serves as attachment for inguinal ligament).

Tip of greater trochanter: From ASIS go along iliac crests and mark some 5 cm arc (or 4-finger-breath) behind ASIS. From here gently descend down and the first bony point felt is tip of greater trochanter, confirm this by gently rotating thigh (Alternately some people may mark it by going along femoral shaft and the place where your thumb dips is tip). Another method is to mark the PSIS and directly descend

The Hip

below where one will encounter posterior border of greater trochanter, then ascend anterior and superior to find the tip of trochanter.

PSIS: Marked at dimple of Venus.

Ischial tuberosity: Patient lateral and hip and knee flexed at right angle feel right in the center of gluteal region and mark the base (most prominent part).

4. What is femoral triangle and how do you mark it?

Ans. Femoral triangle also called Scarpa's triangle lies in the anteromedial aspect of the upper thigh **(Fig. 19)**. It has three borders:

1. Superior border is formed by inguinal ligament that runs from ASIS to pubic tubercle
2. Lateral border is formed by medial border of Sartorius muscle (the longest muscle of body)
3. Medial border is formed by medial border of adductor longus muscle—so this muscle is a part of triangle.

The roof is formed by the fascia lata, while the base is formed by pectineus, iliopsoas, and adductor longus muscle. Adductor longus is palpated as a distinct ridge when legs are abducted.

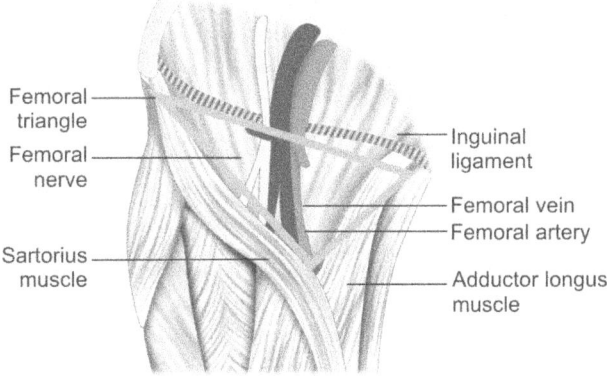

Fig. 19: Femoral triangle.

5. What are the contents of Scarpa's triangle and clinical relevance?

Ans. The femoral/Scarpa's triangle contains femoral nerve, artery, vein, and femoral canal from lateral to medial aspect. Femoral pulsations are palpable just below mid-inguinal point against the femoral head (*See* Narath sign below). This is different from mid-point of inguinal ligament that lies lateral to it. Hip joint center *per se* lies 1.5 cm below and lateral to mid-inguinal point. Commonly femoral artery is punctured here for coronary angiography. Any fullness at base of femoral triangle should be evaluated for femoral hernia or psoas abscess that may point in this region. Other pathological swelling includes that of lymph nodes (inguinal nodes) that may be enlarged in infection.

6. What is Narath sign?

Ans. Absent (or feeble) femoral pulsations due to lack of bony support below (head of femur); seen in old unreduced dislocations, DDH, squeal of septic arthritis, pestle and mortar type TB hip, central fracture dislocation of hip, arteriosclerosis of femoral artery [The Narath sign should not be spoken as positive or negative—always mention that femoral pulses are bilaterally (B/L) comparable or femoral pulses on affected site are feeble/not palpable].

7. How do you look for temperature locally?

Ans. Temperature difference is noted with the dorsum of fingers of dominant hand by first gently touching the unaffected part (corresponding normal part like the other normal hip) → then the affected (pathological) part → then again the unaffected (normal) part.

8. Why do you choose xiphisternum as the bony landmark for measuring apparent length?

Ans. A fixed easily identifiable reference in *midline* of body is required to compare apparent length, the following landmarks are available:
- Suprasternal notch
- Xiphisternum
- Umbilicus
- Symphysis pubis.

The Hip

Landmark 1 lies too high (unexposed) and is quite wide—may give erroneous measurement. Landmark 3 is not fixed as it can move with slightest of hand movement. Landmark 4 lies below the level of hip joint and as a rule no landmark below the hip is chosen. So it is better to choose 2.

9. Why and how do you square pelvis?

Ans. Squaring is done to remove the effect of compensation by body (e.g. the body apparently lengthens a shortened limb), by reversing the deformity produced due to compensation. In an abduction deformity foxed by soft tissue contracture (in late stages) to pull the hip outward; body tries to compensate say by bending the spine. In such case no adduction (movement in opposite direction) will be possible, however some abduction (movement in direction of deformity, unless deformity has reached the limits of ROM) would still be possible. If we pull the hip in adduction the ASIS will further be pulled down further increasing the deformity that we do not want. Squaring is hence done by abducting the limb in fixed abduction deformity and vice versa. Moving the limb this way always first corrects the compensatory deformity (say spine compensation for abduction) then only residual movement occurs at joint. In early deformities, it is usually the muscle spasm that produces compensation if there is no destruction in joint.

10. What are the fallacies of squaring pelvis?

Ans. Squaring is not possible for:
- Absent ASIS due to previous surgery
- Fixed pelvic obliquity/scoliosis
- Malformed pelvis
- Deformed pelvis, e.g. following trauma
- Ankylosing spondylitis with sixed spinal and hip deformities.

11. What does apparent length measure?

Ans. As such nothing specific! It is only a rough guide and a confirmation to visual appearance of shortening/lengthening. Interpretation is possible only in conjunction with true length. As such apparent lengthening generally indicates abduction deformity so one can proceed with this guide in further examination.

12. What do you understand by abduction and adduction deformities?

Ans. These are coronal compensatory mechanisms of body for limb length inequality. Abduction deformity denotes apparent lengthening and adduction deformity denotes apparent shortening.

Simple deformities: These are present in early stages only; these can only be detected while examining the patient standing! And they often go away on lying down—that's why not fixed. (*They are referred to as "adduction/abduction deformity"*). Movement in direction opposite to deformity may still be possible as the deformities are not fixed.

Fixed deformities: Over time without treatment, the deformities become fixed due to soft tissue contracture whereby "movement is still possible in the direction of deformity but not in the other direction". (*They are referred to as "fixed abduction/adduction deformity"*).

Lastly limb may get ankylosed in one of the deformities and there it is called *"fixed in abduction/adduction".*

They are measured by squaring pelvis or by Kothari's parallelogram.

13. What are various compensatory mechanisms and what is their importance?

Ans. Compensation for hip deformity occurs at:
- Spine (often lumbar)
- Pelvis (coronal tilt or flexion/extension)
- Hip joint itself (coronal deformity)
- Knee
- Ankle
- Foot.

They are physiological response of body to a pathological condition and must not be thought of as a disorder. These compensatory mechanisms help body by:
- Concealing the deformity
- Maintaining equilibrium while standing/walking by shifting center of gravity
- Stabilizing the joint (remember they *"fix"* the joint)
- Making up for the loss in limb length.

The Hip

14. Can all deformities around hip be compensated?

Ans. No, there is a limit to compensation for rotational deformities which often remain revealed unless very mild. Only coronal and sagittal plane deformities are corrected, that to only for a certain extent.

15. How much shortening can be effectively compensated without producing ankle equinus?

Ans. Approximately one and a half inch (around 3–3.5 cm).

16. What is the difference between attitude and deformity?

Ans. Attitude is the habitual (mostly compensatory) position of limb or posture of body identified at inspection that is adopted by the patient to ease discomfort. It is spoken in anatomical terms of arrangement of parts of body usually at a referring joint like the lower limb appears in flexion, abduction, and external rotation at hip. In general, if there is no deformity that has developed then attitudes can be corrected to neutral position albeit with discomfort to patient. Passive or active correction will not produce compensatory deformity in other part of body.

Deformity is the disfigurement, mishappening, malformation or distortion in body part or joint that cannot be replaced to normal/neutral position of the limb or body. Neither the patient nor examiner can correct the deformity to neutral by passive or active manipulation without producing compensatory deformity in the "associated" part. For example, if one wants to correct the flexion deformity by pressing the thigh against couch then lumbar lordosis will increase.

17. OK, so what is the difference between deformity and contracture?

Ans. Simply, contracture would produce deformity but deformity does not always result from contracture and it can also arise from primary bone/joint pathology like ankylosis or degeneration, congenital absence of bone/part, etc. Contractures usually develop with long-standing deformities. Both are clinical findings and you try to find cause of deformity whether it is due to contracture or primary bony/joint pathology.

Practical Orthopedic Examination Made Easy

18. What is Thomas test?

Ans. Test for indirectly revealing and measuring flexion deformity at hip or iliopsoas tightness **(Fig. 20)**.

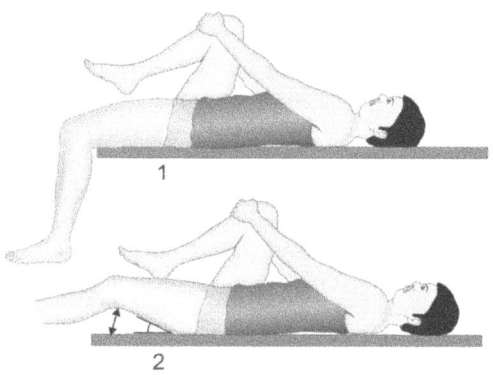

Fig. 20: Thomas test for determining flexion contracture at hip joint and measuring further flexion.

19. What are the prerequisites of performing Thomas test?

Ans. The following should be observed:
- General prerequisites of examination
- Unilateral deformity (bilateral measured by modification)
- No bony ankylosis in other hip/knee
- Other hip should be painless, ipsilateral hip should not be very painful
- No fixed pelvic/spinal deformity.

20. How do you perform this test?

Ans. Stand on right side of couch or better a firm/hard bed, explain the procedure. Patient lies supine in his comfortable position. First do the inspection part by kneeling below and bringing your eye level with couch looking for a gap between patient's lumbar spine and bed. Presence of light on the other side indicates that spine is not in full contact with the couch and there is flexion deformity (not findings). Pass your hand behind back volar side up to confirm the gap. Manipulate the asymptomatic limb by holding just below knee to flex the hip and knee to fullest by touching the chest thus obliterating

The Hip

lumbar lordosis, which is confirmed by back of patient touching your volar hand and pressing against it. Ask patient to hold the knee in same position. Check for ischial tuberosity movement simultaneously and it should not rise off couch (this denotes overflexion). One should not further force the unaffected limb against chest to try and "reveal" more deformity as it instead increases pelvic obliquity exaggerating lumbar lordosis. Passively gently extend the affected limb by pressing down at knee to correct any overcorrection if present; also correct any accidental abduction at hip and measure the angle (couch as horizontal reference) after reconfirming obliteration of lordosis (visually). Alternate method—ask patient to flex both limbs so that both knees touch chest. Then ask to release the affected limb while holding the normal knee to chest.

(*Passing hand beneath the back only checks for the presence of lumbar lordosis, inability to pass the hand means obliteration of the same. Do not insinuate your hand again while measuring the flexion deformity as, one it is uncomfortable and two it may reproduce the deformity as the patient may try to adjust your hand out of respect thus decreasing the exact measurement!*)

21. What will you do for bilateral deformity?

Ans. I will do the test in prone position (modification)—both lower limbs dangling off the couch. Support both thighs and obliterate lumbar lordosis in direct vision then measure the flexion deformity from imaginary horizontal parallel to floor. Other more practical way is to test in lateral position and obliterate lumbar lordosis.

22. What precautions you should take care of and what are the drawbacks of this test?

Ans. One should not allow overflexion and lifting off pelvis. There should be no abduction in the affected limb while measuring deformity—it spuriously reduces the deformity.

Drawbacks:
- Exact flexion contracture cannot be commented, if adduction/abduction deformity coexists
- Not comfortable for a patient with already painful hip

- If the ipsilateral knee is painful or ankylosed, then the test is difficult (painful) and inaccurate (ankylosed)
- Inaccurate in obese (thigh is stopped by abdomen and prevents further correction of deformity—pushing further increases pelvic obliquity rendering test void) and uncooperative patients
- Difficult to do prone test for bilateral deformity
- Rule out rectus contracture before performing the test.

23. What is the principle behind Thomas test?

Ans. Fixed sagittal plane deformity at hip is compensated by pelvic extension (flexion deformity) and vice versa. This is produced by increase (for hip flexion deformity) or decrease (for extension deformity at hip—uncommon) in lumbar lordosis which also shares the compensation. The combined effect allows a patient to walk with feet touching the ground in conjunction with knee flexion. While we flex the normal hip the deformity in pelvis first gets corrected (something akin to squaring pelvis) then lumbar lordosis is corrected simultaneously revealing the deformity.

24. Can we test by manipulating affected hip?

Ans. Of course we can, it will be similar to squaring pelvis but the patient with painful hip will be hurt and also such a maneuver will make him apprehensive. This is what is done in alternative maneuver described above.

25. Why do you keep the other limb flexed?

Ans. To keep the pelvis fixed in corrected position.

26. What are the causes of false-positive Thomas test?

Ans. Wrong technique is the most common cause.

Others are:
- Fixed pelvic obliquity in scoliosis and polio
- Exaggerated lordosis in obese individuals
- Malformed pelvis.

27. What other information you may derive from Thomas test?

Ans. If the affected hip goes into abduction while performing Thomas test then it indicates iliotibial band tightness possibly a contracture. Perform Ober's test to confirm then.

The Hip

28. Does the true length measurement change with hip position?

Ans. The line ASIS → medial malleolus passes lateral to hip joint so moving from full abduction to adduction increases the limb length measure. In full abduction as the measurement is done from the "starting point", ASIS that lies lateral to true position of femoral head, the measured length will come smaller than true length. However, if same measurement is repeated in full adduction then because ASIS is at a higher level than femoral head so the measured length gets erroneously longer. This difference usually is 1–2 cm when measured from full abduction to adduction. Also flexion deformity gives erroneous limb shortening, hence mirrored limb position (unaffected limb kept in same position as that of affected limb due to deformities for measurement) with squaring of pelvis is recommended.

29. What are the movements of pelvis?

Ans. Internal movements (within bones—minimal), external movements [extension (anterior pelvic tilt)—superior pelvis moves forward flexion (posterior pelvic tilt)—superior pelvis moves backward]. Just to remember one *F*—K's in *F*lexion. Pelvic nutation are the movements that occur at SI joint and are actually movements of the sacrum with pelvis fixed in space. In nutation the top of sacrum moves down and forward in relation to fixed pelvis.

30. How much flexion deformity at hip can be hidden by lumbar lordosis?

Ans. Up to 30°.

31. What are the causes of increased lumbar lordosis?

Ans. The various pathological and physiological causes of increased lumbar lordosis are:
- *Suprapelvic:* Pregnancy, obesity, spondylolisthesis, and constitutional
- *Pelvic:* Congenital defects, rickets, and developmental defects
- *Infrapelvic:* B/L or unilaterally (U/L) flexion deformity of hip and DDH.

32. How do you do Trendelenburg test?

Ans. There are at least four different methods vaguely described in various textbooks. The following is the most standard method studied and described. *(The instructions and sequence is best demonstrated by the examiner to patient himself as verbal orders are difficult to follow).*

- Stand behind patient. Observe the angle between pelvis (line joining iliac crests) and ground. Ask patient to stand on unaffected side first, lifting affected side foot and flexing hip (between neutral and 30°) and knee to clear foot off the ground (this is done to nullify the effect of rectus femoris). Note the position of pelvis. (In some patients to maintain balance either a supporting stick can be used on the hand of weight-bearing hip or examiner can support both shoulders).
- Then ask patient to raise the affected side of pelvis as high as possible. (One may provide support to the patient by holding arm of the weight-bearing side). Correct any tendency to lean over the weight-bearing side by bringing shoulders at same level **(Fig. 21)**.
- Repeat the same on affected side (the side to be tested).

Interpretation: Normally ("negative test") one is able to lift the other side (watch iliac crest) without losing balance for at least 30 seconds and the lift is equal to the abduction possible at that hip.

Gluteal folds have been long propagated as "standard" reference for judging pelvic lift but a lot of limitations arise primarily due to muscle wasting so common in hip disorders. PSIS is a good reference if there is significant gluteal wasting or folds, which are asymmetrical, however it is too near to midline to judge pelvic lift and to be taken as a primary reference.

Alternately, one can less reliably stand in front of patient and support patient's palm. Perform the test the same way but notice the pressure transmitted by patient's palm when they attempt to balance. Increased pressure in opposite side in an attempt to gain support from you suggests positive test.

The Hip

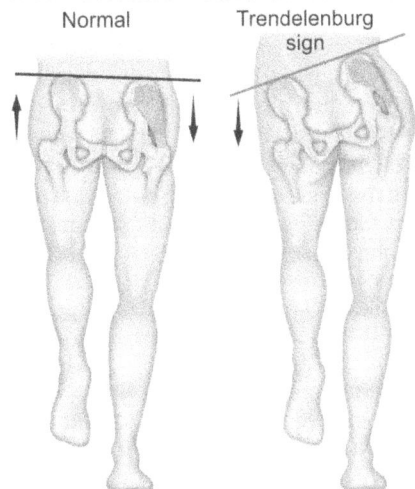

Fig. 21: Trendelenburg test.

33. What constitutes a positive Trendelenburg test?
Ans. Any of the following constitute a "positive test" (abnormal response):
- Maximal elevation not achieved.
- Sustained elevation not achieved (for 30 seconds)—delayed abnormal response.
- Iliac crest not elevated (pelvis parallel to ground).
- Pelvis drops down (opposite iliac crest).

34. What does this test assess?
Ans. It is a screening test to check integrity of "abductor mechanism" comprising head and acetabular socket as fulcrum, neck and trochanteric region as lever (site of effort), abductor [primarily gluteus medius aided by tensor fasciae latae (TFL)] as power, and load is the lower limb distal to trochanteric region. Hip is a class-3 lever. Insufficiency at any level is reflected as a positive test.

35. What can produce a false-positive test?
Ans. Painful hip, poor balance, uncooperative patient, and costopelvic impingement (as in scoliosis).

36. What can produce a false-negative test?
Ans. Use of suprapelvic muscles by patient, use of psoas and rectus femoris, wide lateral translocation of trunk to allow balance over the hip as a fulcrum are some of the trick movements that develop in a patient with weak abductors and they mask Trendelenburg test.

37. What are the prerequisites for doing this test?
Ans. There are a lot of limitations that itself are frequently seen in hip pathologies, so it is not a very reliable test to judge hip abductor mechanism:

- It should not be a very painful hip (spuriously positive).
- There should be no abduction or adduction deformity in any hip.
- Quadratus lumborum must be normal (affected in polio)—this effects a normal Trendelenburg test.
- In obese and patients with medial shift of lower limb mechanical axis (like ipsilateral genu varum deformity) the test may be pseudo-positive. Here the work of abductors is greatly increased and they may not sustain the pelvis straight due to mechanical disadvantage.
- Sacroiliitis may produce a positive test.

38. Who described Trendelenburg test?
Ans. It was originally described by "Duchenne de Boulogne" in 1867 but was rediscovered by Friedrich Trendelenburg in 1895 for assessment of DDH.

39. What are the causes of a positive Trendelenburg test?
Ans. *Gluteus medius paralysis:*

- Polio, L5 radiculopathy, girdle muscular dystrophy, cerebral palsy (and other disjunctive disorders), etc. *Power of 5/5 MRC grade is required for normal response ("negative test") any power less than or equal to 4 will produce positive test.*

Failure of lever:

- Trochanteric avulsion, fracture neck of femur, and coxa vara

Disruption of fulcrum:

- Dislocated hip, DDH or subluxating hips, wandering acetabulum, Perthes disease, SUFE, osteonecrosis, sequelae of septic arthritis.

Gluteal inhibition:
- Painful hip due to arthritis/infection, Sacroiliitis.

40. Is it possible to mask Trendelenburg's sign or resulting gait?

Ans. (*An impractical but a very conceptual question—concept can be utilized in conservatively managing unreconstructible abductor paralysis*). Yes, if one carries a weight of 6–7 kg on the affected side (say carrying a briefcase) while walking, the lurch can be largely obliterated. This is due to shift of center of gravity toward the affected side and hence masking the weakness.

41. How do you test for telescopy?

Ans. Patient lies supine on bed, examiner on right side facing the patient to observe patient reaction also, explain the maneuver to patient first and demonstrate on uninvolved side first to calm him. Fix pelvis by left hand (for examining right hip of patient) so that trochanter is embraced by fingers while rest of hand fixes iliac crest. Flex hip to more than 60° (preferably to 90°) and adduct the limb slightly (to put hip in vulnerable position) by holding the knee with right hand then apply a push-pull force along the axis of shaft and note first the translation of trochanter and secondly crepitus from joint. (*Remember this is a provocative test and offensive one to the patient—be gentle!*) (*Now, whether to push or pull first—do not be concerned, result will not change!*)

42. What are the prerequisites for telescopy?

Ans. Hip and knee should have flexion range of movement; adduction should be possible at hip and firm mattress, ideally a painless hip.

43. What are the causes of a telescoping hip?

Ans. Causes in hip joint *per se:*
- Girdlestone arthroplasty
- Old unreduced dislocation with lax structures
- Developmental dysplasia of the hip
- Pathological dislocation, e.g. TB
- Charcot's joint
- Perthes disease
- Slipped capital femoral epiphysis

- Squeal of septic arthritis
- Osteonecrosis with collapse
- *Tuberculosis of hip*: Mortar and pestle type, destroyed head, and wandering acetabulum

Causes out of hip joint:
- Nonunion fractured neck of femur
- Nonunion fractured intertrochanteric.

44. What are Ortolani's and Barlow's tests?

Ans. Better called Ortolani's test and Barlow's maneuver. These are basically for evaluation of DDH.

Ortolani test (1947); Froelich (1911); LeDamanu (1912): Hips flexed 90° and knees flexed. Start from adducted position and slowly abduct hip whilst exerting pressure over greater trochanter. Reducible dislocated hip gives "clunk of entry" feeling. Usually observed till 3 months of age.

Barlow's maneuver (1962): Modified Ortolani test. His test has two parts, first one similar to Ortolani test but the hips are sequentially tested in 45–60° flexion (involved hip is more likely to be unstable in this position while the other one fixes pelvis). Second part is Barlow test for dislocatable hips—exert outward pressure on hip; if it dislocates but reduces, then it indicates dislocatable but not dislocated hip.

45. What is thickening and broadening of trochanter?

Ans. Thickening of trochanter is identified by holding it between index finger and thumb whereas broadening is observed by palpation over trochanter where it feels more prominent than the normal side. Causes are often same.
- Tumors, cysts, malunited (or uniting or nonunion) intertrochanteric fractures, postoperative (fixation of fractures around hip and osteotomy), infection, and Perthes disease.

46. Discuss interpretation of Bryant's triangle.

Ans. *Shortening of base:* Suggests upriding of greater trochanter seen in coxa vara, coxa breva, destruction of head, nonunion fracture neck femur, old dislocations, Girdlestone arthroplasty, and Perthes disease.

The Hip

Shortening of perpendicular only: Suggests internal rotation of femur or central migration of head—old unreduced posterior dislocation, central fracture dislocation, etc.

Shortening of hypotenuse: It is always associated with shortening of either or both of other lines (*Remember Pythagoras theorem*) (**Fig. 22**).

Isolated shortenings are rare and a combination is often seen:

Base + perpendicular shortening (definite hypotenuse shortening): Central fracture dislocation, neck resorption, head resorption, and protrusio acetabuli.

Base shortened but perpendicular lengthening: Nonunion fracture neck femur, anterior dislocation of hip, SCFE, and Girdlestone arthroplasty.

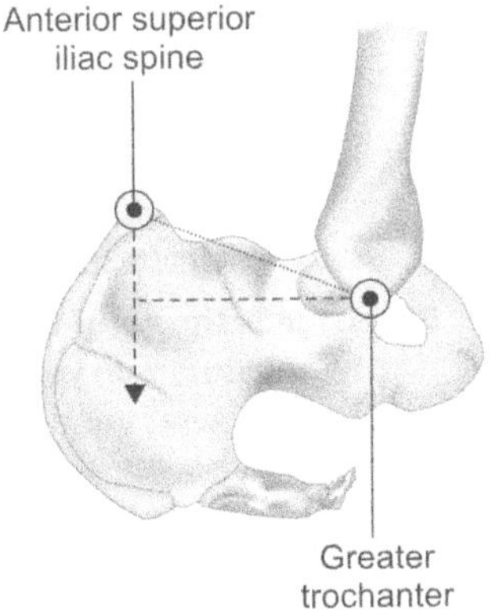

Fig. 22: Bryant's triangle.

Base shortened + lengthened perpendicular: Malunited fractured neck femur.

Lengthened perpendicular + hypotenuse (normal base): External rotation deformity at hip joint.

All lines lengthened: Coxa magna and coxa valga.

47. What are the fallacies of Bryant's triangle measurement?

Ans. Useless in bilateral affections and/or if ASIS cannot be palpated or there is pathology at trochanter (avulsion, surgical removal/advancement, etc.)

The other practical fact is that the lines drawn are quite arbitrary serving as rough measures only so errors in interpretation are easy to occur for mild to moderate deformities.

48. How will you perform bitrochanteric compression test?

Ans. *(This is different from Morris bitrochanteric test: The bitrochanteric compression test is done to elicit deep tenderness in hip joint).* With the patient in supine position, observing the facial expression; both the trochanters are compressed centrally into acetabulum by placing the palm in such a way that the cleft between thenar and hypothenar eminences engages most prominent part of trochanters. Positive test indicates local bony (fracture/neoplasia/infection) or joint (inflammatory) pathology of hip joint/trochanter.

49. **What are the sites of psoas abscess that can be clinically examined?**

Ans. Abdomen (iliac fossae), base of Scarpa's triangle, gluteal region, supratrochanteric region, anteromedial aspect of thigh (sub-sartorial canal and through adductor hiatus), popliteal fossa, lumbar triangle at back, and flanks.

50. **What is the lymphatic drainage of hip "or" what groups of lymph nodes do you examine for hip case?**

Ans. External iliac, internal iliac, paraaortic group of lymph nodes, and also some drainage to deep inguinal group of lymph nodes are present.

51. **What is the nerve supply of hip joint and what is its importance?**

Ans. Variegated nerve supply:
- Femoral nerve via rectus femoris
- Obturator nerve anterior division
- Accessory obturator nerve
- Nerve to quadratus femoris
- Superior gluteal nerve.

Pain of hip joint may be referred to knee joint (via femoral and obturator nerve) and may be the primary presentation in early pathology. Knee joint is also supplied by femoral nerve via vastus medialis, posterior division of obturator nerve apart from sciatic nerve (genicular tibial and common peroneal).

52. **What are the various sites of referred pain of hip joint?**

Ans. Various patterns of referred pain from hip joint observed are:
- *Obturator pattern:* Pain deep in groin radiating to medial thigh.

The Hip

- *Posterior pattern:* Deep in the buttock (most common).
- *Femoral pattern:* Pain from front of joint radiating along anterior thigh. This pain may also be referred to knee joint and sometimes the primary pain at hip joint may not be noticed by the patient. This is commonly seen in osteonecrosis of femoral head and inflammatory conditions like TB hip and Tom-Smith arthritis. In these conditions due to muscular splinting of the hip joint, minimal or no movement occurs at hip so pain at pathology gets masked whilst knee pain is noticed by the patient which is actually a referred pain.
- *Lateral pattern:* Over greater trochanter radiates along lateral thigh to knee.
- Uncommonly pain can also radiate to leg and foot.

53. Which movement is first lost in hip pathology?

Ans. Extension followed by rotations, adduction, abduction, and lastly flexion (this sequence is followed in synovial disorders—increased volume whereas those in which there is direct injury to cartilage; abduction is lost earlier due to adductor spasm—adductors are stronger).

54. What is the position of rest for hip joint?

Ans. This is the position in which the volume of hip joint is maximal—10° each of flexion, abduction, and external rotation.

55. What is its implication?

Ans. Hip pathologies that increase joint volume say due to effusion of collection of pus; present in this deformity position of flexion, abduction, and external rotation to give rest to the joint.

56. What are the criteria for making diagnosis of ankylosing spondylitis?

Ans. *Rome criteria* (1963)—*Ankylosing spondylitis (AS) present if Bilateral Sacroilitis + any of the below:*
- Low back pain with stiffness for >3 months
- Pain and stiffness in thoracic region
- Limited motion in lumbar region
- Limited chest expansion
- History of iritis or its sequel.

[The Rome or New York criteria are asked only by classical examiners while ASAS criteria are the latest followed for diagnosis of ankylosing spondylosis/axial spondyloarthropathy (Kindly see chapter 11 of the book Essential orthopedics principles and practice for details on ASAS criteria)].

Modified New York criteria: Definitive Sacroiliitis (Grade ≥2 bilateral or unilateral 3–4) and any one of the following (definitive ankylosing spondylitis). Probable ankylosing spondylitis if three clinical criterion or radiological criterion present, but no signs or symptoms to satisfy clinical criteria:

- Low back pain ≥3 months' duration improved by exercise not relieved by rest
- Limitation of lumbar spine movements in sagittal and frontal planes
- Chest expansion decreased relative to normal values for age and sex.

BASDAI (bath ankylosing spondylitis disease activity index) detects the inflammatory burden of disease. It can help establish the diagnosis of AS in the presence of other factors like HLA-B27 positivity, persistent buttock or back pain that resolves with exercise, and X-ray and magnetic resonance imaging (MRI) involvement of sacroiliac joints. *(Apart from HLA-B27, two new genes have been associated with AS— ARTS1 and IL23R but clinical significance is not established well).*

57. Who described Kothari's parallelogram?
Ans. Dr Manu Kothari described this alternative maneuver to look for coronal plane deformities at hip joint without squaring the pelvis *(He was a 2nd year MBBS student at that time and retired as professor of anatomy from KEM Mumbai).*

58. What are the common conditions affecting hip bilaterally?
Ans. Bilateral affection of hip is seen commonly in:
- Osteonecrosis of hip (bilateral in 50%)
- Perthes disease (10%)
- Coxa vara (50%)
- SUFE/SCFE (25–30%)
- DDH (30–40%).

The Hip

CASE I: TUBERCULOSIS OF HIP JOINT

Diagnosis: The patient is a 17-year-old male with 6 months old conservatively managed tubercular affection of right hip on antitubercular therapy (ATT) in healing stage. Patient has 2.5 cm of true shortening (supratrochanteric) with flexion deformity of 20°, adduction deformity 15° and internal rotation deformity of 10° with limitation of all movements. Patient is able to do activities of daily living but not his other routine activities.

(*For a tubercular arthritis under treatment mentioning stage is incorrect as disease would have halted and stage altered but for a patient not on treatment mention stage of disease in first line. From here viva can take any direction as this is an open and adequate diagnosis; like—how do you measure flexion/adduction deformity/ true shortening or what is the range of flexion, etc.—this often entails from the fact that there are multiple candidates and a comparison is coherent to mark candidates, hence common questions are legible*).

1. **Why do you think it is tuberculosis of hip?**
Ans.
- Protracted history with insidious onset pain; night cries
- Age group (As a rule <10-year-old patient population commonly affected but any age can be affected; TB spine: TB hip = 10:7)
- Restriction of movements in all direction ("Global" restriction of movements)
- Typical deformity (according to stage and added supratrochanteric shortening later)
- Association with progressive limp that appeared early
- Relief with treatment (typically traction, ATT)
- Wasting and constitutional symptoms (+ history of contacts if present).

2. **What is your differential diagnosis?**
Ans. I will give a differential according to more common possibilities first:
- *Subacute septic arthritis*: Heals quite early with treatment otherwise atypical forms closely resemble TB (TB in Indian subcontinent gets benefit of doubt and is often the first clinical diagnosis).

- *Proximal femoral osteomyelitis with reactive hip involvement*: Thickening/broadening of trochanter, irregular proximal femur, sinuses, reactive effusion give (FABER) deformity.
- *Osteonecrosis of femoral head with early cartilage eburnation*: Limp and deformities appear late.
- *Late-onset Perthes disease*: Less common, less flexion deformity, movements not limited in all directions, and should not respond to treatment.
- *Monoarticular rheumatoid:* Very uncommon, occurs in middle aged/elderly, should not respond to ATT.
- *Nonunion fracture neck of femur:* Trauma, characteristic initial history, treatment history, telescopy, and deformity (flexion and external rotation).
- *Central fracture dislocation of hip:* Movement in one plane is preserved (*however even in TB in Indian patients, flexion is often present due to practice of squatting which is a daily practice*): Trauma is definitely present.
- *Ankylosing spondylitis:* Oops, you are given the whole patient not just a joint—examine in totality (*don't go so close to a tree that you lose the site of forest*).

3. What can be your other differentials?

Ans. Depending on specific symptomatology I will classify my differentials into:
- *Limitation of movements:*
  - Irritable hip.
  - Upper motor neuron (UMN) lesion: Spasms overcome by pressure, not painful, no wasting.
  - Reflex irritation from lymph nodes, etc.
- *Limp:*
  - DDH: Certain movements exaggerated
  - Coxa vara: ↑ external rotation, adduction – external rotation deformity
  - Perthes disease
  - Irritable hip.
- *Pain:*
  - Osteomyelitis and septic arthritis
  - SCFE

The Hip

- Early poliomyelitis
- Irritable hip.

This question has been deliberately added to complete the remotest possibility for TB hip differential and enabling the candidate face examiner's lethal weapon –"And…"

4. Why do you call it healing "or" in other words, what are the signs of active disease?

Ans. There is no rest pain, night cries (starting pains), no joint swelling, Gauvain's negative, characteristic deformity of stage III.

5. How do you stage TB hip?

Ans. Clinical staging (this is the sequence of untreated TB, treatment may arrest it anywhere!):

Stage	Pathology	Attitude
1. Stage of apparent lengthening (due to pelvic tilt to compensate for abduction deformity. >75% pain-free movements, and no true shortening)	Synovitis/effusion	FABER (Flexion, abduction, external rotation)
2. Stage of apparent shortening [pelvic tilt to compensate adduction deformity (spasm), movements restricted beyond 50%, true shortening either none or <1 cm]	Early arthritis	FADER (Flexion, adduction, external rotation)
3. Stage of true shortening. (Fixed deformities, movements restricted to <25%, real shortening >1 cm)	Advanced arthritis	FADER with shortening
4. Stage of aftermath and destruction (wandering acetabulum, pathological dislocation, destruction of head, fibrous ankylosis, etc.)	Ongoing gross destruction	Shortening ↑s further, deformities can vary depending on the final outcome

6. Why do the deformities differ in different stages?

Ans. In stage I, due to effusion and ↑d requirement for space hip goes into FABER deformity; later in stage II, the deformities are due to spasm of muscles. Flexors and adductors are stronger than other groups so characteristic FADER deformity is exhibited. Moreover, irritation of inferomedial joint capsule by debris irritates obturator nerve causing adductor spasm and direct irritation of iliopsoas occurs by underlying swollen and hyperemic capsule. In stage III, there is eburnation of cartilage and generalized spasm increasing bony contact and enhancing destruction but above two groups dominate to maintain FADER deformity.

7. Can you still see flexion, abduction, internal/external rotation deformity in a patient in stage II/III?

Ans. YES.
- Patient treated by prolonged traction
- Patient maintained in hip spica
- Elderly or debilitated patients who prefer to lie in lateral position and continue with initial posture for relief of pain, moreover they have weak muscles
- Destruction of iliofemoral ligament (inverted Y-ligament of Bigelow)
- Patient who continues to bear weight in the initial deformed position.

8. What is the cause of night cries?

Ans. Destruction of cartilage exposes the subchondral nerve endings. Periarticular muscle spasm in awakened position prevents any joint movement so there is no/minimal pain. In the night with muscle relaxation, the splinting effect is taken away and the bony surfaces rub across each other causing severe pain.

9. What will you do next?

Ans. I will get an X-ray of pelvis done anteroposterior (AP) view with radiographs of right hip in AP and lateral projections.

10. What do you expect to see on an X-ray?

Ans. As per the examination, I expect to see involvement of both femur and acetabulum with reduction of joint space, cystic sclerotic lesions in head and acetabulum, acetabular widening and/or destruction of femoral head, upriding of greater trochanter, flexion adduction and external

The Hip

rotation deformity, with or without subluxation of joint and displacement of fat planes.

11. Does this *support* your diagnosis?

Ans. Yes ☺ or No ☹. *(Note: clinico-radiological coherence supports the diagnosis but does not confirm it!)*

12. How do you clinico-radiologically classify TB?

Ans. *Shanmugasundaram classification*:
- Normal hip
- Traveling acetabulum
- Dislocating type
- Perthes type
- Protrusio acetabuli.
- Atrophic type
- Mortar and pestle type

(More commonly in *Adult* the atrophic form; *in children*—normal, Perthes, and dislocation types, while mortar and pestle, wandering, and protrusion types are seen in *both*) **(Fig. 23)**.

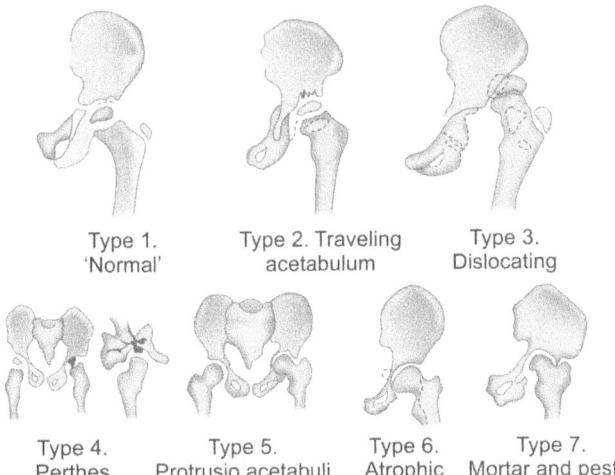

Type 1. 'Normal'   Type 2. Traveling acetabulum   Type 3. Dislocating

Type 4. Perthes   Type 5. Protrusio acetabuli   Type 6. Atrophic   Type 7. Mortar and pestle

Fig. 23: Various clinicoradiological types of tuberculosis (TB) hip as described by Shanmugasundaram.

13. What are the common radiological signs of TB hip?

Ans. Osteoporosis is the earliest sign, "Cat-Bite" lesion in articular margin, ↓ joint space, destructive changes. Bony lamellae undergo osteoporosis in early stages (osteoclasts and Howship's lacunae) later with healing there is osteosclerosis (osteoblastic activity).

14. What are the radiological signs of healing?

Ans. The following are seen in healing TB:
- ↑ in thickness of trabeculae
- ↑ density of bone
- Recommencing of epiphyseal growth.

15. How will you confirm diagnosis?

Ans. *Blood tests (none have been found useful so better to avoid mentioning in examination also, they carry only historical importance):*
- Raised erythrocyte sedimentation rate (ESR) and c-reactive protein (CRP) (only support inflammation nonspecifically anywhere in body)
- *Enzyme-linked immunosorbent assay (ELISA) (WHO shuns its use)*: IgG and IgM response to A60 antigen complex (interspecific antigen and is common to typical and atypical mycobacteria)—sensitivity of 60–80%
- Polymerase chain reaction (PCR) is highly sensitive and specific but osteoarticular TB being paucibacillary yield is often negative *[lots of them are available, still more reliable, and specific is the ribonucleic acid (RNA) testing but is much expensive].*

Skin tests: False positives and negatives are high; strongly positive reaction in previously negative patient is highly suggestive (but hardly found in an adult patient).

(Confirmation is possible only with examining the pathology) Synovial fluid examination/synovial biopsy/bone biopsy:
- ↑ Protein, poor formation of mucin clot, etc. in synovial fluid examination
- Staining (Ziehl-Neelsen) (definite diagnosis)

The Hip

- *Culture*:
  - Provides ultimate diagnosis
  - But is very slow (Rapid alternatives are BACTEC TB-460, BACTEC MGIT960, etc.)
- Histopathological demonstration of caseating necrosis—definitive diagnosis
- *Rapid methods*:
  - Centrifuged samples
  - Thin-layer and gas-liquid interphase chromatography for detection of lipids and long-chain fatty acids—rarely used now
  - Xpert MTB/RIF—best additional primary test for diagnosis
  - Line probe assay (DNA strip test) recommended for multidrug resistance (MDR) rapid diagnosis

Staining requires around 10,000 bacilli/mm^3, culture requires 1,000 bacilli/mm^3.

16. How will you treat this case?

Ans. After ascertaining diagnosis, the aim is to obtain ideal outcome of a painless, mobile, and stable hip. But the patient's disease has already been present for 6 months and is in stage III, so treatment has to be provided according to present situation. I will continue with chemotherapy and advice for heliotherapy, liberal diet, fresh air, restrain from exertion until healing, traction to correct, and maintain deformity with intermittent mobilization.

17. What is the role of chemotherapy and what is the regime?

Ans. Chemotherapy is absolutely essential and should be a combination chemotherapy (at least one of which is bactericidal) and prolonged for long to kill persisters. It is divided into intensive and continuation phases. In general, the intensive phase (aka initial phase) kills the rapidly multiplying extracellular bacteria while continuation phase is aimed at killing the dormant bacteria and preventing recurrence. WHO regime for skeletal TB had been classically considered inadequate and prolonged regimens for 12–14 months have been deployed at various institutions in Indian subcontinent at will. I doubt the practice and adhere to WHO regime for treatment of TB Hip. Currently the WHO recommends 9 months treatment for treatment of osteoarticular TB placing it in the same class as that of HIV-positive TB cases. Intensive phase for 2 months of four drugs (INH, RIF, PZE, and ETH) along with vitamin B6 is given followed by continuation phase for 7 months of two drugs (INH and RIF) + vitamin B6.

(*Please follow your institutional regime if it differs from above or when in doubt you can always bank upon WHO regime, class IV and ignore all above*).

However, [*In Asian sub-continent one is expected to know the whole regime, drugs (first and second line), dosage, side-effects, and interactions for ATT. You should refer to the standard pharmacologic texts for this—it's essential!*].

18. How will you judge response to treatment?

Ans. Clinically, reducing pain and tenderness, general sense of well-being, improving ROM or reducing pain on ROM, reduced tenderness, improvement in deformity (early stages), and improvement in appetite. Serologically, serial ESR demonstrates normalization and reduction in CRP (early to appear). Radiological signs of healing as above.

19. What is the pathology of an untreated hip?

Ans. *Synovial type*: Hypertrophy, congestion, unhealthy hypertrophic granulation tissue formation (pannus) → cartilage destruction → fibrosed and thickened synovium → granulation tissue bridges bony surfaces → fibrous ankylosis.

Bony extension type: Occurs via subperiosteal space or direct metaphyseal spread → cartilage is the only barrier → once breached leads to growth plate destruction → deformities and shortening.

Clinical types of hip joint TB:
- *Granular form*: Common in adults, protracted course, less destruction, and ↓ tendency for cold abscess formation.

- *Caseous type*: Severe constitutional symptoms, more common in childhood, destruction, and abscess common.
- *Tubercular rheumatism (Poncet's disease)*: Asymmetric polyarthritis + focus of infection.

20. What are rice bodies?

Ans. Accumulation of fibrin over worn pieces of articular cartilage produces small soft to firm loose bodies that float in the synovial fluid giving appearance of boiled rice.

21. What is the focus of infection in TB?

Ans. Tubercular arthritis commonly arise from nearby focus of infection that initiates in:
- *Synovial*: It is rare site of initiation and often has protracted course
- *Osseous*:
  - Acetabular side (roof of acetabulum)
  - *Head of femur "Babcock's triangle"*: It is an area which is the watershed between obturator and femoral circulation and bone is weaker in this region. It lies toward the cervical side of lower part of head and proximal part of neck in lower half near epiphyseal line.
  - *Neck of femur*: *See* above
  - Greater trochanteric region.

22. What is the role of traction?

Ans. Traction is used for:
- Overcoming spasm and deformity due to same
- Providing/enforcing rest
- Maintaining length and functional position of limb
- Maintaining joint space (separating capital and acetabular cartilage)
- Correction of deformities (stretching contractures)
  - Pain relief
  - Prevent complication like subluxation and dislocations, wandering acetabulum.

23. How much traction do you give?

Ans. Traction is usually decided on age of patient and 0.45 kg/year of traction is given:
- Give bilateral traction as:
  - Unilateral may increase abduction deformity
  - Pelvic tilt may also increase
- Slight abduction is advisable as:
  - Compensates real shortening
  - Usually a tendency toward adduction is seen in convalescence.

24. What is the role of surgery in TB?

Ans. Surgery is indicated either to obtain tissue for diagnosis and/or do a formal debridement in clinically non-responsive TB. Other type of surgery is done to manage the deformities and provide an optimized outcome:
- *Painless, stable, and immobile (fixed) joint*: Hip arthrodesis
- Corrective osteotomy
- *Painless, unstable, and mobile joint*: Modified Girdlestone arthroplasty
- *Painless, stable, and mobile*: Total hip replacement.

25. What are the indications for surgery?

Ans. The following conditions needs to be managed by surgery in TB hip:
- *Clinically nonresponsive TB hip*: Excision of focus.
- Failure to obtain acceptable outcome (unacceptable deformity) after completion of conservative treatment.
- Painful healed disease due to secondary osteoarthritis.

26. What do you mean by excision of focus?

Ans. Removal of all diseased tissue from the joint which is often the synovium and any obvious bony focus/lesion. The material is thoroughly curetted out and sent for histopathology and bacteriological diagnosis (reconfirm diagnosis). Limb is immobilized in acceptable position following procedure. Surgery should be done in proper ATT cover (6 week–2 months presurgical cover).

The Hip

27. What are the complications of this surgery?

Ans. One or more of the following:
- Fulminant progression of disease
- Osteonecrosis of femoral head
- Pathological fracture of femoral neck
- Slippage of capital femoral epiphysis
- Chondrolysis
- Pathological dislocation of hip.

28. What will you do in this patient?

Ans. As the patient is responding to conservative treatment, I will continue the same till healing then depending on the outcome I will choose a procedure.

29. What do you expect in this patient?

Ans. Patient in stage III of disease is unlikely to have a well-formed painless joint. I expect a painful healed joint with features of secondary osteoarthritis at the end of treatment.

30. What will you do then?

Ans. I will give patient the options (*see* above) and explain in detail the functional limitations and merits of each. Also I will assess the functional demands of patient.

31. What does the patient want?

Ans. Patient belongs to poor laborer family and principally requires joint for doing hard work. I would prefer doing a hip arthrodesis for him.

32. What are the indications of arthrodesis in TB hip?

Ans. Four main indications:
1. Young active adult patient doing hard work and putting lot of stress on joint
2. Failure to arrest disease after 1 year of supervised treatment
3. Relapse and recurrence of pain and deformity after conservative treatment (now with the advent of good total hips and chemotherapy people prefer doing THR)
4. Destructive disease, viz. formation of sequestra in head of femur or acetabulum [again people may prefer total hip replacement (THR)]

In general, a young adult patient with no life limiting (focus on remaining survival) or activity limiting (e.g. rheumatoid arthritis) unilateral hip disease and is not a candidate for osteotomy/mold arthroplasty. Also one who desires a standing work rather than sitting.

33. What are the types of hip arthrodesis?

Ans. *Intra-articular:*
- Central dislocation and internal compression arthrodesis of charnley
- Watson–Jones transarticular nail arthrodesis
- Intramedullary arthrodesis of Onji
- Cobra-plate arthrodesis **(Fig. 24)**.

Extra-articular:
- Iliofemoral arthrodesis of Albee
- Ischiofemoral arthrodesis of Brittain

Pararticular (usually done to augment intra-articular procedure):
- Davis muscle-pedicle arthrodesis.

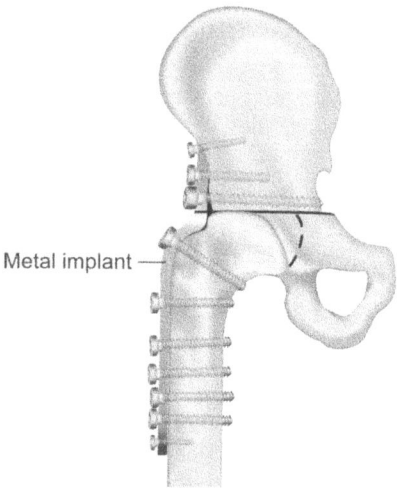

Fig. 24: Intra-articular arthrodesis by Cobra-plate method.

The Hip

34. Which one will you do and why?

Ans. I will do intra-articular arthrodesis using cobra plate for the following reasons:
- Joint debridement can be done simultaneously.
- Large raw surfaces can be carved out to enhance chances of union.
- More secure fixation and one directly addresses the diseased site without changing the anatomy elsewhere.
- In destroyed joints, space can be filled with bone graft with good approximation in intra-articular methods.

35. What is the role of extra-articular arthrodesis?

Ans. These were practiced on the premises that opening up diseased joint will flare up the infection and there was lack of availability of good chemotherapy. However, these procedures destroy the anatomy of hip joint making any future procedure difficult.

36. In what position do you fix joint?

Ans. *Flexion of 30°*: As a general rule, 1° per year of age above 10 years till a maximum of 30° above 25 years of age (rationale is that ongoing compensation develops in children with flexible spine and in adults up to 30° of flexion can be hidden by lumbar lordosis). Flexion provides necessary ground clearance and lets one hide fixed joint while sitting.

Adduction/abduction: Previously favored abduction no longer holds true as it leads to later development of frontal plane knee deformity and also gait is better with hip fused in adduction. Prefer either neutral or 5° of adduction.

Rotation: No objective data but 0–15° external rotation preferred.

37. What is Brittain's method of extra-articular arthrodesis?

Ans. The method consists of first doing a subtrochanteric osteotomy followed by incising ischium just below the acetabulum *through* osteotomy. Then a massive tibial graft is pushed into the defect through osteotomy. Alternatively, in a healed case (ankylosed) with adduction and flexion deformity a subtrochanteric McMurray's osteotomy can be done **(Fig. 25)**.

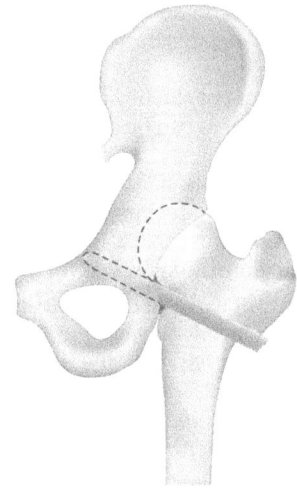

Fig. 25: Brittain's method of hip arthrodesis.

38. What are the contraindications of arthrodesis?
Ans. It should not be done in:
- *Ongoing uncontrolled active infection*: Wait at least 1 year after infection has healed.
- Opposite hip and ipsilateral knee already arthrodesed.
- Severe degenerative changes in lumbar spine, opposite hip, and ipsilateral knee.

39. When can you do THR in TB hip?
Ans. Classsically, the concept was to do THR after 10 years (every examiner must be acquainted to this—safest option). Ambitiously done THR even after 1 year of healed infection under ATT cover gave comparable results (this appears to be a safer choice). Now with the advent of effective chemotherapy, people have attempted THR after 6 weeks of ATT cover under the premises that fixation for spinal TB with ongoing infection has got fair results and change to chronic osteomyelitis and implant failure *per se* due to infection uncommonly occurs (most ambitious choice if you speak may be unacceptable to many!). (*Howsoever difficult this*

The Hip

question and answer seem due to uncertainty—basic principle is that the disease must show good response to ATT and thorough excision of focus must be done else joint will come out with pus!).

40. What is Girdlestone arthroplasty and who described it?

Ans. Girdlestone arthroplasty in essence comprised of extensive debridement of septic joint and surrounding soft tissue with free drainage creating a "type" of excisional arthroplasty. Excisional arthroplasty *per se* was first described by A White (1849). In extensive review of literature, various interesting facts are revealed and there is quite a great misconception for the procedure. Gathorne Girdlestone described his operation in 1923 (not the other oft quoted dates) as a modification of Robert Jone's operation (1921) done for ankylosis of hip joint whereby greater trochanter with its attached muscles used to be attached to resected end of neck to produce pseudoarthrosis. Since then there are as many modifications as there are descriptions.

41. What do you do in Girdlestone arthroplasty?

Ans. The original description as sent by Girdlestone in a telegram to Sir Robert Jones on 15th July 1926 is described below:

- Transverse incision 5 inches long centered 1 inch above trochanter is used to expose deep structures.
- Make two transverse cuts to remove all involved gluteal muscles, trochanter and 3–4 inch wide and 1 inch deep bone is removed from depths (this includes superolateral acetabulum).
- Curette out all carious bone and decide whether to leave bone for ankylosis or remove further to create pseudoarthrosis. [*Here it appears that this procedure was not to create pseudoarthrosis only rather a method to do joint debridement (saucerization for drainage) in long-standing infections of hip with outcome as either ankylosis or pseudoarthrosis*].
- Suture the flaps to periosteum in depths to prevent proud granulation tissue to appear.
- Loosely pack the wound with vaseline gauze.

42. What is the difference between originally described Girdlestone arthroplasty and its modification?

Ans. The most popular modifications are firstly that of Taylor (1950) using Smith-Petersen approach. Additionally, trimming of acetabular rim was done to provide opposing surfaces, pain relief, deformity correction and movements. Nelson (1971) described soft tissue interposition to achieve pseudoarthrosis. The other is that of Grauer et al. (1989) who described four different levels of proximal femoral resections and one by Nagi (1997) who did a subcapital osteotomy and sutured anterior capsule. He reposed the neck back into acetabulum. Basically, now the concept is to retain adequate amount of bone and no acetabular surgery or extensive muscle debridement, using posterior approach.

43. How will you manage a patient of Girdlestone arthroplasty in postoperative period?

Ans. It is again very confusing. The principle is to create stout pseudoarthrosis by fibrous tissue and avoid any lateral impingement. Nagi recommends 6 weeks of postoperative traction. Tuli and Mukherjee (1981) recommend 6-8 weeks skeletal traction and further 6-8 weeks skin traction (total 3 months) followed by walking in caliper for 1 year. It is advisable to put patient on skeletal traction in Thomas splint with Pearson's attachment for first 6 weeks (important to prevent external rotation) in 30-50° abduction with radiographic demonstration of distraction at operative site. After 1st week of surgery, patient should be encouraged to mobilize hip and knee. This will be followed by skin traction for further 6 weeks and then mobilization with bucket top caliper for at least 6 months.

44. What can you do to address the hip instability arising after this osteotomy?

Ans. Instability and shortening arising out of resection arthroplasty can be partially addressed by pelvic support osteotomy of the Milch and Batchelor type.

The Hip

45. What is Milch-Batchelor osteotomy?

Ans. It is a resection angulation osteotomy (RAO/PSO) described as a two-stage procedure by Batchelor and Carry (1943, London).
1. Release of pelvis and restoration of femoral mobility by resecting femoral head and neck
2. Reestablishment of stability by means of particle swarm optimization (PSO) (Schanz). The two stages were combined into one by Milch and Gruca (New York) as traction after stage 1, and immobilization after stage 2 wasted a lot of precious time for mobilization of joint. The essence of osteotomy is "post-osteotomy" angle that should place proximal femur congruent to lateral pelvic wall (mean lateral pelvic wall tilt = 205–210°) else the aim would be defeated. Classically, iliofemoral approach was used sacrificing the nerve to tensor fascia lata. The angulation osteotomy is done at the level of ischial tuberosity. Distal fragment was abducted (virtual lengthening to compensate true shortening) and internally rotated else spontaneous external rotation would again destabilize the pelvic support.

46. What other types of PSO you know of?

Ans. Schanz, Ganz, Lorenz (bifurcation osteotomy), McMurray's, etc.

47. What is the role of PSO?

Ans.
- Surgically shifts the shaft of femur near the center of gravity of the body so that the weight-bearing axis is more along the axis of femur
- Supports pelvis by creating medial fulcrum
- Improves adductor function by causing valgus
- Abduction of distal fragment causes of gain of length.

48. What is Phemister triad?

Ans. Classically described for tuberculosis of hip, which consists of:
- Juxta-articular osteoporosis
- Peripherally located osseous lesion
- Gradual narrowing of joint space.

49. What triangles you know in relation to hip joint?
Ans. Learn the following:
- Babcock's triangle
- *Ward's triangle*: Between primary tensile, primary compressive trabeculae and calcar portion of neck—relevant in osteoporosis and fixation of hip fractures
- *Fairbank's triangle*: Coxa vara
- Bryant's triangle
- Scarpa's triangle (femoral triangle)
- *Abductor triangle*: Formed between gluteus medius, ilium, and neck of femur (displays abductor mechanism).

50. What is the role of manipulation under anesthesia?
Ans. Manipulation under anesthesia is indicated in healing disease with less severe deformities to:
- Attempt gaining mobility of hip while on treatment when articular cartilage is supposedly "preserved"
- Provide a functional position (correcting the deformity) to hip lest it goes in fibrous ankylosis when cartilage is irreparably damaged and functions cannot be regained.

CASE II: NONUNION FRACTURED NECK OF FEMUR (THE UNSOLVED FRACTURE—SPEED)

Diagnosis: The patient is a 52-year-old male with 7-month-old nonunion fracture of femoral neck following trauma treated conservatively. There is 30° fixed flexion deformity with 20° external rotation deformity and 20° adduction deformity and true supratrochanteric shortening of 3 cm. The patient is unable to do his routine activities.

1. What makes you think this is a case of old fracture neck of femur?
Ans.
- Middle-aged (or elderly) patient with history of definite trauma and inability to bear weight following injury (in impacted fractures patient may initially bear weight but with displacement later patient is unable to stand). Examination revealed:
  - Tenderness over mid-inguinal point

The Hip

- FABER deformity with supratrochanteric shortening
- Desault's sign positive
- Telescopy test positive and Trendelenburg's positive
- Active SLRT not possible (unless impacted)
- Bitrochanteric compression test positive
- Active movements not possible or only present with great effort of patient and are ill-sustained with pain.

2. Why is it not nonunion fracture intertrochanteric?

Ans. There should be irregularity over trochanter with broadening and thickening. Tenderness should be at trochanteric region rather than mid-inguinal point.

3. Why is it not old anterior dislocation of hip considering the deformity?

Ans. There is often extension deformity with lengthening in low types of dislocation. Moreover, head is not palpable in the classical sites of dislocation.

4. Why do you think that head is located in this patient?

Ans. Femoral pulses are bilaterally comparable (Narath sign). (*Also see examination for palpable head in dislocated hip*).

5. What will be your differential diagnosis?

Ans. I will put forward the following differentials (*It is always better to speak your answer and diagnosis itself this way—as I presented a very hypothetical and classic case for understanding which is hardly the case in examinations, although I cannot predict or present here all pathological presentations!*):

- Old ununited fracture intertrochanteric right femur
- *Old fracture head of right femur*: Telescopy often absent or minimal
- *Malunited fracture acetabulum posterior wall/superior wall/both*: Very difficult to differentiate but often internal rotation deformity is observed as the hip is unstable and dislocates/subluxates posteriorly—not always true, so it is the closest but rarest differential to be given in examinations (DNB candidates beware).
- *Old treated TB hip with bony changes (wandering acetabulum/mortar-pestle type)*: All said and done traumatic event with typical follow-up should be absent.

6. What are the causes of nonunion in fractured neck femur?

Ans. Nonunion here is predominantly due to combination of mechanical (points 1–4 below) and biological (points 5–10) disruptions:

1. *Morphologic features*: High-fracture angle 60–90° (Pauwels' shear angle)
2. *Displaced fracture*: Garden's III/IV
3. *Fracture comminution*: Posterior comminution (affects adequacy of reduction, angulation, and stability of fixation)
4. Inadequate reduction and stability of fixation
5. Poor bone quality (osteoporosis)
6. *Injury to vascularity*: Direct and tamponade effect (Deyerle)—remember head of femur is already a "hypovolemic bone" (PET studies) even small disturbances put vascularity at risk
7. Absence of cambium layer in periosteum in the neck region, thus the healing is dependent on endosteum only
8. Chondrogenic factors in synovial fluid that inhibit callus formation and consolidation
9. *Lack of hematoma formation*: Synovial fluid prevent hematoma formation
10. Washing away and dilution of osteogenic factors.

Patient's age (It only decides treatment!), gender, osteonecrosis has no influence with nonunion fracture neck femur.

7. Which type of nonunion do you see here?

Ans. Atrophic type.

8. How does duration of nonunion affect planning?

Ans. Increased duration of fracture is counterproductive in the following ways:
- Resorption at fracture ends (resorption begins as early as 3 weeks)
- Contractures prevent adequate lengthening and reduction
- Acetabular cartilage damage.

9. How do you radiographically assess the fracture?

Ans. Poor prognostic factors **(Fig. 26)**:
- ↑ fracture angulation

The Hip

- Osteopenia
- Bone loss
- Osteonecrosis
- Calcar comminution
- Varus angulation

Lateral projection:
- Flexion/extension
- Posterior comminution

MRI/bone scan to look for viability of head.

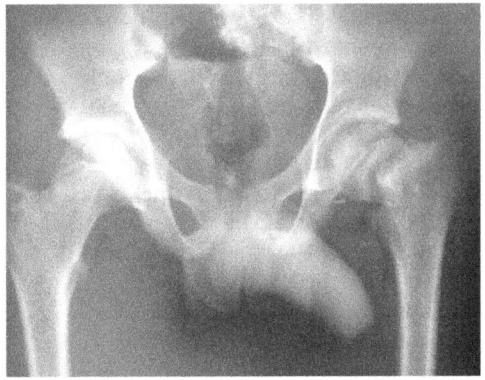

Fig. 26: Anteroposterior radiograph of the pelvis with both hips demonstrating nonunion femoral neck fracture of left side with osteopenia and most of poor prognosticating signs.

10. How do you radiographically assess osteoporosis?

Ans. Singh and Maini index on AP radiographic evaluation of trabeculae:
- *Grade 6 (normal):* All trabeculae present
- *Grade 5:* Loss of trochanteric and secondary tensile, attenuated secondary compressive
- *Grade 4:* Loss of secondary compressive, attenuation of primary tensile
- *Grade 3 (definite osteopenia):* Break in primary tensile
- *Grade 2:* Marked loss of primary tensile
- *Grade 1:* Only primary compressive seen but they are also reduced.

11. When do you call a fracture neck of femur to be a nonunion?

Ans. 3 months following fracture.

12. What is the most standard management for managing fracture neck of femur nonunion?

Ans. There is no standard regime or method for managing nonunion fractured neck of femur that will give uniformly successful results. This is the reason we call it "unsolved fracture".

13. What are the various treatment options available?

Ans. The followings have been successfully practiced (*and should be individualistically given to the patient!*):
- Open reduction and internal fixation (ORIF) with cancellous bone grafting
- ORIF with fibular grafting
- ORIF with vascularized bone grafting
    - Free vascularized fibula
    - Muscle pedicle bone grafting
- Neck reconstruction
- Osteotomy
- Arthrodesis
- Arthroplasty
- Girdlestone type of resection arthroplasty.

14. How do you plan surgery?

Ans. *Clinical assessment:*
- Age of patient
- Presence of osteonecrosis
- *Prior hip symptoms*: Osteoarthritis, etc.
- *Comorbidities*: Smoking, etc.
- Duration from injury
- *Fracture variables*:
    - Site of fracture
    - Fracture configuration.

15. How would you classify nonunion fractured neck of femur?

Ans. *Sandhu et al. (Predictive classification):*
- *Fracture surfaces*:

- Irregular
- Smooth
- *Size of proximal fragment*:
  - 2.5 cm or more
- *Gap between fragments*:
  - Up to 1 cm
  - More than 1 cm
  - More than 2.5 cm.

Three groups (decided on a combination of above)
- *Group three*: Worst results.

16. What are the guidelines for managing this fracture nonunion?

Ans. First look for osteonecrosis (this can be done by getting MRI scan):
- *Osteonecrosis + nonunion:*
  - *<50 years*: Pedicle grafting versus arthrodesis versus osteotomy (McMurray's type)
  - *>50 years*: Arthroplasty.
- *Nonunion + anatomy preserved (NO Osteonecrosis):*
  - *<65 years*: Osteosynthesis
    - ORIF with vascularized grafting
    - ORIF with fibular grafting.
  - *>65 years*: Arthroplasty
- Nonunion with destroyed anatomy (e.g. neck resorption) (NO Osteonecrosis)
  - *<65 years*: Osteotomy (Pauwels' type) (in a subset of younger people <40 years—Neck reconstruction also is a suitable option)
  - *>65 years*: Arthroplasty (*This option has become so favorable that for this situation nearly all patients >40 years are offered arthroplasty! But always remember in exams you should play on side of conserving native head as far as possible. Choose arthroplasty only if arthritis has set-in or there is excessive neck resorption that reconstruction is not possible or patient is too malnourished to bear reconstructive surgery and has sedentary lifestyle*).

17. What are the various muscle pedicle grafts described?

Ans. There are various muscle based grafting techniques described:
- *Muscle pedicle bone grafting:*
    - Quadratus femoris based (Judet, Meyers et al.)
    - Gluteus medius based (Hibbs)
    - Anterior trochanteric bone grafting (Das and Balasubramaniam – modified Hibbs)
    - Sartorius based (Li et al.)
    - Tensor fascia lata based (Bakshi)
    - Gluteus maximus based (Onosun et al.)
- *Muscle pedicle "grafting":*
    - Gluteus medius based (Frankel and Derian)
    - Vastus lateralis based (Stuck and Hinchey)
- *Muscle pedicle periosteal (Myoperiosteal) graft:*
    - Quadratus femoris-based periosteal grafting
- *Combined:*
    - Often used in eastern Asian countries
        - Combined Sartorius + deep circumflex femoral artery based iliac crest
        - Quadratus based + osteoperiosteal anterior grafting
- *Neck reconstruction*:
    - Devising a trough like rectangular box in the region of resorbed neck and filling with bone graft
    - Using cage and autologous cancellous bone grafting.

18. What is the advantage of muscle pedicle bone grafting?

Ans. *Following are the advantages of using these grafts*:
- There is no substitute for original biological joint
- Always give a fair chance to save a salvageable joint
- Vascularized bone graft may additionally take care of osteonecrosis
- Pedicle grafts are less cumbersome than free grafts with comparable results.

19. What are the principles of this grafting technique?

Ans. *Principles:*
- Vascularized grafts are shown to increase the vascularity of devascularized head (Stuck and Hinchey, Frankel, and Derian)

The Hip

- The hypovolemic head is converted into normovolemic head
- Often spontaneous revascularization after ORIF/closed reduction internal fixation (CRIF) stops at anterosuperior region leading to segmental collapse which is taken care of.

20. What is the role of osteotomy in treating nonunion fractured neck of femur?

Ans. Osteotomy alters both mechanical and biological environment around nonunion site which may enhance healing or at least provide relief to the patient (McMurray's concept):
- *Altering mechanics*: Medial shift of line of weight bearing
- *Correction of deformity*: Rotational deformity can be corrected, shortening compensated by apparent lengthening (Pauwels')
- Realignment of limb during movement
- Relaxation of joint capsule
- Increased vascularity
- Psoas relaxation providing pain relief by a mechanism similar to hanging hip of Voss
- Improved congruity of joint surfaces (only if deformed due to osteonecrosis)
- Improved leverage and stability
- Relief of pressure by muscles
- Redistribution of tensile forces at fracture line to compressive forces → *Arm chair effect.*

21. What is the arm chair effect?

Ans. As above (*I understand that this does not explain what one is curious about*). In McMurray's osteotomy, the distal fragment is placed directly under the head so that weight is directly transmitted from head to shaft bypassing neck so tensile shearing forces are converted to compressive forces. Now just imagine and compare yourself getting up from a chair without arms and a chair with arms. In the first instance, forces are concentrated around knee in a tensile manner (unless you support them with your hand) whereas in the second instance, you will get off the chair pushing at the arms which are more or less situated at knee level or sometimes even in front, dissipating in effect the shearing stresses across knee. This is the effect of an arm chair (dissipating the tensile forces at the lateral border of fracture), which was recommended originally for osteoarthritis of knee and hip.

22. What are the various osteotomies described around hip for treating nonunion?

Ans. Classically two landmark osteotomies with various modifications are cited:
1. *Lineal osteotomy*: Medial displacement osteotomy first described by Haas revised by McMurray and Leadbetter
2. Angulation osteotomy described by Schanz with modification by Pauwels'.

23. What is the McMurray's osteotomy?

Ans. It is aptly described as medial displacement oblique intertrochanteric pelvic support osteotomy.

24. What are the principles of McMurray's osteotomy?

Ans. *Conditions for success:*
- Upper end of shaft must be just below the edge of acetabulum
- There must be union between portions of divided femur.

25. For what condition did he describe this osteotomy and what are the prerequisites?

Ans. Osteoarthritis of hip joint with pain, stiffness, and deformity. There should be a minimum of 70° flexion at hip joint (90° ↓ general anesthesia). It should not be done in coxa magna, loss of sphericity of head both in AP and lateral projections, dysplastic acetabulum, subluxation of head, inflammatory disease, and ankylosing spondylitis.

26. How do you do this osteotomy and how to fix it?

Ans. The line of osteotomy goes from the base of greater trochanter obliquely up (10–15°) to exit just above lesser trochanter. After doing medial displacement of distal fragment fixation was done by Wainwright-Hammond spline (plate). By doing adduction it used to tilt the proximal fragment into valgus making the fracture line horizontal.

The Hip

27. What are the disadvantages of this osteotomy?

Ans. It causes shortening, lurching gait, frequent nonunion at osteotomy site, difficult future THR (so it is recommended not to displace by >50%), predisposes to genu valgum of ipsilateral knee.

28. What is Pauwels' osteotomy?

Ans. Pauwels' repositioning valgus intertrochanteric osteotomy replaces the pseudoarthrosis site to remove the shear forces **(Fig. 27)**. The osteotomy is aimed to enhance fracture healing and other benefits like:
- Equalizing limb lengths (virtually)
- Lateralization: Reducing tendency to genu valgum
- Early mobilization by fixing osteotomy.

Planning: Body forces subtend an angle of 16° at hip joint. The anatomical axis is at an angle of 8–10° to body forces, so the pseudoarthrosis site is subjected to forces at around 25°. Subtract this from the pseudoarthrosis angle (vide Pauwels' classification). This gives the wedge angle to be resected at osteotomy site. The same principle applies for Murray's modified osteotomy classically described for pseudoarthrosis of femur neck.

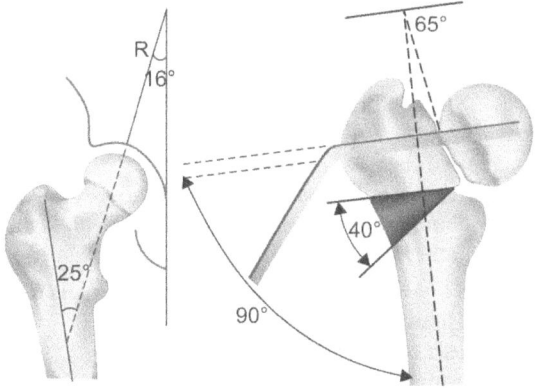

Fig. 27: Pauwels' osteotomy.

29. What is the role of arthroplasty in nonunion fracture neck femur?

Ans. In patients where reconstruction of proximal femur is not possible to retain native head (as in excessive neck resorption with a shell of head only remaining) or with global osteonecrosis of femoral head "or" in patients that are unable to bear with the prolonged restriction of weight bearing and mobilization following surgery (physiologically older patients) one can provide the option of arthroplasty to the patient.

30. What arthroplasty option would you choose?

Ans. In general, for active patients with good lifestyle demanding mobility, I would choose total hip replacement (cemented versus uncemented is a big controversy but I favor cemented) while for malnourished patient having comorbidity or sedentary lifestyle, I would provide option of hemiarthroplasty of hip.

31. Which test would you use to decide instability at hip joint?

Ans. *Telescopy test:* Significant telescopy (>1 cm trochanteric excursion in one direction) is a good indicator of unstable hip, whilst absence of the same does not substantiate stability. Telescopy is seen due to absorbed neck, comminution at fracture site, and tearing of capsule in high-impact injuries.

32. Which other test can you use?

Ans. Due to limitations of telescopic test (*See examination above*) active SLRT (Stinchfield test) can be performed. This test may however be fallacious (false negative) in impacted fragments, capsular contracture, and leverage of distal fragment on acetabular margin. It may be absent (false positive) in a frail patient and cannot be done in hemiplegia or paraplegic patient.

33. What are various closed reduction maneuvers for fracture neck of femur?

Ans. *Maneuvers in extension:*
- Whitman
- Deyerle
- Swiontkowsi.

Maneuvers in flexion:
- *Leadbetter*: Flexion → internal rotation → circumduction to abduction and extension; check by resting heel on palm, if it rests without externally rotation then it is a secure reduction.
- Flynn
- Smith-Peterson method ("gentle Leadbetter" method).

34. How do you make an assessment of alignment?

Ans. Assessment of alignment can be done by any one or a combination of following:
- *Garden's index*: AP—160° and lateral—180°, radiographs required 155-180° acceptable
- *Lowell's S-curves*: Image intensification
- *McElvenny*: "Hat on hook" position
- *Lindequist and Tornkvist criteria of good reduction*: ≤2 mm displacement, AP Garden angulation of 160-175° and lateral angulation of ≤10°.

35. What is the shape of fracture line in fractured neck of femur?

Ans. Spiral.

36. How do you classify fractured neck of femur?

Ans.
- *Garden's classification [complete/incomplete; degree of displacement*—Garden's index—trabecular disposition in AP (160°) and lateral (180°) projections]:
    - Incomplete, Valgus impacted fracture with trabecular displacement (↑ Garden's index in AP, may be normal in lateral)
    - Complete, undisplaced ± impaction
    - Complete, displaced (partial displacement <50%)
    - Complete, displaced >50% and dissociation between proximal and distal fragments so that proximal one realigns with acetabular trabeculae.

Eliasson et al. according to displacement in femoral neck fractures divided fractures into undisplaced (= Garden 1 and 2) and displaced (= Garden 3 and 4) types.

- *Linton's classification*:
    - Fracture in adduction (varus displacement/angulation: Garden's index ↓)

- Fracture in abduction (valgus displacement/valgus angulation)
- Intermediate type.
- *Pauwels' (higher the shear angle more will be the stresses and hence unstable fracture)*:
    - Angle of fracture line <30°
    - Angle of fracture line 30° to 50°
    - Angle of fracture line >50° and < 70°
- *Anatomical*: Subcapital, transcervical, basicervical
- AO
- *Stress fracture neck of femur (Fulkerson and Snowdy)*:
    - Tension stress fracture → superolateral aspect of neck, ↑ risk of displacement
    - Compression stress fracture → inferomedial aspect, ↓ risk of displacement
    - Completely displaced fracture neck of femur displaced.
- *Classification in children (Delbet and Collona)*:
    - *Transepiphyseal*: Involves physis with/without dislocation of femoral head from acetabulum. Flexion, abduction and external rotation deformity.
    - *Transcervical* (most common): Most are displaced and unstable. Osteonecrosis proportional to degree of displacement
    - *Cervicotrochanteric*: 2nd most common, similar to basicervical
    - *Intertrochanteric*: Good fracture.

37. What is the blood supply of femoral head?

Ans. The blood supply to *femoral head* is derived from three primary sources (as described by Crock)—(1) the metaphyseal system, (2) retinacular system, and (3) the foveolar system as follows **(Fig. 28)**:

- *Extracapsular arterial ring [ECA]*: This is the chief system giving rise to both intramedullary and extramedullary arterial systems. The ECA gives less prominent metaphyseal branches to intertrochanteric region which also supply the head through neck (intramedullary

The Hip

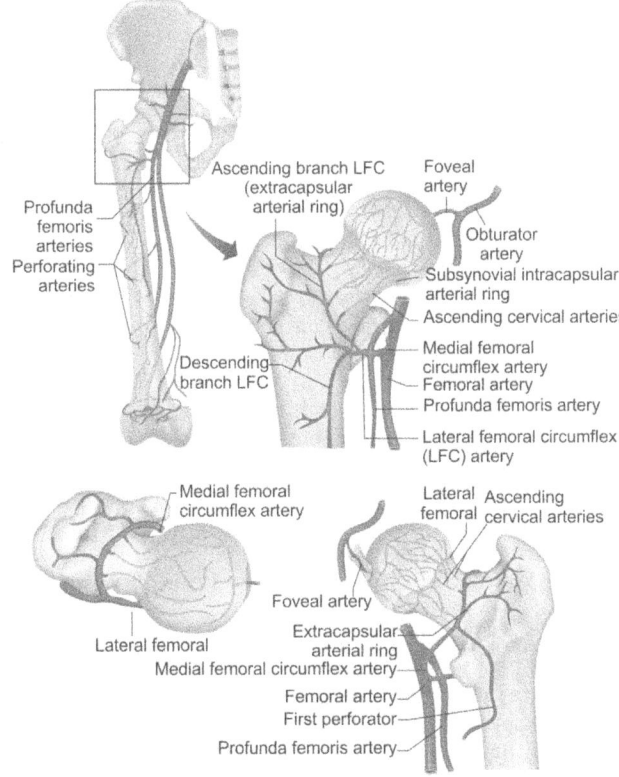

Fig. 28: Labeled diagrammatic representation of blood supply of femoral head.

metaphyseal system). It is located at the base of femoral neck and is formed:

- Posteriorly by branch of medial circumflex femoral artery
- Anteriorly by branch of lateral circumflex femoral artery more often a branch of profunda femoris artery (main branch of femoral artery)
- *Ascending cervical branches* of ECA (aka Epiphyseal arteries of Trueta or retinacular arteries) arise from

ECA (more prominent system) and ascend up the neck partly also supplying the neck in due course:
- Divided into anterior, posterior, medial, and lateral groups
- Anteriorly these vessels penetrate the capsule at intertrochanteric line while posteriorly they pass underneath the orbicularis fibers of the capsule
- Lateral group (*lateral ascending cervical vessels*) is the most important group carrying major portion of blood supply to head and neck of femur

- *Subsynovial intra-articular arterial ring of Chung (Circulus articuli vasculosus of Hunter)* is formed from lateral ascending cervical vessels:
  - Located at the margins of articular cartilage on surface of neck of femur
  - It is either a complete or incomplete ring
  - Provides epiphyseal vessels (that penetrate the head just outside the articular cartilage to supply major portion of head).

- *Artery of ligamentum teres*:
  - Branch of obturator artery (more often) or medial circumflex femoral artery
  - Variable supply in adults
  - Supply head around the region of fovea

The metaphyseal *femoral neck* is supplied by a cruciate shaped anastomosis between:
- Branches from ascending cervical arteries
- Branches from subsynovial intra-articular arterial ring
- Intramedullary branches of superior nutrient artery system
- Metaphyseal vessels from intertrochanteric region. This rich anastomosis makes the neck a very unlikely site for avascular necrosis.

38. How do you look for protrusio acetabuli and what are the various causes of the same?

Ans. Distance between medial wall of acetabulum and the pelvic brim (iliopectineal line) Sotelo-Garza and Charnley (1978, **Figs. 29A to C**):
- *Grade I*: 1–5 mm (mild)

- *Grade II*: 6–15 mm (moderate)
- *Grade III*: >15 mm (severe).

Causes:
- Familial/idiopathic (Otto pelvis)
- Rheumatoid arthritis and juvenile chronic arthritis (JCA)
- Osteoporosis
- Osteomalacia and rickets
- Marfan syndrome (45% have protrusio, 50% of these are unilateral and 90% associated with a scoliosis)
- Pagets disease
- Ankylosing spondylitis
- Osteoarthritis (occasionally)
- Acetabular fractures
- Osteogenesis imperfecta.

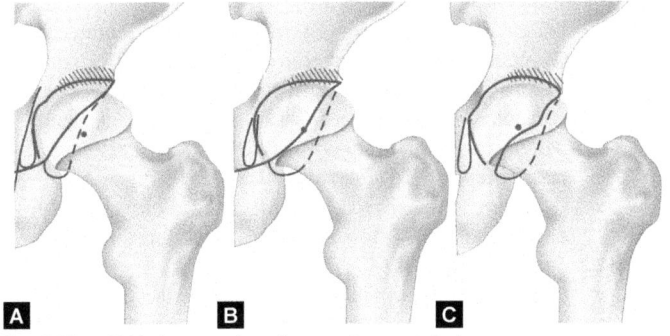

Figs. 29A to C: Various grades of protrusion acetabulum.

CASE III: OSTEONECROSIS OF FEMORAL HEAD

Diagnosis: The patient is a 32-year-old male with right hip flexion deformity of 30°, adduction deformity of 25°, internal/external rotation deformity of 20° with true supratrochanteric shortening of 1.5 cm. The patient is able to perform his routine activities that are but limited by pain and he uses cane in left hand for walking. I would like to give a differential diagnosis of 1. Osteonecrosis, 2,3,4,5...

It is important to understand that osteonecrosis is by itself a differential diagnosis for various disorders nearly all of which have the end result of producing secondary osteoarthritis, however the development of head deformity is an early finding with osteonecrosis with characteristic progression. The deformities are not characteristic and with development of secondary osteoarthritis the movements are also lost early. So as a rule always try to give the diagnosis as a differential diagnosis and be safe.

1. What is your differential diagnosis?
Ans. Typical differential diagnoses include:
- *Tuberculosis of hip*: Old cases of osteonecrosis that develop arthritic hip have restriction of most movements mimicking global restriction of movements as in TB of hip.
- Transient osteoporosis of hip in females (but here true shortening is not a feature).
- Primary osteoarthritis of hip (once the osteoarthritic changes develop in osteonecrosis it would be difficult to discretely make diagnosis of osteonecrosis unless you have already seen radiographs, so clinically 1° osteoarthritis of hip becomes a differential!): deformity of head and sectoral signs absent.
- Old Perthes disease, femoral head deformity due to epiphyseal/other dysplasia with development of secondary osteoarthritis.
- Old femoral head fracture with secondary osteoarthritis or a malunited neck fracture with traumatic osteonecrosis (considering history of trauma is present).
- Monoarticular rheumatoid is as such rare and if mentioned, then should be last as it is a diagnosis of exclusion.
- Extremely rare limited Paget's disease. Yes this is seen and has been reported.

2. Why do you keep osteonecrosis as your first differential?
Ans. *History*:
- Single joint involvement (compare from—ankylosing spondylitis), insidious onset, slow progression

The Hip

- Characteristic course of progression of disease and disability
- No constitutional symptoms
- Deformities do not match with staging of TB hip (viz. even for a possible stage III TB, hip considering the deformity; movements at hip are fairly preserved)
- No history of trauma (for idiopathic case)
- Use of steroids or bodybuilding medications, renal disease, hepatic disease or blood disorder would further strengthen the diagnosis.

3. What are the diagnostic criteria for osteonecrosis of hip?

Ans. For nontraumatic osteonecrosis of hip (Japanese investigating committee, 1990):

Major criteria: There should not be any joint-space narrowing or acetabular changes for 1–3 to be positive:

- Radiological (depression of femoral head, demarcating sclerosis in the femoral head, crescent sign)
- Bone scan (cold-in-hot)
- MRI (low intensity band on T1-weighted image)
- Histology (trabecular and marrow necrosis).

Minor criteria:

- Radiological (depression of femoral head with joint-space narrowing, cystic radiolucency/mottled necrosis, flattening of the superior portion of femoral head)
- Bone scan (cold "or" hot)
- MRI (homogeneous/inhomogeneous low intensity without a band pattern)
- Symptom (hip pain with weight bearing)
- History (corticosteroid or alcohol usage).

Definitive osteonecrosis: ≥2 positive major criteria. *Probable osteonecrosis:* One positive major criteria or ≥4 positive minor criteria, at least one radiological.

4. What are the causes of osteonecrosis of hip?

Ans. *Idiopathic* form (Chandler's disease) is the most common (? *COL2A1* gene mutation/P-glycoprotein or alcohol metabolizing enzyme polymorphism, etc.). The other causes are:

- *Trauma:*
  - Fracture neck of femur
  - Dislocation (posterior >> anterior but one to one case wise incidence is more common in anterior dislocation).
- *Corticosteroids:* "Threshold" cumulative dose of 2,000 mg for prednisolone within 2–3 months, 4.6 fold ↑ in incidence with every additional 10 mg intake.
- *Alcohol:* Consumption of >400 mL/week (this is equivalent absolute alcohol content)—9.8 fold ↑ in incidence (*This value was notably not rounded off—remember the value of "g"*)
  (DRINK YEARS = weekly alcohol consumption × years)
- Coagulation disorders (hypercoagulability)
- Hyperlipidemia
- *Dysbarism:* Does not occur <17 psi, not believed to be a risk factor <30 months
- SLE and connective tissue disorders
- Organ transplantation (metabolic changes and chemotherapy including steroids)
- Liver dysfunction
- Radiation
- *Pregnancy:* Small body frame and relatively large weight gain
- Smoking (>20 pack years, pack years = packs per day × years)
- Hyperuricemia
- Myeloproliferative disorders
- HIV infection.

5. What are various pathogenic mechanisms?

Ans. Direct cellular toxicity, extraosseous arterial, extraosseous venous, intraosseous extravascular, intraosseous intravascular, multifactorial.

6. What is the difference between two most common causes of osteonecrosis?

Ans. Idiopathic and traumatic are the two most common forms of osteonecrosis. In the idiopathic form the lesion is characteristically located in the anterosuperior region. The

The Hip

involvement could be bilateral in more than half of the cases (some texts may say ~ 75%). Post-traumatic cases have often total involvement with isolated joint involvement.

7. How will you confirm your diagnosis?

Ans. I will get the radiographs of pelvis with both hips, involved hip in AP and lateral projections.

8. How much time does it take to be evident on radiographs?

Ans. Perhaps the earliest changes appear by 2 months which are easily discernable by 6 months.

9. How do you stage osteonecrosis?

Ans. Ficat and Arlet classification (4 stage), modified Ficat-Arlet (stage "0", subdivision of stage II), university of Pennsylvania classification **(Tables 1 and 2)**.

	Table 1: Ficat-Arlet (modified) classification.		
Stage	*Symptoms and signs*	*X-ray*	*Bone scan*
0	None	—	? ↓ uptake
I	None/Mild	—	↓ uptake
II	Mild	Altered density A. Sclerosis/cysts/normal joint line, normal head contour B. *Crescent sign* (subchondral fracture), flattening	↑ uptake
III	Mild-to-moderate	Loss of sphericity, collapse	↑ uptake
IV	Moderate-to-severe	↓ joint space, acetabular changes	↑ uptake

Original Ficat's classification did not include sub-classification of stage II.

There are numerous other classification that are regionally followed, association research circulation osseous, Japanese orthoaedic association, Marcus et al., Sugioka, Kerboul et al., Smith et al., etc.

Table 2: University of Pennsylvania classification (Steinberg et al.).

Stage	0	I	II	III	IV	V	VI
Findings	All present technique normal/non-diagnostic Histology + ve	X-ray, CT normal	X-ray—mottled and sclerotic cysts, porosis	X-ray—crescent sign	X-ray—flattening of anterior surface	IV + narrowing of joint space/acetabular changes	Complete joint destruction
Techniques	—	X-ray, CT, Scintigraph, MRI Quantitate—MRI	X-ray, CT, Scintigraph, MRI Quantitate—MRI and MRI	X-ray, CT only Quantitate—X-ray and MRI	X-ray, CT only Quantitate—X-ray only	X-ray, CT only	X-ray, CT only
Sub-classification	NO	QUANTITATION (Stage II–V)					NO
			% area involved	Length of crescent	% surface collapse and dome depression	Location	
			A—<15% (minimal)	A—<15%	A—<15%, <2 mm	Medial	
			B—15–30% (moderate)	B—15–30%	B—15–30%, 2–4 mm	Central	
			C—>30% (severe)	C—>30%	C—>30%, >4 mm	Lateral	

(CT: computed tomography)

The Hip

10. What are the tests for hemodynamic function?

Ans. These tests are for research purpose and not available for population at large, however they are positive in stage "0" Ficat-Arlet/Pennsylvania classification.
- *Intramedullary pressure (at rest = 10–20 mm Hg, rapid saline injection → rises by about 15 mm Hg)*: In osteonecrosis, both increase by 3–4 times of normal
- Venography.

11. Do you know of any classification based on MRI only?

Ans. Schimuzu (1994) MRI grades for treatment:

In general:
- The extent (area of coronal femoral head involvement) determined at the outset does not change
- Lesion <1/4 in extent and medial 1/3 in location (portion of weight bearing surface involved) grade I, rarely collapse
- Lesion up to 1/2 in extent and 1/3–2/3 of weight-bearing surface collapse in ≈ 30% cases (Grade II)
- Lesion > 1/4 in extent and > 2/3 of weight-bearing surface (Grade III) collapse within 3 years in 70% cases.

12. How will you plan treatment based on classification (Steinberg)?

Ans. *Grade 0*: Reassure and treat symptomatically keep in close observation (non-weight bearing/restricted weight bearing has been shown to be of NO benefit, lipid-lowering agents, anticoagulants, and iloprost prostacyclin inhibitor), intravenous bisphosphonates, shock wave therapy, hyperbaric oxygen, pulsed electromagnetic field (PEMF) are all indeterminate. *In general, all lesions in pre-collapse stage (Ficat IIA and below, Steinberg II and below) have good chances with joint-preserving procedures, post collapse stages—the disease is bound to progress; so in any case, a surgical procedure is indicated. Only stage "0" at the present time can be observed—but is hardly ever diagnosed as it is preclinical and preradiological!! So why talk of conservative treatment? Most of idiopathic cases are sequentially bilateral—this treatment is to preserve the opposite hip)*

Grade I: Core decompression, percutaneous drilling (multiple drill holes with 3.2 mm drill bit), muscle-pedicle bone grafting

Grade II (precollapse): Age < 45 years, core decompression with/without bone grafting, osteotomy, muscle-pedicle bone grafting (try to preserve native hip)

Age > 45 years but <60 years—if limited sectoral involvement—osteotomy to derotate the necrotic sector away, global involvement—total hip replacement

Age > 60–65 years—total hip replacement

Grade III (crescent): Younger patients → bone grafting, (?) osteotomy. Older patients → total hip arthroplasty.

(*Bipolar and hemiarthroplasty have been shown to be a POOR performer as of now for various potential but unproven reasons, so an option of bipolar arthroplasty has been intentionally dropped here, its sole indication is probably patient over 70 years of age with poor performance status*).

Late Cases

Steinberg IV-VI/Ficat III/IV: Total hip replacement/osteotomy (?stage IV)/arthrodesis/Girdlestone (nowadays will be considered criminal!). In younger patients, bone grafting (trap door, etc.) still remains treatment of choice (stage IV), some cases might also fit into osteotomy.

If one does not want to follow this complicated version, here is the *simpler one*!

About 70–86% will progress (for nontraumatic one and less for a traumatic etiology but surely spontaneous resolution is remote!), hence there is no role of conservative treatment!!

In general (Ficat classification followed here):

- Core decompression with/without bone grafting → for Ficat IIa or earlier
- Osteotomy → stage II and (?) III
- Trap-door/light-bulb procedures *(nobody does them so keep this option reserved as it was mentioned only in Chapman's orthopedics and not widely known to world)* → stage IIb and III (hardly ever done, better keep quite unless asked specifically, you can score better in stronger fields!)

The Hip

- Arthroplasty/arthrodesis → stage III and IV (avoid arthrodesis in majority – you see, most idiopathic cases are bilateral!)

So here you will find you have maximum choice for stage III Steinberg, but practically speaking this is the most difficult stage to treat.

13. What is core decompression and how you do it?

Ans. Also called "Forage" this procedure is typically used to decompress the hypertensive head by creating a hole extending till necrotic area. This often gives immediate pain relief. It can be done as an:

- Isolated procedure or
- With adjuvant [like electric current stimulation, bone morphogenetic protein (BMP), demineralized bone matrix (DBM)]
- *With bone grafting (non-vascularized/vascularized) Hungerford Technique:* Using Jewett nail starter (12 mm) Ficat (modified)—10 mm window with 8 mm central core made by Michele trephine and two additional channels made by 5–6 mm trephine.

Entry point is just distal to vastus lateralis origin in metaphyseal to prevent stress fracture.

Postoperative: Single hip → PWB walk on two crutches → 3-point gait.

Bilateral cases → partial weight-bearing (PWB) on two crutches → 4-point gait.

14. What is the rationale of core decompression?

Ans. Femoral head is likened to Starling's resistor (thin vessels in unyielding bony channels). Femoral hypertension is relieved by drilling the head and neck. The benefits are thought to arise from:

Biological changes:

- ↓ intraosseous pressure
- Revascularization through channel or (fibular intramedullary canal if used)
- Prevents additional ischemic events.

Mechanical changes:
- Removal of necrotic bone removing the obstruction to revascularization
- Subchondral graft supports the cartilage.

15. What are the various methods of core decompression and bone grafting?

Ans. Suggested first by Phemister, now often used:
- Cancellous (Modified Ficat)
- Cortical (vascularized fibula and nonvascularized strut graft)
- *Muscle pedicle bone graft*: Usually for traumatic osteonecrosis.
- *Osteochondral grafting*:
  - *Trapdoor procedure*: Raise a chondral flap, curette out bone, fill with cancellous graft and struts, replace flap
  - *Light-bulb procedure (Rosenwasser et al.)*: Above through a metaphyseal cortical window.

16. How do you insert fibula?

Ans. Harvest fibula (90–100 mm), split it into two, mallet through the core with canal portion presenting along the wall of the core (split and flip over the graft). This provides a facilitative pathway for revascularization channels.

17. What are the principles of free-vascularized fibular grafting?

Ans. (Urbanik). Harvest cancellous graft from ilium and 13 cm of fibula with vascular pedicle (peroneal artery and branches). Make a core 2 mm wider than fibular girth, insert fibula, and make an anastomosis between peroneal stump and lateral circumflex femoral vessels, stabilize fibula with K-wire. Vastus lateralis should be released to prevent kinking and pressure on lateral circumflex femoral vessels. Iliac graft (Autogenous cancellous) is inserted into the necrotic region and around fibula before inserting fibular graft (it can also be obtained from greater trochanter). Odds favor the use of free-vascularized fibular grafting strongly over nonvascularized bone grafting.

The Hip

18. What is the role of osteotomy?

Ans. *Goals*:
- ↓ in intramedullary pressure/venous hypertension (biological)
- Removal of lesion from weight bearing area (biomechanical)
  - Giving time to heal
  - Decreasing progression.
- Restoration of blood supply (biological)
- Other effects as (*See Q 20 Case II above*).

19. What are the various osteotomy options?

Ans. Following osteotomy principles are described, exact procedure and choice depends on site of lesion, extent of lesion (ideally should be <200° combined necrotic angle), early stages, surgeon's preference:
- Merle D' Aubigne type curved varus osteotomy to load the most lateral portion (at least >20° of normal femoral head laterally and <160° combined necrotic angle required). (*Note: McMurray type varus displacement osteotomy or Pauwels' type varus angulation osteotomy has also been successfully used by some*).
- *Valgus extension osteotomy (Pauwels')*: Moves necrotic portion laterally considerably enlarging the weight bearing surface and loads the capital drop osteophyte (? The osteophyte is well developed only in stage IV).
- *Sugioka's anterior rotational osteotomy*: Moves necrotic area anteriorly (up to 90° rotation can be done), done through trochanteric (hence transtrochanteric, based on vascular pedicle of medial circumflex femoral artery). At least 36° of preserved lateral femoral head should be there with combined necrotic angle <200°. First rotational osteotomy was described by Wagner and Zeiler using a double intertrochanteric osteotomy that could rotate the necrotic fragment by 180°. Posterior rotational osteotomy is also described (Atsumi T) that has theoretically the advantage of medially shifting the medial circumflex femoral artery and relieving tension with posterior rotation. These are very technically demanding with inconsistent results.

- *Flexion intertrochanteric osteotomy (Schneider)*: Places posterior healthy portion into weight-bearing area.
- Valgus flexion osteotomy (Scher and Jakim) with autogenous bone grafting.

    (*If you are confused with Pauwels' osteotomy for was it varus or a valgus angulation osteotomy, then it means you are reading the text well! Pauwel described angulation osteotomy for osteoarthritis hip! Varus osteotomy (Pauwels' I) and valgus osteotomy (rather Valgus extension osteotomy—Pauwel's II were both described by him. This should take away the confusion-Hurray!!).*)

    (*Now a note on which osteotomy to be mentioned in examination Frankly speaking please read the algorithm for planning treatment first. While answering, only mention "osteotomy", if further asked mention, "intertrochanteric osteotomy to unload the necrotic segment"; if still asked then tell that "I will plan osteotomy according to site of femoral head involvement" and bank upon valgus extension/flexion osteotomies or varus osteotomy; others are difficult and one may not have ever seen—see below*).

    (*Just a learning note—osteotomy is better suited for post-traumatic osteonecrosis, in these cases although osteonecrosis extends more distally into femoral head but it responds favorably to joint preserving and revascularization procedures and is often non-progressive*).

20. **How do you plan osteotomy?**
Ans. On X-ray and MRI, I will evaluate the following:
- Look at the site of involvement [anterior—then do a flexion osteotomy, anterosuperior—valgus flexion osteotomy; posterior—extension osteotomy, posterosuperior—valgus extension osteotomy, superior with >30° (now >20°) of preserved head—curved varus or McMurray's type, >36° preservation—rotational transtrochanteric].
- *Whether it satisfies the criteria and prognostic factors:*
    - Kerboul et al. (X-ray, combined necrotic angle – measured sum of necrotic arc measured in degrees from the center on AP and lateral views): Small

The Hip

combined necrotic angles are ≤150°, medium angles are between 151° and 200°, and large angles are >200°.
- Modified Kerboul (X-ray and MRI—central coronal and sagittal cuts used to calculate the combined necrotic angle): grade 1 (<200°), grade 2 (200° to 249°), grade 3 (250° to 299°), and grade 4 (≥300°).

Grade I/small necrotic angles (Kerboul) are ideally suitable for osteotomy.

21. What is Bakshi's procedure?

Ans. Muscle-pedicle bone grafting using either quadratus femoris, tensor fascia lata, sartorius, gluteus medius muscle with multiple drilling of the necrotic fragment. It can be done till stage III (Ficat) in younger patients (Dr DP Bakshi did it in patients up to 60 years old). Internationally, however, the results have not been very acceptable for stages above IIA.

CASE IV: PERTHES DISEASE

The patient is a 7-year-old boy with conservatively managed Perthes disease of (left/right) hip for past 6 weeks **(Fig. 30)**. There is 1 cm of true shortening and patient is able to do his routine activities. *(Duration of disease is unknown to all so it cannot be mentioned and only treatment duration can be mentioned—some can argue that*

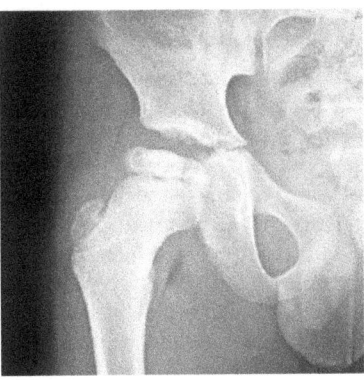

Fig. 30: Radiograph of a patient with healing Perthes disease of right hip.

limp can be taken as disease duration though not everyone agrees. You can mention conservative treatment like traction or abduction cast if applicable.)

If diagnosis is unclear on history and examination, then give a description of case with deformities and restricted movement and present a differential diagnosis.

1. What is Perthes disease?
Ans. It is a self-limited disease of hip in children produced by varying degrees of idiopathic osteonecrosis of capital femoral epiphysis. It is more common in males (M:F = 4:1) and is more common in age range 4 to 9 years. Out of this range some call it atypical Perthes presentation.

2. What are the various synonyms?
Ans. LEGG-CALVE-PERTHES disease, pseudocoxalgia [Calve (France)], arthritis deformans juvenalis [Perthes (Germany)], precoxalgia (Soudart), coxa vara capitalis (Levy), coxa plana (Waldenstrom). Legg was from USA. (*What's in a name?—the one you call rose would smell as sweet by any other name*).

3. Why is it more common in boys and what are gender differences for this disease?
Ans. This is more common in males (M:F = 4:1), peaks at around 6 years. Anterior anastomosis is often incomplete in boys. Females have earlier onset and prognosis is worse. More common in whites than blacks and Indians, possibly due to early establishment of foveolar blood supply in the latter.

4. What are the common associations of Perthes disease?
Ans. As such the disease is idiopathic in nature but while studying its epidemiology and natural course some associations were found, these are by NO means syndromic and are mostly occasional so no concrete "association" has been established. Some patients have undescended testis, groin hernia, hypospadias, pyloric stenosis, congenital cardiac or renal disease. Commonly, however it is noticed that these patients lag behind the normal in height/weight/skeletal maturity and have smaller feet compared to normal child.

The Hip

5. What is the blood supply of head in children?

Ans. The blood supply of femoral head changes over development as follows:
- Till 3 years of age metaphyseal and retinacular are the two major sources of blood supply. There is additional minor supply from ligamentum teres vascularity.
- During growth of head (4-8 years), the metaphyseal vessels are obliterated and retinacular vessels are the only significant source of blood supply which enter as lateral epiphyseal vessels. Lateral epiphyseal vessels are predominantly divided into posterosuperior and posteroinferior, occlusion of former leads to development of osteonecrosis in anterolateral aspect of femoral head (proposed vascular hypothesis for Perthes disease, *Trueta hypothesis*). Being fragile and small in diameter, they are prone to compression and obliteration of blood supply from various reasons that increase intracapsular volume like—transient synovitis, hemarthrosis (traumatic or in hemophiliacs), intra-articular abscess (septic arthritis) and vasculitis (Rickettsial infection). Some other causes identified include Gaucher's disease, Caisson's disease and cretinism that can cause vascular occlusion. In continuation of Trueta hypothesis, it has been proposed that repeated ischemic incidents (2 or more) within a short span of time (4-6 weeks) increases risk of Perthes disease.
- After 8 years' foveolar supply is developed enough and dual channels are established (i.e. retinacular and foveolar). By 16-18 years' growth plate is disappeared and all three groups supply head (i.e. metaphyseal in addition to above).

6. What is Caffey's hypothesis?

Ans. Intraepiphyseal compression of blood supply leads to osteonecrosis. (This may be relevant in Gaucher's and other storage disorders).

7. Why do you call it Perthes disease?

Ans. *There is*:
- Protracted course and insidious onset of limp followed by pain
- Limitation of abduction and internal rotation (painless limp is the usual presentation, limited abduction in flexion is the first usual sign) that is especially more prominent in hip flexion
- Trendelenburg gait/sign ± wasting of thigh muscles/ anterior groin pain/adductor spasm – these are variable
- Minimal shortening (true). Normal knee and spine examination.

TB hip is the closest differential and cannot be adequately differentiated so always give a differential diagnosis. However, flexion deformity is not very prominent in Perthes disease and the patient's clinical findings will not usually fit the stages of TB.

8. What is the other differential diagnosis?

Ans. In the absence of trauma, irritable hip is the other close differential. Other differential diagnosis include TB hip (here movements are restricted in all directions, ESR is raised and Montoux positive), low-grade septic arthritis (fever + raised TLC, quite severe restriction of movements), SUFE, Gaucher's disease, cretinism, and sickle-cell anemia.

9. How will you differentiate irritable hip from Perthes?

Ans. Irritable hip has less strong male dominance (2:1), and occurs in early age group (mean = 3 years). Average duration of symptoms is often less than a week (>6 weeks in Perthes).

10. How will you confirm diagnosis?

Ans. I will get an X-ray done (X-ray pelvis with both hips—AP and X-ray index hip—lateral); the following findings support the diagnosis of Perthes:
- *Lateral subluxation*: CE angle >20°
- *Small femoral capital epiphysis*: Temporary cessation of enchondral ossification in the bony growth center,

The Hip

continued articular cartilage growth as the cartilage receives nutrition from synovial fluid.
- Flattening and loss of sphericity with subchondral fracture (Caffey's sign, typically occurs in anterolateral region as there are maximum weight bearing stresses and bone resorption)
- Increased width of epiphysis
- Gage sign
- Broadening and shortening of femoral neck
- Decreased neck shaft angle: Due to cessation of capital physeal growth exaggerated by trochanteric growth
- Convex growth plate
- Overgrowth of greater trochanter
- Step like irregularities in growth plate
- Metaphyseal rarefaction and cystic changes due to sprouting blood vessels
- Sagging rope sign
- Head within head appearance.

Acetabulum is comparatively well preserved! (Important in differentiating TB hip).

11. Would you need any other investigations for evaluation?

Ans. In view of above signs, I do not need any other investigations to make/confirm diagnosis but for further management of the patient, I need additional information by following investigation(s):
- *Ultrasonography (USG)*: This gives information about synovial effusion and subluxation of epiphysis
- *Bone scan*: It shows decreased uptake on superoanterolateral region of head.
- *MRI*: Single best additional investigation of choice for confirming diagnosis and gathering additional investigation like—subluxation of femoral head, demonstration of osteonecrosis, effusion, revascularization changes, additional pathology in acetabulum, etc. in case, it is not Perthes.

12. What are head at risk signs?

Ans. Clinical head at risk signs:

- *Age > 8 years*:
  - Younger patient has more time for remodeling the defect
  - Acetabulum in older patient loses its potential to develop
  - Older patient due to more weight are likely to damage epiphysis further.
- *Female sex*:
  - Girls tend to skeletally more mature than boys of same age so less remodeling time
  - Age for age, girls tend to be more severely affected.
- Obesity
- *Limitation of range of motion*:
  - Flexion less than 80° and abduction <30°
- Increasing adduction contracture
- Subluxating hips.

Radiographic head at risk signs (Catterall):

- Lateral subluxation of femoral head
- *Calcification lateral to epiphysis*:
  - Indicates extruded cartilage
  - Increased pressure on cartilage by acetabular lip
- *Metaphyseal cysts (Not in original Catterall)*:
  - Metaphyseal changes represent replacement by adipose tissue then fibrocartilage
  - Step like deformity in growth plate due to cartilage necrosis.
- *Gage sign:*
  - "V"-shaped defect in lateral part of bony epiphysis, indicates cartilaginous overgrowth.
- Horizontal growth plate: Due to premature physeal closure.

Scintigraphic head at risk signs:

- Failure of revascularization of lateral column
- Decreased activity of physis
- Anterolateral extrusion of epiphysis

The Hip

- Disappearance of previously present lateral column
- Intense metaphyseal activity.

13. How do you classify Perthes disease?

Ans. The most useful classification is of Herring (Lateral pillar classification for disease severity): Femoral head is divided into 3 columns and classified on the basis of lateral pillar height (middle column is the extent of sequestrum on AP view, epiphysis lateral to it is the lateral column and one medial to it is the medial column).

- *Herring A:* Lateral pillar height normal
- *Herring B:* Lateral pillar height reduced by <50%
- *Herring C:* More than 50% reduction in height of lateral pillar.

Catterall groups:
- *Group 1:* Anterior head of femur, no sequestrum, no crescent sign, and epiphyseal height maintained.
- *Group 2:* Anterolateral ⅓ to ½ femoral head, sequestrum + lateral pillar maintained. (*Subgroup 2½:* Lateral pillar maintained but there is radiolucency).
- *Group 3:* Anterolateral ¾ femoral head involved, subchondral fracture extends to posterior half, lateral pillar not preserved (reverse group 3: Affects ¾ femoral head but in anteromedial region).
- *Group 4:* Entire femoral head, dense sequestrum, subchondral fracture extends throughout the head.

Salter and Thompson:
- Extent of subchondral fracture less than half of femoral head
- Extent is more than half of femoral head.

14. How do you manage the cases?

Ans. Simple algorithm based on age, range of motion, and radiologic staging.
- *Group I:* <6 years old → 50-70% do well. Containment done in rare cases with persistent loss of motion with Herring C/ Catterall III or IV with head at risk signs, Salter and Thompson group "B".

- *Group II:* 6–8 years (Bone age more important than chronological age):
  - Symptomatic treatment for Herring group A, Catterall I/II with no head at risk signs, Salter and Thompson group A with symptomatic treatment and range of motion exercises.
  - Herring group B/C with persistent loss of motion, Catterall III/IV with head at risk signs, Salter and Thompson group B → containment indicated.
- *Group III:* ≥9 years:
  - *As above*: Observation
  - *As above*: Surgical containment.

15. What are the principles of treatment?
Ans. *Principles*:
- *Restoration and maintenance of movements*: By counterpoised split Russell traction, analgesics, serial abduction splintage, adductor tenotomy (<7 years) or adductor + iliopsoas tenotomy (>8 years) may be required if spasm increases discomfort
- Reduce hip irritability
- Prevent ball from extruding/collapsing (containment)
- Regain a spherical femoral head and resumption of weight bearing and full activity.

16. How would you do containment?
Ans. *Bracing or surgical*:
- *Bracing*:
  - Non-ambulatory recumbent weight relieving:
    - Abduction broomstick plaster casts
    - Bivalved hip spica cast
    - Milgram hip abduction orthosis.
  - Ambulatory static affected limb only:
    - Harrison hip containment splint
  - Ambulatory dynamic both limbs:
    - Petrie cast
    - Scottish rite orthosis
  - Ambulatory unilateral orthosis
    - Trilateral socket orthosis.

The Hip

- *Surgical:*
  - *Salter's innominate osteotomy/Elizabethtown osteotomy*: Best done between 6 years and 8 years, <20% epiphyseal extrusion
  - *Femoral varus derotation osteotomy (VDO)*: Best done between 5 years and 8 years and if arthrogram shows head containment in abduction and medial rotation
  - Combination
  - Lateral shelf.

17. What are the prerequisites and contraindications of bracing?

Ans. *Prerequisites*:
- Full range of motion
- Entire femoral head containable
- Motor strength and balance should be adequate
- *Arthrography:* Essential to judge congruency throughout range of motion, rule out hinge abduction.

Contraindications ≡ indications for surgery:
- Persistent/recurrent loss of movements
- Progressive collapse
- Psychosocial problems
- Noncompliant.

18. What is the end-point for bracing?

Ans. Orthosis can be discontinued when:
- Disease enters healing stage
- Increased density of femoral head appears
- Medial segment of femoral head increases in size
- Metaphyseal rarefaction ossifies
- Intact lateral column
- Complete subchondral ossification.

19. What are the prerequisites for Salter's osteotomy?

Ans. *Prerequisites*:
- Nonirritable hip
- Normal or near normal range of movements
- Absence or minimal deformity of head
- Concentric containment can be achieved.

20. What are the advantages of Salter's and VDO osteotomy?

Ans. The exact procedure to be chosen is controversial. Combination of innominate osteotomy and VDO may achieve containment avoiding complications of each (Staheli). The advantages of Salter's osteotomy are:
- Lengthening of extremity
- Anterolateral coverage
- Avoidance of second surgery for plate removal (*see* VDO).

Advantages of VDO:
- Achieves anteversion and coverage simultaneously
- Decompress femoral head
- Decreases stresses across hip joint
- Tends to enhance remodeling process.

21. When should one restrain from surgical containment?

Ans. *Contraindications*:
- Persistent limitation of movements
- Deformed femoral head
- Age < 5 years
- Presence of significant physeal involvement.

22. What are the indications of reconstruction surgeries?

Ans. These surgeries are done to correct residual deformities as follows:
- *Hinged abduction*: If hips are congruent in adduction and have movements beyond point of congruency then—valgus extension osteotomy
- *Malformed femoral head*: Garceau's cheilectomy
- *Large malformed femoral head with "mushrooming"*: Chiari's osteotomy
- *Coxa magna*: Shelf augmentation (Staheli)
- *Femoral epiphyseal arrest (irrelevant overgrowth of greater trochanter)*: Trochanteric advancement. (*Note*: Trochanter tip should be ideally at the level of center of femoral head and 1½ times the distance of radius of femoral head from center of femoral head).

23. What are the causes of shortening in Perthes disease?

Ans. The following account for shortening:
- Fixed flexion deformity

The Hip

- Fixed abduction deformity
- Destruction of femoral head
- Coxa vara.

24. Theoretically can you think of a procedure that can be done in opposite limb (normal) to "contain" the affected hip?

Ans. (*This s a very conceptual question but hypothetical one!*) One can do shortening of normal limb that will produce relative abduction deformity in affected limb and hence effect containment.

25. Why is soft tissue release contraindicated in hinged abduction?

Ans. (Salter's procedure as a rule involves iliopsoas release in Perthes disease). Soft tissue release will enhance the tendency of hinged abduction.

CASE V: CONGENITAL AND DEVELOPMENTAL COXA VARA

Beware of the term adolescent coxa vara, which refers to slipped capital femoral epiphysis actually, also the term "coxa vara" refers to deformity and not diagnosis per se except if it is congenital or developmental.

1. Why do you call it congenital coxa vara?

Ans. *Findings*:
- Deformity (shortening) since birth, painless limp since walking age, progressive increase in deformity
- Associated congenital deformities [DDH, femoral developmental anomalies, craniocleidodysostosis, CACP syndrome (camptodactyly, arthropathy, coxa vara, pericarditis syndrome)]
- Prominent greater trochanter
- Upridden trochanter
- Shortening (progressive)
- Limited abduction
- On flexion the knee points to same shoulder
- Adduction, external rotation deformity
- No telescopy (differentiate from DDH).

2. What is the cause of this deformity?

Ans. Can be divided into following causes:

- *Primary (often bilateral):*
  - *Congenital*: (present at birth and often associated with femoral shortening, cleidocranial dysostosis, etc.)
  - *Developmental (presents later in childhood):*
    - As a part of PFFD (proximal focal femoral deficiency)
    - Multiple epiphyseal dysplasia
    - Achondroplasia
    - Hypothyroidism.
- *Secondary to*:
  - Perthes disease
  - Osteogenesis imperfecta
  - Rickets
  - Infection (Tuberculosis)
  - Paget's disease
  - Osteoporosis
  - Fibrous dysplasia
  - Trauma
  - Severe osteoarthritis
  - Iatrogenic (treatment of DDH).

3. Why does this deformity worries an orthopedician?

Ans. This is a progressive deformity with decreasing neck shaft angle with increasing age and weight bearing and may ultimately lead to pseudoarthrosis of neck. The gait and mechanics of hip are at a disadvantage, producing early degenerative arthritis. The disease has a poor prognosis after 8 years of age.

4. How do you classify congenital coxa vara?

Ans. Severity classification based on angular measurements:

- *Hilgenreiner's epiphyseal (H-E) angle*:
  - *Angle > 60°*: Coxa vara almost always progresses
  - *Angle < 45°*: Deformity almost always corrects over time and observation
  - *Angle between 46° and 90°*: Natural history not clear, correct at the first sign of progression.

The Hip

- *Neck-shaft angle (somewhat less reliable)*:
  - *Angle <100°*: Surgically correct
  - *Angle >110°*: Observe
  - *Angle between 100° and 110°*: Close follow-up and correct if progresses.

5. What do you see on X-ray?

Ans. Following findings are seen:
- Decreased neck-shaft angle
- Shallow acetabulum
- Widened teardrop
- *Fairbank's triangle*: "Y"-shaped defect present in the inferior part of capital physis and adjacent metaphysis, it is a defect in enchondral ossification with cartilage deposition at abnormal place
- Upridden trochanter
- Short femur.

6. What are the goals of treatment?

Ans. Goals are to:
- Restore neck-shaft angle [to around 140° (135–150°) or H-E angle to <45°]
- Reduce shortening
- Reduce abductor lurch.

7. How will you treat this patient?

Ans. The treatment of choice is subtrochanteric valgus osteotomy (*And I suppose the only one practiced!*). This restores neck-shaft angle and provides virtual lengthening to limb. The disadvantage is that there is premature physeal closure in majority even without a direct physeal injury. The typical indication for surgery is (are):
- Neck-shaft angle <90°
- Progressive deformity
- Vertical physis as demonstrated by HE angle >60° (Patients with HE angle 45–60° is closely followed up. Patients with HE angle < 45° are known to have spontaneous resolution)
- Significant limb length abnormality.

CASE VI: SLIPPED CAPITAL FEMORAL EPIPHYSIS

This is a very unlikely case in Asian subcontinent as the disease is quite uncommon here and it is an emergency to treat. If given at all the cases will be of chronic slips.

1. **Why do you call it slipped capital femoral epiphysis?**
Ans. *Findings:*
   - Obese child, intermittent limp with or without pain
   - History of minor trauma followed by typical course
   - Shortening
   - Attitude of flexion, abduction, external rotation with waddling gait
   - Lower gluteal fold on same side
   - Restriction of abduction, internal rotation, and flexion
   - Increased extension, adduction, and external rotation
   - Increased femoral retroversion
   - Increased external rotation with straight leg raising/flexion of hip due to tense posterior capsule
   - When child sits → thigh is held in external rotation and adduction resulting in tendency to cross the leg on uninvolved side.

2. **What are your differential diagnoses?**
Ans. Differentiate from:
   - *TB hip*: Here one finds characteristic deformities with movement restricted in all directions.
   - *Perthes disease*: Mild-to-moderate coxa vara may be difficult to differentiate just on the basis of history but here you will find restricted extension and also the age of onset is earlier in Perthes.
   - *DDH*: Head palpably outside joint, increased movements.

3. **What is SCFE?**
Ans. SCFE [or SUFE (slipped upper femoral epiphysis)] is posteroinferior slip of proximal femoral epiphysis in relation to metaphysis. In correct terminology, it is better defined as an anterosuperior slip of femoral neck relative to epiphysis.

4. How do you classify SCFE?

Ans. The accepted classifications in the order of preference:

- *Stable and unstable slip (it also has a good prognostic value and fairly decides treatment)*:
  - Stable slip is defined as ability of child to ambulate with or without crutches
  - Unstable slip is where the child cannot walk with or without support.
- *Severity of slip (linear displacement of epiphysis relative to metaphysis, angular displacement of epiphysis relative to long axis of femoral neck, % surface contact remaining)*:

	Linear displacement (%)	Angular displacement (degree)	Contact (%)
Preslip	0	0	100
Minimal	<33	<30	58
Moderate	33–50	30–60	39
Severe	>50	>60	22–0

- *Duration of slip*:

	Features	Signs and symptoms
Preslip	Widened physis, no displacement	Unknown
Acute	Displacement	<3 weeks
Acute on chronic	Displacement + remodeling	
Chronic—early	With/without remodeling, physis open	>3 weeks
Chronic—late	Remodeling and closed physis	>3 weeks
Chronic—late with osteoarthritis	Sclerosis; osteophytes, decreased joint space	

- *Direction of slip*:
  - *Varus slip*: Common
  - *Valgus slip*: These patients usually have a relative coxa valga with a more laterally tilted physis.

5. How will you manage this case?

Ans. I will assess and plan treatment after assessing the slip radiologically (AP and cross-table lateral radiograph).

6. What are the treatment goals?

Ans. *Goals*:
- Prevent further slip
- Physeal closure
- Maintain adequate function
- Avoid complications like osteonecrosis and chondrolysis.

Principles:
- All children with SCFE and open physis need treatment
- Simplest procedure that will achieve the goals should be done
- Patients with closed physis primarily require proximal femoral osteotomy for unacceptable gait, functional limitations and cosmetic deformity.

7. What are the treatment options?

Ans. *Stable SCFE*:
- *In situ* fixation: With single 6.5 mm (or 7.0 mm) cannulated partially threaded titanium screw
- Epiphysiodesis
- Proximal femoral osteotomy:
  - *Cuneiform (Fish/Dunn)*: Sort of open reduction, highest complication rate
  - *Basilar neck osteotomy*: Compromise surgery not very popular
  - *Intertrochanteric/Subtrochanteric*: Least complication and manipulates joint from "outside"
- Spica cast immobilization

Unstable SCFE:
- *In situ fixation*: As above without any "intentional" reduction unless the slip is so severe that fixation cannot be

achieved in that case gentle single attempt at reduction to bring the slip in the "chronic" position or a suitable position for fixation can be attempted. Whatever the consensus is toward immediate (within 24 hours)

- Epiphysiodesis (Schmidt technique)
- Cuneiform osteotomy (acute-on-chronic slip)
- Surgical dislocation of hip, open reduction, femoral osteotomy, and fixation of SCFE (Ganz, described recently) – not very much in vogue.

Always explain the risk of osteonecrosis and chondrolysis with procedures, the closure one operates to the physis higher the chances.

8. What will you do for the other hip?

Ans. *There is a lot of controversy in addressing this issue.* In general, it is logical to fix a disease that is known to have grave complications, in spite of the current knowledge that 20–35% are bilateral and majority of surgeries may be unnecessary.

CASE VII: LATE SEQUELAE OF SEPTIC ARTHRITIS OF HIP JOINT

1. Why do you call it sequel of septic arthritis?

Ans. Also known as Tom-Smith arthritis (Tom Smith described acute septic arthritis of hip joint in 1874. The focus of infection could arise from umbilicus, skin or from osteomyelitis of proximal femur that causes hip arthritis due to intracapsular location of the physis. There is frequently chondrolysis that may proceed to dislocation of the hip joint later. The common risk factors include premature delivery, umbilical vein catheterization and femoral vein puncture. The child is septicemic and there is failure to thrive. USG demonstrates capsular distension with superolateral subluxation of femoral head and dislocation. Radiographs show osteopenia of proximal femur and periosteal reaction while later there would be loss of femoral head. Treatment includes urgent decompression of hip and extensive lavage with intravenous antibiotics).

Findings:
- History of infectious arthritis in neonatal/perinatal period or infancy (typically <2 years of age)
- Premature birth
- Shortening (true)
- Increased gluteal creases on the pathological side
- Wasting of the gluteal and thigh muscles
- Abductor lurch with positive Trendelenburg gait
- Absent femoral pulses—Narath sign
- Upridden trochanter and corresponding changes in Bryant's triangle
- Adduction, external rotation deformity
- Hypermobile joint (movements increased in all direction, typically identified by increased extension, abduction and internal rotation)
- Desaults's positive.

2. What is your differential diagnosis?
Ans. DDH (may be bilateral, other congenital abnormalities else difficult to differentiate).

3. What are the various outcomes of septic arthritis hip joint?
Ans. Outcomes of septic arthritis in general! *You were not asked for a specific case—keep your mind open.*
- *Dislocated joint*: Due to destruction of femoral head and acetabular changes
- *Ankylosis of hip*: If the natural history of disease gets halted by treatment or immunity overrides infection
- *Osteomyelitis of femur and persistent infection*: Intramedullary spread of infection
- *Myositis ossificans*: Inflammatory changes in the surrounding muscles, local massage therapy and manipulation
- Contractures and various deformities primarily flexion and adduction
- *Coxa breva*: Due to destruction of growth plate
- *Coxa magna*: Reactive inflammatory hyperemia causing acceleration of growth locally provided infective destruction takes a backseat, or residual hyperemia once infection is controlled by treatment.

4. How do you classify late sequelae of septic arthritis?

Ans. Radiological classification of severity of residual femoral head deformities (Choi modification of Hunka classification below):

Choi classification (four major types and eight subtypes)		
Affected region	**Type**	**Disease process**
Proximal femoral epiphysis and physis	IA: Normal radiographic appearance	Almost normal hip
	IB: Early Perthes like osteonecrotic changes	Mild coxa magna
Proximal femoral epiphysis, physis, and metaphysis	IIA: Symmetric closure of physis	Coxa breva with no change in neck-shaft angle
	IIB: Asymmetric closure of physis	Progressive coxa vara or valga with acetabular dysplasia
Femoral neck	IIIA	Severe anteversion/retroversion with severe coxa vara/valga
	IIIB	Pseudoarthrosis of femoral neck with slipping of epiphysis
Epiphysis, physis, and metaphysis	IVA	Unstable hip with persistent small remnant of neck
	IVB	Complete loss of femoral head and neck

Hunka classification (Fig. 31):
- *Type I*: Minimal or no femoral head changes. The negligible collapse is usually promptly reossified. The course resembles and follows radiologically the pattern of failed Perthes disease
- *Type IIA*: Femoral head deformed, but physis intact
- *Type IIB*: Femoral head deformed, physis fused prematurely so produces deformity of neck as well
- *Type III*: Femoral neck pseudoarthrosis, the head may or may not be vascular

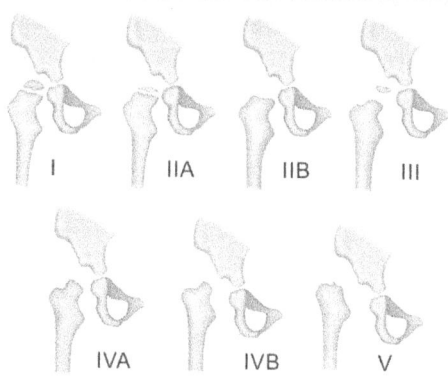

Fig. 31: Hunka classification.

- *Type IVA*: Complete destruction of proximal femoral epiphysis, with a small stable neck segment to maintain articulation
- *Type IVB*: Complete destruction of proximal femoral epiphysis, with a small neck that fails to maintain stable articulation
- *Type V*: Complete destruction of head and neck to the intertrochanteric line with dislocation of the hip.

5. What will you do for this patient?
Ans. I will get an X-ray done to confirm the diagnosis, look for the geometry of hip joint and determining the type.

6. What are the treatment options?
Ans. The treatment options are decided based up on the following factors:
- Age of patient
- Type of sequelae
- Abductor lurch
- Movements and stability
- Limb shortening
- Previous reconstructive procedures.

Algorithm (simplified) for surgical management in accordance with various Choi et al. types:

- *Type I:* Observation, loss of movements restricting function may be dealt with specific soft tissue releases. For type IB containment, procedure can be individualized.
- *Type II:*
  - *Type IIA:* Early—containment (pelvic osteotomy) + trochanteric apophysiodesis; Late—may additionally require correction for leg length discrepancy in the form of epiphysiodesis.
  - *Type IIB:* Realignment osteotomy to restore neck shaft angle + growth arrest of proximal femoral physis to prevent recurrence. Later in life, additionally manage the leg length inequality by contralateral leg epiphysiodesis.
- *Type III:*
  - *Type IIIA:* Correction of angular deformity as above with derotation osteotomy to correct version.
  - *Type IIIB:* Valgus osteotomy with achieving union at pseudoarthrosis by bone grafting.
- *Type IV* (*In general for type IV, one can always safely recommend pelvic support osteotomy of Schanz type, Lorenz or Milch batchelor type*) other reconstructive options are as below:
  - *Type IVA:* Age ≥ 6 years—Ilizarov hip reconstruction osteotomy with distal lengthening.
    - *Age < 6 years:* Trochanteric epiphysis well-formed and hyaline cartilage cover present—open reduction. Modified Harmon's procedure with distal transfer of greater trochanter.
  - *Type IVB:* Age ≥ 6 years—Ilizarov hip reconstruction osteotomy with distal lengthening.
    - *Age < 6 years:* Greater trochanteric arthroplasty, varus osteotomy, and acetabular osteotomy to provide coverage. Failed IVA/IVB procedures are treated with Ilizarov hip reconstruction osteotomy with lengthening.

(One can follow details from chapter 11 of the Essential Orthopedics Principles and Practice, 2nd edition).

7. What are the principles of Harmon's procedure?

Ans. Harmon's neck reconstruction procedure (as described by L'Episcopo and Harmon separately) involved repositioning of cartilage remnant attached to neck into acetabulum facilitated by longitudinal femoral osteotomy (modified Harmon's as described by Choi et al. provides a neck lengthening effect whereby a cartilage graft taken from iliac apophysis is placed into incomplete longitudinal femoral osteotomy). Often additional coverage procedures are required in the form of Chiari osteotomy and additional limb lengthening later is often needed.

8. What are the principles of trochanteric arthroplasty?

Ans. This procedure banks upon the growth potential remaining in the uninvolved greater trochanter and remodeling potential, which theoretically at least moulds toward the shape of femoral head if subjected to pressure and stresses in acetabulum. The osteotomy is done just below lesser trochanter and medial based wedge is removed. Vastus lateralis and medius attachments are retained to prevent devascularization. Abductors are transferred distally. Pelvic osteotomy is required to provide additional coverage.

9. What are the limitations of trochanteric arthroplasty?

Ans. *Limitations*:
- Avascularity of proximal segment
- Gradual loss of correction due to femoral remodeling and straightening
- Abductor weakness
- Stiffness
- Degenerative arthritis of hip
- Difficult future total hip arthroplasty.

10. What is the role of pelvic support osteotomy?

Ans. Better choose Milch-Batchelor osteotomy and describe as dealt in detail elsewhere (*see* Case I). Lorenz bifurcation osteotomy puts proximal end of distal fragment into acetabulum with capsular interposition. These osteotomies provide stability and displace the line of weight-bearing medially without approaching hip joint. Femoro-pelvic impingement may produce later degeneration and pain. In a nutshell, a properly performed PSO:

- Surgically shifts the shaft of femur near the center of gravity of the body so that the weight bearing axis is more along the axis of femur
- Supports pelvis by creating medial fulcrum
- Improves adductor function by causing valgus
- Abduction of distal fragment causes of gain of length.

11. What is Ilizarov reconstruction osteotomy and lengthening?

Ans. This is a one-step reconstruction for stability of hip joint by valgus subtrochanteric femoral osteotomy and lengthening with medialization (to compensate for abduction attitude) distally in experienced and expert hands. The valgus osteotomy is overcorrected to eliminate any further adduction that may impinge on pelvis or cause valgus stress at knee.

CASE VIII: DEVELOPMENTAL DYSPLASIA OF HIP

FINDINGS

- Trochanter upridden and palpated over Nelaton's line **(Figs. 32 and 33)**
- Adduction contracture
- Absent femoral pulses
- Asymmetrical thigh folds (↑ on the side of dislocation)
- Widened perineum (bilateral dislocation)
- Galeazzi's sign **(Fig. 34)**
- Telescopy
- Higher buttock fold on the affected side
- Head palpably out of acetabulum
- Movements—restricted abduction, increased internal rotation
- Positive Trendelenburg's sign
- Positive Barlow's and Ortolani's signs
- Duck-like or Sailor's gait
- Increased lordosis **(Fig. 35)**

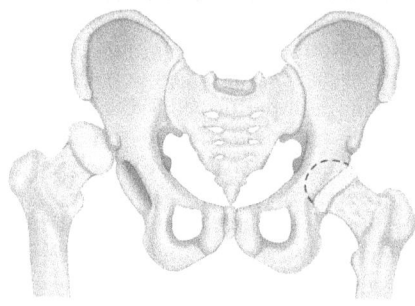

Fig. 32: Upriding of trochanter shortening.

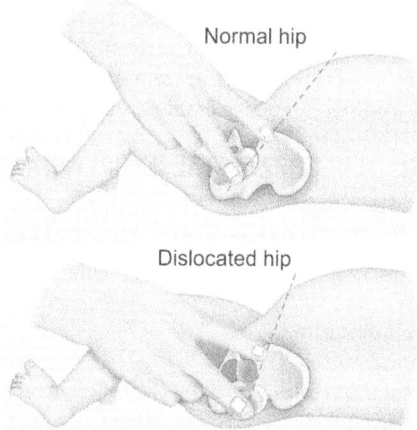

Fig. 33: Trochanter over Nelaton's line.

- Positive impingement test (older child; flexion, adduction, internal rotation produces pain)
- Positive instability test (tests anterior instability; extension, abduction, and external rotation. *Doubtful usefulness*)
- Shortening.

The Hip

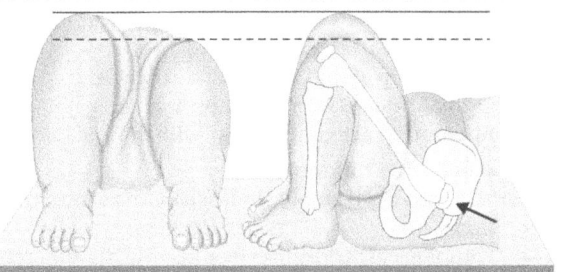

Fig. 34: Positive Galeazzi sign.

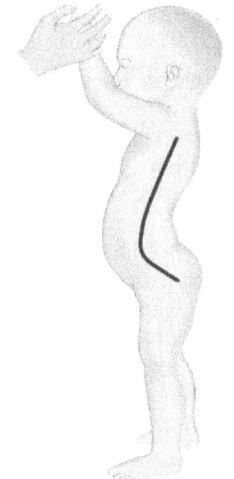

Fig. 35: Increased lumbar lordosis.

1. How do you define DDH?
Ans. Partial/complete displacement of femoral head from acetabulum because of inadequacy of acetabulum. Klisic introduced the term DDH (first "D" → developmental; second "D" represents both displacement and dysplasia but I prefer the latter).

2. What are the Hart's classic signs of hip dysplasia?
Ans. *Three signs*:
1. Limited hip abduction in 90° hip flexion
2. Ortolani's sign (first 3 months only)
3. Apparent shortening of thigh with hip and knee in flexion.

3. What are other differentials?
Ans. *Various other differentials for this condition are*:
- Coxa vara
- Pathological dislocation (septic arthritis, tubercular)
- Paralytic dislocation of poliomyelitis
- Cerebral palsy.

4. Why is it not sequelae of septic arthritis?
Ans. Lack of typical history and restriction of abduction goes against it.

5. What is teratologic dislocation of hip, is your patient having this type?
Ans. These are complex and difficult to treat forms of DDH usually associated with other disorders in genetic syndromes, arthrogryposis or myelodysplasia. The hips in these patients are malformed from early intrauterine period whereby there is complete acetabular malformation and marked displacement of the proximal femur. These patients can be identified clinically as they have irreducible hips on Ortolani test and relatively tight hips due to fixed deformities. No, my patient unlikely seems to have teratologic dislocation as there are no associated identifiable genetic syndromes or arthrogryposis and hip is reducible on Ortolani test.

6. How will you differentiate paralytic dislocation of hip from classical DDH?
Ans. My patient has good power in limbs and no evident spinal abnormalities (spina bifida, etc.)

7. What are common nonsyndromic association of DDH?
Ans. Congenital torticollis, metatarsus adductus, genu recurvatum, talipes calcaneovalgus deformity, and possibly clubfoot.

8. Where is the defect in DDH?
Ans. The primary defect lies in acetabulum (deficient development "dysplasia") whereby a constant defect is seen in the development of acetabular labrum (also a characteristic

of lower forms where hind limbs are rudimentary). The femoral defect is secondary, however soon they become complementary! A ridge of thickened articular cartilage forms over posterosuperior wall of acetabulum "Neolimbus" (Ortolani) over which head of femur rides in and out → clunk or "Scatto" (Ortolani).

9. What are the obstacles for reduction of hip?

Ans. *Obstacles*:
- Pericephalic insertion of capsule
- Ligamentum teres
- Inverted limbus
- Iliopsoas muscle
- Capsular adhesions
- Pulvinar thickness in acetabulum
- Transverse acetabular ligament pulled up along with ligamentum teres.

10. What will you do for this patient?

Ans. I will get an X-ray done to evaluate various parameters, USG, and measurement of angles and for follow-up. If required an MRI (to detail the soft tissue problems).

11. What are the various radiographic findings?

Ans. *Typical radiographic findings include*:
- Broken Shenton's line
- *Perkin's quadrants (Fig. 36)*:
  - Normal hip → lower medial quadrant (Fig. 37)
  - Subluxated hip → upper medial quadrant
  - Dislocated hip → lower lateral quadrant (Fig. 37)
  - High dislocation → upper lateral quadrant
- *Medial gap (distance separating proximal femur and a line perpendicular to lateral margin of ischium)*: Normally <4 mm; 5 mm → suspicious; ≥6 mm → dislocation.

Tear drop: Normally appears by 4–6 months; failure to appear >6 months is pathological (open/closed/crossed/reversed/U-shaped/V-shaped are all associated with DDH.

- *Increased acetabular index*: Tells acetabular dysplasia and its severity. Normal is 27.5° in newborns that reduces to 23.5° by 6 months and 20° by 2 years. Upper limit of normal is 30°.

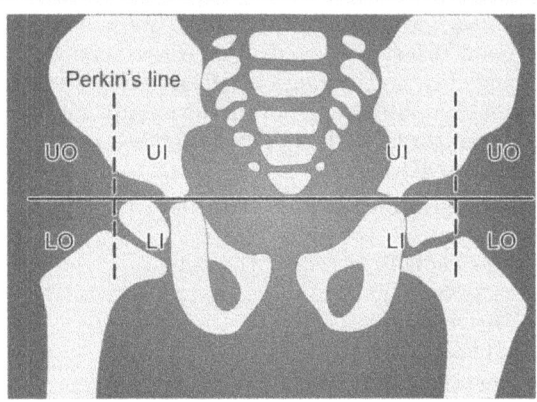

Fig. 36: Perkin's quadrants. (UO: upper outer; UI: upper inner; LO: lower outer; LI: lower inner).

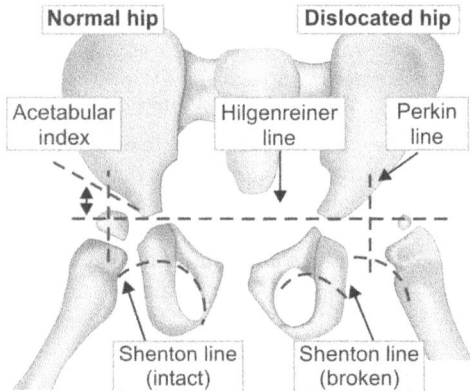

Fig. 37: Illustration showing some of the prominent radiographic comparative features of a normal appearing (right hip, as seen on your left hand side) versus dislocated hip (left hip, as seen on you right hand side).

- *Center-Edge (C-E) angle of Wiberg*: Tells degree of subluxation; decrease or reversal of angle is seen depending upon degree of dislocation; normal is >19° (6–13 years).

The Hip

12. What are the boundaries of teardrop?

Ans. Formed by lateral wall of lesser pelvis medially, wall of acetabulum laterally, curved line inferiorly and upper limit marked by acetabular notch.

13. What is the role of ultrasonography in diagnosis and management of DDH?

Ans. This is now a popular modality to diagnose and follow-up cases of DDH under conservative treatment. Based on specific α and β angles described by Graf **(Table 3)** DDH can be classified and diagnosed. It is better a tool for documenting response to treatment (closed reduction, Pavlik harness, etc.) of DDH.

Table 3: Graf's classification (simplified) (based on ultrasonogram).			
Type	α-angle	β-angle	Description	Treatment
I	>60°	<55°	Normal	None
II	43–60°	55–77°	Delayed ossification	*Controversial*
III	<43°	>77°	Lateral subluxation	Pavlik harness
IV	Immeasurable	Immeasurable	Dislocation	Pavlik harness/ closed/open reduction

14. How do you classify DDH?

Ans. Various types and classification based on etiopathology, radiology, MRI, reducibility, etc. are described. For prognostic and descriptive purposes, the following may be noted:

Klisic subgroups:
- *DDH "at risk"*: Family history, breech, female child, 1st born, oligohydramnios, associated deformities (torticollis, clubfoot, etc.)
- *DDH*: Hypoplastic with limited abduction
- *DDH*: Reducible dislocation with jerk of entry
- *DDH*: Reducible dislocation with jerk of exit

- *DDH*: Subluxation and limited abduction
- *DDH*: Dislocation with limited abduction, femoral shortening, and telescopy.

Etiopathological types:
- *Teratologic type:* Intrauterine dislocation in early fetal life, complete acetabular malformation, marked displacement of femoral head, tight soft tissues, and fixed deformities.
- *Paralytic type:* Associated with arthrogryposis multiplex congenita (AMC), spina bifida, etc.
- *Diastrophic dysplasia:* Mucopolysaccharidosis.

15. What is the direction of hip dislocation in DDH?
Ans. *Depending upon various pathological positions*:
- *In extreme flexion:* Posterior dislocation over acetabular rim
- *Lateral rotation:* Stretching of anterior capsule (seen in neglected DDH with increased anteversion)—anterior dislocation (*I got this case in DNB exam!*)
- *Adduction and flexion:* Lateralization of head and dislocation over posterolateral acetabular rim.

16. What is Ilfeld phenomenon?
Ans. Clinical examination for infantile DDH is difficult and results are poorly reproducible due to various reasons (crying baby, tense baby, hungry baby, hurried/inexperienced doctor, too firm a grip "white knuckle sign of Salter").

17. How will you plan treatment?
Ans. Various factors decide the treatment. Age, type of dislocation (etiopathological, radiologic), and reducibility all have a direct bearing.

Up to 6 months of age:
- USG positive, Ortolani's positive, dislocatable/subluxatable hip (especially >3–6 weeks) → abduction splint like Pavlik harness, Tubingen splint (less chances of osteonecrosis). Assess every 2 weeks. Ultrasonographic examination should be done at least once at the end of 6 weeks when the hip appears to be clinically stable (If reduction is not achieved by 6 weeks it is better to stop

use of harness and switch to other treatment). Brace changes are required to take care of the growth every 3-4 weeks. Once a stable hip has been achieved the harness is weaned off allowing more harness free time in the day.
- Continued use of Pavlik harness beyond 6 weeks in hips that are not concentrically reduced with its use can lead to development of "Pavlik harness disease". In these cases if the dislocation is reducible, the child should be taken up for closed reduction under general anesthesia.
- *For nonreducible hips*: Open reduction is the treatment of choice. The aim of open reduction is to achieve concentric reduction of the femoral head in the acetabulum after correcting the soft tissue interposition.

Over the age of 6 months:
- Abduction/flexion splintage may work for reducible hip till 3-6 months of age but the success rate keeps declining steadily.
- Closed reduction is the treatment of choice for DDH patients above 6 months of age if hip is reducible concentrically on arthrogram. Reduce by gentle traction ("human position" of 90° flexion and mild abduction, higher abduction → osteonecrosis) after arthrogram → successful (head should come at least to the upper edge of acetabulum), hold in spica for 8 weeks → mobilize in abduction splint. Follow every 3 weeks till stability (usually 3-4 months). Multiple cast changes may be needed due to soiling and growth of child.
- Failure to obtain stable concentric reduction by closed method is an indication for open reduction. The open reduction should be associated with capsulorrhaphy. If stability cannot be restored by open reduction alone then additional procedures to improve stability may be needed. Femoral side procedures are needed in the form of shortening to facilitate reduction of hip without undue pressure on femoral head. Proximal femoral varus derotation osteotomy is needed if hip is reducible

only in internal rotation and abduction. Acetabular side procedures are indicated as follows:
- As a rough guide if greater than 30% of head is visible after open reduction then additional procedures are needed to improve stability. Other signs that indicate an inadequate or eccentric reduction are moderate or pronounced limitation of abduction. Instability of reduction with easy dislocation.
- Also acetabular side osteotomies are needed if there is progressive subluxation after either conservative or operative treatment.
- The third indication for ancillary acetabular procedure is uncommon cases where the acetabulum fails to remodel after open reduction.

Management in toddler (2-3 years of age):
- These patients commonly need extensive procedures in combination. Open reduction + capsulorrhaphy + femoral and/or acetabular side procedures are needed.
- When the primary dysplasia exists in acetabulum, a pelvic redirectional osteotomy will be more appropriate. Generally, pelvic osteotomies are indicated only after the femoral head has been concentrically reduced, but the acetabulum is dysplastic, or the joint has failed to develop satisfactorily or the growth potential for acetabulum no longer exists. An upper age limit of 8 years is generally assumed after which acetabular dysplasia does not remodel even after open reduction.
- The femoral osteotomy for correcting rotation/anteversion is generally associated with shortening of femoral length to decrease pressure on the reduced femoral head, thereby diminishing the chances of avascular necrosis.

Management of neglected cases (>3 years of age):
- The treatment is directed to correct the identified adaptive pathology that is unique to individual cases with guarded prognosis.
- Primary femoral shortening should accompany the open reduction and capsulorrhaphy with or without pelvic

The Hip

osteotomy. The capsular dissection is necessary to produce lasting results; rarely tendon of piriformis muscles and gluteus medius may have to be released to bring the femoral head down to the level of acetabulum. Additional acetabular coverage may be needed.
- A varus angulation may be produced in the distal shaft additionally if required.

18. What is the role of Pavlik harness?

Ans. Usually the first choice during 1–6 months. The harness works on the mechanism of "dynamic flexion-abduction of hip". In supine position, the hip goes into abduction giving relief to the child when a reduction is affected. This further relaxes adductors (that are also relieved by sleep) further maintaining the reduced position and abducts the hip still more. Hips must be flexed >90° with proximal metaphysis pointing to triradiate cartilage and child must lie supine (*Note: hip need not be reducible on clinical examination before application of harness, however chances of reduction of high dislocations are much less!*). Reduction obtained → continue for 6 weeks otherwise discontinue. Appearance of notch above acetabulum and improved acetabular development (↓ acetabular angle) indicate success. Four patterns of dislocation are seen with the use of Pavlik harness:

1. *Superior:* Additional flexion required
2. *Inferior:* Reduce flexion
3. *Lateral:* Gradual reduction can be anticipated
4. *Posterior:* Difficult to treat, usually requires adductor release.

19. What are the contraindications of Pavlik harness?

Ans. *Do not use if:*
- Child is in walking age
- Hip cannot be centered toward triradiate cartilage with 90–110° flexion
- Dislocation develops several weeks after birth
- Dislocation associated with muscle imbalance:
  - Meningomyelocele
  - Down's syndrome, Marfan syndrome, etc.

20. What is the role of arthrogram?

Ans. Good investigation to assess the depth and stability of reduction. Width of medial dye pool indicates the likely stability of reduction. Fair reduction has 5-6 mm of dye pool. Poor reduction has >6 mm with difficult to hold reduction.

21. How will you do open reduction?

Ans. *Indications:*
- Femoral head lying persistently above triradiate cartilage
- Arc of reduction and redislocation <25°
- Femoral head remains laterally displaced >6 weeks (because of hourglass constriction)
- Previous failed reduction.

Either use median adduction approach as described by Ferguson or by Ludloff's incision or by anterior approach ("Bikini" incision). Anterior approach preferred for high dislocations, expected difficult reduction, and significant growth difference. This additionally allows pelvic osteotomy and anterior capsular reefing. Clear all the obstacles for reduction and hold the reduction with K-wire. Assess stability of reduction; if stable but inadequate coverage for head [age between 2 years and 8 years → do a pelvic osteotomy (Salter/Pemberton), age >8 years → needs acetabular procedure like Ganz's, Steel's or Dega's osteotomy]. If unable to reduce with adequate stability then plan for additional procedure like femoral shortening/derotation and assess coverage as above.

22. What are the advantages of femoral osteotomy?

Ans. It reduces chances of osteonecrosis, chondrolysis (by reducing pressure on femoral head), and redislocation.

23. What are the complications of combining acetabular procedure with femoral shortening?

Ans. Posterior dislocation particularly if derotation also done simultaneously.

24. What is the upper age of reduction of hip?

Ans. Difficult guidelines! In general unilateral cases have significant gait asymmetry and functional limitation than bilateral

The Hip

also complication rate is higher when both hips must be reduced:

- So for unilateral dislocation reduction can be attempted up to 9–10 years of age
- For bilateral cases, results are very unsatisfactory >8 years of age and probably the natural outcome of untreated bilateral dislocation is better than the results of treatment.

25. What are the indications of Salter's and Pemberton osteotomy?

Ans. The following are the indications:
- Failure to achieve stable reduction by open method due to acetabular incongruity or deficiency
- Progressive subluxation of hip after either conservative/operative treatment
- Failure of acetabulum to remodel.

Salter's type of osteotomy is done for rotational stabilization (if acetabulum has abnormal direction) and capsular reefing; Pemberton osteotomy is indicated in acetabular dysplasia (abnormal shape).

26. What are the indications for Salter's osteotomy?

Ans. This osteotomy can be done from 18 months to 8 years of age for unilateral cases and up to 5 years for bilateral cases. The acetabular roof is directed forward, downward, and laterally to stabilize hip in functional position.

Indications:
- Failure of acetabular angle to improve within 2 years following reduction
- Persistent mild-to-moderate dysplasia at 5 years.

27. What are the prerequisites and where do you do this osteotomy?

Ans. *Prerequisites:*
- Concentric reduction of hip joint
- Good range of movements
- Mild-to-moderate dysplasia only.

Site: Just above acetabulum running transversely from anterior inferior iliac spine to greater sciatic notch, lower fragment displaced forward, downward, and outward.

28. Where is the hinge of rotation for this osteotomy?

Ans. Pubic symphysis.

29. What are the disadvantages of this osteotomy?

Ans. *All procedures have some!*
- *Unstable osteotomy:* Requires fixation
- Correction limited by the size of graft
- Defect created in posterior acetabulum with narrowing of joint space.

30. What is Pemberton osteotomy?

Ans. Pemberton incomplete pericapsular osteotomy achieves stabilization by rotating the anterosuperior portion of acetabulum forward, laterally and downward. Posterior portion remains undisturbed. The osteotomy is often done in the presence of moderate to severe acetabular dysplasia but there should be adequate remodeling duration left so it is done for ages from 18 months to 6–7 years.

31. Where is the hinge for this osteotomy?

Ans. Triradiate cartilage.

32. What is Chiari osteotomy?

Ans. Chiari osteotomy is a medial acetabular displacement osteotomy over intact hip capsule for inadequacy to obtain concentric reduction. The osteotomy is aimed at:
- Deepening acetabulum
- Displacing the femoral head medially to reduce stresses
- Covering a subluxed head but not a dislocated head Over time, hip capsule transforms into fibrocartilage. The indications for the osteotomy are as follows:
    - Symptomatic patient in adolescent age up to middle age
    - Femoral head has little to no support
    - False acetabulum is not too high.

33. How does Chiari osteotomy differ from Salter's or Pemberton's osteotomy?

Ans. Salter's and Pemberton's osteotomy alter the orientation of acetabulum in order to cover the anterolateral defect present in these cases, whereas Chiari provides a new lateral extension to existing acetabular roof.

34. What is Shelf procedure?

Ans. Staheli shelf procedure is also described for hip that are not concentrically reducible. Shelf is made from outer table of ilium over supero-antero-lateral aspect of femoral head and augmented with ample graft.

35. What are the various palliative procedures?

Ans. These procedures are indicated in symptomatic patients where reduction is no longer possible by either closed/open reduction methods. Arthrodesis, arthroplasty, and osteotomy, all have their own indications as discussed briefly. Arthritic pain in a young heavy laborer can be managed by arthrodesis. Osteotomy of Schanz type to align the proximal fragment with pelvis and distal fragment parallel to weight bearing axis.

(For details on various osteotomies and preference of procedure better read from Chapter 32 of the book Essential Orthopedics Principles and Practice, 2nd edition).

CASE IX: POLIOMYELITIS AFFECTION OF HIP

1. What will you do for paralytic hip instability?

Ans. First, I will assess whether it is a complete dislocation, incomplete dislocation or hip subluxation. Assessment of muscle power is also important as the abductors and extensors are often involved leading to flexion and adduction contracture in unstable hip.

2. What is incomplete dislocation?

Ans. The hip dislocates in adduction and flexion but is otherwise stable in abduction. This often presents as "snapping hip".

3. How will you manage complete dislocation?

Ans. For a true dislocation, I would like to determine whether the cause of dislocation lies within the joint (viz. coxa valga) or periarticular soft tissues (muscle paralysis/ligament stretching) (type one Somerville). In the other type, the dislocation is secondary to pelvic obliquity/scoliotic deformity.

4. How will you manage first type?

Ans. I will correct deformity by traction to gradually gain abduction and reduce the hip joint till acetabular level. Deformity in hip joint proper needs osseous correction, so I will do varus osteotomy and correct anteversion for coxa valga. Simultaneous adductor contracture needs adductor tenotomy and other weak muscles also need management. If the hip is not reducible then after release of contractures I will make Staheli shelf to provide a superior support for the head. If everything else fails, hip arthrodesis can be done. The second type needs specific correction (spinal deformity) by addressing the causative factors.

5. How will you manage hip contracture?

Ans. The deformity at hip is typical of iliotibial band contracture producing FABER deformity. This is supplemented by iliopsoas, sartorius, and rectus femoris. The deformity and compensatory mechanisms due to iliotibial band and tensor fascia lata (TFL) contracture are progressive and should be promptly corrected. There are two methods of correction:

1. *Stretching*: Suitable for mild deformities, causes pain, damages tissues, and is unreliable for moderate to severe deformities. Hence for these deformities prefer option "2"
2. *Release of muscles and soft tissue*: Soutter's or Ober's release at hip and Yount's release (iliotibial band) at knee. Soutter's release primarily is aimed at correcting flexion deformity by releasing flexors of hip; additional correction can be achieved by releasing iliopsoas, anterior joint capsule, and abdominal muscles from crest. Ober's addresses the FABER deformity by releasing iliopsoas, rectus, sartorius, gluteus medius, and minimus and TFL and joint capsule. Campbell release and transfer of iliac crest is another option.

6. How will you manage abductor and extensor weakness?

Ans. The gluteus medius and maximus weakness needs to be addressed primarily for abductor and extensor weakness, respectively. Gluteus maximus weakness produces extensor lurch and increased lumbar lordosis, whereas the medius weakness produces Trendelenburg gait.

Gluteus maximus paralysis: Difficult to compensate by transfer due to lack of powerful muscles. Erector spinae transfer (Ober's) or posterior shift of TFL origin can be done to produce some functional compensation.

Gluteus medius paralysis: There are two muscles commonly used for compensating the paralysis:

1. External oblique transfer (Thomas, Thompson) to greater trochanter and adductor release (or transfer): This has following advantages over iliopsoas transfer:
   - Synergistic transfer
   - Maintaining power around hip joint
   - Preserving ilium for other bony procedure, if needed
   - Additional of external muscle power.
2. *Iliopsoas transfer*: Works for combined medius and maximus paralysis. Sharrard's modification of mustard operation is often used. Here psoas along with whole of the iliacus muscle is transferred to outer surface of ilium and tendon is attached to greater trochanter which now acts as abductor and extensor.

CASE X: OLD UNREDUCED DISLOCATIONS AND FRACTURE DISLOCATION

FINDINGS

History

- Trauma (significant and often high energy)
- Treatment with failed reduction/neglected/traction.

Examination

- FADIR in posterior dislocation (commoner ones)
- Supra trochanteric shortening
- Wasting
- ASIS often high due to adduction deformity
- Absent femoral pulse on the pathological side with preserved distal pulses

- Round, bony hard, globular (spherical) smooth swelling palpable in gluteal region
- Crepitus
- Movements often only present in sagittal plane (flexion)
- Inverted/reversed Bryant's triangle
- *Sciatic nerve injury (foot drop):* Try to find out if it was associated with injury (tingling and loss of sensation with injury) or it developed after attempted treatment (traction or failed reduction). Always perform complete neurological examination of the lower limb in these cases and report the normality/abnormality as the case may be.

1. What are your differential diagnoses?
Ans. *The above characteristic findings (the pathognomonic palpable head in gluteal region) are often absent in other disorders:*
- Pathological dislocation (TB of hip and septic arthritis)
- TB hip with destruction of head (will have painful global restriction of movements in active stage or fibrosis ankylosis or hypermobile unstable hip in healed disease)
- Avascular necrosis (AVN) of hip with destruction of head will have secondary osteoarthritis, and often external rotation deformity
- Old unreduced fracture neck of femur (external rotation deformity and limited shortening).

2. What will you do next?
Ans. I will confirm my diagnosis radiologically (X-ray pelvis AP projection and AP and cross leg lateral of involved hip).

3. What will you find on X-rays?
Ans. The following are the characteristic and ancillary findings:
- Loss of congruity of femoral head and acetabulum
- Broken Shenton-minard line
- Proximal migration of trochanter
- Smaller obturator foramen (flexion deformity)
- Smaller ilium (rotation of pelvis)
- Less prominent lesser trochanter
- Adducted femur.

The last few signs are ancillary signs of flexion and internal rotation of hip.

The Hip

4. What are the causes of chronic old unreduced posterior dislocation of hip?

Ans. *Various causes*:
- Inability to identify/Quack treatment
- Incarcerated acetabular or femoral head fragment (types III, IV, and V)
- Buttonholing of femoral head through capsule
- Inversion of labrum and obstruction to reduction
- Incarceration of piriformis
- Posterior unstable acetabular fractures (type II, III, and IV).

5. What are the complications of hip dislocation that you will keep in mind for managing the patient?

Ans. The complications of hip dislocation are:
- *Early*:
  - Sciatic nerve injury
  - Injury to superior gluteal artery and nerve—causes gluteal atrophy and arterial injury may cause exsanguination, threatening life of patient.
  - Irreducible dislocation (*see* above).
- *Late*:
  - Osteonecrosis of femoral head
  - Myositis ossificans
  - Osteoarthrosis of hip joint.

6. What will you do next?

Ans. I will get CT scan of the pelvis to assess associated fractures of acetabulum, MRI to look for vascularity of head and condition of acetabular soft tissues.

7. How will you manage the patient?

Ans. The patient will be assessed on the basis of associated injuries (classify as per Thompson and Epstein classification of posterior dislocation of hip) and vascularity of head and medical condition of patient (fitness for major interventions and preoperative ambulatory status).

8. What is the Thompson and Epstein classification?

Ans. Classified posterior dislocation of hip on the basis of fractures of acetabulum and femoral head fractures:

- *Type I*: With no or minor acetabular fracture
- *Type II*: With a large chunk of posterior wall of acetabulum
- *Type III*: With comminuted rim fracture of acetabulum
- *Type IV*: With rim and floor fracture of acetabulum
- *Type V*: With fracture of head.

9. How will you treat the patient?

Ans. *Type I:* <3 months old with viable head → closed reduction ↓ GA → (if fails then) Gupta's heavy traction method

Type I: >3 months old with viable head → Gupta's method versus open reduction (preferred) using anterior or anterolateral approach

Type II: <3 months (viable head) → reconstruction of acetabulum and open reduction (preliminary heavy traction often required)

Type II: >3 months (viable head) → arthroplasty versus arthrodesis (as while trying open reduction the acetabular cartilage will often be damaged irreparably in an attempt to curette the soft tissues)

Type III: As for type II

Type IV and Type V: Viable head → reconstruction and open reduction must be tried for young patients for older patients → arthroplasty is better

Nonviable head (any type any duration): Arthroplasty is the procedure of choice versus arthrodesis.

10. What is Gupta's method for closed reduction with traction?

Ans. Gupta and Shravat devised the method for closed reduction of hip <3 months old using traction and abduction. Apply skeletal upper tibial traction with 18 kg weight and sedate the patient. When head comes at or below the acetabular margin then gradually abduct the limb and reduce weight @ 3.6 kg every 4th day. Once the reduction is achieved then traction with 7 kg weight is maintained for 2 weeks. Patient is allowed no weight bearing (NWB) for 4 weeks followed by gradual weight bearing to full weight bearing after 3 months. The aim is to obtain concentric reduction.

11. Why the duration of 3 months is critical?

Ans. After 3 months, soft tissue often develops inside the acetabular cavity that prevents reduction of head by closed methods.

12. What is the role of arthrodesis?

Ans. Arthrodesis is a good proposition for young patients. However, achieving solid bony union is often difficult in the setting of osteonecrosis.

CASE XI: MALUNITED/OLD NEGLECTED FRACTURE INTERTROCHANTERIC

Unusual case but given commonly in endemic areas like eastern India. Importantly concepts of intertrochanteric fixation and methods are assessed rather than the case itself.

Read times: 4-6 times (DNB and MS candidates).

Diagnosis: This is a 68-year-old female with 6 months old malunited fracture of right proximal femoral region** most likely intertrochanteric (or a pathological fracture if known!). There is 30° adduction deformity, 40° external rotation deformity, and 2.5 cm of true supratrochanteric shortening of right lower limb. *(Should you mention coxa vara in diagnosis? → probably not as this is specifically a radiological finding of reduced neck-shaft angle. Clinically it is evident as shortening with abduction deformity and reduced abduction with prominent trochanter, that's it).*

FINDINGS

- Externally rotated limb at hip, adduction attitude may be seen in long-standing (>3 months) malunions
- Shortening (supratrochanteric)
- Prominence at the region of greater trochanter
- Broadening and irregularity over greater trochanter
- Prominent trochanter (that may be posteriorly displaced)
- External rotation deformity and adduction deformity at hip
- Decreased abduction, external rotation and, extension at hip
- Movements often painful in all directions due to impingement of soft tissue

- Trendelenburg positive (usually in old age muscle power is weak and long-standing muscle inhibition because of pain producing hypotrophy and varus at fracture manifests as positive Trendelenburg's sign)
- Able to do active SLRT (malunited fractures should not hamper SLR)
- Telescopy negative (do only if painless!)
- Shortening of base of Bryant's triangle, increased hypotenuse, and perpendicular.

Important note: Old neglected intertrochanteric fractures are commonly pathological. History taking and examination should incorporate finding the primary cause of fracture. Traumatic neglected cases as may be found in remote areas are less likely to be kept in exams as they are rare.

1. Why do you call this an intertrochanteric fracture malunion, would you like to present any differentials that have been excluded?

Ans. See above for findings in support of intertrochanteric fracture malunion. Differentials include:
- Malunited basicervical fractured neck femur** (really cannot be differentiated from malunited IT fracture so never commit specific diagnosis as neck of femur fracture or intertrochanteric fracture rather use term like "region").
- Malunited subtrochanteric fracture.
- Congenital coxa vara.
- Neoplastic pathology [cyst/giant cell tumor (GCT)] at greater trochanter.
- Fibrous dysplasia and associated proximal femoral deformity (like shepherd crook deformity).
- Sequelae of septic arthritis of hip.
- Sequelae of Perthes disease.
- Old-healed rickets.
- Achondroplasia.
- Paget's disease.
- Cretinism.
- Neglected dysplastic dislocation of hip.

The Hip

2. What will you do next and why?

Ans. I will get X-ray of the involved hip in anteroposterior and lateral projections to look for configuration and status of fracture (union). I will also look for any primary pathology (neoplasia/osteoporosis) that might be responsible for the fracture. I would also like to get X-ray of pelvis with both hips for comparison from uninvolved hip. X-ray of spine can be obtained, if there is associated symptomatology from the region (in old cases, there may be compensatory/degenerative scoliosis).

3. What pathology do you suspect?

Ans. Osteoporosis, osteomalacia, and neoplastic pathology (metastasis mainly, primary tumor at the region are uncommon for this age).

4. What are the problems to patient?

Ans. Shortening, Trendelenburg lurch, reduced movements, pain (if recent), and hip arthritis in long run.

5. How will you manage this patient?

Ans. *Malunited fracture*: Assess the movements at hip. If the movements are reasonably preserved and muscle power is regained then I will discuss with the patient corrective surgical options versus conservative method.

Initial trial with shoe raise for compensation of shortening will be provided. Universal shoe raise of 2.5 cm is generally adequate. Patient is also instructed hip abduction and extension exercises and allowed full weight-bearing walk with compensation of shortening. If the patient is satisfied, then no further intervention is needed, else one can explain surgical procedures.

Patient will gain limb length with corrective valgus osteotomy, abductor lurch will improve and pain due to abnormal transfer of forces across the hip joint will be relieved. Patient will have to, however, be bedridden for a week and slowly regain movements over a month to full weight-bearing walk and usual complications of surgery, viz. infection, nonunion, etc. With conservative management, there is a high chance for development of hip degenerative arthritis.

Old-neglected fracture (>3 weeks old): If the fracture is <6 weeks old (mobile on fluoroscopy), I will provide the option of open reduction of the fracture with bone grafting and fix using sliding hip screw. The patient can then be started on graduated hip mobilization and muscle-strengthening program.

For fracture >6 weeks old (not mobile on fluoroscopy), I will explain the pros and cons of osteoclasis and fixation + bone grafting versus wait for fracture union and graduated muscle strengthening program and delayed osteotomy. Osteotomy will be usually planned after around 1 year for fracture to consolidate.

(For valgus osteotomy details, kindly see the case for fracture neck of femur above).

6. How will you manage a fresh intertrochanteric fracture?

Ans. After assessing the medical condition of the patient and discussing the willingness for surgery, I will treat the patient as follows.

For stable intertrochanteric fractures. I will use sliding hip screw.

For an unstable fracture pattern. I will preferably use an intramedullary fixation.

7. What are the clinical differences between intra- and extracapsular fracture of proximal femur?

Ans. In intracapsular fractures of proximal femur, the external rotation deformity and shortening is lesser due to capsular restriction. Unfortunately, the complications of treatment are more in the form of nonunion and osteonecrosis in these patients.

8. How do you define an unstable intertrochanteric fracture?

Ans. *Presence of any or combination of*:
- Four part fracture
- Medial cortical comminution (loss of calcar support)
- Reverse obliquity of main fracture line

The Hip

- Large and separate posterior greater trochanteric fragment
- Subtrochanteric extension.

9. How will you fix a stable intertrochanteric fracture?

Ans. I will use sliding hip screw [or dynamic hip screw (DHS), AO].

There are a lot of devices mentioned in the literature like variable angle sliding hip screw, talon compression hip screw, Medoff plate, percutaneous compression plate, etc. but speak only those in exams that you have seen or used and can defend for further questions!

10. How do you reduce an intertrochanteric fracture?

Ans. The patient is placed on a fracture table after anesthesia and traction is applied under fluoroscopy. Additionally, commonly internal rotation is needed. The reduction is assessed in both anteroposterior and lateral projections.

11. What are the causes of failure of closed reduction?

Ans. Comminution at fracture site, severe osteoporosis, laxity of soft tissues in frail elderly patient, and malposition of fracture table are causes of nonreducible fractures. In such cases, commonly the shaft fragment sags below on lateral projection. One should ensure that the foot holder is in line or just below the level of hip, else placing it too high will angulate the femur posteriorly. This is also a problem, if iliopsoas tendon is attached to the proximal fragment in very oblique fracture lines that exit below lesser trochanter. In such cases, one may utilize Korean maneuver of pushing the proximal fragment down using a Steinman pin.

12. What is the entry point for lag screw used in sliding hip screw system?

Ans. Approximately 2 cm below the vastus lateralis ridge.

13. What is the ideal position of lag screw?

Ans. The lag screw should be placed in center-center position of femoral head. Previous recommendations of inferior and posterior placement of the screw to prevent superior and anterior cutout no longer hold true as they actually increase the TAD (Tip apex distance). Eccentric placement of screw also places more rotational stress at the fracture site and may cause early failure.

14. What should be ideal angle of barrel plate used?

Ans. First, understand that for unstable fractures, there is usually a posteromedial defect. Second, the joint reaction forces are transmitted at around 160°. Now Barrel plates are available in angle ranging from 130° to 155°.

Posteromedial fragments are most difficult to reduce even partially. When a larger angle plate is used one is actually putting the screw eccentrically (mean neck-shaft angle is 129°) so that the head will be in valgus reduction to produce a center-center screw position. This valgus reduction increases the medial gap and makes the construct unstable. Also it is difficult to negotiate the guidewire off the medial cortex to center it in the head. For such unstable construct, some form of osteotomy is required to improve medial loading. Otherwise the load to failure of these angle construct is higher for stable fractures as the bending forces are minimal (screw nearly parallel to resulting forces) and fracture is perpendicular to the forces due to valgus reduction.

When one uses the 135° barrel plate (as is commonly practiced), the posteromedial opening is less and one comfortably places the screw at the center of head reducing the potential of iatrogenically displacing the anatomical fracture reduction. Although the bending moment is higher than larger angle barrel, but it is preferred for anatomical reduction.

15. What is TAD?

Ans. TAD is tip apex distance first referred by Baumgaertner. The distance is sum total of the distance in mm of screw tip to apex of the medial femoral head curve in anteroposterior and lateral radiographs after magnification correction. Ideal range is 11 mm to 25 mm, but surgeons tend to achieve TAD < 20 mm **(Fig. 38)**.

The Hip

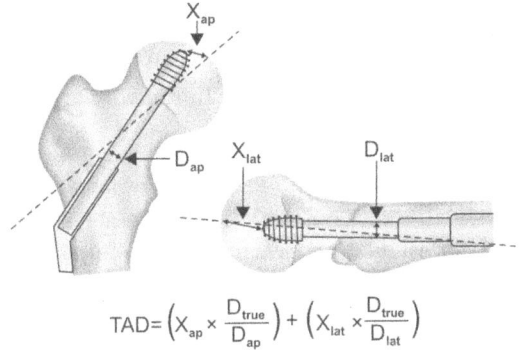

$$TAD = \left(X_{ap} \times \frac{D_{true}}{D_{ap}}\right) + \left(X_{lat} \times \frac{D_{true}}{D_{lat}}\right)$$

Fig. 38: Diagrammatic representation of tip-apex distance.

16. Why do you call this a lag screw?

Ans. The screw slides in the barrel plate and has no other fixed end. By itself, it cannot produce compression. The screw only acts to facilitate collapse. Compression is aided by separate compression screw put at the rear of lag screw.

17. When should you avoid giving compression at fracture site?

Ans. In osteoporotic fractures and weak bones, there is a high chance of the screw pull out from cancellous bone so compression should be avoided.

18. When should you put short barrel plate?

Ans. Barrel length is chosen to facilitate optimal sliding and collapse of the fracture without letting the screw jam inside barrel under bending moment (vertical force). The larger the length of screw outside the barrel, higher is the bending moment at screw barrel junction jamming the screw. Again, if a smaller length screw is put, then screw may touch the barrel before complete fracture consolidation has occurred. Short barrel length (25 mm) is used for screw lengths ≤80 mm while otherwise standard barrel length (38 mm) is preferable.

19. What is the thread length for DHS lag screw?

Ans. The thread length for standard DHS lag screw is 22 mm, thread diameter is 12.5 mm, and shaft diameter is 8 mm.

20. What are the options for intramedullary fixation of fracture IT?

Ans. Gamma nail (second and third generation), proximal femoral nail (short and long and PFN-a), intramedullary hip screw, trochanteric hip screw, and trochanteric antegrade nail.

21. Can all unstable intertrochanteric fractures be managed with intramedullary fixation?

Ans. No. Intramedullary fixation is typically suitable for subtrochanteric extension, reverse obliquity fracture, and medial cortical comminution hampering medial support. IT fractures, where there is no lateral wall support, are also good candidates for intramedullary fixation. Fractures with large posterior fragment or four-part fractures where greater trochanteric fragment is not localized or reduced well, are not well suited for intramedullary fixation due to entry point problems. These are better fixed with tension band wiring of greater trochanter fragment and additional trochanteric stabilizing plate with a sliding screw fixation. Alternatively, dynamic condylar screw or condylar blade plate can be used but patient has to delay weight-bearing. *(DCS or CBP provide a prosthetic lateral wall of metal, it is unclear how well a support can these provide!)*

22. Why you do not use DHS for fixation of reverse oblique fracture?

Ans. DHS is unable to resist the medial displacement tendency of distal shaft fragment. With continued fracture consolidation, the proximal fragment has no good screw purchase (lag screw only is meant for controlled collapse and not fracture fixation) and has constant abductor pull. The distal fragment has constant adductor pull from muscles. Now the fracture line (reverse oblique slanting upward medially) is such that it will not resist medial displacement of the distal shaft fragment so the fixation will surely fail. Intramedullary device is best suited to fix the fracture. Dynamic compression screw (DCS) or condylar blade plate (CBP) can be used provided, there is no medial comminution (medial continuity and contact is imperative), else they will fail ultimately in varus collapse.

23. What are the pros and cons of using intramedullary implant?

Ans. *Advantages:*
- Ability to fix majority of fractures.
- Short surgical time and less blood loss for unstable fractures (no difference comparing to DHS fixation for stable IT fractures).
- Smaller moment arm so better able to bear tensile forces and lesser calcar strain is produced. A sliding hip screw produces 1.5 times the calcar strain of a normal femur while intramedullary implant produces <10% of strain.
- Better controls collapse as the bending moment at lag screw for nail is lesser than DHS.
- Biomechanically the nail construct is stiffer (so more stable) than DHS for torsional and bending forces.

Disadvantages:
- Abductor injury while insertion.
- Difficult revision by arthroplasty if fails.
- Anterior thigh pain due to impingement of unlocked nail tip.
- Curvature mismatch of nail and femora may produce iatrogenic fracture.
- Stress concentration at tip of nail predisposing to fracture.
- Costlier implant.

24. What is "Z-effect" and reverse Z-effect?

Ans. "Z-effect" and "reverse Z-effect" are complications that arise from fixation of unstable proximal femoral fractures with PFN having two screws (newer version has single blade). Z-effect is lateral migration of caudal screw, varus collapse, and perforation of femoral head by superior screw while reverse Z-effect is lateral migration of cephalic screw, varus collapse, and femoral head cutout by inferior screw.

The cause is not fully elucidated, however, varus fixation of fracture, severe medial comminution, inappropriate entry point, and poor bone quality have been provisionally implicated.

25. Do you know of any intraoperative procedure to stabilize an unstable fracture?

Ans. There are various osteotomies, which can be done to improve the contact between fragments (in unstable fractures) and load transmission and were devised to be used with fixed-angle nail plate design like the *Smith-Petersen nail plate*:
- Dimon-Hughston medial displacement osteotomy
- Sarmiento valgus osteotomy
- Wayne County lateral displacement reduction. There is no evidence to support the use of these osteotomies with sliding hip screw. Instead, one should aim at obtaining an anatomical reduction and fixing with a standard device.

26. What are the mechanisms of failure of DHS?

Ans. DHS fails primarily if the fracture is not consolidated and stabilized whence instability still remains at the fracture site by virtue of fracture configuration and screw has either jammed or slide to limit has already occurred. In this instance, the construct behaves like a fixed-angle nail plate device failure involved any of the four modes:
1. Penetration of the nail through head into hip joint.
2. Pulling out of plate and shaft screws (varus collapse)
3. Cutout of lag screw superiorly through head
4. Bending and break at barrel plate junction.

27. What is the role of arthroplasty for treatment of unstable intertrochanteric fractures?

Ans. Due to higher failure rates for fixation of unstable intertrochanteric fractures and difficult revision following failed fixation many surgeons have resorted to arthroplasty as primary treatment modality. The modality has become increasingly popular and promising. Both cemented and cementless; hemi- and total hip arthroplasties have been used with comparable or better outcomes in terms of *postoperative complications*. Cone prostheses (cementless) are

The Hip

more popular as there is a higher chance of cementless stems subsiding into the wider femoral canal following osteolysis. The treatment is, however costly and requires specialist.

28. Would you like to do anything for poor bone quality?

Ans. I will start the patient on pharmacotherapy for osteoporosis with calcium, vitamin D and oral bisphosphonates. If the patient is willing I will prefer intravenous bisphosphonate to avoid adverse effects with the use of oral compounds and ensure compliance. I will avoid putting compression screw during surgery.

29. What are the management options for poor bone purchase in osteoporosis?

Ans. Using bone cement in femoral head to improve lag screw purchase can be done else implants specific to minimize screw cut-out should be used like:
- Delta bolt.
- Spiral blade instead of screw.
- Injecting cement into the screw tract before putting the screw.
- Talon compression hip screw.

30. Can you start the bisphosphonates at fracture healing?

Ans. I will start the bisphosphonate (either alendronate or zoledronic acid) at the earliest. I will take care to make the patient calcium replete for 3–4 days before starting bisphosphonates. There is no evidence till date to delay bisphosphonate therapy. They do not delay callus. Real concern is sequestration of bisphosphonates at the fracture healing site so that with reduced systemic drug efficacy may be lost. There is no answer to this but one can use weekly bisphosphonates to allow frequent body loading with the drug rather than giving yearly administered drugs.

31. Can you start parathormone at acute stage and with surgical procedure?

Ans. rPTH has been found to improve bone healing in animals. It can be systemically or locally administered. Locally administered drug has been found to improve implant anchorage.

32. How do you classify intertrochanteric fractures?

Ans. The question has been put in last as there is no consistently followed classification. Instead, usually the surgeons see a fracture and recall a matching "type" from various classifications. The commonly followed is Evans (1949) as it differentiates stable from unstable types and is easy. AO/OTA classification has been found to be more consistent if regularly followed.

Evan's classification for intertrochanteric fracture:
- *Type I:* Undisplaced two-fragment fracture
- *Type II:* Displaced two-fragment fracture
- *Type III:* Three-fragment fracture without posterolateral support (displaced greater trochanter fragment)
- *Type IV:* Three-fragment fracture without medial support (displaced lesser trochanter or posteromedial calcar fragment)
- *Type V:* Four-fragment fracture without posterolateral and medial support (combination of Type III and type IV)
- *R:* Reversed obliquity fracture.

3

The Knee

EXAMINATION POINTS FOR A KNEE CASE

HISTORY

- *Pain*: Onset, duration, severity, character (aching—degenerative and tumor; throbbing—infection), progression (insidious—degenerative and mechanical; acute—traumatic and infection), diurnal variation (morning—inflammatory; evening—mechanical and degenerative; night—inflammatory and tuberculosis), activity related (degenerative viz. osteoarthritis), radiation (usually to calf—degenerative and mechanical), pain after prolonged flexion (patellar disorders; "theater sign"), bar- or vice-like pain suggests patella baja (low-riding patella), pain at other sites (inflammatory, referred pain from lower back), previous history/episodes.
- *Deformity*: Varus (rickets, osteoarthritis, post-traumatic, etc.), valgus (rickets and rheumatoid arthritis), recurvatum (poliomyelitis and generalized joint laxity), flexion (effusion, infection, sequelae, scurvy, and hemophilia), triple deformity (tuberculosis), bizarre (Charcot's), broadening (hemophilia and arthritis—osteophytes), patellar (alta, baja pronounced as *baha*), lateral (subluxed/dislocated, small, double—bipartite), deformity at other joints especially hips (congenital) and small joints (inflammatory).
- *Swelling*: When? (Onset and duration), How? (Traumatic or atraumatic—infection, inflammatory, and tumor), How long? Associated symptoms? (Fever, pain, etc.) Previous aspiration "recurrent"—straw colored (hydrarthrosis—inflammatory,

osteoarthritis, loose body; all due to synovial irritation), pus (pyarthrosis—septic arthritis), blood-colored (hemarthrosis—hemophilia and traumatic), amber colored [pigmented villonodular synovitis (PVNS)]. Long-standing painless swelling may be meniscal cysts and benign tumors, viz. osteochondroma (painless), painful swellings—tumors (malignant) and hematoma in soft tissues.

- *Laxity (English = Laxity; French = Instability or Instabilitè)*: Specifically enquire about "going out" of knee—anterior cruciate ligament (ACL) tear, patellar dislocation or subluxation (subluxation usually presents with anterior knee pain). Symptom of "giving way" (knee failing to provide support fully—sort of apprehension ± pain) especially on walking on uneven surfaces usually indicates "interposition" (meniscus, cartilage—free bodies, synovial membrane, etc.); "cartilage damage"; "muscle weakness" (polio and neuropathy), "generalized joint laxity" (*Marfan syndrome, etc. See Chapter 5; Case II*).
- *Locking (inability to extend fully—free flexion)*: "True locking" also called meniscal locking is usually due to meniscal tear but may also be caused by loose bodies—"funny" feeling in joint (joint mice) or ACL stump. "False locking" also called patellar locking rather "catching" may also be caused by hypertrophied fat pad.
- *Limitation of movement or stiffness*: Painful (inflammatory, degenerative, and traumatic, tumors), painless "mechanical" (soft tissue—contractures of muscles, tendon, fascia, postoperative, inadvertent—total knee replacement, arthrodesis; bony—malunited fractures, tumors, and osteophytes). *Intra-articular (usually painful, bony, and sudden stop—firm end point, postsurgical); extra-articular (developmental, painless, and soft-end point).*
- Other clinically relevant features:
    - *Noise from joint:* Crepitus, snapping syndromes, "thud" of discoid meniscus, and "clunks" and "clicks" of menisci.
    - Evaluation for IKDC score.

EXAMINATION

General and systemic examination: Rickets, hypermobility syndrome (Down syndrome, Larsen syndrome, Marfan syndrome, and

Ehlers–Danlos syndrome), hemophilia, rheumatoid, dysplasia, and myopathy.

LOCAL EXAMINATION

Prerequisites

- *Position, lighting, and draping:* Examine both knees (limbs) together. Expose from flanks to ankle for examination of knee joints. Examine in ambient day light. Adequately drape the patient to avoid embarrassment.
- Firm couch for supine examination.
- Examine the patient first in standing position then the gait and lastly in "lying down" position (may require prone position also for some tests). However, if the patient has significant pain in standing or walking then postpone it till the end.
- Keep other ("normal") joint in same position for comparison, e.g. valgus in a knee with flexion contracture should be commented only by observing the normal joint in same degree of flexion. (*Ideally speaking varus is definitely pathological and can be commented upon even in a flexion deformity; however, it is less well-accepted for valgus deformity.*)
- Be gentle and always explain to the patient what you are going to do and what you expect. Warn if it is going to be painful and be sorry if it hurts.

Inspection

Patient standing (kneel down in front of patient to look head on):

- *Attitude:* "Front and side"—extension at knee joint and hip joint with foot plantigrade planted fully and patellae looking forwards.
- *Alignment:* Patient looking to horizon and you looking head on (i.e. "front only")—knee and medial malleoli barely are touching each other with great toe pointing forwards. (Always speak of "normal alignment" and not as normal joint as there is inbuilt varus in recurvatum deformity.)
    - Genu valgum
    - Genu varum
    - Windswept deformity.

Now inspect joint from "all around":

- *Swelling:* Generalized, localized (tumor, bursitis, meniscal cyst, Baker's cyst, Osgood–Schlatter disease, Sinding-Larsen-Johansson syndrome, Jumper's knee—patellar tendinitis, and Hoffa's disease), thickened synovial band seen as swelling at side (meniscal tear).
- Effusion (fullness of peripatellar fossae)
- *Skin:* Neurofibromatosis
- Scars
- Sinus
- *Patella and extensor apparatus:*
    - Bipartite patella (swelling at superolateral aspect)
    - Squinting patella (increased femoral anteversion)
    - Frog-eye patella (patella facing out—femoral condyle hypoplasia, subluxed patella, increased Q-angle, etc.)
    - Patella magna (osteophytes) and breva (hypoplasia)
- Wasting especially of vastus medialis.

Gait: Inspection of gait has been described in **Box 1**.

Examination in sitting position:
1. Patella alta and baja
2. J-sign (bony or soft tissue pathology at trochlea—trochlear dysplasia, internal femoral torsion, tense lateral retinaculum)
3. Dynamic patellar tracking (N-straight line) and patellar tilt.

Box 1: Inspection of gait.

Examine from anterior and posterior perspectives:
- Valgus thrust gait (single joint—osteoarthritis, malunited tibial plateau fracture)
- Valgus thrust with circumduction (both joints affected)
- Varus thrust gait (osteoarthritis, malunited tibial plateau fracture, lateral ligament complex injury)
- Varus recurvatum thrust (posterolateral laxity)
- Duck-footed (slew-footed) gait (increased femoral anteversion).

Lateral perspectives:
- Antalgic gait
- Stiff knee gait
- Flexed knee gait.

Examination in supine position: Confirm above findings report any change in findings as correction of version and deformity (correction denotes intra-articular deformity). Special attention to effusion and flexion deformity should be given as small amount may be hidden in standing.

Palpation

Anterior aspect:
- *Temperature and effusion:*
  - Fluid shift (visible fluid wave ≈ 15 mL)—mild effusion.
  - Palpable fluid wave (cross fluctuation ≈ 30 mL)—moderate effusion.
  - Ballotable patella sign (patellar tap test)—gross effusion.
  - Transillumination
  - Palpate synovium (from above below feel for thickened bands/doughy thickenings which "rolls" under the finger).
- *Patella and extensor apparatus:*
  - Patellar facet tenderness (push patella medially—feel undersurface)
  - Patellar/quadriceps tendinitis (Jumper's knee)
  - Apical patellar tenderness and bipartite patella (base)
  - Patellar glide/shift test (measured in quadrants, Sage sign) and tracking **(Fig. 1)**
  - Patellar lift ("push and lift", N = none on lateral side, minimal over medial aspect <10°)
  - Patellar grind test (push patella over femur with palm and flex the joint)
  - Fairbank's apprehension test (glide patella laterally in knee joint flexed to 30°—positive if patient is apprehensive and tries to protect patella) **(Fig. 2)**
  - Tibial tubercle.
- Wilson's test (osteochondritis dissecans)—lift ankle → flex knee 90° → extend knee → pain due to ACL impingement.

Medial aspect:
- Joint line tenderness [90° flexion—typically elicited medially; laterally obscured by iliotibial band (ITB)]
- Pes anserinus bursa and meniscal cysts
- Medial collateral ligament (MCL)—both femoral and tibial ends.

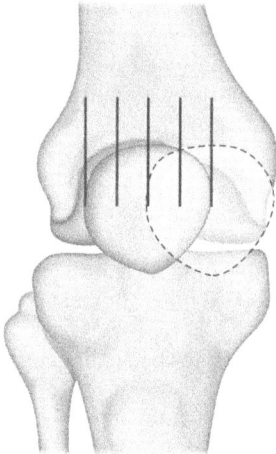

Fig. 1: Patellar shift/glide test—glide of patella less than 1 quadrant medially indicates tight retinaculum while glide more than 2 quadrants laterally indicates lax retinaculum/medial patellofemoral ligament (MPFL) medially.

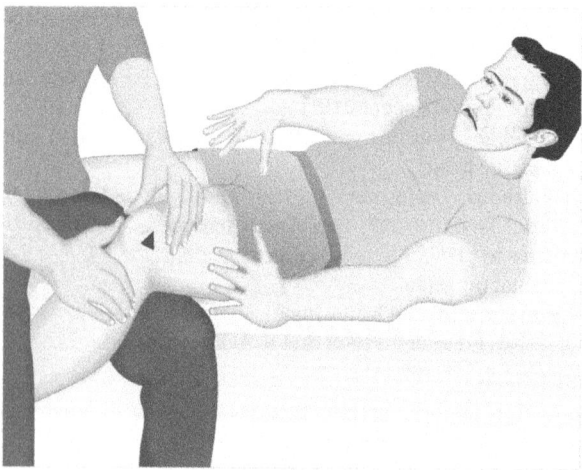

Fig. 2: Fairbank's apprehension test for patellar instability.

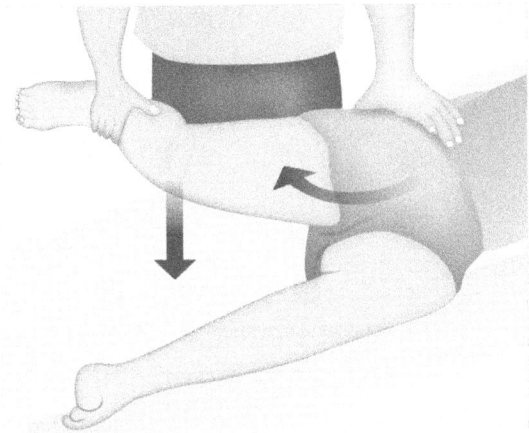

Fig. 3: The Ober's test.

Lateral aspect:
- Lateral collateral ligament (LCL) and meniscal cysts
- Iliotibial band and Gerdy's tubercle
- Ober's test (lateral decubitus position; knee flexion to 90° → hip abduction 40° → hip extension as permitted → gentle hip adduction; tests ITB contracture). Inability to adduct the hip so that the knee touches the couch down indicates a tight ITB **(Fig. 3)**.
- Allis' test (Galeazzi sign)—differentiate femoral and tibial shortening.

Posterior aspect (prone):
- Confirm and measure flexion deformity
- Baker's cyst (most prominent in extension) and other swellings (aneurysm, lymphadenopathy, etc.)
- Craig's test (Ryder method).

Manipulation and Special Tests

Tests for Menisci (Figs. 4A to C)

- *McMurray (MM) test:* Fully-flexed knee; external rotation at hind foot + varus stress → extend knee; LM—internal rotation + valgus; patient feels pain and examiner feels click (uncommon):

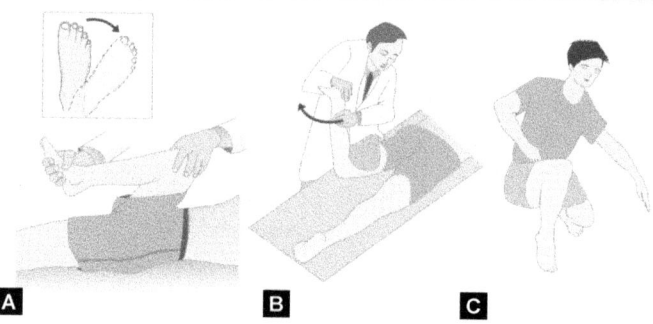

Figs. 4A to C: Tests for meniscal tear/pathology. (A) McMurray test; (B) Apley's test; (C) Childress test.

Pain in initial, middle, and late extension "suggests" involvement of posterior, middle portion, and anterior horn).

- *Apley's distraction/compression test:* Prone patient; stabilize thigh with your knee → pull leg up in 90° flexion → rotate foot internally and externally: Painful → abandon test—no pain → perform in compression; medial joint line pain—MM tear and vice versa.
- *Cabot's maneuver:* Figure of "4" produces lateral joint line pain.
- *Childress' test:* In deep squat walk, patient feels respective joint line pain in fully flexed knee in meniscal tear; retropatellar pain suggests patellofemoral arthritis.
- *Passive extension test* (Bounce home test)—respective joint line tenderness during forced extension of knee after maximal active knee extension.

Tests for Stability (Table 1)

- *Valgus and varus laxity* (**Figs. 5A and B**):
  - Valgus and varus stress test
    - In extension—damage to MCL and posteromedial capsule (valgus stress); LCL and posterolateral ligament complex (varus stress)
    - In 20° flexion—more specific for MCL/LCL.
  - Cabot's position
  - Henri Dejour "frog position"—simultaneous evaluation of both knees lateral structures.

The Knee

- *Anterior laxity:*
  - Lachman test and Trillat modification (*see* details below in case on ACL injury)
  - Anterior drawer test in neutral, internal, and external rotation.
  - Pivot shift test of McIntosh and Galway:
    - Trace pivot shift "pivot glide" of Henri Dejour
    - Dejour's test (pivot shift in extension)

		Table 1: Tests for stability.		
Test	**Method**	**Interpretation**	**Grading**	**Comments**
Lachman test	20–30° flexion: Hold femur with left hand; right hand holds tibia (thumb on tibial tuberosity—"Trillat") (compare) Watch end-point and anterior translation (Gerdy's tubercle/medial condyle)	Soft endpoint: ACL tear Firm with ↑ translation ↑ incomplete tear <2 mm translation + firm endpoint −ve test	In normal knees the difference in anterior translation is <2 mm. If the difference is >10 mm then also consider possible MCL tear. Grade I—"feel" of +ve test. Grade II—visible anterior translation. Grade III—passive subluxation of the tibia with the patient supine. Grade IV—ability of the patient to actively subluxation the proximal tibia	First described by Torg. Sensitivity = 0.86 Specificity = 0.91 Best negative predictive value Overall better test to rule out and rule in ACL tear

Contd...

Practical Orthopedic Examination Made Easy

Contd...

Test	Method	Interpretation	Grading	Comments
Anterior drawer test	90° flexion Hold leg with both hands—thumbs on anterior tibial plateau. Index fingers check hamstrings. Watch anterior translation and endpoint (compare)	Do *External rotation*—↑ anteromedial rotatory instability, ? MCL tear *Internal rotation*—normally decreased translation, ↑–? Significance	<2 mm— insignificant 2–5 mm = nearly N >5 mm* = abnormal	Sensitivity = 0.2 Specificity = 0.88 *Limitations:* <ul><li>Acute injury—painful</li><li>Door stopper effect of menisci</li><li>Hamstring spasm and checkrein effect</li><li>Normal ↑laxity in 90° flexion</li></ul>
Pivot-shift test	Internal rotation of leg + valgus at knee → flex knee. "Pivot" = Gerdy's tubercle "Axis" = PCL	Visible or palpable shift of Gerdy's tubercle (reduction of tibia) posteriorly at around 20–30° flexion	Dynamic test—"NO" grades (you start from a posterior subluxed femur to reduce tibia over femur)	Sensitivity = 0.18–0.48 Specificity = 0.97–0.99 Best positive predictive value *Limitations:* <ul><li>Flexion deformity</li><li>Acute injury</li></ul>

*Ensure PCL is not torn else false increase in translation
(ACL: anterior cruciate ligament; PCL: posterior cruciate ligament; MCL; medial collateral ligament)

- Hughston's jerk test
- Losee test
- Flexion rotation drawer test.
- *Posterior laxity:*
    - Godfrey's sign—posterior tibial sag in 90/90 position

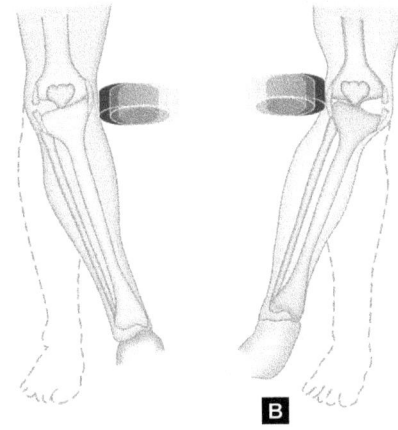

Figs. 5A and B: (A) Varus stress test; (B) Valgus stress test.

- Müller's test
- Posterior drawer test and drop-back phenomenon
- Quadriceps active drawer test of Daniel.
- *Posterolateral instability*:
  - External rotation recurvatum test (varus recurvatum test)
  - External rotation test
  - Reverse pivot shift test.
- *Anterolateral rotatory instability (ALRI)*:
  - Slocum's test.

Measurements

- *Linear measurements*:
  - Apparent length
  - True length
  - Femoral and tibial length
  - Intermalleolar (genu valgum) and distance between two knees (genu varum).
- *Circumferential measurements*:
  - Quadriceps wasting (15 cm from knee joint line; >2 cm is significant).

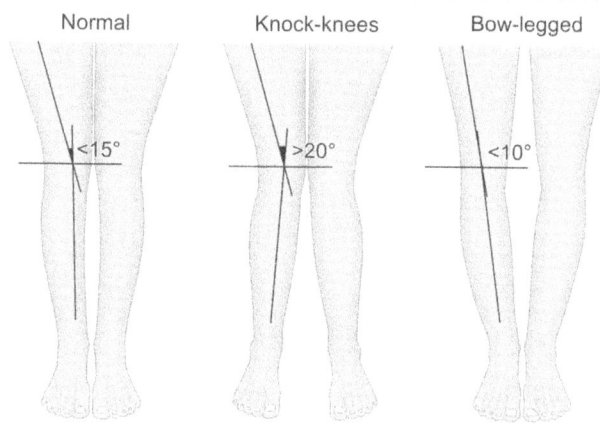

Fig. 6: Q-angle of knee in normal, valgum and varum dispositions.

- *Angular measurements:*
  - Varus and valgus at knee
  - Q-angle **(Fig. 6)**
  - Tuber sulcus angle.
- *Torsional measurements:*
  - Tibial torsion
  - Femoral anteversion.

Neurological and vascular status (At least offer to examine)
- Palpate lower limb pulses (compare)
- Sensory and motor distribution of tibial, common peroneal, and femoral nerves
- Reflexes (knee, ankle, and tibialis posterior).

CASE I: RECURRENT DISLOCATION OF PATELLA

Diagnosis: The patient is a 20-year-old female/male with recurrent/habitual dislocation/subluxation of R/L patella with 5 cm circumferential wasting of thigh muscles. There is increased femoral anteversion/tibial external torsion/patella alta/tight lateral retinaculum.

The Knee

COMMON POSITIVE FINDINGS

History [anterior knee pain especially on climbing stairs or dancing with feeling of instability and fall on maneuvers involving partial knee flexion and rotation like pivoting, dancing, and turning on stairs; sensation of give-way; past recurrent falls; and history of multiple thigh injections in past (for habitual dislocation)]

- *Standing:*
  - Varus/valgus
  - Squinting/frog eye patella
  - Patella alta
  - ↑ pronation of foot
- *Sitting:*
  - Tracking—"J-sign"
  - Lateral tilt (patella tilts down laterally)
- *Supine:*
  - ↑ Q-angle
  - Patellofemoral crepitus and effusion
  - Lateral tibial tubercle (positive Bayonet sign)
  - Hypoplastic femoral condyle
  - Medial patellar or femoral condyle tenderness [especially look for insertion point of medial patellofemoral ligament (MPFL)], retinacular tear also may cause medial tenderness
  - Retropatellar tenderness
  - Quadriceps atrophy (look for cord like band on superolateral aspect indicative of quadriceps contracture in cases of habitual patellar dislocation)
  - Patellar glide (>2 quadrants laterally/or <1 quadrant medially—Sage sign) lateral laxity is positive in MPFL incompetency
  - ↓ Patellar lift
  - Fairbank apprehension test
  - Ober's test (HDP)
  - Ely's test (HDP and quadriceps contracture) *(See Chapter 2; examination points; special tests).*

1. **What do you understand by obligatory dislocation and persistent dislocation of patella?**

Ans. The term obligatory dislocation of patella is similar to habitual dislocation of patella (HDP) where patella dislocates laterally every time the knee flexes (sort of a habit of patella dislocation). Persistent dislocation of patella is one of the subtypes of chronic patellar dislocation where the patella remains in dislocated position always, i.e. even with knee in extension the patella is laterally dislocated (also called permanent patellar dislocation). Persistent/permanent patellar dislocation differs from obligatory in the manner that patella is always dislocated in the former irrespective of knee position while in the latter the patella is placed in trochlea in knee extension while it dislocates with knee flexion.

2. **What is the difference between recurrent and habitual dislocation/subluxation of patella?**

Ans.
- In recurrent dislocation of patella (RDP), there is tendency of patella to dislocate/subluxate (abnormal tracking) making patient "insecure". Patella does not always dislocate/subluxate with flexion. In HDP, patella comes off the joint with every flexion and patient is less bothered (habitual).
- Habitual dislocation of patella is a subgroup of chronic patellar dislocations (other one being permanent). Mostly recurrent dislocation follows traumatic event or is developmental (increased femoral anteversion or external tibial torsion) whereas habitual cases are most often than not due to congenital deficiencies or quadriceps myofibrosis.
- In RDP, flexion occurs to full range without dislocation patella whereas in HDP patellar dislocation is "required" to complete flexion at knee joint so it is an example of "compensatory" pathology to pursue a physiological function.
- Secondary deformation of tibia (external torsion and valgus at knee) may develop in habitual dislocation of patella due to tight ITB/quadriceps contracture while these are predisposing factors for RDP. Fixed extension contracture of knee may be a finding at birth in HDP.
- Recurrent dislocation/subluxation cases report to hospital (that is why kept in examination) usually during

The Knee

adolescence while many habitual cases present either during first decade or not at all till late (neglected—remember they take it as a habit!).

3. What factors may lead to recurrent patellar dislocation?
Ans.
- *Bony*: Patella alta, patella breva, trochlear dysplasia (shallow trochlea), genu valgum, genu recurvatum, hypoplastic femoral condyle, external tibial torsion, and increased femoral anteversion. Many of these conditions increase Q-angle (tibial extortion, femoral intorsion, genu valgum, laterally placed tibial tuberosity, contracted lateral retinaculum, and coxa vara).
- *Soft tissue*: Vastus medialis obliquus hypoplasia, vastus lateralis hypertrophy, lax medial retinaculum, tight lateral retinaculum, deficient medial patellofemoral ligament, and hypermobility syndrome.
- *HDP (Please see Case III)*: Quadriceps contracture (multiple intramuscular injections), hypoplasia of patella, femoral dysplasia/hypoplasia, and ITB contracture.

4. What are the restraints for patella?
Ans.
- *Static*: Shape of patella, trochlea, retinaculum, patello-femoral distance, medial capsule, patella-femoral and patella-tibial ligaments. Medial patellofemoral ligament (MPFL) has an important role in stabilizing patella and contributes to 60% stability of the articulation. Injury to this ligament along with medial capsule is responsible for most of the cases of recurrent dislocation of patella. Competency of MPFL is what is commonly assessed by glide test.
- *Dynamic*: Vastus medialis obliquus (pulling patella medially at 50–55°).

5. How do you measure tibial torsion clinically?
Ans. Clinical assessment of tibial torsion can be done by thigh-foot angle test **(Fig. 7)**. Here the patient lies prone and knee is bent to 90°. The angle made by the axis of foot to thigh gives idea of tibial torsion. Normally, this is 8–10°, angle more than 30° indicate increased tibial torsion. Tibial torsion can also

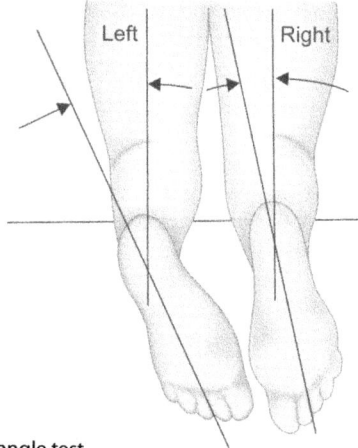

Fig. 7: Thigh-foot angle test.

be measured by dropping a plumb line with patient seated and comparing from other side.

6. What is Q-angle?

Ans. Q-angle (short for quadriceps angle) represents the mean vector angle of quadriceps pull on patella. It represents the dynamic "instability" of patella—the greater it is the more unstable patella will be! **(Fig. 8)**. First described by Brattstrom, it is clinically measured by intersection of lines formed between center of patella and anterosuperior iliac spine (ASIS) and that between patellar center and tibial tuberosity (*in standing position*). Prerequisites are that patella should be centered in trochlea otherwise in an already dislocated patella angle will be falsely reduced (so measure it in 15-20° flexion of knee with relocated patella). Various factors outlined in Q2 can cause ↑ Q-angle. N values (supine) 8–10° in males and 15°±5° in females while in standing 14° for males and 17° for females is normal. Q-angle >8° in sitting position is abnormal. To remove the effect of femoral rotation tubercle sulcus angle can be measured. In sitting position with knees flexed 90° intersection of line joining tibial tuberosity and center of patella and perpendicular to patellar center gives tubercle

The Knee

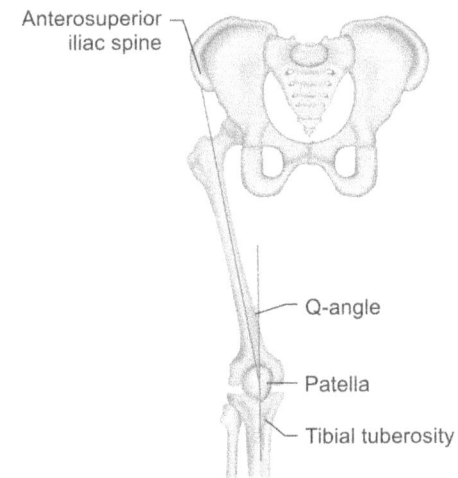

Fig. 8: The Q-angle.

sulcus angle. N is <5° in males and <8° in females. An increase in this angle also signifies lateral shift of tibial tuberosity.

Increased Q-angle leads to patellar subluxation, chondromalacia patellae, and excessive foot pronation.

7. What is J-sign?

Ans. J-sign denotes one of the forms of abnormal dynamic patellar tracking (maltracking) **(Fig. 9)**. Normally patella glides in a straight line with minimal sideways shift at the end of extension in the trochlear groove, however, due to various reasons (see above) patella may have excessive lateral shift (sort of subtle lateral subluxation) at the end describing an inverted "J" trajectory. Other forms of maltracking include subluxation (positive congruence angle even after 10° of flexion, tilt (tilt angle < 80°) and combination of above. Dynamic patellar tracking is judged in sitting position while patient extends knee from 90° flexion to full extension as above. Active patellar tracking is checked in full extension asking the patient to contract quadriceps and observing patellar shift which should be more superior than lateral.

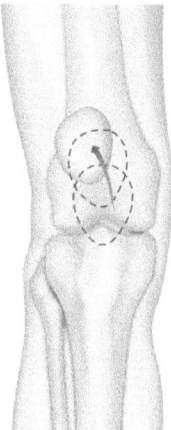

Fig. 9: The J-sign.

8. Can you classify patellar instability?
Ans. Yes, it is based on two factors: (1) Patella alta—Insall-Salvati index < 1.3 and (2) Generalized joint laxity.
- *Grade I:* (1) and (2) absent
- *Grade II:* (1) absent; (2) present
- *Grade III:* (1) present; (2) absent
- *Grade IV:* (1) and (2) present.

9. Now after clinical assessment what will you do and why?
Ans. I would like to get roentgenograms of involved and normal knees in anteroposterior (AP), lateral, and axial (infrapatellar/axial/skyline—like Merchant's view) views and MRI scan for associated soft-tissue injuries. AP view may show osteochondral fragment and loose bodies.

Axial view demonstrates:
- Tilt angle (angle between lateral patellar facet and femoral condyle—always open laterally minimum 8°)
- Congruence angle ($N = 6°$) **(Fig. 10)**.

Lateral view demonstrates:
- Trochlear flatness ("Y" sign or "crossing" sign where trochlear and lateral condylar shadow merge, N = parallel)

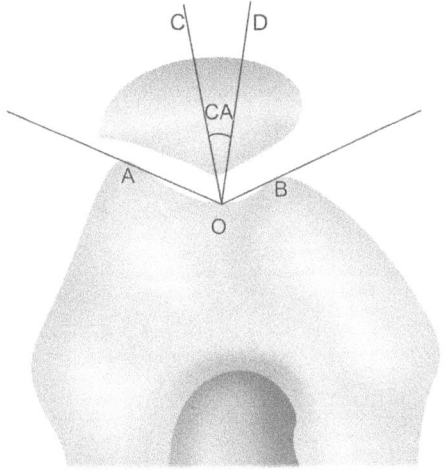

Fig. 10: Congruence angle (CA) as a measure of trochlear depth.

- Trochlear convexity ("X" sign—lines cross)
- Patellar height.

MRI scan demonstrates capsular injury, MPFL injury, osteochondral injury, and free fragments in the knee. Other associated meniscal or ligament injury can also be identified/documented for further management.

10. How do you access patellar height?

Ans. *On lateral X-ray plate:*
- *Insall-Salvati ratio:* Diagonal patellar length/patellar tendon length **(Fig. 11)**.
- *Modified Insall-Salvati ratio:* Articular patellar length/distance from articular surface to tibial tuberosity.
- *Blackburne-Peel ratio:* Articular patellar length/distance from articular surface to tangent from tibial plateau.
- *Blumensaat line:* In 30° knee flexion, line extending from intercondylar notch should touch lower pole of patella. Patella above this line—alta and below—baja is considered nonreproducible by many.

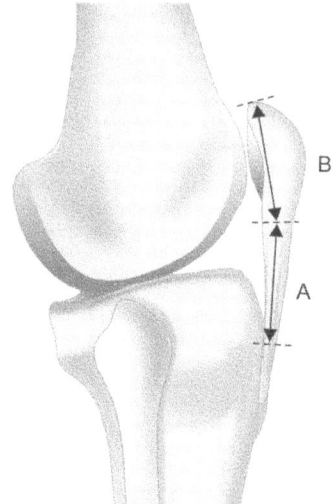

Fig. 11: Insall-Salvati ratio = A/B.

11. How will you manage acute injury?
Ans. *In acute stage*:
- PRICE (pain control, rest, ice, compression, elevation)
- In addition TENS.

In repair phase:
- Restore range of motion (ROM), neuromuscular control, muscular strength, and muscular endurance.

In maturation phase:
- Functional progression back to activity
- US, massage, joint mobilization, and fascial stretching.

12. How will you manage this case?
Ans. The answer should be based upon assessment of:
- Q-angle and Insall-Salvati ratio
- Skeletal maturity and activity level (athlete)
- Presence of associated pathology such as osteochondral fracture, chondromalacia, and MPFL insufficiency.

The Knee

In general the simplest procedure that achieves realignment and patellar stability should be done.

- Recurrent subluxation, normal Q-angle, tight lateral structures—lateral retinacular release (arthroscopic or open)
- Above + medial laxity—Insall medial imbrication, Madigan
- Above but Q-angle > 20°—Roux-Goldthwait/Galeazzi (skeletally immature); Elmslie-Trillat (skeletally mature)
- Above + distal malalignment—Hughston and modified Elmslie-Trillat
- Athlete requiring rapid resumption of activity—repair MPFL and vastus medialis in addition to lateral release
- MPFL injury and insufficiency—MPFL reconstruction
- Patient with chondromalacia—Fulkerson type osteotomy
- Insall-Salvati ratio > 1.2—Simmons procedure
- Skeletally immature patient—3-in-1 procedure [medial imbrication, lateral release + patellar tendon hemitransfer (transfer of medial 1/3rd of patellar tendon to medial collateral ligament), especially if Q-angle is increased or the tibial tubercle-trochlear groove (TT-TG) distance is raised].

13. What is "critical angle"?

Ans. It is the angle of knee flexion at which patella dislocates laterally. Lower the critical angle, severe is the bony restraint deficiency or contracture of soft tissues or both.

14. Why do you see wasting in RDP?

Ans. Quadriceps inhibition.

CASE II: ANGULAR DEFORMITY OF KNEE (GENU VARUM AND GENU VALGUM)

Diagnosis: The patient is a 16-year-old male/female with 17° genu varum/valgum deformity of R/L/both knee(s) most probably secondary to *"etiology"* (idiopathic/rickets/epiphyseal dysplasia/trauma/tumor/infection, etc.). There is increased femoral anteversion (genu varum) with 2 cm lengthening/shortening and 4 cm wasting of quadriceps muscle.

COMMON FINDINGS

Standing:
- Genu varum/valgum **(Figs. 12 and 13)**
- External (valgum)/internal (in toeing) rotation of foot
- Patella subluxation/dislocation (lateral in valgum)
- Flat feet (valgum).

Gait:
- Abnormal foot progression angle
- Varus/valgus thrust gait
- *Stigmata of associated disease:*
  - Rickets
  - Dysplasia (acral shortening)
  - Cerebral palsy
  - Ligamentous laxity.

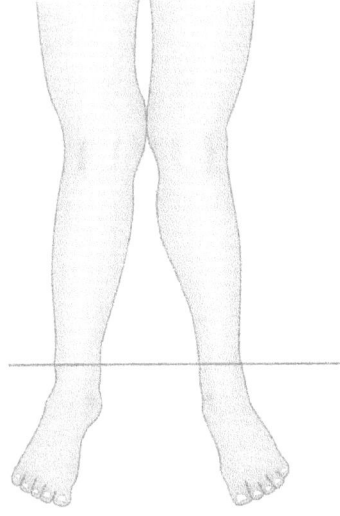

Fig. 12: Genu valgum.

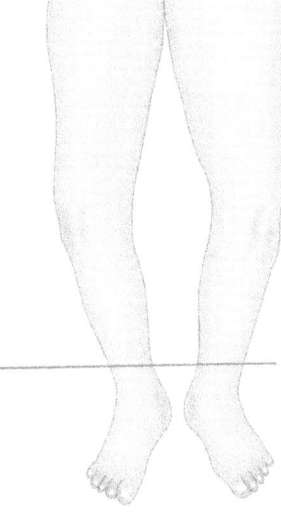

Fig. 13: Genu varum.

The Knee

Supine:
- Increased hip external rotation in extension and tibial intorsion (varum)—measure thigh-foot angle. (For demonstration of deformities in supine position, *remember* to rotate the limb so that patella faces ceiling. This unmasks various torsional deformities of bones and reveals true joint deformities and malalignment.)
- Ober's test.

1. How do you define genu varum/valgum?

Ans. These are angular deformities (coronal malalignment) of lower limb; some centers include it under orthopedic cosmetology. Valgum (knock-knees) or varum (bow-legs) refer specifically to abnormal coronal "alignment" in which the leg is shifted away from midline (valgum-medial angulation) or towards it (varum-lateral angulation). In a normal person standing with heels/knees touching each other, ASIS, center of patella, center of malleoli, and second toe/web are in a straight line, deviation of this line to inside of knee is varus at knee and vice versa. Up to 1 cm separation can be allowed for soft tissue in obese patients.

2. How do you measure these?

Ans. Measured in standing position. Two methods:
1. *Femorotibial alignment*: Angle formed between lines joining ASIS to center of patella and line joining center of intermalleolar line to center of patella. Subtract normal valgus from the measured alignment (7° for males, 8° for females > 7 years) for a valgus malalignment and add the same for varus. Varum or valgum is said to exist if the angle is outside two standard deviations from the normal for males and females for that age.
2. Measure the intermalleolar distance in centimeters (normal < 10 cm) using measuring tape for valgus, and distance between two knees for varus (normal < 8 cm) **(Fig. 14)**. It can also be expressed in "finger-breadth" albeit crudely. For unilateral deformities, measure from midline (plumb line from nape of neck).

The first method is more specific and reproducible; however, it is limited by age factor and charts are not readily available. Second method although crude but

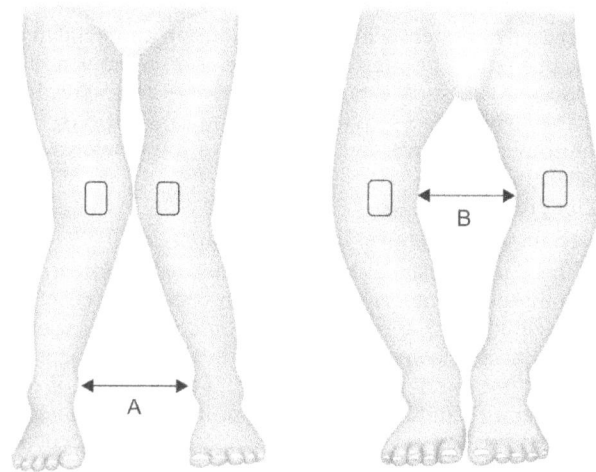

Fig. 14: Measuring (A) intermalleolar and (B) intercondylar distances.

can be readily pursued to judge the progression of deformity. Also distance in centimeters is not absolute for all—same distance is much more significant for a short statured person.

3. What else will you look for?

Ans. I will also look for ligamentous laxity. If the deformity significantly increases on weight bearing (standing) compared to that evident on supine examination then ligamentous laxity is present. I will also look for signs of generalized ligamentous laxity (*See Chapter 5—Case on unstable shoulder for criteria and Beighton score*).

4. OK your cases did not have generalized ligamentous laxity, but do you know of any tight structure that can produce angular deformity at knee?

Ans. Yes, iliotibial band contracture can produce genu valgum similarly contracture of quadriceps can cause genu valgum while gracilis contracture can cause genu varum. I tested for tight iliotibial band by Ober's test and gracilis contracture by Phelps test.

The Knee

5. What are the causes of unilateral and bilateral deformity?

Ans. *Unilateral angular deformity of knee occurs in:*
- Post-traumatic—fracture of tibial/femoral condyle with subsidence, injury to physis causing growth disturbance from intraphyseal tethering or physeal damage
- Infective—damage to hemiphysis (causes deformity in same direction so lateral physeal damage will create genu valgum), hyperemic overgrowth of contralateral side of physis
- Neoplastic—exostosis by itself or its management causing physeal injury, chondroblastoma affecting the physis
- Idiopathic.

Bilateral deformity develops in:
- Idiopathic—this is the most common cause of bilateral deformities
- Physiological—see below
- Metabolic—rickets
- Congenital and syndromic—epiphyseal dysplasias, osteogenesis imperfecta, and Paget's disease
- Inflammatory—rheumatoid arthritis—genu valgum and osteoarthrosis—genu varum
- Paralytic disorders—postpolio residual paralysis and Charcot's disease.

6. How do you differentiate if the deformity is in femur or tibia?

Ans. Supine position in a relaxed patient, flex the knee fully (heel touching ischial tuberosity is normal alignment):
- If the deformity disappears altogether, then it should have been in femur
- If it persists it should be tibial
- If it is partially corrected then it could be in both.

This is because the nonweight-bearing posterior femoral condyles are usually relatively spared (Hueter-Volkmann law) of deformity (unless it is epiphyseal/metaphyseal dysplasia/trauma, etc.). In full flexion, the tibia is in articulation with posterior femoral condyles; if the deformity is tibial it persists; however, if femoral it corrects. There is usually only a partial correction in dysplasia. Patient can also be made to squat to demonstrate this. This method is usually applicable for metabolic and some developmental causes only. Ideally it should be assessed radiologically. Usually the deformity is in femur in genu valgum while the deformity is in tibia in genu varum.

7. What is physiological malalignment?

Ans. Child is born with genu varum (physiologic) which due to persistence of tight posterior capsule of hip (external rotation) and internal tibial torsion. This overcorrects to physiologic valgus by 24–36 months of ambulation. Valgus should correct to adult levels by 7 years of age. In females, the valgus sometimes keeps correcting up to 16 years also. So varus should be pathological after 2–3 years of age and valgus after 11 years of age (>2 SD of normal physiologic alignment). [*Heath CH, Staheli LT. Normal limits of knee angle in white children—genu varum and genu valgum. J Pediatr Orthop. 1993;13(2):259-62.*]

8. What are the signs of rickets?

Ans.
- *Infant rickets symptoms:*
  - Deformed skulls
  - Late-closing fontanels
  - Rib-breastbone joint enlargement
  - Delayed milestones
- Knobby enlargements on the ends of bones
- Distorting pelvis under weight
- Spinal curvature
- Restlessness
- Lack of sleep
- Retarded growth
- Mental retardation
- Thin top of skull (craniotabes)
- Thin back of skull
- Bossing (frontal bossing)
- Harrison's groove
- Beading where rib joins cartilage (rachitic rosary)
- Bowed legs
- Knock-knees

The Knee

- Weak muscles (floppy-baby syndrome and rickety myopathy)
- Pot belly and widening of perineum
- Deformed chest (pigeon chest)
- Weak ribs
- Abnormal teeth development
- Tooth decay
- Fragile bones if untreated
- Fractures if untreated (especially greenstick fractures)
- Double malleoli sign
- Windswept deformity (tackle deformity)
- Tetany spasms.

9. What would you do next?

Ans. I would like to get an anteroposterior and lateral views of both lower limbs fully including femur and tibia in standing position. If not possible then I will get orthoscanogram/computed scanogram of both lower limbs. [*Remember for genu varum radiographs are indicated only if child is short (dwarfism), asymmetric deformity, age > 3 years, and progressive deformity*].

10. What do you see on X-rays?

Ans. *Look for:*
- Confirmation of diagnosis
- Site of disease
- Degree of malalignment (magnitude in degrees—tibiofemoral angle, mechanical axis, and metaphyseal-diaphyseal angle for differentiating *tibia vara* from genu varum > 16° = tibia vara)
- Associated disorders and assessment of physes
  - *Signs of rickets:*
    - Rarefaction of the provisional zones of calcification
    - Irregularly frayed and cupping metaphysis
    - Deepened physes and rarefaction of the margins of the epiphyses
    - Diffuse rarefaction of the shafts with thinning of the cortex and coarsened texture
    - In healing rickets—zones of provisional calcification become denser than the diaphysis.

11. What would you do to confirm the location of disease "or" what if the malalignment is not very clear on X-ray?

Ans. Measure CORA (center of rotation of angulation)

This reveals:
- Site "apex" of deformity (femoral/tibial/metaphyseal/disphyseal sometimes at joint line)
- Number of deformity in complex deformities/both femoral and tibial involvement
- Magnitude
- Planning guide
- Reveals additional deformities like bowing of bones and torsional deformities.

12. How will you manage this case?

Ans. Reply only after considering age, deformity magnitude and deformity site, and activity of underlying disease process.
- *Age*: In general *varus* malalignment should be corrected ASA underlying disease is settled because varus would not correct itself with age and is deemed as a progressive deformity. Bracing for genu varum is not favored but for tibia vara as special case bracing can be undertaken for children ≤3 years, Langenskiöld grade up to II (? III), medial physeal slope < 50°, and metaphyseal-diaphyseal angle between 10° and 15° [surgical treatment is indicated for grade ≥ III, failure of orthotic management (up to 1 year), medial physeal angle > 60°, obese child, female gender, and late-onset tibia vara]. Genu *valgum >15° in female >11 years and male >12 years should be corrected.* Osteotomy for genu valgum is indicated by some at age >12 years female and >14 years for male. (*Note: The females mature early for skeletal age. This is partly in controversy to the finding that genu valgum may correct in them till 16 years of age (see above), but I am afraid, that is the way it is!*) (*Another query needs to be addressed—What is 2 SD from normal. It is 5° but varies regionally. This means 7 or 8 + 5 = 12 or 13, but the guidelines of 15° takes into account the error during measurement and the gray zone of regional differences so that unnecessary surgeries are avoided.*)

The Knee

- Take into account the *growth spurts left* for the patient as deformity progresses rapidly during growth spurts. If patient can wait, then do it after both growth spurts are crossed. However, if deformity is severe and disabling or progressing rapidly then correction may be undertaken after explaining the parents and patient appropriately.
- *Deformity site*: Better assessed by CORA—do intervention ideally at the site "apex" revealed by CORA.
- *Deformity magnitude*: Severe deformities put limb at risk of shortening (closed osteotomy) and neurovascular damage (open osteotomy). Usually up to 25° of (mild) deformity correction is successfully accepted [≈2.5 cm shortening (closed) or 2.5 cm excursion for neurovascular bundle (open)]. More severe deformities (*moderate*: 25–40° and *severe*: >40°) can be treated by staged surgery or simultaneous femoral and tibial compensatory osteotomies (viz. open lateral femoral and closed medial tibial for genu valgum)/Ilizarov method.
- *Underlying disease*: If active, (viz. rickets) then first treat the disease then only operate as if done in active disease the intervention may fail (nonunion) or the deformity may recur.

The stages of healing rickets and their impacts:

1. *Acute stage:* The normal rounded physis is replaced by cloudy area with indistinct center(s) of ossification. Metaphysis is splayed and periosteum may be thickened.
2. *Second stage:* Mottled, irregular epiphysis; broader and ragged metaphysis; and periosteal thickening disappears.
3. *Third stage:* Epiphyseal shadow is denser and regular in outline and a dense line appears at the metaphysis due to deposition of calcium.
4. *Fourth stage:* Clearly defined bone and normal calcium content. Metaphysis may still be broadened.

    Any osteotomy or surgical procedure must *not* be done before *stage three* has appeared.

13. What are the advantages and disadvantages of your method?

Ans. Often the answer rests finally on open/closed wedge osteotomies **(Fig. 15)**. "Usually" but not always (you can

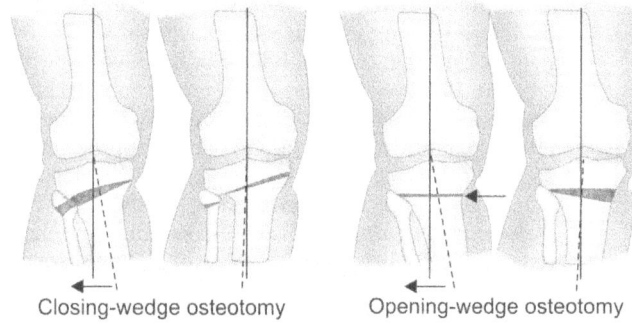

Fig. 15: Closing-wedge and opening-wedge osteotomy for genu varum.

always defend your answer—till you remain logical of course) it is deemed better to do a lateral procedure in femur and medial on tibial side (*remember to mention partial fibulectomy with your chosen open/closed tibial osteotomy*).

Opening-wedge osteotomy:
Advantages:
- Avoids shortening and hence a second procedure to correct limb lengths.
- Open lateral femoral osteotomy avoids vascular complications associated with closed medial femoral osteotomy for genu valgum.
- Open medial tibial osteotomy for genu varum averts the possible neurological complications of lateral closed osteotomy of tibia.

Disadvantages:
- Need for graft with associated complications like nonunion, graft displacement, and graft site morbidity.
- Need for fixation to hold the osteotomy in desired position and maintain correction.
- Collapse of graft and losing correction.
- Stretching neurovascular bundle and morbidity.
- Delayed weight bearing.

The Knee

Closing-wedge osteotomy:
Advantages (apart from above):
- Periosteal splint at apex of osteotomy is a good stabilizer.
- Compression of osteotomy site with weight bearing.

Disadvantages:
- Shortening
- Medial femoral closing-wedge osteotomy needs careful protection of vessels
- Visualization and fixation of lateral tibial closing-wedge osteotomy is hindered by fibula and also requires protection of common peroneal nerve.

14. What precaution will you take before performing osteotomy and how will you fix your osteotomy?

Ans. Apart from taking into consideration as above, I will first perform derotation (as decided by intorsion or extorsion) and then decide the amount of wedge required for removal as derotation frequently reduces the amount of wedge required grossly. Plate and screw (DCP, LCDCP, LCP, condylar blade plate, DCS, and L-plate), Puddu plate (has metallic wedges of varying sizes to hold osteotomy and prevent collapse—open osteotomy), thick K-wires, crossed Steinmann pins and POP cast, external fixator, and POP cast only. *(I am not sarcastic but please choose your option.)*

15. What other osteotomies you know of and what are the complications?

Ans. Dome osteotomy **(Fig. 16)** (Barrel-Vault osteotomy—additional rotational component can be corrected, avoid bump at the site of osteotomy, and minimal alteration of true limb length), oblique osteotomy, proximal tibial osteotomy with physeal resection (tibia vara), intraepiphyseal osteotomy and elevation of medial tibial articular surface (tibia vara), and progressive lateral opening osteotomy (genu valgum). Complications apart from above include infection, implant failure, nonunion, loss of reduction, recurrence, chronic pain, and compartment syndrome (prevent by doing simultaneous fasciotomy of anterior compartment).

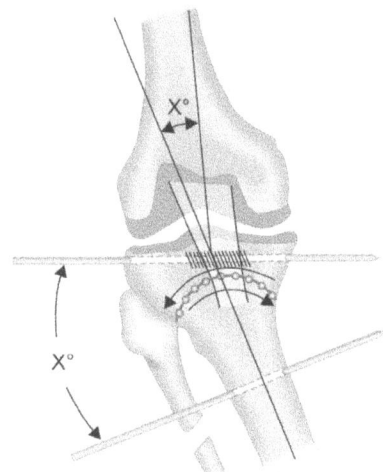

Fig. 16: Dome osteotomy—the cut is made in dome fashion and distal part is rotated to align the limb.

16. **Are there methods other than osteotomy?**
Ans. Yes, hemiepiphysiodesis, hemiphyseal stapling, Ilizarov ring fixation system "corticotomy" and gradual correction, and callotasis (that may be done with an external fixator).

17. **What are the disadvantages of hemiepiphysiodesis/hemiepiphyseal stapling?**
Ans. Hemiepiphysiodesis is a permanent method whereas hemiepiphyseal stapling is a temporary measure. First of all, it is not a corrective method rather it is a compensatory measure controlling the physiologically normal side! Disadvantages are complete arrest and hence production of opposite deformity, asymmetric physeal arrest producing complicated deformities, breakage/extrusion and joint penetration of staples, overlying bursitis, and second surgery for removal. They are suitable in only a small group of patients (in a narrow age group range and mild-to-moderate deformity up to 15°). It can be done only in patients in whom growth potential exists and may have to be repeated or followed with

The Knee

other procedures (for under correction/overcorrection due to unexpected physeal fusion). Results and correction are unpredictable; also there is risk of compensatory overgrowth and recurrence of deformity after removal of staples. Stapling is more often indicated in genu valgum as there are infrequent; if at all any associated rotational deformities of bones.

18. How much correction do you aim to achieve?

Ans. A tricky question! Ideal is to correct exactly the amount of deformity as has been measured which should be true for "all static" deformities. However, it is nice to understand that no amount of varus is acceptable at knee whereas to err on side of added valgus can be accepted unless the patient is obese where knees may rub each other during walk and will be unacceptable (remember, deformities anywhere in body in the direction of physiologic bow/angulation can be accepted and remodeling is possible). Further for progressive deformity like *tibia vara* where physeal defect can somewhat be countered by valgus, "overcorrection" ($\approx 5°$) should be done, this also holds true for stapling. In general otherwise, undercorrection of deformities is commonly practiced as any overcorrection (so called "malcorrection") will get magnified as the child grows, whereas magnification in the direction of original deformity is less disheartening to patient and parents and can be recorrected.

19. What is pseudo valgum and varum?

Ans. Excessive femoral anteversion and compensatory tibial extorsion produces appearance of genu valgum. Femoral anteversion only or with tight posterior hip capsule without tibial compensation appears like genu varum in supine position.

20. What is hemichondrodiastasis?

Ans. Asymmetrical physeal lengthening ("distraction") by fixator to correct angular deformities.

21. What deformity(ies) does iliotibial band contracture produce?

Ans. Early in the course tight ITB produces hip abduction deformity causing apparent lengthening, but later true shortening is the rule.

- *At lumbar spine:* Ipsilateral lumbar scoliosis and increased lumbar lordosis
- *At pelvis:* Pelvic obliquity due to abduction contracture
- *At hip:* Flexion, abduction, external rotation (FABER)
- *At knee:* Genu valgum and knee flexion contracture
- *At leg:* External tibial torsion with or without knee subluxation
- *At Ankle and foot* (Secondary deformities): Talipes equinovarus and heel varus
- *Whole leg:* Shortening (true), initially there may be apparent lengthening due to abduction contracture at hip and pelvic obliquity.

22. What is Blount's disease?

Ans. This is a physeal growth abnormality of the posteromedial proximal growth plate of tibia that fails to grow due to various portended reasons. Abnormal growth (lack of it) causes tibia vara (not genu varum) radiologically characterized by beak-shaped metaphysis and medially flattened epiphysis.

CASE III: QUADRICEPS CONTRACTURE

Diagnosis: The patient is a 7-year-old male/female with quadriceps contracture of R/L side with restricted flexion, patella alta, and patellar hypoplasia. There is associated subluxation of the knee (anterior) and habitual subluxation of patella. Patient is unable/able to perform activities of daily living.

(*Note:* Arguments may be raised to present it as a case of habitual dislocation of patella, but remember that habitual dislocation of patella is "secondary" to primary quadriceps contracture—*ask from history if patellar subluxation developed later.*)

COMMON FINDINGS

Presents in one of these forms (at birth—stiff extended knee, congenital recurvatum, congenital dislocation; as toddlers—progressive painless loss of flexion at knee; later childhood—habitual dislocation of patella; and in adults as painful knee due to habitual patellar dislocation and arthritis). In acquired form there is history of multiple injections in thigh muscle with later development of gradual progressive painless loss of knee flexion and inability to squat/sit cross-legged.

Standing

- Genu recurvatum
- ↑ Lumbar lordosis, flexion at hip (to relax rectus)
- Posterior knee (femoral condylar) prominence (knee subluxation)
- Lateral patellar subluxation
- Patellar hypoplasia and patella alta
- Reduced knee creases
- Scars of previous surgery/injections
- Wasting.

Gait

- Stiff knee gait
- Walk with internal rotation of leg
- Valgus thrust gait.

Sitting

- Dimple over thigh (tethering of quadriceps)
- Lateral position of tibial tuberosity and Bayonet sign.

Supine

- ↓ Knee flexion
- Habitual dislocation of patella
- Ober's test
- Positive Ely's test (prone).

1. What are the causes of muscle contracture formation?

Ans. The causes of muscle contractures can be divided into:
- Idiopathic (congenital or birth related like in torticollis)
- Ischemic—ischemic myositis and fibrous degeneration as in VIC
- Traumatic—post-traumatic myositis and ectopic ossification
- Infective as in osteomyelitis with tethering of muscle to bone
- Postsurgical—scarring/muscle engulfment in callus

- Injection related—injections of irritative drugs that cause exquisite tissue reaction may induce fibrosis causing fibrosis.

2. What is the most common cause of quadriceps contracture?

Ans. In children and adolescents acquired form due to multiple injections (antibiotics, tetanus antiserum, etc.) in quadriceps is the most common cause. Other causes are infusions into thigh, idiopathic (congenital), surgical (e.g. plating for fracture femur), fracture femur causing malunion/tethering of muscle, infection (osteomyelitis in which muscle has adhered to bone), and myonecrosis (postmyositis). In adult, postsurgical intervention is the most common cause. It is a "progressive" disease in children with ongoing fibrosis, especially idiopathic forms. The muscle most commonly affected is vastus lateralis (in postinjection cases; idiopathic/congenital form—intermedius). Vastus medialis is least involved. The congenital form arises out of still elusive pathology and is deemed to resemble sternocleidomastoid tumor of torticollis, contracture akin to those in clubfoot and Sprengel shoulder, localized arthrogryposis congenita, and Seddon's ellipsoidal infarct of VIC (however, this has distinct etiopathology and pathogenesis). Natarajan (Kini Memorial Oration, 1968) showed that vastus intermedius inherently has a precarious blood supply and additional infusions/injection into it may further jeopardize the vascularity and hence induce fibrosis due to injury.

3. How will you differentiate contracture of vastus lateralis/intermedius from rectus femoris?

Ans. In both the former there is limitation of knee flexion range of motion, however, in rectus femoris contracture there is additional positive Ely's test and concomitant flexion at hip. It should be noted, however, that combined contractures are difficult to assess.

- *Vastus intermedius only:* ↓ knee flexion + genu recurvatum and hyperextension
- *Vastus lateralis only:* 1 + genu valgum and lateral patellar subluxation
- *Rectus femoris only:* 1 + positive Ely's test + hip flexion

The Knee

- *Combined:* 1 + 2 + 3 + quadriceps wasting (vasti) and cord like tightened rectus on flexion
- *Gracilis contracture (uncommon):* Positive Phelps test.

4. Why do you give your diagnosis as quadriceps contracture and why is this not habitual dislocation of patella?

Ans. The habitual dislocation of patella is a consequence of progressive contracture of quadriceps muscle. So primary pathology is quadriceps contracture that produces knee stiffness, genu recurvatum, and habitual patellar dislocation where conspicuous dislocation of patella is a part of natural history of disease of quadriceps contracture.

5. What are your differentials?

Ans. I will suggest following differential diagnoses:
- *Chronic dislocation of patella* [permanent (congenital) type—stiffness never precedes dislocation, presents at birth, permanent and irreducible, and "flexion" contracture]
- Genetic and syndromic—Larsen syndrome, Down syndrome, arthrogryposis multiplex congenita (AMC), Nail-patella syndrome, Rubinstein–Tyabi, and Ellis–Van Creveld syndrome and diastrophic dysplasia, patellar aplasia/hypoplasia
- *Arthrogryposis multiplex congenita*
- *Congenital dislocation of knee* [present at birth, hereditary, more in females (3 times), one-third bilateral, round condyles, absent suprapatellar pouch, absent or hypoplastic cruciates, quadriceps contracture—acquired, hamstrings, and ITB—subluxed anterior, associated abnormalities common: developmental dysplasia of the hip (DDH), congenital talipes equinovarus (CTEV), AMC, Larsen, cleft lip and palette, imperforate anus, etc.]
- Patellar aplasia
- Congenital genu recurvatum
- Postpolio residual paralysis
- Congenital quadriceps hypoplasia (localized muscle dysplasia of unknown origin).

6. Where else can you find similar affections?

Ans. Postinjection contracture of deltoid (Shanmugasundaram) and gluteus maximus extension contracture of hip.

7. What will you do next?

Ans. I will get AP and lateral views of knee along with AP view of pelvis and femur are required. I will access and look for primary pathology (?infection and fracture) and secondary developments in joint [viz. patellar displacement (alta), patellar hypoplasia, genu recurvatum, fragmentation of superior/inferior pole of patella, flattening of femoral condyles, anterior tibial subluxation/dislocation on femur, and degeneration of knee joint and arthritic changes].

8. How do you plan surgery?

Ans. Factors to consider (Thompson):
- Whether rectus femoris is also involved
- How well can this muscle be isolated during surgery?
- How well can the muscle be developed after surgery? Aim for at least 0–90° of flexion ROM (critical arc) at knee joint.

Options:
- *Only rectus femoris involved:* Sasaki type rectus release.
- *Early stage with no joint changes:* Only proximal quadriceps release (Sengupta)—this procedure is indicated in early contractures without bony involvement. There is less postoperative morbidity and extensor lag and minimal or no incidence of knee hemarthrosis.
- *More extensive involvement:* Thompson/Payr type quadricepsplasty*—the success of procedure depends on rectus femoris sparing, if this muscle is spared or can be well dissected from scar then Thompson's procedure achieves desired outcome. Also, one should be diligent in postoperative stretching and functional rehabilitation of rectus to maximize good outcome.
- *Genu recurvatum:* Supracondylar femoral osteotomy
- *Arthritis and extensive involvement:* Arthrodesis.

9. What precautions will you take perioperatively?

Ans. Explain to the parents for sure that there would be some degrees of extensor lag following quadricepsplasty that may, however, resolve later (hence proximal release was devised).

---

*Simultaneous patellectomy is indicated if the deep surface of patella is grossly involved.

During surgery, obtain as much hemostasis as possible to avoid recontracture and hemarthrosis. Immobilization should be done in flexion [90° (Sengupta), 50° less than that obtained on table (Thompson)] for 2–3 days followed quickly by continuous passive motion.

10. What is the pathology you try to address during surgery?

Ans. Commonly there is fibrosis of the vastus intermedius (idiopathic) or lateralis (injection associated) that causes muscle shortening. The rectus femoris is commonly spared but it may get tethered to femur in suprapatellar pouch region in later cases. Vastus lateralis fibrosis may also be associated with contracture of extensor expansion and its adherence to the femoral condyles causing stiffness of the knee and lateral patellar subluxation. In late cases, shortening of the rectus femoris may develop along with intra-articular adhesions and fibrosis of patellofemoral joint. All these need to be addressed depending on the stage and individual case.

11. How will you manage habitual dislocation of patella?

Ans. Habitual dislocation of patella (HDP) conceptually differs from RDP. Managing HDP on lines of RDP will aggravate the disease. In HDP, restricted flexion is hardly seen and hence is quietly accepted by patient. In early cases, management of quadriceps contracture with/without medial retinacular plication and sartorius reinforcement may give success otherwise in late cases with patellofemoral arthritis patellectomy and reconstruction of extensor mechanism may be undertaken. Restricting patella from dislocating prevents flexion also from occurring *(See Chapter 3; Case I: Recurrent dislocation of patella).*

CASE IV: EXOSTOSIS (OSTEOCHONDROMA ICD 10: C40-C41; ICD-O: 9210/0)

Diagnosis: The patient is a 14-year-old male with 4 × 3 cm pedunculated swelling over distal femur on medial aspect possibly solitary exostosis (if multiple then rephrase sentence with multiple

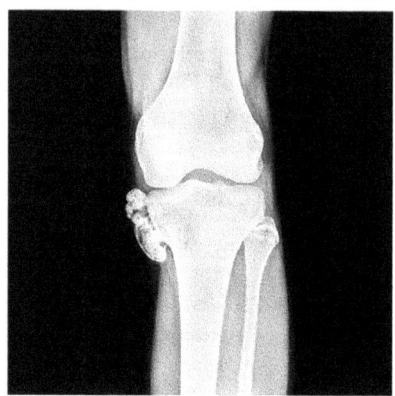

Fig. 17: Solitary exostosis.

exostoses and do not use the term "possibly") **(Fig. 17)**. There is true shortening of 2 cm and genu valgum/varum (multiple forms).

COMMON FINDINGS

Inspection

- Lump in metaphyseal region of bones
- Joint deformity
- Patellar subluxation
- Associated swellings
- Shortening.

Palpation

- Nontender bony hard spherical/ovoid lump 4 × 3 cm arising from femoral metaphyseal region (metaphysis is a radiological term so better call it "distal femur") over medial aspect. The swelling is directed away from the knee joint. Surface is irregularly bosselated with distinct edge. Swelling is arising from underlying bone and is pedunculated/sessile. Overlying skin is free from swelling. The swelling is noncompressible/reducible/pulsatile and there is no fluctuation. There is no abnormal mobility (fracture) and no distal neurovascular deficit
- Examine patella
- Examine other swellings.

Movements of Adjacent Joint

Measure:
- Genu valgum
- Shortening
- Q-angle.

1. Is this solitary or multiple?

Ans. Look for other swellings typically around shoulder, elbow, wrist, scapula (vertebral border), ankle, cristal border of ilium, and medial and lateral ends of clavicle (neurocentral synchondroses of vertebrae are also a common site but cannot be clinically examined).

2. Why do you think it is exostosis?

Ans.
- Hard painless lump present for long duration in a skeletally immature patient.
- The swelling is arising and located at the growing end of bone.
- Swelling is growing (directed) away from the growing end of bone (growing ends of bones are "towards the knee and away from elbow")
- Characteristic findings and underlying bone is not showing clinical signs of involvement (tenderness/irregularity/scalloping).
- There are no signs of aggressive tumor/neoplasia (like shiny stretched skin, raised local temperature, dilated veins, and fungation).
- Swelling is pedunculated (not true for sessile ones).

3. What are the other names for this swelling?

Ans. (Solitary) osteochondroma, biotrophic osteoma, osteocartilaginous exostosis; (Multiple) hereditary multiple exostoses (HME), osteochondromatosis, diaphyseal aclasis (Sir Arthur Keith), metaphyseal aclasis (Greig), dyschondroplasia, and hereditary deforming chondrodysplasia.

4. Is this a true tumor of bone "or" what is the process of development "or" pathogenesis?

Ans. No, this is a developmental disturbance of bone growth (developmental enchondromatous hyperplasia) typically affecting bone remodeling (Keith) hence representing failure of normal "tubulation" of bone (Jansen). Tendency of disease is usually inherited (doubtful for solitary form) and present at birth, but manifests itself only after 7–8 years of age during growth spurt. The growth of swelling stops with physeal closure (cartilage may grow to form sarcoma later but of course!). It affects bones that grow by combined enchondral and membranous ossification. Bones growing "only" by enchondral or only membranous ossification are very uncommonly involved. Exostoses arise at those parts where cartilage ossification comes to be surrounded by subperiosteal bone (i.e. at the growing ends). Somehow the peripheral cartilage cells from growth plate begin to grow centrifugally instead of longitudinal growth making a bump on side of bone. From irregularity of ossification process, cartilage cells fail to ossify. Henceforth if central cartilaginous cells are involved they form enchondroma, but if peripheral ones are involved they form exostoses.

Various theories have been advanced—isolation of islet of cartilage cells, defective anchorage of germinal cartilage cells, physical stress theory (focal embryonal cells at tendon insertions converted into hyaline cartilage), clonal/neoplastic theory (three loci isolated: *EXT* Genes for HME—*EXT1* is in **8**q23-q24, *EXT2* is on **11**p11-p12, and *EXT3* is on chromosome arm **19**p). (It is not mandatory to remember all these theories as hardly ever they have any impact on management—examiners also will never nail you for not remembering these; they are only mentioned here for comprehensiveness. You will not be forgiven, however, if you do not know the first paragraph!)

5. If it is a defect of remodeling then why it does grow?
Ans. The inner surface of cartilage cap (hyaline cartilage resembling growth plate, normally <3 mm) is involved in enchondral ossification and is responsible for growth in size. Swelling arises from physeal plate but with time and longitudinal growth of bone is shifted to metaphysis.

6. What is the mode of inheritance?

Ans. Hereditary multiple exostoses HME is inherited as autosomal dominant trait with variable expressivity and high penetrance although sporadic forms are also known to occur; may also occur with metachondromatosis, Langer–Giedion syndrome, and trichorhinophalangeal syndrome type II (TRP II), and DEFECT 11 syndrome. Male:Female for HME = 1:1 and for solitary = 2:1. Boys are somehow more severely affected by the disease.

7. What is your differential diagnosis?

Ans. *For HME*: Trevor's disease[®] (dysplasia epiphysealis hemimelica, single osteochondroma affecting single lower limb typically on the medial side and causing limb deformity due to overgrowth of cartilage), multiple epiphyseal dysplasia[®], dominant carpotarsal osteochondromatosis of Maroteaux, multiple enchondromatosis[®], and bizarre parosteal osteochondromatous proliferation (BPOP)—the Nora lesion.

For solitary osteochondroma: Organized subperiosteal hematoma[®], traumatic osteoma ("rider's bone[®], of adductor magnus, and traumatic osteoma of brachialis), Pellegrini-Stieda disease[®], parosteal osteosarcoma[®], myositis ossificans[®], nonossifying fibroma, soft-tissue ossifying lipoma, pedunculated lesions hardly have any differentials, and sessile lesions are often confused with above. (Again we do not have perverted memories and cannot remember all of these; the common ones are marked with[®]).

8. What will you do next "or" how will you confirm your diagnosis?

Ans. I will get the AP and lateral roentgenographic views of the extremity.

9. What would you see on X-ray?

Ans. *I would like to confirm my diagnosis*: The lesion may be sessile or pedunculated. Outgrowth usually arises from metaphysis of a long bone with stalk continuous with the cortex and oriented away from epiphysis. Outline is well demarcated. The medullary canal is typically continuous with the parent bone (important to differentiate from parosteal osteosarcoma). Sessile swellings arise as plateau like irregular swellings with variable (smooth to irregular) outline. Cartilage cap may form a bump in soft-tissue shadow. *(Computed tomographic scans may be required for evaluation of axial lesions and detailed study. MRI may be helpful in demonstrating continuity of medulla with parent bone, cartilage cap, and malignant degeneration.)*

10. **What are the complications of exostoses "or" what are the operative indications for exostosis?**

Ans. These are also the usual presenting features apart from cosmetic deformity:
- *Mechanical:*
    - Locking knee
    - Muscular restriction
    - Subluxation/dislocation of joints (proximal and distal radioulnar joint and distal tibiofibular joint)
    - Reduced or loss of movements
    - Large pelvic osteochondromas may obstruct parturition.
- *Compression:*
    - Musculotendinous
    - Neurologic
        - Paresthesia
        - Paralysis
    - Vascular
        - Vessel displacement
        - Stenosis/occlusion
        - Pseudoaneurysm
- *Growth:*
    - Angular deformity (genu valgum, varum, manus varus, and cubitus valgus/varus)
    - Cosmetic deformity.
- *Trauma:*
    - Fracture
        - Nonunion (fibrous)
        - Infarction of cartilage cap
        - Ischemic necrosis
    - Bursitis.
- *Malignant degeneration:*
    - Benign
        - Chondroma

- Malignant
  - Chondrosarcoma
  - Osteosarcoma
  - Malignant fibrous histiocytoma.

11. What are the causes of sudden onset of pain developing in a previously painless exostosis?

Ans. The following are the causes of sudden onset of pain in exostosis:
- Malignant degeneration
- Overlying bursitis
- Fracture
- Neural impingement
- Infarction of cartilage cap and ischemic necrosis.

12. When do you suspect malignant transformation in exostosis?

Ans. *Clinically*:
- Continued growth of lesion after skeletal maturity
- Sudden appearance of pain in adulthood
- Sudden enlargement of pre-existing lesion in an adult.

Radiologically:
- Stippled calcification or variable mineralization of cartilage cap
- Soft-tissue mass in vicinity
- Loss of distinctive bony margin
- Cap size > 1.5 cm measured by USG or MRI (only raises suspicion; there is no one-to-one relationship).

13. How does this tumor differ from *de novo* tumors?

Ans. Malignant degeneration (uncommon complication 0.5–50% in HME—lower value probably true, <1% in solitary form) is more common in central lesions (pelvis, scapula, ribs, and vertebra). They have a better prognosis than *de novo* lesions and rarely ever metastasize.

14. How will you treat this case?

Ans. *Frame your answer considering following facts:*
- Majority of lesions are asymptomatic and incidental findings. Small lesions can be left alone and followed

under surveillance. Avoid surgery unless necessary in skeletally immature patients where lesion is close to physis as there is risk of physeal injury.
- Prophylactic excision is indicated for lesions in vicinity of prominent vessels to prevent aneurysm formation and pelvic ones in females.
- Symptomatic or unsightly lesions and those with complication (see above) are excised extraperiosteally.
- Secondary deformities in limb (particularly in HME) require corrective osteotomies and/or reconstruction (distal and/or proximal radioulnar joints and distal tibiofibular joint).

15. How do you excise an exostosis?

Ans. Resection of exostosis is done extraperiosteally (complete extraperiosteal resection), flush with the parent bone or by marking a window of normal bone at the base (wide marginal excision is needed if malignant degeneration is suspected) along with overlying bursa. Some people prefer wide marginal excision in all cases.

16. What do you mean by extraperiosteal resection?

Ans. No attempt is made to elevate the periosteum or perichondrium and the lesion is resected *en masse*. Care should be taken not to cut through cartilage and in sessile lesions the cartilage at the exostosis–host bone junction should be removed. After excision, examine the mass for completeness of excision and send for histopathology. Assessment of bone defect is made as in excising sessile lesions enough cortex may be removed to weaken the underlying bone that may require support in POP cast/slab.

17. Why do these lesions recur?

Ans. Incomplete excision especially of cartilage cap is the most common cause of recurrence. Abnormal cartilage remnants at the excised margins (base of original tumor) have been described so it is recommended to cauterize the margins after excision of tumor), if an attempt is made to cut through cartilage during surgery or a biopsy is attempted from the lesion pre-operatively (core and trephine biopsies are not advised—do an excision biopsy as above straight away) are known causes of recurrence.

18. What are the techniques for deformity correction?

Ans. Underlying principles of deformity are same. For knee deformity please see Case II above.

Forearm deformities are predominantly due to growth abnormality of ulna; radius is less commonly deformed leading to ulnar subluxation of carpus (manus varus). Restriction of rotation is due to exostosis growing into interosseous membrane, sigmoid notch of radius, and excessive bow of bones. Cubitus valgus may develop secondary to radial head dislocation. Masada et al. classified forearm with HME **(Table 2)**.

Type	Ulna	Radius
I	Short, with distal osteochondromas	Bowed
IIa	Short, with distal osteochondromas	Radial head dislocated, with proximal osteochondromas
IIb	Short, with distal osteochondromas	Radial head dislocation
III	Relatively unaffected	Short, with distal osteochondromas

Table 2: Classification of forearms with HME.

Operative techniques for correction of deformity:
- Distal radius hemiphyseal stapling
- Radial head excision
- Differential forearm lengthening
- Derotational osteotomy of both bones.

CASE V: POLIO KNEE

Diagnosis: The patient is an 11-year-old female/male with postpolio residual paralysis with genu recurvatum deformity of 30° at R/L/(bilateral) knee for past 5 years and quadriceps weakness.

1. Why do you call it postpolio residual paralysis?
Ans.
- Flaccid paralysis
- Only motor involvement
- Not present since birth
- Involved muscle groups in a limb without preference to extensors/flexors or proximal/distal
- Nonprogressive paralysis.

2. What are your differential diagnoses?
Ans.
- *Meningitis*:
  - Meningoencephalitis (mumps and coxsackie)
  - Pyogenic meningitis (modified by antibiotic chemotherapy)
  - Tubercular meningitis.
- *Infective polyneuritis (Guillain-Barré syndrome)*: Paresthesia common, bilateral symmetrical paralysis, and increased CSF protein.
- *Myopathy*: Develops often during adolescence, specific muscle groups involved, and progressive disorder.

3. How many types (serotypes) of polio virus you know of?
Ans. Three types (genre: *Enteroviridae*, family: Picornaviridae, RNA (+) virus, isolated first by Karl Landsteiner)
- *Type I:* Mahoney (PV1)—most common
- *Type II:* Lansing (PV2)—least common, most commonly causes paralytic polio
- *Type III:* Leon (PV3)—vaccine associated paralytic polio transmits by feco-oral route. Can infect only humans, higher primates, and old world monkeys with CD155 Ag. Humans serve as reservoir. Infects upper and lower oropharynx, CNS (bulbar type and central brain stem nuclei), spinal type (ventral horn cells), gut, and meninges. Immunity is heterogenic to all types (i.e. no cross immunity—2nd infection possible). Incubation period range 3–35 days.

4. How many types of polio infection you know "or" is paralytic polio a common form of disease?
Ans. Different types of polio infection are given in **Table 3**.

The Knee

Table 3: Types of polio infection.	
Form	**Proportion of cases**
Asymptomatic (abortive polio)	90–95%
Minor illness (abortive polio)	4–8%
Nonparalytic *aseptic meningitis*	1–2%
Paralytic poliomyelitis: - Spinal polio - Bulbospinal polio - Bulbar polio - Encephalitis	0.1–0.5% 79% of paralytic cases 19% of paralytic cases 2% of paralytic cases Spastic paralysis and seizures

5. What are phases of symptomatic disease?

Ans. *Three phases:*

1. *Acute phase* (5-10 days): Stage of onset of paralysis usually 2-3 days after fever begins
   - Preparalytic—fever, headache, neck rigidity, painful spasm, and muscle tenderness
   - Paralytic—if brainstem affected (bulbar polio) respiratory muscle paralysis.

   Progression ceases when fever settles, acute phase terminates 48 hours after fever normally (may last up to 2 months).

2. *Convalescent phase* (may last 18 months): Spontaneous recovery
   - Aims to eliminate deforming tendency, restore ROM and train coordination, rebuild muscle power by hot packs, passive movements, positioning (spine firm mattress or Dunlop pillow with intermittent prone position; lower limbs—knees in slight flexion and foot in splint; upper limb—felt sling), muscle re-education, stimulation for standing reflexes, pool therapy (Hubbard tank bath).

3. *Chronic phase* (residual paralysis)—aims to prevent or correct deformity.

6. What orthopedic apparatus are used during convalescent phase and residual phase?

Ans. Apparatus is required to protect weak muscle, prevent deformity, and support limb.

Upper limb:
- *Abduction shoulder splint:* Now rarely given for deltoid paralysis and protection from effects of gravity and shoulder subluxation
- Cock-up wrist splint
- Spinal brace for axial involvement (often severe cases).

Lower limb:
- *Below knee appliances:* For deformity correction and prevention—bar on the side of deviation and strap at the angulation (for genu valgum: outside bar and inside T-strap)
- Weight-bearing caliper.

7. What is the aim of orthopedic procedures in residual stage of disease?

Ans.
- Correction of soft-tissue contracture
- Improvement of function and prevention of deformity by tendon transfer and stabilization procedure
- Correct limb length discrepancy
- Eliminate external supports.

8. How do you grade muscle power?

Ans. MRC grading (Medical Research Council, Great Britain)
- Total paralysis
- Barely detectable contracture/flicker
- Not enough power to act against gravity
- Strong enough to act against gravity
- Still stronger with activity against resistance (not normal)
    - 4 (+) good resistance but not normal
    - 4 (0) resistance moderate
    - 4 (–) resistance weak and easily overcome
- Full power.

9. What are the causes of genu recurvatum in polio knee?

Ans. It is a progressive deformity.

Two types:
1. Caused by structural bony and articular changes following quadriceps paralysis
2. Relaxation of soft tissues on posterior aspect of knee joint.

10. What are the differences in the two types?

Ans. In the *first type,* primary pathology is in quadriceps but hamstrings and triceps sure are normal so there is loss of anterior soft-tissue support with maintained posterior support. Gradually tibial condyles get elongated posteriorly with reversal of posterior tibial slope. Posterior bow of upper metadiaphysis and subluxation then develops. This is due to patient walking with hyperextension of knee using anatomical knee locking or hand to knee gait. The prognosis for correction of deformity is excellent and should aim at (Irwin):

- Restoration of limb alignment [Irwin proximal tibial posterior closing wedge osteotomy, Storen modification of Campbell osteotomy, and flexion femoral osteotomy of Mehta and Mukherjee (1991)]
- Rectification of cause of deformity [anterior transfer of hamstring (biceps femoris and semitendinosus) tendons to strengthen quadriceps].

The *second type* of knee is due to relaxation of posterior capsular structures and weakness in calf and hamstring muscles. This type is often also associated with calcaneovalgus foot deformity. The hamstrings often subluxate anteriorly and become extensors of knee. There may be flattening of femoral condyles. Prognosis is less certain after correction of this type as no muscles are available for transfer, underlying cause cannot be corrected and deformity can recur. Bracing for up to moderate deformities prevents progression, but has to be discarded later. Perry outlined the principles for successful surgical correction:

- Fibrous tissue mass must be of sufficient strength to withstand stretching force generated.
- Healing tissues must be protected.
- Alignment at ankle be at least neutral or should be achieved so before surgery.

"Triple tenodesis of knee" for paralytic genu recurvatum is often the only option for these patients.

11. How will you manage quadriceps paralysis?

Ans. Hamstring tendon transfer (semitendinosus and biceps femoris). As such the muscles available for transfer are hamstrings, tensor fasciae latae, and sartorius but the latter are insufficient to replace quadriceps function.

12. Why do you transfer semitendinosus with biceps femoris?

Ans. To prevent lateral dislocation of patella.

13. What are the prerequisites for this transfer "or" what will you look for before doing this transfer?

Ans. The power of hip flexors (to clear foot off ground) and abductors along with triceps surae (climbing stairs) must be adequate. There must not be any ankle equinus (to prevent postoperative hyperextension at knee). Flexion contracture at knee must be released before transfer.

14. How would you prevent postoperative hyperextension from developing after tendon transfer?

Ans. Assuring adequate power in triceps surae preoperative, preventing immobilization of knee in hyperextension, and correcting talipes equinus before resuming weight bearing. After tendon transfer hyperextension should be prevented otherwise it becomes a progressive deformity and genu recurvatum ensues.

15. How do you treat flexion contracture of knee joint?

Ans. Flexion deformity (contracture) develops either due to tight ITB or due to powerful hamstrings in the setting of weak quadriceps. Various treatment options with respect to the severity of deformity and etiology are as follows:
- *Only tight ITB:* ITB release and lateral intermuscular septum division (Yount).
- *Tight hamstrings (contractures 15-20°):* Posterior hamstring lengthening and capsulotomy or wedge plaster cast treatment.
- *Deformities up to 40°:* Initial treatment in reverse dynamic traction then as above or femoral osteotomy (for combined ITB and Hamstring tightness).
- *More severe deformities:* Supracondylar extension osteotomy along with posterior release either in single stage (up to 70°) or in two stages (>70°); often 5-10° of recurvatum is aimed at.

The Knee

16. What is flail knee?

Ans. When there is weakness of both extensors and flexors leading to instability in all directions the knee is called flail knee. For such knee no muscles are left that can stabilize the joint for day-to-day activities. Management involves using a long brace with lock or if preferable to a heavy labor—arthrodesis of knee joint.

17. What will you do for bilateral flail knee?

Ans. Options are providing locking knee brace on both sides or better an arthrodesis on one side and locking knee brace on other. It is prudent to give the patient an "arthrodesis trial" by putting the limb in cylinder POP cast.

18. What is the role of total knee replacement for paralytic polio knee?

Ans. Typically indicated for pain relief for arthritic changes. Quadriceps strength of 3/5 is a prerequisite for this procedure as TKR does not allow hyperextension and patient may not be able to walk. Results are poor even for pain relief for quadriceps power <3/5. Total constrained prosthesis is often advised.

CASE VI: INJURY TO ANTERIOR CRUCIATE LIGAMENT

1. What is your diagnosis?

Ans. Anterior instability of the knee joint due to anterior cruciate ligament (ACL) tear.

2. What are the points in favor of your diagnosis?

Ans. *Symptoms*:
- Pain
- Swelling
- Popping or snapping sensation
- Feeling of give way
- Instability.

Signs:
- Anterior drawer test—positive
- Pivot-shift test—positive
- Lachman test—positive.

3. What is your differential diagnosis?
Ans.
- *Posterior cruciate ligament (PCL) tear*: This can mimic ACL tear due to presence of false positive anterior drawer and reverse pivot shift test.
- Constitutionally lax ACL (compare from other side).

4. What is the cause of false negative drawer test?
Ans. The drawer test can falsely negative due to:
- Hemarthrosis and hamstring spasm in acute injury, knee cannot be flexed till 90°.
- Door stopper effect of the posterior horn of medial meniscus.

5. How do you grade instability?
Ans. Grading of instability is done as follows:
- 1+ joint surface separate 5 mm or less (forward subluxation of tibia under femur)
- 2+ joint surface separate 6–10 mm
- 3+ joint surface separate > 10 mm.

6. Which is the most sensitive test for diagnosis of ACL tear?
Ans. Lachman test **(Fig. 18)**.

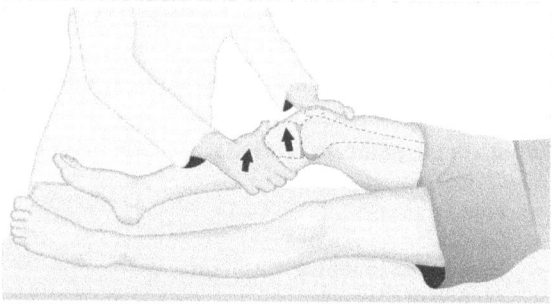

Fig. 18: Lachman test.

7. What are the advantages of Lachman test?
Ans.
- Highly specific for ACL rupture
- Not hampered by posterior horn of meniscus

- Not hampered by hemarthrosis
- Less painful because the muscles are relaxed
- Not hampered by sprained or partially ruptured medial collateral ligament
- Performed in functional position of flexion of knee. Can be performed when there is a fracture close to knee.

8. What are the various modifications of anterior drawer test?

Ans. Weatherwax described a modified anterior drawer test in which the lower leg is supported in the examiner's axilla (**Fig. 19**). It is relatively difficult to establish a specific position of tibial rotation with this technique, but anterior displacement is easily recognized.

The Noyes test can be performed from the same initial position without significantly changing the hand position. Varus and valgus laxity also can be tested by slightly adjusting the placement of the fingers.

Feagin recommends performing 90° drawer tests with the patient in the sitting position. Gravity pulls the tibia downward and helps to relax the muscles. The advantages claimed are that anterior displacement of the tibia can be more easily perceived and confirmed and that the rotational response of the proximal tibia (medial and lateral compartmental translation) also can be evaluated using this technique.

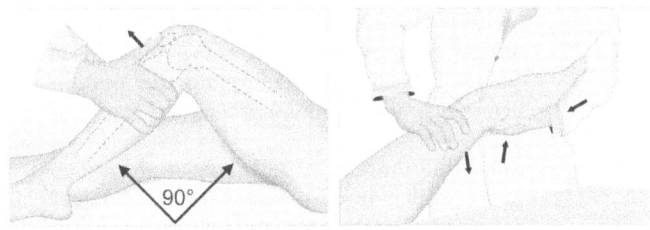

Fig. 19: Anterior drawer test—Classical and Weatherwax modification.

9. What is the significance of "endpoint" in stress testing?

Ans. There are two discernible endpoints in stress testing for disruptions of ligaments about the knee:
1. "Hard" implying a firm, definite stop

2. "Soft or mushy" a less distinct and less sudden stop. Following are the types of endpoints and their interpretations:
   - Firm endpoint with hemarthrosis—implies an acute partial rupture
   - Firm endpoint without hemarthrosis—implies an old partial rupture or elongation
   - Soft endpoint with hemarthrosis—complete rupture
   - Soft endpoint without hemarthrosis—old complete rupture and acute complex ligamentous injury.

10. **What is "door stopper" effect of meniscus and its role in diagnosis of ACL tear?**

Ans. With knee flexed to 90° for classic anterior drawer sign, medial meniscus, being attached to tibia, abuts against acutely convex surface of medial femoral condyle and has "door-stopper" effect, and hindering anterior translation of tibia. With knee extended; however, the relatively flat weight-bearing surface of femur does not obstruct forward motion of meniscus and tibia when anterior stress is applied.

11. **What is the significance of performing anterior drawer test in doing in different degrees of rotations of tibia?**

Ans.
- 90° flexion with internal tibial rotation
  - *(Nil)* Iliotibial tract and PCL intact. The test is not made positive by rupture of the ACL and posteromedial structures, because the internal rotation "locks" the joint by tightening the posterolateral ligaments, the iliotibial tract, and especially the PCL.
  - *(Slight)* Rupture of ACL. Injury of arcuate complex and iliotibial tract, possible lesion of medial and posteromedial structures.
  - *(Marked)* Rupture of ACL and PCL. Lateral and posterolateral structures and lesion of iliotibial tract.
- 90° Flexion with neutral tibial rotation
  - *(Nil)* Medial and lateral capsuloligamentous structures intact. ACL may be torn.

The Knee

- *(Slight)* Lesion of medial and/or lateral structures. Possible rupture of ACL. With a firm endpoint, a PCL ligament rupture must be excluded.
- *(Marked)* Rupture of ACL and lesion of medial and posteromedial and/or lateral and posterolateral structures. Possible rupture of PCL.

■ 90° Flexion with external tibial rotation
- *(Nil)* Medial and posteromedial structures intact.
- *(Slight)* Rupture of medial and posteromedial structures.
- *(Marked)* Rupture of ACL, medial, and posteromedial structures.

12. How do you classify knee instabilities?
Ans.
- *Single plane instability simple or straight:*
  - One plane medial
  - One plane lateral
  - One plane posterior
  - One plane anterior
- *Rotatory instability:*
  - Anteromedial
  - Anterolateral
    • In flexion
    • Approaching extension
  - Posterolateral
  - Posteromedial
- *Combined instability:*
  - Anterolateral-anteromedial rotatory
  - Anterolateral-posterolateral rotatory
  - Anteromedial-posteromedial rotatory.

13. What is single plane instability and what is its significance?
Ans. Single plane instability is the one that is present only in single sagittal or coronal plane that can be tested by appropriate stress testing.

One-plane *medial instability with the knee in full extension* is apparent when, as the abduction or valgus stress test is performed, the knee joint opens on the medial side.

This indicates disruption of the medial collateral ligament, the medial capsular ligament, the ACL, the posterior oblique ligament, and the medial portion of the posterior capsule.

One-plane *medial instability* detected in 30° of knee flexion indicates a tear predominantly of the medial compartment ligaments.

One-plane *lateral instability with the knee in extension* is apparent on adduction or varus stress testing when the knee opens on the lateral side; that is, the tibia moves away from the femur. This indicates disruption of the lateral capsular ligament, the lateral collateral ligament, the biceps tendon, the iliotibial band, the arcuate-popliteus complex, the popliteofibular ligament, the ACL, and, often, the posterior cruciate ligament. One-plane lateral instability detected only with the knee in 30° of flexion may be present in minor lateral complex tears or may be normal when compared with the opposite knee.

One-plane *posterior instability* is apparent when the tibia moves posteriorly on the femur during the posterior drawer test. This indicates disruption of the PCL, the arcuate ligament complex (partial or complete), and the posterior oblique ligament complex (partial or complete).

One-plane *anterior instability* is present when the tibia moves forward on the femur during the anterior drawer test in neutral rotation. It indicates that disrupted structures include the ACL, the lateral capsular ligament (partial or complete), and the medial capsular ligament (partial or complete).

The anterior drawer sign is positive in neutral rotation when the ACL is disrupted with immediate or subsequent stretching of the medial and lateral capsular ligaments. In this type of instability, the test becomes negative as the tibia is internally rotated because in this position the PCL becomes taut.

14. What are the rotatory tests to diagnose ACL and other ligamentous disruptions?

Ans. Slocum anterior rotary drawer test, jerk test of Hughston and Losee, lateral pivot-shift test of MacIntosh, flexion rotation drawer test of Noyes, external rotation recurvatum test, reverse pivot-shift sign of Jakob, Hassler, and Staeubli, tibial external rotation test, and posterolateral drawer test are the rotatory tests to diagnosis ligamentous disruptions.

15. What investigations will you do?

Ans.
- X-rays may show bony avulsions of tibial spine.
- MRI—edema in ACL substance or avulsions from tibial or femoral ends.

16. What will you do to treat the patient?

Ans. I will do arthroscopic ACL reconstruction using quadrupled hamstring tendon graft. The treatment options available include nonoperative management, repair of the ACL, either isolated or with augmentation, and reconstruction with either autograft or allograft tissues or synthetics.

(Young athletic patients with complete ACL tear are treated with arthroscopic ACL reconstruction whereas old patients with partial ACL tear can be managed conservatively. In these two extremes the surgeon has to decide the treatment.)

17. What are the various autografts for ACL reconstruction?

Ans. The most common current graft choices are bone-patellar tendon-bone graft and the quadrupled hamstring tendon graft.

18. What are various graft options for ACL reconstruction?

Ans. *Autograft*:
- Patellar tendon (bone-patellar tendon-bone)
- Hamstring tendon
- Semitendinosus
- Gracilis
- Central quadriceps
- Achilles tendon
- Multiple looped
- Fascia lata/Iliotibial band
- Meniscus
- Reharvested patellar tendon.

Allograft:
- Patellar tendon
- Hamstring
- Fascia lata/Iliotibial band
- Achilles tendon
- ACL
- Tibialis anterior
- Peroneal tendon

Synthetic:
- Gore-Tex
- Dacron
- Carbon filaments
- Polyester

Engineered graft:
- Fabricated collagen.

19. What is the ideal tunnel position for arthroscopic ACL reconstruction?

Ans.
- Tibial tunnel should be centered in the posteromedial aspect of the tibial footprint or 5–7 mm in front of PCL. This point is along the line drawn from the posterior edge of anterior horn of lateral meniscus to the medial tibial eminence.
- Femoral tunnel placement should be at 10:30 position for right knee or 1:30 for left knee.
- The femoral tunnel should embrace the posterior cortex.

20. What is the difference between single and double bundle techniques and which one is better?

Ans. In single bundle technique one tunnel is drilled each in femur and tibia for fixing the graft; however, in double bundle technique two different tunnels are drilled for fixation of ACL bundles. Though it was thought that the rotational stability would be better with double bundle technique, but clinical differences have not been substantiated.

21. What types of exercises are preferred in patients with ACL reconstructed knees rehabilitation?

Ans. Closed chain exercises.

22. What are closed chain exercises and what is their rationale?

Ans. Resisted quadriceps exercises put strain on the ACL, particularly in terminal extension if the limb is not bearing weight, these are called open chain exercises (the foot is in air and the chain is hence open). In an effort to protect the graft (reconstructed ACL) during quadriceps exercises, it has been suggested that the foot be in contact with the couch (making the chain closed). The knee joint is thus so loaded that during movements the graft is protected from shearing stresses and perhaps the contours of the joint help stabilize the knee and protect the graft, these are also called as closed chain exercises.

[I strongly encourage the reader to go through Chapter 34 of the book Essential Orthopedics Principles and Practice, 2nd edition (Varshney MK, Jaypee Publishers) for learning details of surgical technique, different fixation methods for the ACL grafts, and addressing controversial issues].

CASE VII: INJURY TO POSTERIOR CRUCIATE LIGAMENT

1. What is your diagnosis?
Ans. Posterior instability of the knee joint due to PCL tear.

2. What are the points in favor of your diagnosis?
Ans. *Symptoms*:
- Pain
- Swelling
- Popping or snapping sensation
- Feeling of give way
- Instability.

Signs:
- Posterior drawer test—positive
- Reverse pivot-shift test—positive
- Lachman test—positive
- Absence of normal proximal tibial step (1 cm) when traced along femoral condyles anteriorly
- Telltale signs as scar mark of injury over proximal leg
- Godfrey's sign (posterior sagging of tibia).

3. What is the differential diagnosis of PCL tear?

Ans. ACL tear can mimic PCL tear due to presence of false positive posterior drawer and pivot-shift test.

4. What is the cause of false negative drawer test?

Ans. In acute injury with hemarthrosis and hamstring spasm, knee cannot be flexed till 90°.

5. What investigations will you do?

Ans.
- X-rays may show bony avulsions of tibial spine.
- MRI—edema in PCL substance or avulsions from tibial or femoral ends.

6. What will you do to treat the patient?

Ans. (*The reconstructive outcome may not be as productive for PCL as for ACL reconstruction hence the guidelines are quite different*)

Guidelines:

Acute PCL avulsions:
- Large bony fragment—treat with either arthroscopic or open screw fixation.
- *Small fragment (nonfixable):*
  - Posterior tibial translation <10 mm—quadriceps exercises and rehabilitation
  - Posterior tibial translation >10 mm—PCL reconstruction
- Young athletic patients with complete PCL tear are treated with arthroscopic PCL reconstruction whereas old patients with partial PCL tear can be managed conservatively.

Chronic PCL avulsions/tear:
- Isolated PCL deficiency is asymptomatic then rehabilitate → improvement → continue and watch for degenerative changes → PCL reconstruction if progresses. If fails to improve with rehabilitation then perform arthroscopic PCL reconstruction in young symptomatic grade III tears. Associated injuries should be simultaneously treated like medial collateral ligament repair/reconstruction; fixation of fibular tip fracture, etc. In later middle age

with degenerative changes of the knee set in (identified on arthroscopy or MRI) explain the need for arthroplasty that may not be ameliorated by performing PCL reconstruction at this stage.
- *Chronic posterolateral instability (+):*
  - Get AP hip to ankle radiograph in extension
    - Normal alignment → rehabilitate → no relief → perform posterolateral corner reconstruction (PCL + LCL + popliteofibular ligament) [choice varies from nonanatomical (biceps tenodesis, proximal bone block advancements, extracapsular sling, etc.) versus anatomical reconstruction (LaPrade or Larson style reconstruction)].
    - Varus alignment → perform valgus osteotomy → relief → rehabilitate otherwise do posterolateral corner reconstruction (if still symptomatic and degenerative changes absent); else consider arthroplasty (degenerated joint).

7. **How will you reconstruct PCL and what are various options?**

Ans. The treatment options available include nonoperative management, repair of the posterior cruciate ligament either isolated or with augmentation, and reconstruction with either autograft or allograft tissues or synthetics *(See Case VI above)*.

[I strongly encourage the reader to go through Chapter 34 of the book Essential Orthopedics Principles and Practice, 2nd edition (Varshney MK, Jaypee Publishers) for learning details of injury patterns, classification, and grading of PCL insufficiency, combined ligament injuries, surgical technique, management of posterolateral corner injuries, and addressing controversial issues].

CASE VIII: TUBERCULOSIS OF THE KNEE JOINT

Diagnosis: My patient is a 11-year-old male with tuberculosis of the right knee. There is flexion deformity of 40° with posterior and lateral subluxation of tibia on femur and lateral rotation with abduction. There is joint effusion and patient is on antitubercular treatment for 2 months (± traction), presently unable to do his activities of daily living with the right lower limb. The patient walks with cane support. [If sinus or abscess is observed in vicinity then this also should be mentioned along with surgical intervention for biopsy, etc. if done (seeing scar mark and obtaining history).]

HISTORY

Insidious onset recurrent episodes of swelling and later pain in single knee. Gradual development of stiffness over a period of few months. Gradual increase in swelling and stiffness of joint with pain. Night cries, constitutional symptoms, antituberculous treatment (ATT), etc. History of TB contacts.

FINDINGS

- Flexion deformity of knee
- Triple deformity (flexion, posterior, and lateral subluxation of tibia on femur)
- Knee effusion
- Sinus and discharge are quite characteristic
- Wasting of muscles of thigh
- Boggy, spongy, and doughy knee swelling due to synovial proliferation
- Secondary infection of the joint (if sinus present) may cause local rise in temperature
- Joint line tenderness
- Restricted movements
- Hamstring spasm
- Regional lymphadenopathy.

1. What is your differential diagnosis?

Ans.
- Juvenile rheumatoid arthritis
- Subacute septic arthritis of knee joint
- Acute exacerbation of inflammatory (rheumatoid) arthritis of knee
- Monoarticular rheumatoid arthritis of knee joint
- Recurrent hemarthrosis in hemophilia.

2. **What is triple deformity of knee?**
Ans. Classically described for tuberculosis of knee. However, it is also found in various long standing chronic diseases like rheumatoid arthritis and in ITB contracture.

   Deformity components:
   - *Flexion deformity at knee* (due to chronic nature of diseases and synovial effusion knee is commonly kept in position of maximum joint space—30° which persists to produce flexion deformity of knee).
   - *Posterolateral subluxation of tibia* (most of chronic destructive diseases joint subluxates laterally—reasons are not clear; one explanation could be that in rheumatoid disease which commonly affects females there is already more physiological valgus which leads to increased stresses over lateral joint compartment, other more plausible one is that in destructive diseases there is exaggeration of the physiological alignment—remember there is a physiological valgus and posterior tibial slope in a normal knee joint).
   - *External rotation of tibia over femoral condyles*—various reasons; quadriceps pull, popliteus action, ITB, etc.

   Sometimes *quadruple deformity complex* is described where *genu valgum* is added as a component of deformity (however, this is not a primary pathomechanism and develops secondary to tibial subluxation).

3. **What causes this deformity?**
Ans. Pull of the hamstring muscles due to spasm on a knee joint where ligaments have been destroyed posteriorly subluxates tibia. Patients lying supine also help in posterior sag of the tibia aided by gravity. Presence of tight and strong ITB laterally causes lateral subluxation as medially there are no such strong structures that become incompetent over time by the disease process.

4. **How common is tuberculosis of the knee joint?**
Ans. Tuberculosis of the knee joint is the third most common site of tuberculosis after TB spine and hip joint. It is common in children though it can occur at any age.

5. What are the pathological stages of TB knee?

Ans. The disease passes through stages of synovitis (mostly the focus of infection also) → early arthritis (stiffness, flexion deformity, and effusion) → late arthritis (loss of movements and subluxation of tibia) → deformity and complications.

6. Where do you look for synovial thickening?

Ans. Synovial thickening is best palpated under the vastus medialis and rolled over the edge of medial femoral condyle as a boggy or doughy band of tissue. The muscle extends till very near patella normally but with knee disease it becomes atrophic so there is only soft tissue remaining through which hypertrophied synovium can be characteristically palpated. On lateral side presence of thick retinaculum and iliotibial band preclude such luxury of identification.

7. What is the lymphatic drainage of knee joint and where do you palpate for it?

Ans. The primary drainage of knee is to popliteal nodes efferents from which pass towards deep inguinal lymph nodes through femoral blood vessels. Inguinal nodes also receive direct lymphatics from skin over anterior aspect of the knee joint so if there is an active sinus in the region inguinal lymphadenopathy may precede popliteal lymphadenopathy. The usual consistency of tubercular lymphadenopathy is that of matted, elastic to firm mass that is not very tender or warm to touch.

8. What are the similarities and dissimilarities in TB knee and TB hip?

Ans. *Dissimilarities*: TB of the hip usually has initial focus in the bone (osseous focus) either on the femoral or acetabular side while knee joint TB is predominantly synovial to begin with (uncommonly juxta-articular subchondral focus is found in femur/tibia/patella). Bony destruction is more conspicuous in the TB hip producing various types (*see* Case on TB hip) while in knee joint the destruction of ligaments and spasm of surrounding muscles produce early deformity while bony destruction is not as conspicuous.

The Knee

Similarities: Both the diseases tend to occur in children and pass through stages of synovitis → early arthritis → late arthritis → destruction and complication. Formation of pannus is seen in both the diseases that erodes the articular cartilage and with time settles in between to produce fibrous ankylosis.

9. Can TB knee joint develop bony ankylosis?

Ans. Yes, in cases where there is secondary pyogenic infection of the knee joint (say traveling through sinus), the joint will rapidly get destroyed and will develop bony ankylosis with healing.

10. What will you do next and why?

Ans. I will get X-ray of the patient done (see all orthopedicians are fascinated with radiographic findings despite being clear that this is tuberculosis of knee! So always ask for X-ray after finishing with clinical part!). The radiographs will demonstrate the bony deformities and destruction of the joint. Presence of cystic-sclerotic regions will support chronic infection.

11. Does this confirm your diagnosis?

Ans. No, the radiographic findings only support my diagnosis of an inflammatory process that is causing joint and bone destruction.

12. How will you investigate the case?

Ans. I will do CBC, ESR, and CRP to confirm inflammatory process and to identify its chronicity. Mantoux text is an indirect test to identify tubercular infection (but has no definite reliability only supportive evidence). I will also perform serology for HIV infection as tubercular infection is common amongst them and it is also needed for invasive procedure. I will perform synovial fluid examination and biopsy to confirm my diagnosis.

13. How will you take synovial biopsy?

Ans. Personally, I prefer arthroscopic biopsy under direct vision to improve the yield and also synovectomy can be done simultaneously to improve patient symptomatology and morbidity.

14. How will you manage this case?

Ans. For the presented patient after arthroscopic biopsy and debridement I will attempt deformity correction at knee by providing "double" traction. As soon as the investigations (histopathology and synovial fluid examination) are available I will continue ATT if corroborative.

15. What is the role of traction?

Ans.
- Traction counters muscle spasm preventing progression of deformity and over time with increasing linear distal weight the deformity is also corrected.
- The articular surfaces are pulled apart so pain reduces from friction of free nerve endings.
- It also immobilizes the patient and gives rest so further damage to joint does not occur with weight bearing.

16. How long will you continue this treatment?

Ans. Usually once the deformity is corrected and patient is comfortable with antitubercular therapy I will start mobilization. Commonly 2–3 months are needed for deformities to fully correct. Initial mobilization consists of gentle knee bending and ROM exercises with quadriceps building and as pain is tolerable patient is mobilized partial weight bearing with crutches.

17. What if the patient does not improve?

Ans. I will wait for 6–8 weeks completion of ATT then if the progress is not good then I will proceed to formal/arthroscopic (choose the one you feel comfortable) knee debridement and send the tissue for line probe assay and Xpert-MTB test for identification of multidrug-resistant (MDR) tuberculosis.

18. What is the role of arthrodesis in TB knee?

Ans. This is indicated in patients with old disease that have persistent pain due to arthritis and residual fixed deformities that make the knee unfit for function and activities of daily living. Even after fibrous ankylosis the patient can still continue to have pain and if the demands are of heavy labor in job then arthrodesis is the best method to make him pain free.

19. What is the role of total knee arthroplasty in knee joint and what precautions will you take?

Ans. This method reconstructs the joint into functional painless mobile joint and is the preferred option in adult patient (preferably > 50 years) with old disease that has healed. Patient should be free of infection and collateral ligaments and extensor apparatus should be intact for favorable outcome. Due to risk of reactivation of disease I would keep the patient on 4-6 weeks ATT before doing arthroplasty and will continue full 6 months course.

4
Foot and Ankle

The foot and ankle is a difficult topic for examination and in itself is a speciality topic. The cases are often short cases but long cases of a polio foot can be presented.

Read times: 3–5 times, 5–7 times for polio foot; MS and DNB candidates.

EXAMINATION POINTS FOR FOOT AND ANKLE CASES

HISTORY

- *Age:* Congenital talipes equinovarus (CTEV) present since birth, talipes equinovarus (TEV) secondary to polio, neural tube defects, etc. appear later. Congenital vertical talus (CVT) noticed at walking age around 1 year.
- *Sex:* Boys are common in CTEV.
- *Pain:* Duration, site, radiation, type, character, aggravating factors, relieving factors, diurnal variation, and postural variation.
- *Swelling:* Duration, onset (preceding trauma, fever, other joints involvement, and morning stiffness), progress (always increasing as in tumors, regressive as in trauma or increase with on and off reduction as in infection), aggravating factors (walking in subtalar arthritis), relieving factors (antibiotics in infection or chemotherapy in tumors), effect of any treatment received, and diurnal and postural variation. Associated with deformity in other foot.
- *Limp:* Onset, duration, painful or painless, and progressive or not.

- *Instability:* Duration, onset (post-traumatic), unilateral or bilateral (ligament laxity), on even or uneven surfaces (in stiff subtalar joint).
- *Deformity:* Onset [at birth (CTEV) or appeared later (acquired clubfoot)] (appears at around 1 year in CVT) (after an episode of fever and myalgia with weakness of limb muscles in polio), progress (congenital is less progressive than acquired), any treatment received (casts and surgeries), and response to any such treatment.
- *Associated diseases:* Fever with myalgia and weakness of limbs in polio.

EXAMINATION

General Examination

Examine hip and spine for congenital hip dislocation, myelomeningocele, spinal dysraphism, arthrogryposis multiplex congenita.

Local

Prerequisites
- Patient must be sitting at edge of table with legs hanging freely.
- Entire lower limb from lumbosacral spine to tips of toes must be examined.
- Examine foot during gait, standing, and in nonweight-bearing position.
- Neurological examination of lower limbs should be done as deficits produce different deformities of foot and toes.
- Footwear examination **(Fig. 1)**.

Inspection
Gait
Antalgic, short limbed, foot drop, equinus, and stiff 1st metatarsophalangeal (MTP) joint.

Anterior aspect:
- *Alignment:* Great toe (hallux valgus/varus) **(Fig. 2)**, other toes (claw, hammer, and mallet), relations of forefoot, midfoot, and hindfoot **(Fig. 3)** with respect to each other and lower leg (include tibia vara and rotation).

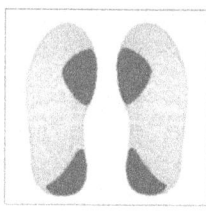 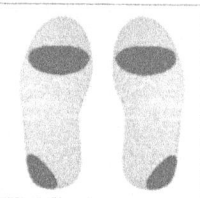 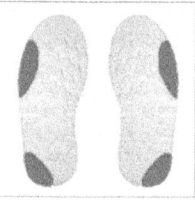

"Pronation" outsole is worn on the inside edge

"Neutral"

"Supination" outsole is worn on the outside edge

Fig. 1: Examination of shoe.

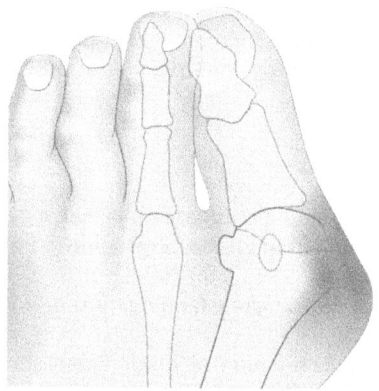

Fig. 2: Hallux valgus.

- *Condition of skin:* Any discoloration, ulcers, dilated veins, and edema (pitting or nonpitting and up to what level).
- *Toes:* Notice transverse skin creases at interphalangeal (IP) joints (sometimes lost in polio). Also note thickened cornified skin over dorsum (heloma durum) seen in toe deformities. Toenail deformities in fungal infections. Paronychia (seen as swelling around base and sides of nail). Ingrown toenail.

Foot and Ankle

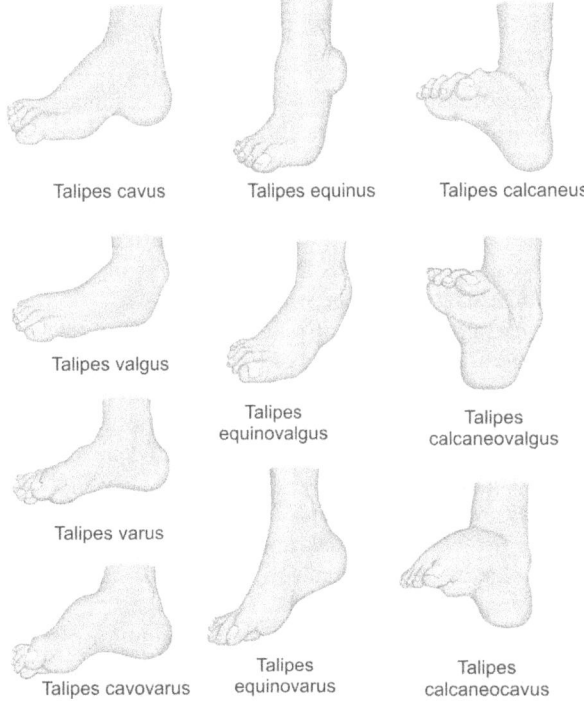

Fig. 3: Various deformities of foot and their clinical appearance.

- Osteophytes medially over 1st MTP joint is called bunion and over lateral aspect of 5th MTP joint is called bunionette.
- Tendons of extensor hallucis longus (EHL) and extensor digitorum longus (EDL) are visible over foot and anterior aspect of ankle by active contraction of muscles. (Remember pneumonic for structures medial to lateral is The Himalayas Are Not Dry Places—stands for tibialis anterior, EHL, anterior tibial artery, anterior tibial nerve, EDL, and peroneus tertius).
- *Relation of medial and lateral malleoli:* Normally lateral is below and posterior to medial malleolus.

- *Any swelling over malleoli:* Seen in trauma and tendinitis.
- Anterior crest of tibia and subcutaneous border may show swelling and deformities.

Lateral aspect: Visualize lateral malleolus, 5th metatarsal base, tendo-achilles, and peroneus brevis tendon. Note for any swelling.

Posterior aspect:
- *Alignment:* Varus/valgus of hindfoot. "Too many toes sign"—more than 2 toes visible from behind means abduction of forefoot, usually associated with pes planus.
- *Heel:* Size (any broadening), pattern, and position.
- Tell patient to stand on tips of toes (windlass effect-inversion and increased height of medial longitudinal arch).
- Plantar fat pad, calcaneal tuberosity [abnormally increased prominence of superior aspect is Haglund's deformity or pump bump **(Fig. 4)**].
- *Retrocalcaneal bursa:* Bursitis.
- *Achilles tendon:* Tendinitis, rupture (2–6 cm above insertion), and swelling at level of malleoli is seen in tendonitis and over whole length is seen in rupture.
- *Calf atrophy (compared to normal):* Residuum of CTEV, TA rupture or prolonged immobilization.

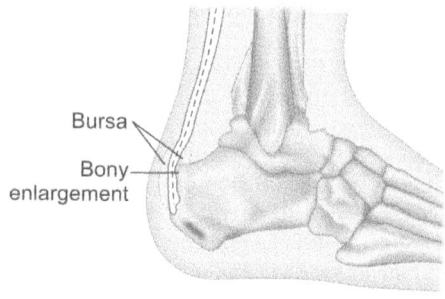

Fig. 4: Haglund's deformity.

Medial aspect:
- *Medial longitudinal arch:* Cavus or planus or rocker bottom deformity (in diabetics or improperly treated CTEV).
- *Bony prominences:* Medial malleolus, head of 1st MT, calcaneal tuberosity, and navicular tuberosity (prominent in accessory navicular).
- Tibialis posterior (TP) tendon made visible by active contraction. Remember pneumonic for structures underneath flexor retinaculum of ankle: The Doctors Are Never Happy—stands for (from anterior to posterior aspect) tibialis posterior, flexor digitorum longus (FDL), posterior tibial artery, posterior tibial nerve, and flexor hallucis longus (FHL).

Plantar aspect:
- Callosity suggests point of weight bearing. Normally seen over metatarsal heads and lateral margin of foot. Painful calluses over MT heads are seen in toe deformities like claw toes and hammer toes with hyperextension of MTP joints.
- Corns are localized thickening of skin over pressure areas. Two types—hard or soft.
- *Ulcerations:* Diabetes and abnormal bony prominences.
- Warts or fungal infections (taeniasis).

Palpation
Anterior
- Local rise of temperature.
- *Tenderness:* Over anterior tibial crest (in stress fractures). Over talar dome: Palpated anterolaterally with maximal passive plantar flexion at ankle (in OCD). Over navicular in Kohler's disease. Over talonavicular joint in osteoarthritis. Also palpate cuneiforms and metatarsals (stress fracture especially in 2nd and 3rd MT). Over 1st MTP joint in bunions, gout, and septic arthritis. 2nd MTP joint (Freiberg's infarction).
- Tenderness in interdigital spaces suggests Morton's neuromas (commonest between 3rd and 4th metatarsal heads).
- *Swelling:* Over stress fractures. Osteophytes over joints. Effusion of joint: Cross fluctuation can be demonstrated between anterolateral and anteromedial swellings in full plantar flexion.

Also seen between posterolateral and posteromedial swellings in full dorsiflexion. In between anterior and posterior swellings, it is seen in neutral position.

- *Tendons (whether they are taut, tenderness, lump or any gap seen in ruptures, diffuse swelling, and crepitus):* Tibialis anterior, EHL, EDL, and peroneus tertius.
- Toes palpated for corns and ingrown toenails.
- Tinel's sign over deep peroneal nerve (at site of dorsalis pedis artery) present in anterior tarsal tunnel syndrome.

Lateral

- Lateral malleolus, anterior talofibular ligament and calcaneofibular ligament for swelling and tenderness.
- Peroneal tendons (cannot distinguish longus and brevis separately).
- Calcaneum, its tuberosity (in Sever's disease) and calcaneocuboid joint.
- Over sinus tarsi in subtalar arthritis.
- Over fibular shaft: Stress fractures.

Posterior

- *Over gastrocsoleus:* In tendo-Achilles rupture, tenderness, gap, and swelling are felt 2–6 cm above TA insertion.
- *Over posterior tuberosity of calcaneum:* Tender swelling in retrocalcaneal bursitis.

Medial

- Medial malleolus and subcutaneous border of tibia
- Head of talus (by eversion of foot)
- *Navicular tuberosity:* Tender swelling seen in accessory navicular
- Tendons of FHL, FDL, and TP
- Tinel's signs over posterior tibial nerve and medial and lateral plantar nerves.

Plantar

- *Callosities:* Tender
- Sesamoids for tenderness
- *Plantar fascia:* Tenderness at calcaneal attachment in fasciitis, tenderness on hyperextending toes, and painful nodules
- *Plantar fat pad:* Tenderness.

Range of Motion

Ankle: Dorsiflexion (normal 20°) and plantar flexion (normal is 50°)—tested with forefoot in inversion and hindfoot neutral. Leg is held with one hand and foot is grasped such that head of talus is gripped in hand to exclude any movement at the subtalar and midtarsal joints. If there is equinus deformity, assess passive dorsiflexion with knee extended and flexed. *(In isolated gastrocnemius contracture, more dorsiflexion is possible with knee flexed as it relaxes muscle arising above knee. In isolated soleus contracture, knee position does not affect range of dorsiflexion. If both muscles are involved, slight increase in passive dorsiflexion is noted with knee flexed but still it is not within normal range).*

Subtalar joint: Inversion (normal is 40°) and eversion (normal is 20°). Examined with patient prone (hold dorsum of foot with one hand such that head of talus is stabilized between thumb and index, hold calcaneum with thumb and index of other hand and perform movements).

Forefoot: Abduction and adduction (normal is jog). With calcaneum stabilized in neutral position.

Great Toe: Extension (normal is 70°) and flexion (normal is 45°) at MCP joint. Flexion (90°) and extension (0°—neutral) at IP joint.

Lesser toes: Flexion and extension (normal is 40°) at IP joint and at MCP joint (40° and 0°, respectively). Also test for adduction (movement towards 2nd toe) and abduction of toes.

Test for muscles individually:
- Grossly ankle plantar flexors are tested by toe walking.
- Ankle dorsiflexors by heel walking.
- Evertors by walking on medial border.
- Invertors by walking on lateral border.

Measurements

- *Longitudinal:* True and apparent length of whole limb, heel length (from tip of medial malleolus vertically down to point of heel), foot length both medial (back of heel to tip of great toe), and lateral (back of heel to tip of 5th toe).
- *Circumferential:* At thigh, calf and foot (at height of medial longitudinal arch).

- Broadening of ankle seen with calipers is seen in inferior tibiofibular diastasis.

Distal neurovascular deficit:
- Palpate for anterior tibial (in between tendons of EHL and EDL), dorsalis pedis, and posterior tibial (behind FDL 1 fingerbreadth behind medial malleolus) arteries.
- Complete neurological examination of lower limb.
- *Sensory examination:* Sural (lateral border of foot and ankle), deep peroneal (1st web space), superficial peroneal (dorsum of foot), saphenous (medial leg), posterior tibial (plantar aspect of heel), and digital nerves (adjacent sides of interspace).

Lymphadenopathy: Inguinal and popliteal.

Special tests: (All done with leg hanging freely at edge of table).
- *Anterior drawer test:* Grasp just above ankle with one hand and hold heel with the other. Gently pull heel forward with an internal rotatory movement to foot. Observe for amount of anterior translation and prominence of talar head anterolaterally. Difference of 3–5 mm in laxity between two sides with a soft end point or skin tenting anterolaterally by talar dome is significant. It tests anterior talofibular ligament.
- *Inversion stress test (varus stress)* **(Fig. 5):** It tests calcaneofibular ligament. Maximally dorsiflex ankle and apply inversion

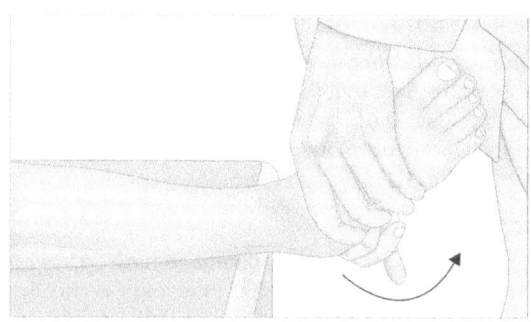

Fig. 5: Inversion stress test.

stress to calcaneus. Abnormal inversion of talus at ankle (not movement at subtalar joint) compared to opposite side is significant (no definite numeric criteria).

- *Peroneal tendon instability test:* Rotate ankle from maximal dorsiflexion to eversion to plantar flexion to inversion. Palpate posterior to lateral malleolus. If peroneal tendons subluxate or dislocate anterior to malleolus, suggests instability.
- *Thomson's test*
- *O'Brien's needle test*
- *First metatarsal rise test:* Done for tibialis posterior tendon. Patient is made to stand. From patient's behind, rotate leg into external rotation. If 1st metatarsal rises off ground, it suggests tibialis posterior insufficiency. Normally, it remains in contact with ground (The test can also be performed in other way—rose test: on dorsiflexing great toe, tibia rotates externally).
- *Morton's test:* Compress 1st and 5th metatarsal heads together. If a neuroma is present, he will complain of pain in affected interspace.
- *Homan's test **(Fig. 6)**:* Pain in calf on passive dorsiflexion of ankle suggests DVT.

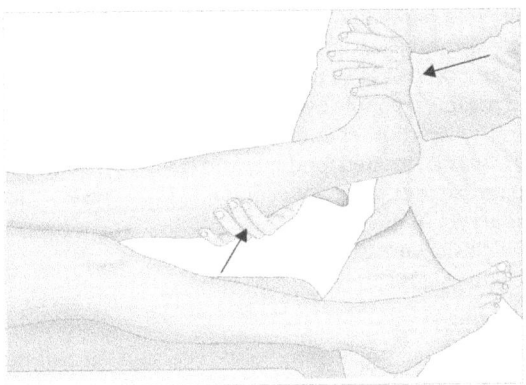

Fig. 6: Eliciting Homan's sign.

- Pain behind heel on toe walking suggests pre-Achilles bursitis and on heel walking suggests post-Achilles bursitis. Pain on both suggests Achilles tendonitis.

CASE I: CONGENITAL TALIPES (LATIN—TALUS = ANKLE; PES = FOOT) EQUINOVARUS

The diagnosis is quite evident however, one will be judged based on the ability to distinguish it from paralytic conditions at least theoretically and clarity of approach towards management.

Read: 4-6 times (MS and DNB candidates).

Diagnosis: The patient is a 4-year-old male child with idiopathic neglected clubfoot deformity of both feet without any associated spinal dysraphism or syndromic association. [It is expected that the candidate looks for and includes associations of CTEV in diagnosis if found like—DDH, radioulnar synostosis, undescended testis, cleft lip/palate, syndactyly/polydactyly, constriction bands, etc. (see below for various syndromes)].

FINDINGS

Foot

- Small foot; stretched thin skin on dorsolateral aspect and thrown into creases along the medial aspect
- Scars and callosities (if patient is ambulatory)
- Head of talus palpable over foot
- Lateral convex border and medial concavity with furrows
- Heel ("small") rotated medially and drawn up (empty heel) with deep crease over posterior aspect
- *Ancillary findings:*
  - Extrinsic/intrinsic type
  - Genu valgum.

Gait: "Stumbling" gait.

ROM: Ankle, knee, inversion, and eversion at subtalar joint. Other examination (a very important question—what else would you like to examine?):
- Hip for DDH
- Spine for dysraphism (meningomyelocele)

Foot and Ankle

- Cerebral palsy
- Arthrogryposis multiplex congenita (AMC)
- Polio—tight ITB (always check)
- Cleft lip, palate, exomphalos, and congenital hernia
- Sensation of foot
- Examine the power of gluteus maximus and quadriceps femoris in particular as weakness of above can lead to compensatory equinus at ankle.

Differential diagnosis: Congenital dislocation of ankle and tibial hemimelia.

1. Why do you call it congenital?

Ans. The deformity is present since birth and following points in **Table 1** should help you answer this question better.

Table 1: Difference between congenital clubfoot and acquired clubfoot.	
Congenital clubfoot	*Acquired clubfoot*
Deformity since birth	Naipe
Bilateral (≈50%), 70% male	Naipe
Deep medial crease commonly present	Naipe
Small and wider foot	Often not
"Absent" heel	Maintained heel
Atrophied calf with cylindrical leg	General lower limb involvement with calf maintaining shape
Internal tibial torsion present	Not present unless grossly neglected for long
Other congenital abnormalities may be present	Typical cause for deformity is evident
Neurological examination normal	Motor/sensory/combined deficit
Achilles attached medially	Not so (*Naipe*)

2. What are the causes of acquired clubfoot?

Ans. Acquired deformity is seen in patients with cerebral palsy, postburn contractures, postpolio residual paralysis,

VIC of calf muscles (say after snake bite), leprosy, and post-traumatic foot deformity.

3. Is congenital form always idiopathic?

Ans. No, the idiopathic form is the most common form of CTEV but it can also be seen with AMC (arthrogryposis multiplex congenita), spinal dysraphism, syndromic (see below), and cerebral palsy.

4. What are the deformities in clubfoot?

Ans. CTEV is a deformity in which foot is turned inwards to varying degrees with *[more precise but clinically impractical definition is—rotatory subluxation of talocalcaneonavicular joint complex (otherwise called subtalar complex) with talus in plantar flexion and subtalar complex in medial rotation and inversion]*:

- Equinus at ankle
- Varus and internal rotation of heel (*varus of heel is equivalent to inversion at subtalar joint*)
- Forefoot adduction with supination
- Cavus of midfoot
- Internal torsion of tibia (*this is controversial and probably secondary deformity—better avoid it unless pressed to answer*)
- Other:
  - Atrophy of calves and smaller circumference than other side
  - Smaller foot.

[Please note that first three typically describe CTEV (Q: thence should be—what comprises CTEV) however if you are asked a specific question like deformities in clubfoot then answer all of above]

Le Noir's proposed joint malalignment as the cause of deformities (ankle equinus, subtalar inversion, Chopart and Lisfranc adduction).

5. Is there any difference in deformities between congenital and acquired forms?

Ans. Yes, in congenital forms varus component of deformity is most prominent while in acquired form equinus is more evident.

6. How do you look for equinus, heel varus, and adduction deformities?

Ans. The evaluation of deformities appears arbitrary in most of the texts. I am presenting the concepts from standard protocol podiatric examination that should be acceptable to many.

Heel varus (frontal plane alignment of calcaneum): Normal alignment of calcaneus is neutral—the line of attachment of tendo-Achilles to center of heel is perpendicular to horizontal reference line. Look at the foot of child (preferably making him stand on ground) from behind. Assess the alignment as above. If the line is directed inwards then it indicates heel varus (*Note: Heel varus/valgus is same as heel inversion/eversion*).

Supination of foot: While observing the foot from behind, two curved depressions concave outwards are obvious above and below the lateral malleolus. These curves are symmetrical in a normal foot. If the curve below the lateral malleolus is shallow/flat/convex outwards then it indicates supinated foot. Similarly exaggeration of curve indicates pronated foot.

Equinus: If patient is able to stand then make him stand on ground with knee in extension otherwise passively dorsiflex the foot to maximum possible. A normal patient will stand with plantigrade foot (ball of great toe and heel simultaneously touching the ground). In equinus deformity the patient will not be able to touch the heel or the heel and great toe ball are not in the same horizontal plane. For quantification measure the distance between center of heel and great toe, else measure the angle foot makes with perpendicular to long axis of foot. [Grading (*subjective I—cannot walk on heel, II—smaller heel with appearance of cavus, III—splaying of forefoot with exaggeration of II, and IV—clawing of toes with III*).]

Forefoot adduction: While examining from behind, heel masks quite a substantial amount of foot (in front) and barely great (medial) and little (lateral) toe prominence are observable, which are equal on medial and lateral aspects.

In forefoot adduction great toe is very prominently seen in totality and lateral aspect is empty.

Cavus: Observe both the medial longitudinal arch height and curve congruence. In pes cavus the arch becomes high and is acutely curved up posteriorly. One can measure the distance of floor to apex of arch to quantify the same. To make cavus more prominent one can ask the patient to stand on toes. (Cavus is exaggerated due to windlass effect—whereby due to forced dorsiflexion of MTP joint the plantar fascia is stretched.)

To get an understanding of foot scoring one should read the FPI (foot posture index)—which is graded from −12 to +12. The relevance to CTEV is not there, but the basics of observation can be understood.

7. What is supination and pronation of foot?

Ans. *Supination is a combination of:*
- Adduction at fore foot
- Internal rotation and plantar flexion at ankle
- Inversion at subtalar joint
- Medial arch elevation.

Pronation is a combination of:
- Forefoot abduction
- Hindfoot eversion
- Dorsi flexion at ankle
- Depression at medial arch.

8. What is meant if equinus at ankle corrects with knee flexion but appears on extension?

Ans. It implies that the contracture is in the gastrocnemius component of gastrocsoleus complex. If there is partial correction then either there is additional ankle stiffness or soleus contracture of lesser magnitude than that of gastrocnemius.

9. Can you tell the etiology of idiopathic CTEV?

Ans. *Still elusive!* Some theories are as follows:
- *Intrauterine packaging defect:* (Excessive packing—primi; large baby; and oligohydramnios)

Foot and Ankle

- *Neuromuscular defect (Isaacs):* Spina bifida; AMC
- Fetal developmental arrest in fibular stage (Bohm)
- Germ-plasm defect (manufacturing defect)
- *Defective cartilage enlarge of talus* (Irani Sterman)
- Retracting fibrosis "Crimp" (Ippolito and Ponseti)
- Anomalous tendon insertion (Inclan)
- Myoblast in medial fascia (Zimny et al.)
- *Heredity:* Polygenic multifactorial trait—1:35 chances if sibling affected; 1:3 if other twin affected. Deletion of chromosome 2 (2q 31-33) related to *CASP10* gene (Heck et al.), and Edward's syndrome
- *Infective pathogens (Carney et al.):* Enteroviruses—conflicting evidence
- Electromagnetic radiation and toxins (maternal and/or paternal smoking, drugs, "ecstasy" use during pregnancy)
- Amniocentesis has been considered to increase chances of clubfoot deformity
- *Vascular theory:* Absent anterior tibial artery in patients or posterior tibial artery in parents.

(I agree it is too much; and is always bad—to pass in exam concentrate and learn other things rather than wasting time to learn all of these—same for next Q)

10. What syndromes are associated with CTEV?
Ans.
- AMC
- Streeter's dysplasia
- Prune belly syndrome
- Tibial hemimelia
- Mobius syndrome
- Freeman-Sheldon syndrome (whistling face)
- Diastrophic dwarfism
- Larsen syndrome
- Down syndrome
- Opitz syndrome
- Pierre Robin syndrome
- Fetal alcohol syndrome.

11. What are types of clubfoot?

Ans. Unexpected question! If asked at all:

Remember—primary (idiopathic) and secondary types (muscular type—AMC; osseous type—tibial hemimelia; neuromuscular; CP, polio, trauma, etc.) are actually "varieties" of clubfoot.

Clinical types (Kawashima and Uhtoff 1990) are given in **Table 2**.

Other types for severity classification viz. nonrigid/rigid/teratologic and Goldner's subtypes are better unmentioned as they are not standardized and hardly used.

	Table 2: Clinical types of clubfoot.	
	Type I (Extrinsic/Nonrigid)	**Type II (Intrinsic/Rigid) (Fig. 7)**
Foot	Normal size; mild varus, medial and lateral border of foot are only slightly deviated	Smaller; marked varus, medial border is very concave while lateral border is convex
Heel	Normal size can be brought down with ease; minimal varus	Small; elevated; cannot be brought down with ease; marked varus
Creases	Normal	Deep medial, posterior and plantar creases(s)
Telescopy	Absent	Present
Calf muscles	Muscles are not much atrophied	Atrophied cord like wiry muscles
Foot palpation	<ul><li>Talar head not palpable</li><li>Rare callosities if at all</li><li>Distance between navicular and medial malleolus is appreciable</li></ul>	<ul><li>Talar head is prominent and palpable</li><li>Callosities common</li><li>Navicular and medial malleolus appear touching due to deformity and there is minimal gap if at all</li></ul>

Foot and Ankle

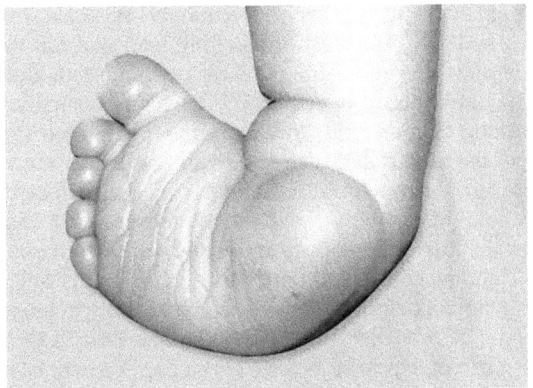

Fig. 7: Rigid clubfoot.

12. What are the aims of treatment?

Ans. Aim is to obtain a pain free, supple, and plantigrade foot with good function and cosmesis that does not require any special footwear for ambulation.

Objectives of correction are to correct the deformity early, correct deformity fully, and develop the muscle power of the limb sufficiently to maintain correction.

13. What is the manipulative correction technique for clubfoot?

Ans. There "are" two popular manipulative techniques using POP cast:
 1. Kite and Lovell's
 2. Ponseti's.

It is just a matter of preference and comfort as to who uses which one! (I would prefer 2 in practice and especially exams!)

The third one uses adhesive tapes for maintaining reduction after manipulation—Dimeglio/Bansahel modified French technique.

14. What is Kite's manipulative correction of clubfoot?

Ans. Generally described as sequential correction of deformities in the order adduction of forefoot → inversion at subtalar joint → varus at heel → equinus at ankle (remember A→I→V→E). However, if carefully read and followed kite's method also did simultaneous correction of deformities. The correction was achieved by pushing navicular laterally putting counter pressure at calcaneocuboid joint. The forefoot is grasped and distracted with the same hand pushing the navicular while the hand giving counter at calcaneocuboid joint holds the heel. Whatever most importantly get the forefoot deformity corrected so that it points outward 20° followed by hindfoot deformity which is key stone to function of deformed foot and must be brought into a vertical plane *before* correcting ankle equinus. (Why?) Dorsiflexion to correct equinus before correcting inversion locks the subtalar joint decreasing the chances of further correction and the foot may break in midfoot region!—Rocker bottom deformity.

15. When to begin?

Ans. Day "1": Manipulation by mother. Thumb rests on talus and press forefoot into abduction repeat at least six times in a day. Correction achieved around talus (*Talus is least displaced but most deformed bone*). *Do not try to untwist the foot*—it increases cavus. As soon as possible begin POP cast correction according to institutional policy serial weekly/fortnightly casting in manipulated position.

Nowadays, with frequent use of ultrasonography the deformity can be identified in utero at 18–20 weeks of gestation (TEV foot at 9–10 weeks corrects to normal by 18th week), so parents can be counseled for manipulative correction pre-emptively.

16. What defines the end of treatment?
Ans.
- No adduction/inversion deformity
- Hollow on dorsum of foot previously occupied by talar head
- Passive movement to full calcaneovalgus position
- Child is able to evert and dorsiflex foot voluntarily to about right angle
- "Squat test".

17. What is Ponseti method of correction of clubfoot?

Ans. *1st phase:* Manipulative casting technique to simultaneously correct the deformities beginning from pronation and correcting equinus in end **(Fig. 8)**. The concept of this technique is relaxation of collagen and atraumatic remodeling of joint surfaces. Simultaneous correction is achieved at talonavicular, calcaneocuboid, and talocalcaneal joints. To begin, the "pronation twist" is corrected by supinating the forefoot to bring it in alignment with hindfoot. The tarsal bones distal to talus are then abducted in *supinated foot* so that navicular comes in front of talus and cuboid in front of calcaneous and calcaneous glides below talus into corrected position. Remember foot is not pronated (sort of untwisting) rather correction is achieved simultaneously by moving Lisfranc joint (tarsometatarsal), naviculocuneiform joint, Chopart joint (midtarsal), and subtalar joint by above technique of abduction in foot in supination and equinus (using talar head as fulcrum) **(Fig. 9)**. Above knee casts are applied every 5–7 days. A total of about 70° of abduction is achieved before last cast is applied. Equinus is corrected at the end. Percutaneous Achilles tenotomy is done just before

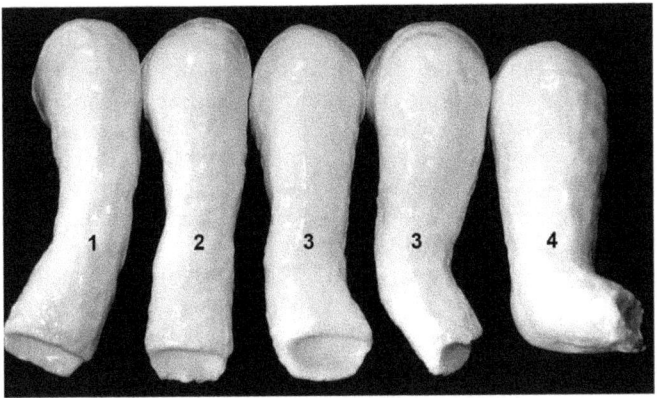

Fig. 8: Ponseti corrective casts for manipulative correction of foot deformity.

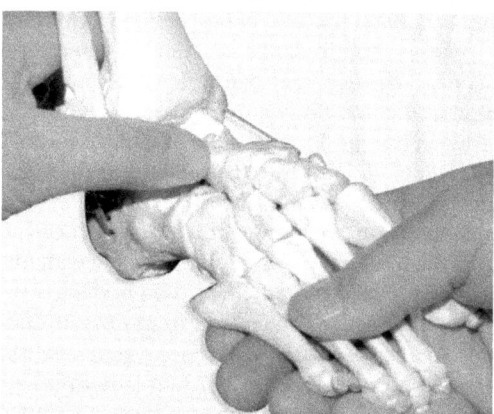

Fig. 9: The reduction and correction of deformities is attempted around the talus using its head as fulcrum.

the application of last cast that heals in about 3 weeks. This is followed by physiotherapy and immobilization of foot in POP cast in corrected position (Pirani et al.).

2nd phase (maintenance): To prevent relapse correction is maintained in foot abduction bar (3 months following manipulation 14–16 hours a day in "night and naps" till 3 years or as accessed by physician) with feet in 70° abduction and 15° dorsiflexion (without Dennis-Browne plates). For unilateral deformity keep normal foot in 30° outward rotation and neutral dorsiflexion.

Some say that the order of correction of deformities in Ponseti is C (cavus) → A (adduction) → V (varus) → E (equinus), but the method originally described corrected all of them simultaneously (after correcting pronation twist); even equinus which if residual was corrected with tenotomy.

18. What is accelerated Ponseti protocol?

Ans. Here casts are applied at 5 days interval and there is low threshold for Achilles tenotomy.

Foot and Ankle

19. What is Kite's error?

Ans. Kite considered that the forefoot is in absolute adduction and emphasized that lateral deviation (abduction) of forefoot by putting pressure on calcaneocuboid joint (fulcrum) laterally holding the heel will correct adduction deformity (Kite's error—this prevented abduction of calcaneum which is in adduction). However, actually the whole foot is in adduction with forefoot in relatively more adduction than hindfoot. This error was rectified in Ponseti method of manipulative correction where simultaneous abduction is done at Lisfranc, calcaneonavicular, Chopart line, and subtalar joint laterally putting pressure at talus head without touching heel. Total of 70° abduction is thus achieved.

Also heel varus does not correct by everting calcaneum, he did not realize that calcaneum will not evert if not laterally rotated.

The other mistake was application of below-knee casts that would leave the gastrocsoleus complex uninhibited that would prevent correction of equinus deformity.

20. What are the advantages of Ponseti method of correction?

Ans. The Ponseti method is favored by most of the surgeons because:

- It is more acceptable due to reduced number of cast and manipulation settings—reduces treatment cost also.
- Results are consistent and progress measurable on developed scores. More so specific guidelines are available as to further progress of treatment in case the correction is slow to achieve or fails to progress after a while.
- Less recurrence and high rate of correction by manipulation.
- Rate of surgical treatment is very less and mostly is in the form of tenotomy, major surgical correction is required in less than 2%.
- Being easy to practice it can be used to train internists, physiotherapists, and nonorthopedic faculty practicing in remote regions to provide correction.

21. **What is the basis of Ponseti method of correction of deformity? Or how is it possible to achieve stable correction in a deformed foot? Or why the deformity does not recur after stable correction?**

Ans. The Ponseti deformity correction realizes benefit from abnormal type of collagen found in these patients. The collagen is unusually cellular and has wavy architecture (crimps) when looked under microscope. This wavy structure allows correction by stretching and ability to correct the deformity. Surprisingly it has been found that once the "slack" (crimp) is stretched out in plaster it reappears after 5–7 days allowing further correction of deformity. With sequential POP casts the newly formed soft tissue and collagen provide stable foot in corrected position and does not spring back as the collagen remodels in corrected position.

22. **How do you apply casts?**

Ans. 2" roll for age <2 months and 3" rolls for age >2 months. Use eversion tug principle and apply snugly fitting cast with only sufficient cotton (not overstuffing cotton which presses out with time losing correction). Cast should not show your fingers and should be smooth enough. Casts should be applied up to groin with knee in 90° flexion to relax gastrocsoleus complex and aid in equinus correction also it prevents cast from slipping out.

23. **Can you use any other method?**

Ans. "Strapping/taping" in circumstances where cast correction is difficult/impossible viz. premature infant with multiple anomalies, monitored infant in intensive care—feet required for blood sampling or IV drug infusions.

The Bansahel/Dimeglio modified French technique especially uses adhesive tapes that are used to temporarily immobilize the foot following manipulation by skilled physiotherapist for 30 minutes. This is followed by continuous passive motion during sleep. The technique is practiced daily for 2–3 months followed by alternate day manipulation; while continuing strapping till ambulation. The technique

Foot and Ankle

is quite labor intensive (physiotherapist is needed daily) and engaging for the family. The cost run is quite high and rate of surgery still exceeds 40%.

24. What is spurious correction?

Ans. Apparent correction without actual correction or development of unrelated deformities due to faulty manipulation:
- Rocker bottom foot
- Bean-shaped foot
- Skewed foot
- Fractures
- Flat top talus.

25. How will you manage this patient?

Ans. I will get a true AP and lateral X-ray done to confirm diagnosis and for scoring foot (viz. Dimeglio scoring and classification). AP: Talocalcaneal angle = 20–50° (normal), CTEV <20°; tarso-1st metatarsal angle—up to 30° valgus, varus angulation is seen in CTEV. Lateral: Talocalcaneal angle = 25–50°, <25° in CTEV.

Radiographic assessment is feasible and advised for neglected clubfoot (take weight-bearing radiographs); however, in infants the radiographs are difficult to assess and mostly do not guide treatment.

I will correct the foot by Ponseti method of manipulative cast correction. Score foot by Pirani scoring **(Fig. 10)**:

Scores six clinical signs (A, B, C, D, E, F)

0—normal

0.5—moderately abnormal

1—severely abnormal

Midfoot score (MS): Three signs comprise the MS, grading the amount of midfoot deformity between 0 and 3.
1. Curved lateral border [A]
2. Medial crease [B]
3. Talar head coverage [C]

Hindfoot score (HS): Three signs comprise the HS, grading the amount of hindfoot deformity between 0 and 3.
1. Posterior crease [D]

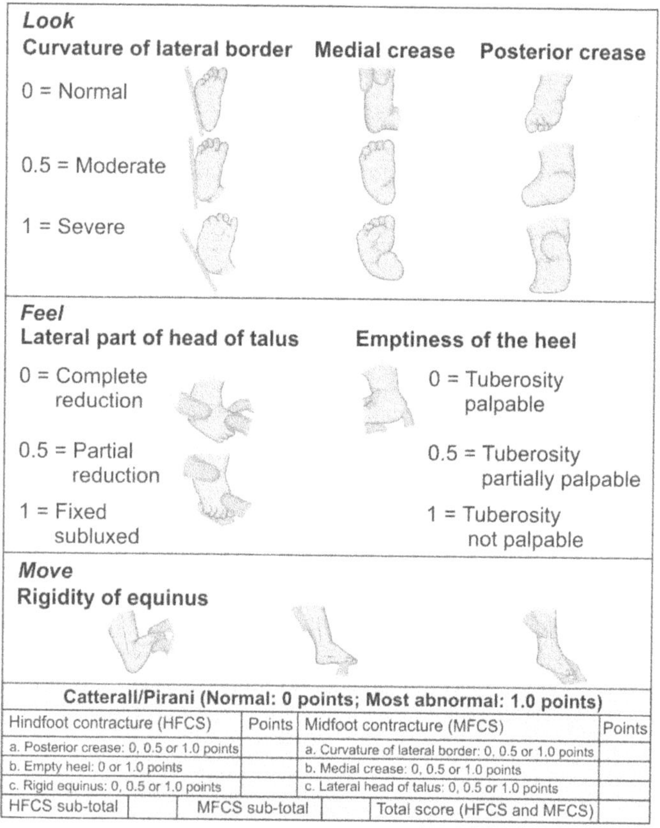

Look

Curvature of lateral border **Medial crease** **Posterior crease**

0 = Normal

0.5 = Moderate

1 = Severe

Feel

Lateral part of head of talus

0 = Complete reduction

0.5 = Partial reduction

1 = Fixed subluxed

Emptiness of the heel

0 = Tuberosity palpable

0.5 = Tuberosity partially palpable

1 = Tuberosity not palpable

Move

Rigidity of equinus

Catterall/Pirani (Normal: 0 points; Most abnormal: 1.0 points)

Hindfoot contracture (HFCS)	Points	Midfoot contracture (MFCS)	Points
a. Posterior crease: 0, 0.5 or 1.0 points		a. Curvature of lateral border: 0, 0.5 or 1.0 points	
b. Empty heel: 0 or 1.0 points		b. Medial crease: 0, 0.5 or 1.0 points	
c. Rigid equinus: 0, 0.5 or 1.0 points		c. Lateral head of talus: 0, 0.5 or 1.0 points	
HFCS sub-total	MFCS sub-total	Total score (HFCS and MFCS)	

Fig. 10: The Pirani score card.

2. Rigid equinus [E]
3. Empty heel [F]

Tenotomy will be done if HS > 1 and MS < 1 and head of talus is covered.

Treat as above and plot score on graph—roadmap of Ponseti treatment.

If deformity not corrected then soft-tissue release will be required.

Foot and Ankle

26. What is soft-tissue release for clubfoot?

Ans. Indications include: Neglected clubfoot (<4 years), resistant clubfoot or deformity(ies), and relapse/residual deformities.

Very infrequently required for Ponseti method of correction of clubfoot. Residual or resistant deformities can be corrected by specific releases (most commonly posterior for equinus).

Various releases are described for clubfoot and include posterior release, posteromedial release, extensile posteromedial release, combined posteromedial and posterolateral release, complete subtalar release, etc. Timing of release is an issue. French do release within few weeks to months of age capitalizing on the remodeling potential of growing foot. Turco; however, considers adequate time to be 1–2 years as the anatomical details are clear, under-overcorrection are not magnified as foot grows, better somatotypic assessment can be done and correction is maintained by ambulatory child. Simon's considers 8 cm as good criteria and not age.

Soft-tissue release must address all pathoanatomic structures:

Turco described one stage posteromedial release. Carol emphasized plantar fascial release and calcaneocuboid joint osteotomy as forefoot adduction and supination were not addressed by Turco. Goldner emphasized on correction of talar rotation by complete release of tibiotalar joint leaving subtalar joint to prevent valgus overcorrection. McKay and Simons described "complete subtalar release" which was actually a peritalar release with release of interosseous ligament and talonavicular and calcaneocuboid joints.

Posterior release only for persistent equinus; full posteromedial plantar and lateral release if all deformities persist.

27. What structures do you release in posteromedial soft-tissue release (PMSTR) of McKay (modified)?

Ans. *Incisions:*
- *Turco's:* Hockey stick posteromedial incision
- *Cincinnati:* Circumferential incision
- *Caroll's two incision technique:* Posteromedial and a small lateral incision over subtalar joint.

Medial release:
- Posterior and medial subtalar joint capsule (preserve interosseous ligament)
- Talonavicular joint capsule
- Spring ligament
- Y-ligament
- Medial calcaneocuboid joint capsule
- Knot of henry
- Abductor hallucis
- Lengthening of posterior tibial tendon, FHL, and FDL
- Plantar fascia, quadrates plantae origin

Posterior release:
- Ankle joint capsule
- Subtalar joint capsule
- Achilles tendon Z-lengthening
- Posterior talofibular ligament

Lateral release:
- Lateral subtalar joint capsule
- Peroneal tendon sheath
- Calcaneofibular ligament
- Lateral talocalcaneal ligament
- Extensor digitorum brevis origin, calcaneocuboid ligament, inferior extensor retinaculum, and cubonavicular ligament may be released in resistant cases.

Structures preserved: Dorsal structures, medial neurovascular bundle, deep deltoid ligament, and interosseous ligament.

Talonavicular joint with subtalar joint is often fixed with smooth K-wires.

28. What are the complications of operative treatment?
Ans.

- Neurovascular damage, bony damage, physeal damage, and wound dehiscence
- *Undercorrection:* Most commonly due to inadequate postoperative maintenance
  - Equinus
  - Heel varus

Foot and Ankle

- Forefoot adduction
- Cavus.
- *Overcorrection:*
  - *Valgus overcorrection:* Caused by cutting interosseous ligament/aggressive casting. Treatment requires medial column shortening and lateral column lengthening and medial translation of talus
  - Forefoot abduction
  - Calcaneus deformity
  - Pes planus.
- *Skew foot:* Forefoot adduction and hind foot valgus
- AVN talus/navicular
- Sinus tarsi syndrome
- *Dorsal navicular subluxation:* Produces a short cavovarus foot. Caused due to incomplete release or loss of talonavicular reduction. Treat by midfoot release with repeated plantar release and TA lengthening.
- *Dorsal bunion (hallux flexus):* Occurs due to loss of depressing strength of peroneus longs on 1st metatarsal as compared to dorsal long and short toe flexors with weak plantar flexion. Treat by 1st ray realignment and dorsal FHB transfer as toe extensor with MTP joint release.

29. What do you understand by terms neglected, resistant, recurrent, and relapsed clubfoot?

Ans. *Neglected clubfoot:* When the patient does not receive treatment (conservative/operative) by walking age—typically 9 months.

Recurrent clubfoot: When one or many or all deformities recur "during" the course of treatment—typically during manipulative correction, which was/were successfully corrected previously.

Relapsed clubfoot: When one or many or all deformities recur after successfully achieving correction of all deformities, i.e. after end of treatment.

Resistant clubfoot: Better called persistent clubfoot—when correction is not obtained in any or all of the deformities by manipulation/surgical methods (commonly due to inappropriate technique).

Untreated clubfoot: When the child has not received any treatment till date, this includes neglected clubfoot.

Incompletely treated clubfoot: This term is used for patients who stop treatment at any stage during treatment (say during manipulative correction or even later during maintenance phase).

Most common *persistent deformities* are forefoot adduction and supination whereas true *recurrent deformity* is most commonly equinus.

30. What is the role of tendon transfer in clubfoot?

Ans. Indicated for poor foot positioning during walk or excessive inter foot progression angle or muscle imbalance. Commonly done either to correct evertor insufficiency or triceps surae insufficiency. Minimum age for tendon transfer is 5 years.

Anterior tibial tendon transfer: Done for dynamic inversion/supination of midfoot when there is "relative" evertor insufficiency and patient bears weight on lateral aspect of foot. *Split type (SPLATT—split anterior tibialis transfer)*: Lateral arm rerouted from retinaculum subcutaneously to cuboid or lateral cuneiform. *Entire tendon*: Inserted just lateral to midline in a comfortable tarsal bone—provides dorsiflexion and eversion without excessive abduction (power lost by 1 grade).

Transfer for calcaneous gait (triceps surae insufficiency): Overlengthening of TA is best prevented than treated—diagnose as early as possible. Peronei, tibialis posterior (TP) or long toe flexors can be used. Peroneus brevis split and rerouted into calcaneal tuberosity with tenodesis of distal stump to longus to prevent evertor insufficiency. Tibial anterior transfer is not recommended as it leads to dorsiflexion paralysis and high stepping gait.

31. What is the role of bony procedures and when will you do them?

Ans. Please note that algorithms may differ from person to person. Simplified versions of different bony procedures for different deformities are given in **Table 3**.

Table 3: Different bony procedures for different deformities.

Deformity	Age	Treatment
Metatarsus adductus	>5 years	Metatarsal osteotomy
Hindfoot varus	<2–3 years	Mod McKay procedure
	3–10 years	Dwyer osteotomy (heel varus) Dillwyn-Evans (if medial column is short) Lichtblau (if lateral column is long)
	10–12 years	Triple arthrodesis
Equinus		Posterior release (mild-moderate deformity) Lambrinudi procedure (severe deformity) Excision of a portion of talar head/navicular Distal tibial dorsiflexion osteotomy (salvage)
Cavus	>6 years	Japas V osteotomy Akron midtarsal osteotomy (dome osteotomy) Transmidtarsal osteotomy (Köse et al.)
All three deformities	>10 years	Triple arthrodesis
Persistent intoeing gait	If persists for >2 years	For a and b—supramalleolar
a. True internal tibial intorsion	Following correction	osteotomy just proximal to distal tibial physis correcting 35° external rotation
b. Medial spin of hind-foot in ankle mortise		For c – Evans/Lichtblau
c. Medial deviation of forefoot due to talar neck deviation		

Contd…

Contd...

Deformity	Age	Treatment
Neglected clubfoot or secondary clubfoot	Cuneiform tarsectomy	Adult patients
	Adult patients	Patients with myelomeningocele can be modified for patients with severe, resistant idiopathic clubfoot
	Wedge tarsectomy	▪ Hardly ever done ▪ Neglected clubfoot 8–11 years. Remove dorsolateral based wedge

Principles and brief description:
- Older the patient more likely is the need for combined procedure
- 2–3 years are good candidate for modified McKay procedure
- >5 years (some say >4 years) almost always require corrective osteotomies.

Dwyer osteotomy: Originally a medial opening wedge (taken from tibia) osteotomy—may increase equinus.

Modified to lateral closing wedge osteotomy that reduces wound healing problems, equinus, improves chances of union. Overall advantages preserve subtalar motion, do not hinder with future procedure and can be combined with other procedure.

Dillwyn-Evans (lateral column shortening): Originally a 4-stage procedure (first 3—soft-tissue releases and 4th one—calcaneocuboid fusion after partial excision). Now done in single stage, may produce hindfoot stiffness in long run.

Lichtblau procedure (lateral column shortening): Essentially a calcaneocuboid arthroplasty (preferred for a too long lateral column). Excise distal part of anterior calcaneal process or take wedge from calcaneum—creating calcaneocuboid pseudarthrosis. Less stiffness.

Foot and Ankle

Triple arthrodesis: May be done as two stages (↑ bone resection but ↑ chances of AVN) or a single stage procedure (↓ AVN). Essentially a modified Lambrinudi type triple arthrodesis, here most of correction is done around calcaneus and not around talus (as in Lambrinudi). Aimed to correct deformity and maintain (>10 years), it is the ultimate salvage procedure. Can be used for neglected clubfoot and varus/valgus overcorrected foot. Crucial not to undercorrect—slight valgus and pronation is favored. Most difficult joint to fuse is talonavicular joint as stresses are concentrated at this joint and mobility is marked.

32. What is JESS fixator?

Ans. Joshi's external stabilization system (JESS) developed by Dr BB Joshi (Mumbai). *Fractional, differential distraction* used to *sequentially* correct deformities. Distraction continued until approximately 20° of dorsiflexion and overcorrection of the forefoot deformities was achieved. Maintained in this overcorrected position for twice as long as the distraction phase by casts/braces. It may require soft-tissue release simultaneously or before fixator application.

33. What is the role of Ilizarov fixator?

Ans. Uses the principle of *distraction histogenesis* to differentially correct the deformities. Correction slows enough to protect soft tissues; correction at the focus of deformity, *simultaneous* three-dimensional, multilevel correction; deformity correction without shortening the foot. Can be applied even in patients with failed previous procedures.

34. Do you know of any other nonoperative treatment for clubfoot apart from Ponseti's?

Ans. Montpellier and Dimeglio method of adding continuous passive motion (CPM) during earliest portion of treatment (usually 1st month of life).

Botox (botulinum toxin) injection into tendo-Achilles.

35. What are characteristics of CTEV shoes?

Ans. Robert Jones shoes are pronation shoes that have:
- Straight inner border to prevent forefoot adduction with medial containment bar

- Outer shoe raise (outflare) to prevent foot inversion
- *No* heel (high counter) to prevent equinus.

They not only maintain correction and prevent relapse of deformities but may also correct mild residual deformities in a flexible foot.

36. Can you name some Indian authors associated with work in CTEV?

Ans.

- Dr RL Mittal—local rotational skin flap for neglected clubfoot and extensive soft-tissue release for posteromedial contracture
- Professor B Mukhopadhyaya—neglected clubfoot "Patna procedure"
- Professor Duriaswamy—(SJH—insulin injection) induction of CTEV in chick embryo
- Dr BB Joshi—JESS.

37. What is Dennis-Browne splint?

Ans. Better called Dennis-Browne bar also known as abduction bar **(Fig. 11)**. It consists of a metal (original) or a polypropylene bar with shoes attached to ends over foot plate (aluminum) rotated outwards of midline. The shoes are open-toe high top with straight medial border and the foot is strapped using adhesive tapes. Shoes are placed in 70° external rotation in bilateral cases while for unilateral cases

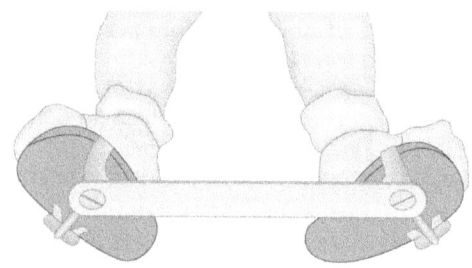

Fig. 11: Dennis-Browne bar with shoe.

Foot and Ankle

the clubfoot side is placed in 75° of external rotation and normal side in 45° external rotation. The bar should be of sufficient length that the feet are abducted equal to the level of shoulders.

Modified splints are made of polypropylene and are light; shoe is made of soft canvas with rigid medial border and is secured with Velcro straps. Problems with original splint were weight, pressure sores, injury to infants and parents and crib.

38. When do you start bracing and what is the schedule of wearing brace?

Ans. Brace is applied immediately after removal of last corrective cast. If tenotomy was done then this comes to around 3 weeks. The brace is worn full 24 hours in a day for 3 months followed by full night time wear and gradually reducing (2 hours every month) day wear to 4–6 hours so as to have a total of 12–14 hours wear in a day. Even when the child is ambulatory this schedule is followed till age of 4–5 years of age.

39. What is arthrogryposis multiplex congenita?

Ans. Arthrogryposis refers to a physical finding (not a diagnosis) of having joint contractures present at birth seen in large group of disorders. Arthrogryposis is defined as multiple congenital contractures affecting two or more areas of the body. The ill-propagated concept of AMC being myodystrophy is incorrect and both myopathic and neuropathic forms are commonly seen in equal frequency. This term finds varied uses as a noun to describe specific diseases [arthrogryposis multiplex congenita (AMC)], and as an adjective, "arthrogrypotic", to refer to rigid joint contractures. Some 65 distinct syndromes and 300 disorders can be grouped under the broad term "arthrogryposis" [conditions caused by environmental agents, single gene defects (autosomal dominant, autosomal recessive, and X-linked recessive), chromosomal abnormalities, known syndromes, or unknown conditions].

[Details on splints and manipulative cast schedule should be read from Chapter 31 of the book—Essential Orthopedics Principles and Practice, 2nd edition]

For further reading one may read Dimeglio classification.

CASE II: CONGENITAL VERTICAL TALUS

Diagnosis: The patient is a 1-year-old male child with bilateral rigid flatfoot most probably due to congenital vertical talus with foot size of 11 cm (medially and laterally) without any associated spinal or lower limb abnormality.

1. Why do you call it congenital vertical talus?
Ans. *History:*
- Deformity in foot present since birth (often noticed when patient starts to walk)
- Toeing out when walking
- Difficulty to fit shoes.

Examination:
- Severe uncorrectable equinovalgus deformity of hindfoot.
- Rocker bottom foot (loss of medial longitudinal arch with prominent rounded talar head as lowermost part of arch).
- Forefoot is abducted, pronated and dorsiflexed with fixed dorsal subluxation of navicular over talar head.
- Lateral toes are outward looking and everted.
- Soft tissues (tendons of tibialis anterior, long toe extensors, and 3 peronei) on dorsolateral side of foot are contracted.
- Deep creases inferior and lateral to lateral malleolus.
- Tendo-Achilles contracture.
- Callosities beneath anterior end of calcaneus and along medial border of foot superficial to talar head.
- Tendons of peroneus longus, brevis, and tibialis posterior are tight and may come to lie anterior to malleoli (acting as dorsiflexors rather than plantar flexors).

Essential components of deformity:
- Fixed equinus at ankle
- Fixed dorsal dislocation of navicular over talar head).

Foot and Ankle

Always additionally examine spine (for meningomyelocele and neurofibromatosis), hips and knees (equinovalgus may be compensatory to knee deformity).

2. What are the various differential diagnoses that you will consider?

Ans.
- Flexible flat foot
- Inflammatory and infective foot disorders
- Neurological like AMC and meningomyelocele
- *Compensatory:* Tight tendo-Achilles with/without equinus deformity and external rotational deformity of lower limb.

3. What will you do next?

Ans. I will do anterior and plantar flexion stress lateral views along with the routine PA and oblique projections.

4. What do you see on X-rays?

Ans. Calcaneum is in equinus. Talus points vertically downward with its long axis almost parallel to that of tibia. Navicular is dislocated dorsally over talar head **(Fig. 12)**.

In maximally plantarflexed (stress) view, navicular dislocation can be reduced in flexible flatfoot but not in congenital vertical talus (CVT). Talus remains vertical. Both talar—1st metatarsal angle and tibiotalar angle do not correct.

In maximally dorsiflexed (stress) view, equinus at calcaneum is fixed.

I will also measure the various angles as discussed here—angles:

Lateral view:
- Increased talocalcaneal angle
- Disrupted talar—1st metatarsal angle
- Line along long axis of talus and calcaneum passes inferior to cuboid (normally crosses cuboid).

AP view:
- Increased talar—1st metatarsal angle (shows marked forefoot abduction)
- Increased talocalcaneal angle.

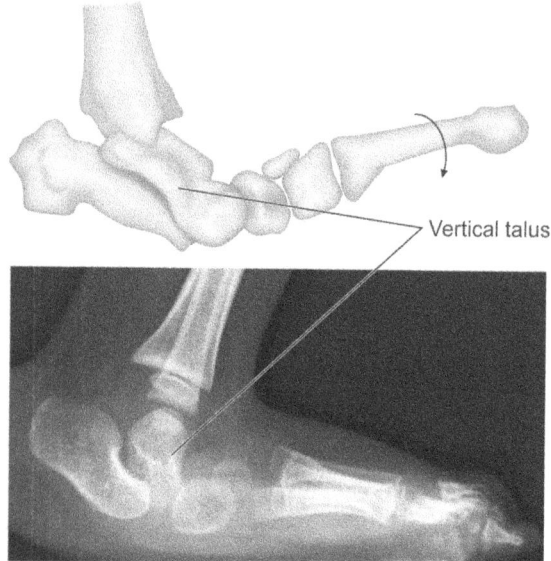

Fig. 12: Pictorial representation and lateral radiograph of patient with congenital vertical talus where the talus seems to be digging into mid tarsal joint and is vertically oriented nearly parallel to tibia. Calcaneum is also seen in equinus.

5. **Why do you use 1st metatarsal for angles and not navicular, though navicular is the one dislocated?**

Ans. Because navicular ossification center appears at 3 years. Till then 1st metatarsal is taken for calculation.

6. **What syndromes are associated with CVT?**

Ans.
- CDH, CDK, and CTEV of opposite foot
- Myelomeningocele, sacral agenesis, and caudal regression syndrome
- Spinal muscular atrophy
- Neurofibromatosis

- Trisomy 13–15, 18
- AMC
- Prune belly syndrome
- Marfan's syndrome
- Multiple pterygium syndrome.

7. How do you classify CVT?
Ans. *Lichtblau types:*
- *Teratogenic*: Associated with CDH, often bilateral with + family history, and very rigid deformities.
- *Neurogenic:* Myelomeningocele, neurofibromatosis—less rigid.
- *Acquired type:* Intrauterine malposition.

8. What is oblique talus?
Ans. Condition where all deformities are present but navicular can be reduced over talar head in plantar flexion.

9. How do you treat CVT?
Ans. In initial stages, serial corrective casts are applied. Aim is not to correct the deformities (which is impossible), but to make skin and soft-tissues supple. Forefoot is pulled into plantar flexion and inversion while calcaneus is dorsiflexed and heel cord stretched. Surgery is the definitive treatment.

10. When do you operate?
Ans. Surgery is to be done at the earliest possible time, preferably before 6 months of age.

11. What are the surgical modalities?
Ans. Modality used depends on age of presentation; however, the following four aspects are to be essentially followed:
1. Talonavicular joint reduction—the main aim
2. Tendo-Achilles lengthening with/without capsulotomy of ankle and subtalar joints. (Remember distal transverse cut in TA is made laterally in CVT because foot is in valgus while it is made medially in CTEV as foot is in varus.)
3. Long toe extensors (EHL, EDL, peroneus tertius, and tibialis anterior) lengthening with Z-plasty with calcaneocuboid reduction.
4. Dynamic sling of tibialis anterior through a drill hole in talar neck—to prevent plantar flexion.

Depending upon age the various modalities are:
- *1–4 years:* Open reduction and realignment of talonavicular, calcaneocuboid, and subtalar joints. Navicular excision, partial talectomy, and decancellation of tarsal bones may be required for reduction in children older than 3 years. Lateral column lengthening may need to be added to navicular excision.
- *4–8 years:* Open reduction (as above), soft-tissue release, and extra-articular (Grice-Green) subtalar arthrodesis. May use intra-articular arthrodesis with screw fixation (Dennyson-Fulford) as well. A gap of 6–8 weeks is usually given between release and arthrodesis. Some surgeons perform talonavicular reduction with subtalar bone-block in one stage followed 6–8 weeks later by posterior release and tibialis anterior sling.
- *More than 12 years:* Triple arthrodesis.

Open reduction can be done in single stage or two stages.

In one-stage surgery, use either Cincinnati incision or combined lateral (for tendo-Achilles and calcaneocuboid reduction) and medial incision (for talonavicular reduction).

[Kumar, Cowell and Ramsey technique uses 3 incisions, i.e. medial, lateral (over sinus tarsi), and posterior (for TA).] In two-stage surgery, 1st stage consists of dorsolateral release, i.e. reduce forefoot over midfoot. Second stage is posterolateral release, i.e. reduce midfoot over hindfoot.

Reduction is held with threaded K-wires across talonavicular and subtalar joints.

Attempt to reconstruct talonavicular ligament should be done. Long leg cast with knee flexed and joints reduced is applied for 2 months. Then wires are removed and another long leg cast is applied for 1 month. A short leg cast is continued for 1 more month after which an ankle-foot orthosis is applied for 3–6 months.

12. Which ligaments are released in the soft-tissue surgery?
Ans.
- Talonavicular capsule
- Tibionavicular ligament
- Interosseous talocalcaneal ligament and superficial part of deltoid ligament

- Calcaneocuboid
- Calcaneofibular
- Plantar calcaneonavicular (spring).

13. What are common complications of CVT?

Ans.
- AVN of talus—when operated
- Callosities in untreated/inadequately treated cases
- Residual feet pain.

CASE III: POLIO AFFECTION OF FOOT AND ANKLE

Polio foot in particular is a difficult topic. Basic understanding of deformities and their causes are essential to initialize the viva session. The treatment of polio depends on deformities present. Always look for muscles that are active and suitable for transfer for the muscles weak or paralyzed.

Diagnosis: The patient is a 10-year-old male/female with postpolio residual paralysis (PPRP) of left/right lower limb with equinovalgus deformity which is partly correctable with shortening without trophic ulcers.

1. Why do you say it is polio?

Ans.
- Asymmetric, patchy, and lower motor neuron type paralysis acute flaccid paralysis (AFP)
- Nonprogressive
- No sensory loss
- Prior paralytic poliomyelitis with evidence of motor neuron loss, as confirmed by history of the acute paralytic illness, signs of residual weakness and atrophy of muscles on neuromuscular examination, and signs of nerve damage on electromyography (EMG).
- A period of partial or complete functional recovery after acute paralytic poliomyelitis, followed by an interval (usually 15 years or more) of stable neuromuscular function.
- Symptoms that persist for at least a year.

(*Remember paralytic limbs are colder than their counterparts.*)

2. What are the differentials?
Ans. Myopathy, neurological disorder or injury.

3. What is critical arc of motion?
Ans. 15° dorsiflexion (minimum required for heel strike and squatting) to 15° plantar flexion (minimum required for push off).

4. What is ideal age for tendon transfers and bony procedures in polio?
Ans. Wait for at least one and a half years after the paralytic attack, i.e. after convalescent stage has passed off and residual stage has started. The following principles apply:
- Tendon transfers in skeletally immature patients
- Extra-articular arthrodesis between 3 years and 8 years
- Triple arthrodesis after 10–11 years
- Ankle arthrodesis after 18 years.

Ideally tendon transfers should be done after 5 years when the child can be trained adequately for rehabilitation. Results are, however, better after age of 10–11 years. This should be supplemented with bony procedures (especially arthrodesis) which should be done before or along with tendon transfers. Bony blocks to prevent opposite motion may be necessary with tendon transfers, especially in children. This is because in pediatric patients, growth along with slight muscle imbalance even after tendon transfers causes recurrence of deformities. For example, if tendon is transferred to cause dorsiflexion of ankle, then posterior bony block to prevent plantar flexion may be done simultaneously.

First the plantar and dorsiflexion movements are to be balanced before inversion and eversion. Among the two, plantar flexion strength is to be regained first. If sufficient muscles are not available for transfer, then joints are to be arthrodesed. For example, if invertors and evertors are not available, do triple arthrodesis so that only plantar and dorsiflexors are needed to be balanced.

It is better to be too tight than to be too loose when attaching tendons to new locations.

Foot and Ankle

It is better to wait for 3 weeks in upper limbs and 4-6 weeks in lower limbs for physiotherapy to start after tendon transplants.

Surgical stabilization of joints (arthrodesis) is ideally done after skeletal maturity.

You should know the actions of groups of muscles namely tibialis anterior, tibialis posterior, long toe dorsiflexors, long toe plantar flexors, and peronei. Transfer to midline if only plantar and dorsiflexion are to be balanced. If you need eversion, transfer it laterally and transfer medially if inversion is needed. For example, if you need to transfer a muscle to gain dorsiflexion and eversion, transfer it to dorsal tarsus (to gain dorsiflexion) and among the tarsal bones, laterally (to gain eversion). Deformity progresses till bone and soft-tissue growth ceases. Any splint/passive stretching cannot prevent development of a deformity. It can only slowdown the process.

5. Do you prefer tendon transfers or excision of stronger muscles? Why?

Ans. Transfers are preferred because excision causes further atrophy of paralytic part. If excised, 7-10 cm of tendon is to be excised to prevent reunion by fibrous tissue.

6. Which is the most common deformity in polio foot?

Ans. Most common is equinovalgus (tibialis anterior paralyzed) followed by calcaneocavovarus and then equinovarus. (Valgus is more common than varus.)

7. What is the aim of treatment in foot surgery in polio?

Ans. Aim is to get a foot which is:
- Stable—no abnormal varus/valgus in hindfoot and ankle on weight bearing
- Plantigrade—even distribution of weight on hindfoot, midfoot, and forefoot on weight bearing
- No significant fixed deformity—without any inversion-eversion deformity, with foot to be able to be brought to right angle passively
- Adequate muscle power—>3 power in active dorsi and plantar flexors of ankle, i.e. sufficient power to clear the toes off the ground.

8. What is Peabody's classification of polio foot?
Ans.
- Limited extensor-invertor insufficiency
- Gross extensor-invertor insufficiency
- Evertor insufficiency
- Triceps surae insufficiency.

9. How do you manage limited extensor-invertor insufficiency?
Ans. Weakness of tibialis anterior is the main feature producing equinus and cavus or planovalgus.

Treatment includes transfer of EHL to base of 1st metatarsal along with plantar fasciotomy. It may be reinforced by peroneus tertius to same site. Planovalgus of long standing duration often becomes fixed may require triple arthrodesis. Fixed equinus may additionally require tendo-Achilles lengthening.

10. What is gross extensor-invertor insufficiency and how to manage it?
Ans. There are two types of extensor-invertor insufficiencies:
1. *Type A:* Weakness of tibialis anterior and toe extensors (EHL and EDL) with a normal tibialis posterior
2. *Type B:* Weakness of tibialis anterior, toe extensors (EHL and EDL), and tibialis posterior.

Treatment for Type A:
- Deformity is equinus or equinovalgus.
- Prefer transfer of peroneus longus to 1st cuneiform. Another option is peroneus brevis transfer that may be attached to dorsum of foot in midline (when TP and peroneus longus balance each other) or over 4th ray (when TP is strong) or 1st or 2nd ray (when peroneus longus is stronger than TP).

Treatment for Type B:
- Transfer of both peroneus longus and brevis to dorsum of foot.
- In both the above triple arthrodesis may be combined if bony deformities are fixed.

11. What is evertor insufficiency and how do you manage it?

Ans. Evertor insufficiency is characterized by weakness of peronei. Treatment depends on extent of weakness:

- *Mild:* EHL transfer to 5th metatarsal base.
- *Moderate:* Tibialis anterior transfer to cuboid with EHL transfer to 1st metatarsal. Tibialis anterior may be transferred more medially if tibialis posterior is also weak so that it balances peroneal weakness.
- *Complete:* Tibialis posterior to cuboid (anterolateral aspect) or lateral cuneiform.

Triple arthrodesis may be combined with any of the above. Split tibialis anterior transfer may be used as well.

12. How do you treat triceps surae insufficiency?

Ans. Earlier you treat this muscle imbalance, the better is the result.

- *Calcaneus deformity:* Posterior transfer of tibialis anterior through interosseous membrane along with transfer of EHL to dorsum of foot, usually 1st metatarsal base. Most successful operation that restores heel to toe gait and tip toe walking.
- *Calcaneovarus (peronei weak and strong TP—produces varus):* Transfer both TP and flexor hallucis longus to calcaneus.
- *Calcaneovalgus (TP weak with strong peronei):* Transfer peronei to calcaneus.
- *Calcaneocavus (both TP and peronei are strong and intact):* Transfer both peronei and TP to calcaneus.

Triple arthrodesis is done if deformities are uncorrectable and associated with bony deformities.

13. What joints are fused in triple arthrodesis? What are commonly used types?

Ans.

- Aim is to reduce the number of joints that the paralyzed muscles have to stabilize.
- Angulatory or rotatory deformities of knee and leg should be corrected immediately after this procedure; otherwise there will be recurrence of deformities.

- The most important joint in the tarsus, determining the mobility of ankle and tarsal complex, is the talonavicular joint and hence any procedure should tackle this joint.
- A stable ankle with no varus-valgus instability is an absolute requirement. Or else, there may be recurrence of deformities or residual instability of ankle and foot complex. If anterior structures around ankle are found lax as in a forced plantar flexion X-ray, then either tendon transfers anteriorly to reinforce dorsiflexors or ankle arthrodesis should accompany triple arthrodesis. Other contraindications include unstable knee joint, painful OA of ankle, severe trophic ulcers and age less than 11 years.
- Ideal position of foot after triple arthrodesis:
  - Hindfoot in 50 valgus
  - Transverse tarsal joints in 0–50 abduction and forefoot in <100 varus
  - The medial border of foot should be straight
  - The heel and 1st and 5th metatarsal heads should be in the same plantigrade plane and heel should be in exact mid position (mild valgus will not harm but varus will definitely).
- Incisions include Kocher, Ollier, and anterolateral exposure to ankle with/without accessory medial incision over talonavicular joint.

Types:

1. *Hoke* (1921): Subtalar arthrodesis with resection, reshaping, and reimplantation of the *head and neck of the talus* with *posterior displacement*. (Remember there is reimplantation of talar neck and posterior displacement of entire foot which is less than Dunn's type.)
2. *Dunn* (1922): Subtalar arthrodesis with excision of *navicular and part of head and neck of talus* with *posterior displacement* which depends on the amount of bony resection. (Remember navicular is completely excised and not reimplanted and posterior displacement is more than Hoke's and depends on amount of bony resection.) Both Hoke's and Dunn's types cause posterior

Foot and Ankle

displacement and hence increase lever arm posteriorly helping weakened plantar flexors of ankle. Both did not emphasize calcaneocuboid joint fusion initially. Both are especially useful with weakened plantar flexors of ankle.

3. *Ryerson* (1923): Arthrodesis of subtalar, talonavicular, and *calcaneocuboid* joints. Correct hindfoot varus by bony cuts on either side of subtalar joint. Forefoot varus-valgus and abduction-adduction by cuts on talonavicular and calcaneocuboid joints. This method is particularly useful when plantar and dorsiflexors of ankle balance each other.

4. *Lambrinudi*: Similar to Ryerson except that a break is created in tarsal bones into which reshaped talar head and neck is fitted to correct the forefoot equinus. Calcaneus remains in equinus at ankle, but equinus deformity is corrected at subtalar joint. By locking the talus in equinus at subtalar joint and realigning rest of tarsus over talus, correction is achieved.

5. *Siffert, Forster and Nachamie*: Dorsal cortex of navicular is excised. Inferior part of talar head and neck is removed such that the superior part along with attached soft tissues anterior to ankle joint remains as a beak into which remaining navicular is locked. Stapling may be required to maintain this alignment. *Complications include:* Pseudarthrosis of joints (most common complication and talonavicular joint is most common joint), residual deformities like supination of forefoot and varus-valgus at hindfoot and midfoot, avascular necrosis of talus, varus-valgus imbalance at ankle, osteoarthritis of ankle, and painful foot (pseudarthrosis and callosities).

14. What is the appearance of foot after triple arthrodesis?

Ans. Ideal foot after triple arthrodesis (Hoke and Thomson):
- Looks natural in shoes
- No external rotation on long axis of foot when standing or walking
- No need for brace

- Appears natural when bare
- Weight is evenly distributed over plantar surface
- Axis of ankle is at right angle to that of foot and well forward
- No pain
- Patient can control ankle joint motion.

15. Define hammer toe, claw toe, and mallet toe.

Ans.

1. Hammer toe is hyperextension of metatarsophalangeal (MTP) and distal interphalangeal joints (DIP) with hyperflexion of proximal interphalangeal (PIP) joint (usually involves single digit and associated with callus on dorsum of PIP joint).
2. Claw toe means hyperflexion at both interphalangeal joints with hyperextension at MTP joint (usually involves many toes and associated with callus on dorsum of PIP joint and tip of toe). The term claw toe is most likely derived from the affected toe's similarity in appearance to the claw of an animal or talon of a bird **(Table 4)**.

Table 4: Deformities of MTP, PIP, and DIP joints.			
Deformity	**MTP Joint**	**PIP Joint**	**DIP Joint**
Hammer toe	Dorsiflexed or neutral	Plantar flexed	Neutral, hyperextended, or plantar flexed
Claw toe	Dorsiflexed	Plantar flexed	Plantar flexed
Mallet toe	Neutral	Neutral	Plantar flexed
Curly toe	Neutral or plantar flexed	Plantar flexed	Plantar flexed

16. What are types of clawing?

Ans. Two types:

1. *Swing phase:* Due to weakness of ankle dorsiflexors, long toe extensors substitute for them. So during swing phase, when ankle dorsiflexors are to be active, long toe extensors contract producing clawing. It is more marked when tendo-Achilles is contracted.

2. *Stance phase:* Due to weakness of triceps surae, long toe flexors are used to substitute them. So during push off phase of stance, when plantar flexors of ankle (triceps surae) are to be active, long toe extensors contract producing clawing.

17. How does clawing present?
Ans. *Common presentation of clawing:*
- Pain at the dorsal PIP joint from an impingement of the toe on the shoe.
- Callus or erythema over the dorsal PIP joint (friction with shoe).
- Patients may report pain at the tip of the toe (pressure against the point of the distal phalanx). There may be callus at the tip of the toe and a malformed nail.
- Pain from MTP joint due to synovitis (following persistent hyperextended position and instability).
- Callus or soft corn on the medial border of the claw toe (seen in clawing of the fourth or fifth toe but is less common, impingement of the lateral claw toe on the adjacent toe).
- *Metatarsalgia:* Increased pressure beneath the metatarsal head and distal migration of the plantar fat pad with hyperextension of the MTP joint.

18. How do you treat clawing?
Ans. Foot deformities should be corrected before surgery for clawing, as clawing correction may be unnecessary after foot deformity correction. Add surgery for clawing if necessary after above. It depends on type of clawing:
- In swing phase clawing, first restore active dorsiflexion of ankle and correct equinus deformity. Add surgery for clawing if necessary after above.
- In stance phase clawing, restore active plantar flexion and correct cavus.

Indications: Pain due to clawing.

Contraindications: Poor vascularity to the toe and poor skin quality.

Splint used for postoperative immobilization is Lambrinudi splint: It has felt pads on which plantar surfaces of toes rest and wires to hold onto the toes.

Surgical procedure:

Girdlestone-Taylor procedure: Transfer long toe flexors onto dorsal expansion of extensor tendons. This enables long toe extensors to act as intrinsic muscles of foot in producing active plantar flexion of MTP joint while extending IP joints. This surgery is more useful when clawing is primarily due to weakness of intrinsic of foot (swing phase).

19. What is the mechanism of great toe clawing?

Ans. Clawing of great toe is caused by insufficiency of dorsiflexors of ankle with normal long toe extensors (EHL) or long toe flexor (FHL) that try to overcome respective weak ankle dorsiflexor (tibialis anterior) or plantar flexor (triceps surae) and in the attempt produce secondary clawing of great toe.

20. How do you treat great toe clawing?

Ans. *Modified Jones procedure:* Done for clawing associated with tendo-Achilles contracture. It consists of attachment of EHL into the 1st metatarsal neck and arthrodesis of interphalangeal joint. Distal part of EHL is attached to soft tissues over dorsum of the proximal phalanx.

Dickson-Diveley procedure: For clawing caused by insufficiency of plantar flexors of ankle and persists after appropriate foot stabilization and tendon transfers to restore active plantar flexion of ankle. It consists of three steps: Transfer of EHL to FHL around the medial side of 1st metatarsal head, arthrodesis interphalangeal joint, and then suture distal part of EHL to soft-tissues over proximal phalanx.

21. What is the difference between Jones and modified Jones procedure?

Ans. *In modified Jones procedure:*
- Two incisions are used
- IP joint arthrodesis is done
- Excision of tendon sheath.

22. What are advantages of modified Jones over Jones?
Ans.
- Less chances of hypertrophic scar
- Less chances of pseudarthrosis at interphalangeal joint
- Regeneration of EHL is less likely.

23. What is clawfoot and how to treat it?
Ans. Cavus of foot with clawing of toes due to intrinsic tightness is clawfoot (*equinus of forefoot is called cavus*). It may be associated with severe ulcerations beneath metatarsal heads.

- *Mild and correctible:* Metatarsal bar on shoes with metatarsal pad during day and a splint with metatarsal bar for use at night can be used.
- *Mild, not correctible:*
  - Peroneus longus to peroneus brevis transfer (Bentzon)
  - Arthrodesis of IP joints of all toes.
- *Moderate:*
  - Steindler's fasciotomy
  - Dwyer's calcaneal osteotomy
  - Japas V osteotomy of the tarsus.
- *Severe:*
  - Anterior tarsal wedge resection
  - Hoke/Dunn triple arthrodesis along with TP transfer to dorsolateral tarsus.

24. What is Steindler's fasciotomy?
Ans. It is done for cavus deformity along with other procedures or as a single operation. The structures released are:
- Plantar fascia
- *Extraperiosteal stripping of following muscles:* Avoid periosteal stripping to prevent bone formation that may cause pain on weight bearing:
  - Abductor hallucis
  - Flexor digitorum brevis
  - Abductor digitorum brevis.
- Long plantar ligament.

If deformity is not corrected, insert Steinmann pin longitudinally into calcaneum from tip of heel. Apply corrective below knee cast.

25. What is Japas osteotomy? What are the advantages?

Ans. V-shaped osteotomy of tarsus often done to correct moderate cavus in children of 6 years or older.

Advantages: No shortening, widening of foot. No bone is excised.

(*Teaching note:* Apex of V is proximal and at the highest point of cavus, usually within the navicular. One limb of V extends laterally through cuboid to lateral border of foot and the other through medial cuneiform to medial border. The proximal border of distal fragment of osteotomy is depressed plantarward while the metatarsal heads are elevated, thus lengthening the plantar surface of foot. Plantar fasciotomy should be done.)

26. What is dorsal bunion?

Ans. It is a deformity where MTP joint of great toe is flexed with dorsiflexion of 1st metatarsal and plantar flexion of great toe. A small exostosis is formed on dorsum of 1st metatarsal head. MTP joint may even subluxate. The plantar part of joint capsule and flexor hallucis brevis may both contract.

Three types:
1. Weak peroneus longus with a strong tibialis anterior—causes unopposed dorsiflexion of 1st metatarsal and cuneiform. Plantar flexion of great toe is secondary to create point of weight bearing. Most commonly due to improperly planned peroneus longus transfer away from its normal insertion.
2. Due to paralysis of all muscles controlling foot except triceps surae and long toe flexors which are strong. They become active in push off phase causing active plantar flexion of toes including great toe. Flexor hallucis brevis adds to effect.
3. Along with hallux rigidus and flatfoot with rocker-bottom deformity.

27. How do you manage dorsal bunion?

Ans. General guidelines are as follows:
- If bunion is flexible—correct muscle imbalance between ankle motors.

- If rigid—do "Lapidus" procedure. Imbrication (double breasting) of dorsal capsule of the 1st metatarsophalangeal joint along with capsular release on plantar aspect. Transfer of tibialis anterior from 1st metatarsal to 2nd and 3rd cuneiform. Transfer of FHL to base of 1st metatarsal through a tunnel passing from plantar to dorsal aspect so that FHL now acts as a plantar flexor of 1st metatarsal. Plantar-based wedge osteotomy of cuneiform-metatarsal with/without naviculocuneiform joints to correct dorsiflexion of 1st metatarsal.

28. How do you treat equinus deformity of ankle in polio?

Ans. When plantar flexors are stronger than dorsiflexors or contracture secondary to posture and gravity in a flail foot.

It is treated by tendo-Achilles lengthening without posterior capsular release of ankle and subtalar joint. This should be accompanied by tendon transfers to restore active dorsiflexion of ankle and a surgery which is either of:
- *Campbell's posterior bone-block:* A bone-block is constructed on posterior aspect of talus and calcaneum such that it will impinge on tibia to restrict plantar flexion of ankle.
- Lambrinudi arthrodesis
- Pantalar arthrodesis
- Ankle joint arthrodesis.

29. What is pantalar arthrodesis? What are the indications?

Ans. Surgical fusion of ankle, subtalar, talonavicular, and calcaneocuboid joints (i.e. triple + ankle arthrodesis; *pan = whole*). The foot is preferably fused in neutral or slight valgus at hindfoot, equinus at ankle (5° for males and 15° for females). Equinus may be adjusted according to shortening (increase for a shorter leg).

Indications:
- Equinus or calcaneus with lateral instability of foot and whose leg and foot muscles are not strong enough to control foot and ankle when only foot is stabilized.
- Recurrence after Lambrinudi or Campbell's procedure.

Contraindications:
- Fixed flexion deformity.
- Uncontrolled recurvatum deformity of knee—functioning hamstrings or triceps surae.

It can be done in one-stage (Steindler) or two-stage (Liebolt and King). In the latter, foot stabilization is done first by Hoke's triple arthrodesis followed by ankle arthrodesis.

30. How do you treat talipes equinovarus?

Ans. Equinovarus occurs with weak peronei and (normal or weak) ankle dorsiflexors with comparatively stronger tibialis posterior, and triceps surae. Removal of this strong TP is essential in management.

Treatment depends on age of patient:
- *Skeletally immature:* Braces (double bar, with inner iron and outer T strap with 90° ankle stop with footpiece attached to leg in external rotation), serial corrective casts, tendo-Achilles lengthening with/without posterior capsular release of ankle/subtalar joint, and Steindler's release.
- *Skeletally mature:* Triple arthrodesis with/without Steindler's release. If deformity is not fully corrected, then 4–6 weeks later, tendo-Achilles lengthening with Jone's transfer can be done.

Both the above age groups should be treated with muscle balancing operations.
- Most common is anterior transfer of tibialis posterior (through interosseous membrane as by Ludloff or around medial surface of tibia as by Ober) onto anterolateral tarsus. If there are no functional ankle dorsiflexors for transfer, then combine triple arthrodesis or posterior bone-block simultaneously with TP transfer.
- If triceps is weak, transfer TP posteriorly to calcaneus.
- If TP itself is weak, transfer tibialis anterior to midline dorsally or slightly lateral.
- Tibial external rotational deformities more than 30° should be corrected by derotational osteotomies of tibia and fibula.

Foot and Ankle

31. How do you treat paralytic talipes cavovarus?

Ans. This deformity is due to strong tibialis posterior and long toe flexors or due to strong foot intrinsic muscles in an otherwise flail foot.

Treatment is by:
- Excision of short toe flexors with a segment of plantar fascia along with motor branches of lateral plantar nerve
- Excision of motor branches of medial and lateral plantar nerves (Garceau and Brahms).

32. How do you treat equinovalgus?

Ans. This is due to weak tibialis anterior and/or tibialis posterior associated with strong peronei and strong contracted triceps surae. Forefoot goes into abduction and pronation.

Treatment depends on age:
- *Skeletally immature:* Correction of deformity with
  - Double bar brace with 90° ankle stop and inside T-strap, shoe with medial arch support, and medial heel wedge.
  - Wedging casts
  - Tendo-Achilles lengthening may be required.

  Once correction is achieved, then extra-articular subtalar arthrodesis (Grice-Green) with anterior transfer of peroneus longus and brevis (4-6 weeks later) is done. Tendo-Achilles lengthening may be required along with this to correct equinus. Ideal age is 4-12 years.

  In isolated tibialis anterior paralysis with valgus deformity, transfer peroneus longus or EDL to first cuneiform.

  In isolated tibialis posterior paralysis: Peroneus longus/FDL/FHL/EHL is transferred through sheath of tibialis posterior onto plantar aspect of navicular.
- *Skeletally mature:* Triple arthrodesis with/without TA lengthening followed 4-6 weeks later by anterior transfer of peroneus longus and brevis tendons and Jones operation.

33. How to treat a calcaneus (calcaneocavus) deformity?

Ans. Weakened triceps surae along with normal ankle dorsiflexors causes calcaneocavus.

In skeletally immature patient: Ankle brace with posterior elastic strap or shoes with elevated and posteriorly extended heel can be used. Early tendon transfers are the rule.

In skeletally mature patient, plantar fasciotomy and triple arthrodesis (preferably Hoke's or Siffert's) should be done.

Tendon transfers are a rule. It should be done at earliest possible time in both the above age groups. Options include peronei and tibialis posterior. In addition, tibialis anterior can be transferred posteriorly into calcaneus if EHL and EDL are normal and are transferred to the proximal aspect of dorsum of foot. FHL can be transferred if above muscles are not strong enough.

When sufficient muscles are not available for transfer, pantalar arthrodesis is the option.

CASE IV: TENDO-ACHILLES RUPTURE (FIG. 13)

Getting a case with acute rupture is quite unlikely and one must prepare for neglected injuries. A theoretical knowledge of various causes and diagnoses will be legible to pass. One should have a clear idea of management.

Read: 2–3 times (DNB candidates), MS candidates are very unlikely to get this case in preference for other examination cases.

Diagnosis: The patient is a 47-year-old male with 3 month old neglected rupture of tendo-Achilles of left side.

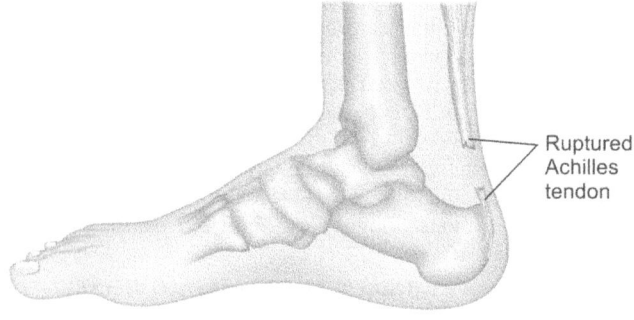

Fig. 13: Tendo-Achilles rupture.

Foot and Ankle

FINDINGS

History

- Sudden onset pain over back of ankle associated with snap and inability to walk
- Acute onset swelling
- Previous history of minor trauma
- No treatment taken
- Laborer.

Examination

- Scar mark, tenderness, and bruise (acute cases)
- Palpable gap/irregularity (old cases) on posterior aspect of lower leg in the region of tendo-Achilles
- Inability to toe-walk
- Positive:
    - Thompson-Simmonds calf squeeze test **(Fig. 14)**
    - O'Brien's needle test
    - Copeland sphygmomanometer test
    - Matles knee flexion test **(Fig. 15)**
- Weakness of gastrocsoleus and painful plantar flexion (especially when resisted).

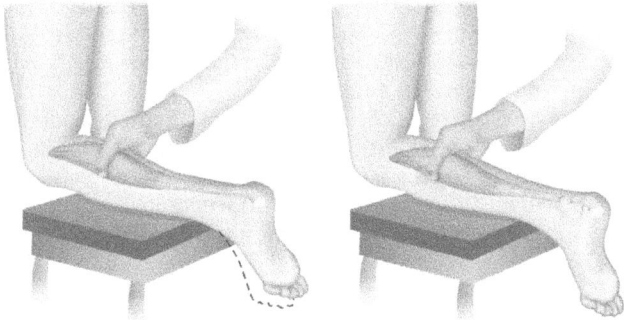

Fig. 14: Thompson test. On the left side is a normal patient where squeezing of calf produces plantar flexion at ankle, while on the right is a patient with torn Achilles tendon where there is absence of plantar flexion with squeezing of calf.

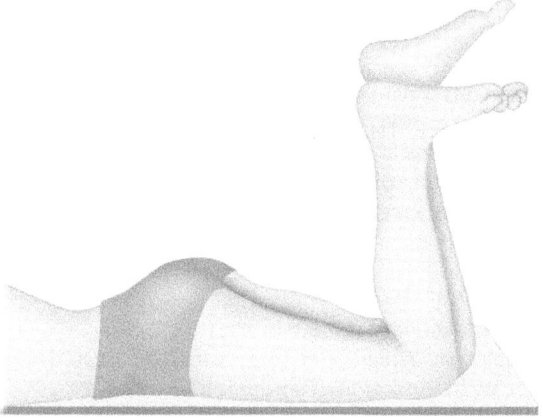

Fig. 15: Matles knee flexion test. In resting position with patient prone and knee bent to 90°, the foot with torn Achilles tendon shows increased dorsiflexion.

1. How do you test for tendo-Achilles discontinuity?
Ans. Apart from history and local palpable gap and plantar flexion weakness, the special tests that help diagnose the discontinuity of tendo-Achilles are:

- *Thompson-Simmonds-Doherty test:* Patient prone—squeeze the calf muscle of patient—passive plantar flexion of foot demonstrates continuous tendon. [*After 7 days (neglected cases) due to intervening scar formation the test may be falsely negative*]
- *Needle test of O'Brien:* Insert a hypodermic needle 10 cm above the insertion of tendo-Achilles so that its tip is just inside the tendon. Alternately plantar and dorsiflex foot. If the outer portion of needle points cranially on dorsiflexion the tendon is supposed to be intact.
- *Sphygmomanometer test:* Wrap the cuff around calf region and inflate it to 100 mm Hg, if then on dorsiflexion of foot pressure rises to 140 mm Hg then it indicates intact tendon.
- *Knee flexion test:* With patient prone ask the patient to flex knee to 90°, neutral position or dorsiflexion of ankle suggests torn tendon.

Foot and Ankle

- *Reverse Silfverskiold test (not very popular):* With knee in full extension (ankle dorsiflexion here is solely restricted by tendo-Achilles) measure the range of dorsiflexion at ankle (more on injured side compared to the normal side).
- *Single leg heel raise test:* Ask the patient to stand on injured leg with heel raised (not possible with torn Achilles tendon).

2. What are the fallacies of Thompson test?

Ans. A positive Thompson-Simmonds test is supposed to clinically demonstrate complete rupture; in particular dependent on integrity of soleal part of the tendon. O'Brien however demonstrated that rupture of gastrocnemius part also produces a positive test and hence described the needle test. Conversely also in cases where the gastrocnemius aponeurosis is separate from soleus; the Thompson test may be falsely positive as the "squeeze" has predominant effect on gastrocnemius muscle belly rather that soleus. The treatment decisions are often based on whether tear is complete or partial and whether soleus is involved rendering Thompson test insufficient.

3. Why is 10 cm chosen as a point for O'Brien test?

Ans. The following reasons explain the rationale:
- In type-I junction (gastrocnemius aponeurosis separate from soleus) the gastrocnemius tendon joins the soleal tendon 12 cm proximal to insertion. In type-II junctions (gastrocnemius inserting into soleus itself) the tendon is composite from beginning. In any case the tendon is a single unit some 10 cm proximal to insertion.
- At the same level the plantaris tendon is comfortably medial to Achilles tendon while the sural nerve migrates laterally preventing false negative test or nerve injury, respectively.

4. What is tennis leg?

Ans. Rupture of gastrocnemius musculotendinous junction is called tennis leg; other types of rupture are complete Achilles tendon rupture and partial tears.

5. Why is the tendo-Achilles called so?

Ans. According to the famous legend Achilles was the warrior of Homer's Iliad who was made invincible by his mother by immersing him in the river Styx holding his heel which remained untouched by water and hence vulnerable. This tendon being the strongest tendon and "location" resemblance in paradox has been so labeled.

6. What is the blood supply of this tendon?

Ans. Three sources (deriving vascularity from both posterior tibial and lateral peroneal artery):
1. Musculotendinous junction
2. Surrounding connective tissue
3. Bone-tendon junction.

The vascular supply is disputably precarious in mid-portion or 2–6 cm from insertion of tendon, and skin directly posterior to the tendon is relatively sparsely supplied.

7. Where does the rupture commonly occur and what are the causes of rupture?

Ans. The weak area of tendon is supposed to be 2–6 cm above insertion, where the vascularity is supposed to be precarious; however there is no site preference with trauma. Various causes listed are as follows:
- Collagen disorders (genetic)
- Inflammatory and autoimmune mechanisms
- Degenerative and repetitive trauma
- Drugs (corticosteroids and fluoroquinolones)
- Exercise induced hyperthermia within tendon
- Mechanical theory (eccentric loading/sudden loading with incomplete synergism of agonist muscles/inefficient plantaris which is not able to maintain tension in tendo-Achilles)
- Ischemic injury to tendon (age related, vasculitis and collagen disorders, torsional ischemia due to vasoconstriction of intratendinous vessels).

8. What are the various pathogenic mechanisms?

Ans. Various factors lead to development of weakness of this tendon that ultimately fails under load. The various pathological changes that have been proposed finally leading to weakness and hence rupture of tendon are tendinosis, paratendinitis, and paratendinitis with tendinosis. The term tendinosis describes various degenerative changes within tendon (hyaline, mucoid, myxoid, fatty, fibrofatty, etc.) that may arise out of various above listed causes. Often tendinosis is not symptomatic and is realized only on rupture of tendon. Repetitive trauma or inflammatory conditions produce paratendinitis which may be later accompanied with tendinosis and is often painful before rupture.

9. What will you do next for this patient?

Ans. I will confirm the diagnosis (only if there are atypical findings on clinical examination) by radiological investigations.

10. What are the findings on plain X-ray?

Ans. *Lateral projection shows:*
- Loss of posterior border of Kager's triangle or complete disappearance (fat filled triangular space in front of tendo-Achilles) is suggestive of torn tendon.
- Toygar's sign involves measurement of angle of posterior skin-surface seen on lateral projection. With disappearance of triangle the angle increases to 130–150° **(Fig. 16)**.

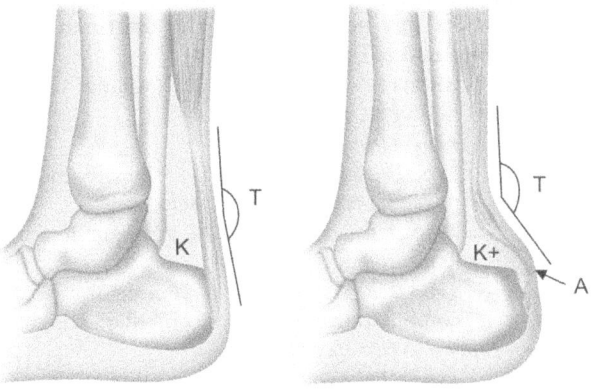

Fig. 16: Toygar sign.

- Exostosis growing into the tendo-Achilles is identified well on radiographs that may be the site of injury (fracture). Osteoporotic bones are weaker than the bone-tendon junction. Same is the case with Haglund deformity.

11. What is the most specific and sensitive investigation to diagnose a tendon rupture?

Ans. MRI (contrast enhanced is better if infection is suspected).

12. How will you manage this patient?

Ans. After confirming complete rupture of Achilles tendon a symptomatic patient with disability needs surgical reconstruction. I will mobilize the gastrocnemius and soleal components of the complex and after flexion of knee and plantar flexing the ankle, try to approximate the ends without tension and do an augmentation with plantaris tendon (or turn down of two flaps of gastrocnemius aponeurosis). Nowadays, I have instead switched to augmentation with FHL tendon regularly to improve the outcome especially delayed outcome because late failure and recurrent tears are common. If the ends cannot be approximated then I will use the peroneus brevis dynamic tendon transfer (rather "splint") of White and Kraynick for reconstruction of tendon.

13. Are there any guidelines for the treatment of chronic Achilles tendon rupture?

Ans. Classifications exist but are not popular and couture treatment is often practiced:
- *Myerson's classification:*
  - *Type 1 defect:* 1–2 cm long → End-to-end repair and posterior compartment fasciotomy.
  - *Type 2 defect:* 2–5 cm → V-Y lengthening with or without tendon transfer.
  - *Type 3 defect:* >5 cm → Tendon transfer alone or combined with V-Y advancement and augmentation.
- *Kuwada's classification:*
  - *Type I:* Partial tear → Conservative management
  - *Type II:* Complete tear → 3 cm defect → end-to-end repair

- *Type III:* 3–6 cm defect → debride + tendon transfer ± augmentation
- *Type IV:* >6 cm defect → debride + tendon graft ± augmentation

(Confused! Better not be—leave apart others; the authors themselves did not evaluate utility of the classifications. Be assured you will not be asked these unless you are getting Gold medal!)

14. **How do you manage acute tears?**
Ans. Simply if the tendon ends can be approximated then I will use an end-to-end suturing with modified Kessler method and plantaris augmentation. If the ends cannot be approximated then I will use complex reinforcement method such as Lindholm's technique with turn down gastrocnemius aponeurotic flap with plantaris augmentation. Postoperatively I will immobilize the repair in above knee cast in flexion at knee and plantar flexion at ankle. After 2 weeks sutures are removed and further immobilization in below-knee cast is done which is followed by gradual dorsiflexion of ankle over further 2 weeks and protected mobilization.

15. **What other methods are available for repair of tendon?**
Ans. Fascial reinforcement, artificial tendon implants, Marlex, and collagen prostheses.

16. **Do you know of any other method of repair?**
Ans. Percutaneous method of Ma and Griffith.

17. **What is the role of nonoperative treatment?**
Ans. Constant fight between supporters of nonoperative versus operative treatment remains unabated. With more recent publications the disparity has more clouded. It is for a surgeon's preference and to his experience to decide between the two. A combined conservative and orthotic regime has recently been reported with excellent results. These methods are based on the premises of not injuring the already precarious blood supply to tendon through anterior mesentery and paratenon and are definitely (and should be) used for partial tears.

18. Do you know any popular surgeon who suffered from Achilles tendon rupture?

Ans. John Hunter in 1767 suffered complete tear while dancing. He treated himself with calf bandaging and raising shoe heel with excellent results.

19. Why is rerupture common after repair or reconstruction?

Ans. Native Achilles tendon is rich in type-I collagen while the healing tendon has high percentage of weaker and poorly organized type-III collagen less resistant to stretch.

20. What factors determine good healing of tendon?

Ans. Preservation of paratenon, good approximation, and prolonged immobilization in equinus position are important for good healing of tendon.

CASE V: FOOT DROP

This is a common case that is kept as short case for examination in orthopedic viva voce, fibular nerve neuropathy is the most common mononeuropathy of lower limb and unfortunately for unknown reasons it is the most common nerve injured in various surgical procedures.

Diagnosis: My clinical diagnosis is a 37-year-old male with non-recovering, complete peroneal (in revised terminology the term peroneal has been replaced by "fibular" and this latter should be preferred) nerve palsy of right leg for past 3 years following injury to proximal leg region [or knee dislocation or postgluteal injection or postsurgical (THR) or spine surgery or leprosy, whatever tell the reason].

Note: Foot drop is a clinical finding and not a clinical diagnosis so it should not be presented as a diagnosis.

FINDINGS

In history the patient has complains of limp and need to unusually raise the foot of involved limb to clear the ground. The patients also complain of catching of toe with ambulation. There is associated sensory loss over dorsum of foot.

- Weakness or absent dorsiflexion at ankle—foot drop

Foot and Ankle

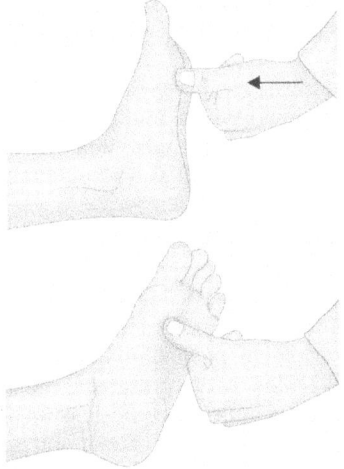

Fig. 17: Duchenne's test.

- Weakness/absent great toe and other toe extension
- Weakness of foot eversion
- Equinus contracture
- *Positive Duchenne's test (Fig. 17):* Ask the patient to plantarflex the foot while pushing up on first metatarsal. Excessive supination of foot indicates superficial fibular nerve (L4-S1) injury.
- Sensory loss over dorsum of foot (superficial) or 1st web space (deep branch)
- High-stepping gait/slapping foot gait.

1. Why do you call it complete peroneal (fibular) nerve palsy?
Ans. The patient has involvement of both superficial and deep components of fibular nerve.

2. What do superficial and deep fibular nerves supply?
Ans. The deep fibular nerve supplies all muscles of anterior compartment of leg namely tibialis anterior, extensor digitorum longus, and extensor hallucis longus along with

peroneus tertius (fibular tertius muscle). It takes sensations from the skin between 1st toe and 2nd toe (the first web space).

The superficial peroneal (fibular) nerve supplies fibular (peroneus) longus and brevis muscles of the lateral compartment of leg and takes sensations from lower two-thirds of anterolateral leg and whole dorsum of foot except the first web space.

3. How do you clinically differentiate deep and superficial fibular nerve palsy?

Ans. In superficial peroneal (fibular) nerve palsy the eversion of foot is lost while dorsiflexion at ankle and of toes will be preserved while in deep fibular nerve palsy ankle dorsiflexion will be lost while preserving the foot eversion. This is uncommon as both are commonly involved (unless there is injury distal to bifurcation of common peroneal nerve).

4. What are the causes of fibular nerve palsy?

Ans. Trauma is the most common cause of common peroneal nerve palsy; however other causes are as follows:
- *Iatrogenic:* Knee arthroplasty, knee arthroscopy, hip arthroplasty, birth trauma, casts, other knee surgeries (correction of genu valgum, HTO), traction, varicose vein surgery, and intravenous injections/infiltrations
- *Trauma:* Knee injury and fractures of femur, tibia, fibula, tibiofibular syndesmosis injury, knee dislocation, and gun-shot wounds
- *Other:* Bony exostosis, severe varus at knee, ganglion, baker's cyst, lacerations, hemangioma, hematoma, synovial cysts, and weight loss.

5. What is anterior tarsal tunnel syndrome?

Ans. This refers to compression of deep fibular nerve under inferior extensor retinaculum that commonly presents as paresthesia in 1st web space of foot.

6. What are the causes of foot drop?

Ans. The foot drop can be broadly categorized into three groups:
1. *Neurological:*
    - Injury or neuropathy of common peroneal or sciatic nerve

Foot and Ankle

- Disk prolapse at L4–L5 level
- Common peroneal nerve compression at fibular head/leprosy
- Multiple sclerosis
- Charcot-Marie-Tooth disease.

2. *Muscular:*
   - Injury to dorsiflexors of foot/toes and tibialis anterior tendon injury
   - Muscular dystrophy and polio

3. *Anatomic:*
   - Compartment syndrome
   - Habitual cross-legged sitting
   - Charcot joints.

7. What will you do next?

Ans. I would like to get nerve conduction studies of leg, radiographs of knee, and blood investigations to rule out other causes.

8. What will nerve conduction studies tell you—only support diagnosis?

Ans. No, apart from supporting diagnosis they will help me determine regeneration of nerve fibers, assess site of lesion, and assess damage to nerve. Electromyogram additionally will help me in identifying peripheral neuropathy, myopathy, nerve radiculopathy, motor neuron disease and peripheral nerve compression, etc.

9. How will radiographs help you?

Ans. Radiographs will help me in looking for site of injury (fractures, osteotomy, etc.), exostosis if any, and Charcot's joint.

10. Will you do anything else?

Ans. Yes, I will evaluate for diabetes mellitus, liver function tests, renal function tests and vitamin B12 levels to look for metabolic causes. Also, if hematoma/aneurysm/ganglion or baker's cyst is suspected then I will get ultrasonogram done.

11. How will you manage this case?

Ans. As the nerve palsy is nonrecovering and complete so conservative management does not have a role. I will assess and discuss the functional requirements of the patient. The patient wants improvement in gait and dorsiflexion at ankle.

I will correct equinus contracture at ankle by tendo-Achilles lengthening and provide dorsiflexion motor by Bridle procedure.

12. What is the role of bony procedures?

Ans. Bony procedures like Gill posterior bone-block can be done to prevent foot drop during walk in paralytic foot (polio).

13. If there is no acceptable motor, what will you do?

Ans. I will explain the need of arthrodesis for providing painless foot with correction but no movements. I will prefer ankle arthrodesis unless there are arthritic changes in intertarsal joints.

5

The Shoulder

For most of the candidates the shoulder joint will be an unexpected case and for this reason most are not required to know a lot about the same. An unfortunate DNB candidate is "at risk" of getting one and will be expected to know at least some important points. What follows gives a very comprehensive examination schema of the joint (more than enough for all) and a brief review of concepts for cases.

Read times: 6–10 times (DNB candidates, MS candidates may either skip or read 2–3 times). This is a difficult case (difficult both to understand and present, especially the unstable shoulder).

EXAMINATION POINTS FOR A SHOULDER CASE

HISTORY TAKING

- *Pain:*
  - *Onset:* Acute (infective and traumatic); insidious (inflammatory, subacute, and chronic infections like TB).
  - *Duration*: Protracted course in inflammatory process and adhesive capsulitis, TB.
  - *Radiation*: To back of shoulder, axilla, and outer aspect of upper arm.
  - *Aggravating factors*: Movements aggravate most of the painful conditions.
  - *Character*: Throbbing severe in pyogenic infections and traumatic conditions.
  - *Relieving factors*: Rest, massage, and analgesics (duration of relief, complete and incomplete relief should be specifically asked).

- *Relation to trauma*: Dislocations, fractures, and fracture dislocations may be a cause of recurrent instability (also enquire the treatment given and duration of immobilization and postinterventional physiotherapy to judge the stiffness and instability).
- *Movements*: The movements that aggravate pain [early abduction—supraspinatus tear; painful arc—supraspinatus; flexion—biceps; and internal rotation (reaching back)—subscapularis].
- *Fever*: Association is helpful for infective conditions.
- *Swelling*: Spontaneous onset (infective, PVNS, reactive effusion, inflammatory, hemophilia, degenerative, etc.) or related to trauma (hemarthrosis).
- *Limitation of movements*: Onset (spontaneous over a period—adhesive capsulitis and subacute infections), treatment related (post-traumatic and postsurgical).
- *Lack of power*: Recurrent subluxation/dislocations and dead arm syndrome.
- *Instability*: Voluntary/involuntary, associated with which movement, direction, how frequent, onset and duration, and associated neurological injury/weakness.

Also ask for causes of radiating pain (gastric/duodenal affections, diaphragmatic affections, and cardiopulmonary and mediastinal disorders) and polyarthralgia.

Past history: Diabetes, hypertension, neurological disorders (epilepsy), hematological disorder, and tuberculosis.

EXAMINATION

General for ligamentous laxity *(See Chapter 5: Case II; Q 11)*.

Inspection

- *Attitude (carriage/posture)*:
  - *Anterior dislocation of shoulder*: Elbow kept away (abduction) and slightly in front and external rotation with support of the opposite hand
  - *Posterior dislocation*: Adduction and internal rotation
  - *Deltoid contracture*: Abducted arm and drooping of shoulder

The Shoulder

- *Klippel-Feil syndrome*: High webbed neck
- *Sprengel shoulder*: Scapula higher than uninvolved side
- Lateral scapular slide (in throwing athletes) scapula of dominant side drawn away from midline
- *Prescapular abscess*: Shoulder kept in flexion and abduction (away from irritating pus)
- *Pyogenic arthritis*: Flexion mild abduction and slight external rotation.

- *From front (compare from other side)*: Sternal notch, sternoclavicular joint, clavicle and its contour, supra/infraclavicular fossae, acromioclavicular (AC) joint, preglenoid fossa, anterior axillary fold, coracoids prominence, deltoid mass and shoulder contour, pectoral muscle, sternocleidomastoid muscle, and alignment of chin to suprasternal notch.
- *From behind*: Midline and alignment of nape of neck to both shoulders, trapezius, medial border of scapula (winging due to serratus anterior weakness or sometimes due to rhomboids and trapezius also), spinous process of scapula, angle of scapula, supra/infraspinatus fossae, posterior axillary fold, "soft spot" (1 cm medial and 2 cm inferior to angle of acromion) to look for swelling.
- *From top*: AC joint and contour of shoulder.
- *From medial aspect*: Swelling of lymph nodes and sebaceous gland infection.
 At all the sites examine the skin for (SEADS)—swelling, erythema, atrophy (of appendages), discoloration, suppuration (scars and sinuses).

Palpation

Note for temperature rise and superficial tenderness then proceed to regional and deep palpation as below:
- *Anteriorly*: Sternoclavicular joint, clavicle, AC joint, and acromion (for os acromiale), subacromial bursa (tenderness just anterior to acromion), long head of biceps (for tendinitis—palpate along 1-4 cm in front of acromion anteriorly with 10° internal rotation of shoulder), myositis mass, pectoralis major tendon (by pressing both palms together), supraclavicular fossa

(for brachial plexus injury and "burners/stingers" due to mild involvement of plexus).
- *Lateral aspect*: For deltoid mass and step deformity due to inferior subluxation of shoulder.
- *Posterior aspect*: Soft spot for swelling.
- Medial aspect for pulsations of axillary artery.

Movements

- *Anterior flexion (forward flexion)*: Normally up to 160–180°.
- *Abduction*: Look for scapulohumeral rhythm while patient does abduction, after 90° abduction patient externally rotates the arm. Shrugging of shoulder with abduction often indicates chronic rotator cuff insufficiency. Note for painful arc where abduction is relatively painless in the initial few degrees of abduction and the pain is reported during further arc and may again abate in terminal degrees (suggests supraspinatus impingement/partial tear). Inability to initiate abduction is due to supraspinatus insufficiency while inability to maintain abduction denotes deltoid insufficiency.
- *Adduction*: Ask patient to take the limb forward and also compare the cross-chest adduction.
- Internal rotation in 0° abduction and 90° abduction (normal = 45°): "Apley scratch test" is more functional to evaluate internal rotation although it also requires some extension (normal IR is up to 80°). In Apley scratch test, ask the patient to try and reach back and note the internal rotation in terms of the spinal level reached with thumb (normal = T7 for women and T9 for men).
- *External rotation in 0° abduction and 90° abduction:* In abduction the "neutral position" is while forearm is pointing directly in front with elbow flexed (normal ER is up to 90°).
- *Total active elevation:* The patient is instructed to raise the arm "in plane of scapula" which is some 20–30° from sagittal plane.
- *Scapular protraction*: Ask patient to bring forward scapulae in "hunched position" by shrugging the shoulders forward.
- *Scapular retraction*: Ask patient to pull back the shoulders in "attention attitude": Alternate retraction and protraction may elicit "snapping scapula" syndrome.

Test for muscle power: Latissimus dorsi (climbing rope maneuver or hanging on beam maneuver), serratus anterior (push against wall—winging of scapula), deltoid (palpate the shoulder contour while asking patient to actively abduct shoulder), trapezius ("shrugging shoulder"—*one does it many times in exams!*), rhomboids ("attention attitude"), pectoralis major (asking patient to press both the palms together in front); other muscles as below.

Measurements

- Apparent length [from seventh cervical spine to radial styloid (patient standing)]
- Arm length (from angle of acromion to lateral epicondyle)
- Mid-arm circumference
- Anterior and posterior axillary folds
- *Palpate pulses* (radial, ulnar, brachial, and axillary).

SPECIAL TESTS

- *Rotator cuff pathology*:
    - *Neer's impingement sign*: Passively do maximal forward flexion of shoulder which reproduces the pain due to approximation of anterolateral acromion with rotator cuff and greater tuberosity **(Fig. 1)**.

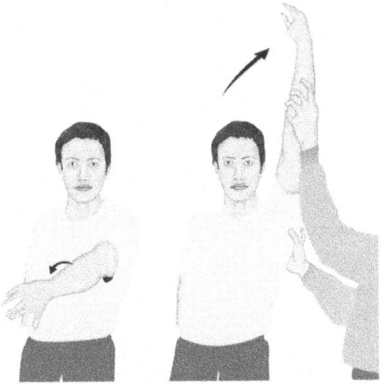

Fig. 1: Neer's impingement sign and test.

- *Neer's impingement test*: Inject local anesthetic in subacromial bursa and repeat the test, pain disappears.
- *Hawkins impingement reinforcement test (Hawkins and Kennedy)*: Passively forward flex the shoulder to 90° and then internally rotate while maintaining the shoulder position **(Fig. 2)**. Pain produced indicates rotator cuff pathology or subacromial bursa involvement and is due to rotation of greater tuberosity and subacromial bursa into the acromion and coracoacromial ligament arch. Similar pain can be produced due to rare coracoids impingement.
- *Drop arm test*: Passively abduct the arm to fullest and then ask the patient to slowly bring the arm down **(Fig. 3)**. After few degrees of retrieval the arm suddenly drops down like a dead limb. Positive in extensive rotator cuff tear and deltoid paralysis.
- *Subscapularis liftoff test of Gerber (lumbar lift-off test)*: Ask patient to reach his back and try to lift the hand away from back. Pain produced in this maneuver at lesser tuberosity suggests subscapularis tendinitis and inability to perform this test or weakness suggests subscapularis inefficiency.

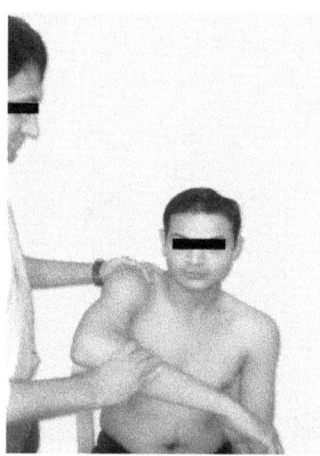

Fig. 2: Hawkins–Kennedy test.

The Shoulder

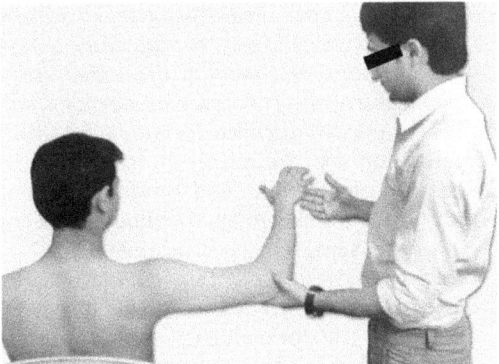

Fig. 3: Drop arm test.

- Belly press maneuver for subscapularis if patient cannot internally rotate shoulder.
- *Jobe's test*: For supraspinatus—ask patient to abduct arm to 90° and then bring it in 30° forward flexion (from coronal plane) followed by internal rotation (like "emptying a can of water"). This maneuver produces pain in supraspinatus tendinitis. Further in the test, power of muscle can be tested by asking patient to push the elbow to ceiling and examiner actively resisting it.
- *Passive rotation test*: Passively rotate the shoulder through full range of external and internal rotation in 90° abduction while palpating the front area of shoulder. Popping sensation can be felt in hypertrophied subacromial bursa and torn irregular rotator cuff.
- *Test for infraspinatus and teres minor*: Ask patient to forcefully externally rotate while arm is by the side of the body, resistance to this maneuver can be applied and may produce pain at the greater tuberosity in tendinitis of these muscles.
- *Tests for shoulder instability:*
  - *Anterior instability (provocative tests)*: It is good to remember the sequence in which these tests are done (apprehension test

→ *augmentation test* → *relocation test* → *release test*) *as this is a continuous array of test that should be done in a single sitting. Note, however, should be made that the position for performing this array of test is supine and not sitting/standing as had been advised discretely for individual tests.*

- "Apprehension test" (originally given by Rowe and Zarins and renamed by Silliman and Hawkins): Patient *supine*—abduct (90°), externally rotate the shoulder, feeling of giving way (apprehension) is taken as positive **(Fig. 4)**.
  - *"Augmentation test" of Silliman and Hawkins:* To above test, apply anteriorly direct force, i.e. extend shoulder if previous test does not elicit apprehension—positive if patient resists or "apprehends".
  - *Relocation test (of Jobe)*: If above maneuver produces pain instead of apprehension then apply a posteriorly directed force—relieves pain (indicates instability) this can be further tested.
  - *Release test of Silliman and Hawkins*: Release the posterior force that relieved pain—patient again complains of pain/apprehension in a positive test.
  - *Load-shift test*: Load the glenoid with humeral head and do anterior-posterior shift to assess laxity.

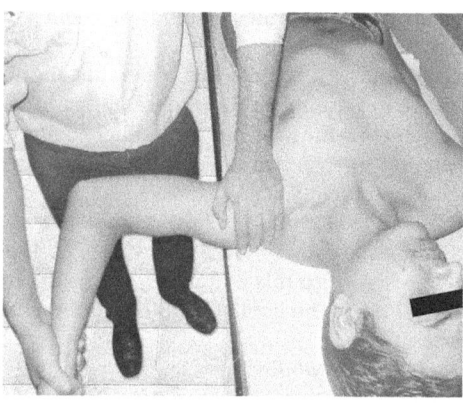

Fig. 4: Apprehension test and relocation test.

- Anterior and posterior instability:
  - *Drawer test "shoulder Lachman test" of Gerber and Ganz*: With patient supine, hold proximal humerus in mild abduction and pull and push it forward and backward after stabilizing scapula with other hand and grade the instability. Grade "0" = no translation, "1" = translation up to glenoid rim but not over it, "2" = translation beyond rim with spontaneous reduction, and "3" = dislocation and locking of head **(Fig. 5)**.
  - *Modified drawer for posterior instability*: Forward flex the arm and apply axial load along humerus to subluxation the head out of glenoid—pain and palpable shift suggest posterior labral tear.
  - *Jerk test*: With patient seated abduct the arm to 90° and apply a downward force, then adduct the arm till front of scapular plane when head may subluxate then abduct the arm behind scapular plane when head reduces with a jerk.
  - *Circumduction test*: Perform circumduction in abduction while palpating the posterior aspect for subluxation of head.
  - *Posterior apprehension test of O'Driscoll*: Arm positioned as in Hawkins test—produces pain and is relieved by injection of local anesthetic.

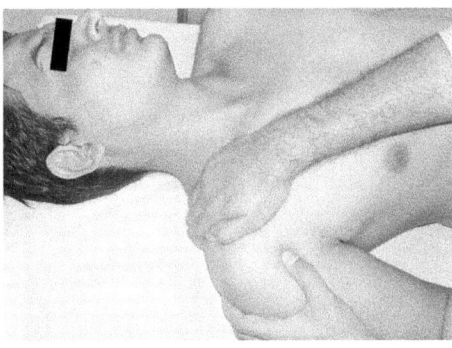

Fig. 5: Drawer test.

- *Posterior subluxation test of Clarnette and Miniaci*: Axially directed force along arm in adduction, 70–90° flexion and internal rotation with the other hand feeling for posterior subluxation of head.
- Inferior instability:
  - *Feagin maneuver*: Place the abducted arm of patient on your shoulder and apply an inferiorly directed force to subluxation the head inferiorly.
  - *Sulcus sign "inferior drawer test" of Neer*: Pull the patients arm downward while it is by the side of patient's body, formation of a sulcus beneath acromion suggests inferior laxity or multidirectional instability **(Fig. 6)**. Grade "1" = 1 cm, "2" = 2 cm, "3" = 3 cm; >2 indicates a capacious capsule and specific laxity of rotator interval.
- Multidirectional instability:
  - Compression rotation test for glenoid labrum
  - O'Brien's test for superior labral injuries
  - Snyder's biceps tension test
  - Sulcus sign >2.

- *Tests for dislocated shoulder:*
  - *Hamilton ruler test*: Keep a straight ruler along lateral aspect of arm—in a normal person it does not touch the acromion angle, but in dislocated shoulder it does. This will also be positive in any affection of head of humerus.

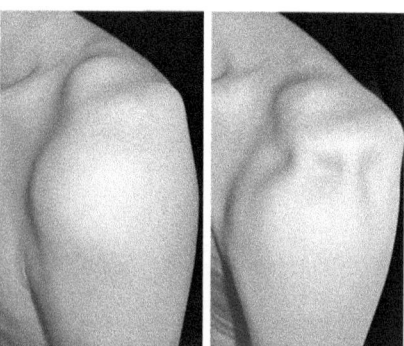

Fig. 6: Sulcus sign.

- *Callaway's test*: Girth of shoulder is normally symmetrical—increases in effusion, suppuration, and dislocation of shoulder.
- *Duga's test*: The elbow cannot be brought to the midline of body.
- *Bryant's test*: In anterior dislocation of shoulder the anterior axillary fold is elongated.

- *Tests for thoracic outlet syndrome:*
  - *Adson's test*: Abduct the arm by 30° and ask patient to take a deep breath while palpating the pulse (feel the character and compare with other side), then ask the patient to tilt his head towards the same side—reduction or diminution of pulse suggests thoracic outlet syndrome.
  - *Wright's maneuver*: In the above test abduct the shoulder to 90° and externally rotate the arm.
  - *Roos test*: Abduct the arm and flex elbow to 90° then externally rotate the shoulder so that the hand faces up. Ask patient to clench and release fist 15 times. Paresthesia/pain/cramps/weakness suggest thoracic outlet syndrome.
  - *Halsted's test*: While patient standing with arm by the side ask patient to turn the head to other side and extend the neck. Give a downward traction and feel for diminution/obliteration of pulse.
  - *Hyperabduction test*: Abduct and hyperextend both the arms (behind the body) simultaneously. Feel for diminution of pulse on affected side.

- *Tests for biceps tendinitis*:
  - *Yergason test*: Arm by side and elbow flexed to 90°. Patient is asked to flex elbow and pronate while examiner resists. Pain is felt on anterior aspect of shoulder.
  - *Speed test*: Forward flex the arm and extend the elbow fully. Supinate the upper limb and apply a downward force with patient resisting against it **(Fig. 7)**. Pain is felt in the region of bicipital groove.

- *Tests for SLAP lesion (superior labrum anterior to posterior):*
  - *O'Brien's test*: Tested by asking patient to resist when their limb is in 90° flexion and 10° adduction with thumb pointing down. Production of pain is positive which relieves with thumb pointing up.

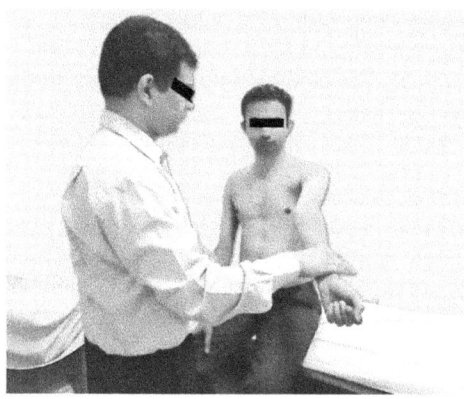

Fig. 7: Speed test.

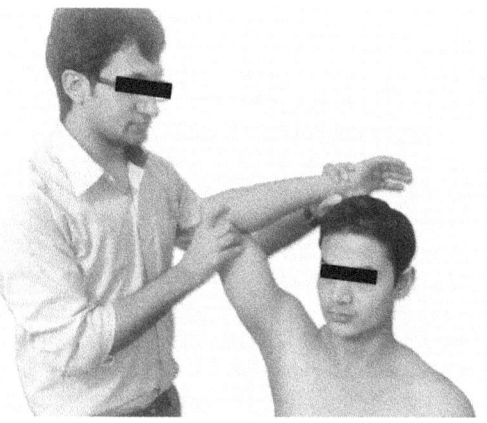

Fig. 8: Crank test.

- *"Crank test" of Liu et al.*: With arm in 160° of abduction in scapular plane apply an axial force with forced internal and external rotation (*like Apley's grinding test for menisci*) **(Fig. 8)**.

CASE I: TUBERCULOSIS OF SHOULDER JOINT

1. **What findings support the diagnosis of tuberculosis in this case?**

Ans. *History:*
- Young adult to middle aged male (TB shoulder is not at all common in children, also this type of TB is one where often a pulmonary focus can be found)
- Insidious onset pain
- Rapidly accompanied by loss of movements and stiffness
- Gradual progression over time of both complaints
- Exacerbation in night and partial relief with analgesics
- Constitutional symptoms—evening rise of fever, night sweats, weight loss, loss of appetite, asthenia, etc.
- Negative history—trauma, polyarthralgia, cervical spondylosis, and exertion associated pain.

Examination:
- Wasting
- Tenderness (deep joint)
- Spasm of surrounding muscles
- Painful limitation of movements in all directions
- Shortening of arm.

Swelling and abscess formation or sinuses are usually absent in TB shoulder as the dry form is much more common than the wet form.

2. **What is your differential diagnosis?**

Ans. Periarthritis (adhesive capsulitis), primary osteoarthritis of shoulder, osteonecrosis of humeral head, secondary osteoarthritis, and rheumatoid arthritis.

3. **What are the foci of infection in TB shoulder?**

Ans. Glenoid process, humeral head, and synovium.

4. **How do you classify TB shoulder?**

Ans. *Clinical types:*
- Caries sicca (dry form—no abscess formation, pus accumulation or sinus formation)
- Wet suppurative form (swelling and sinus formation common).

Dry form is much more common of the two and has an onset commonly in middle-aged patients. Wet form is less common and is seen in younger patients who are often nutritionally deficient and compromised.

Staging TB shoulder is often not productive as the stages progress so fast that often the patient would be first seen or diagnosed in advanced arthritis or ankylosis stage. Hardly if ever one would see a patient in synovitis stage.

5. How would you establish the diagnosis?

Ans. *Please see Chapter 2: Case I.*

6. What are the radiological features?

Ans.
- Generalized osteopenia around shoulder
- Reduction of joint space
- Involvement of both the humeral head and glenoid fossa
- Lytic lesions in humerus and/or glenoid, later healing stages show lytic-sclerotic regions
- Reduction of subacromial space (in sicca form; it may increase in wet form)
- Wet form often presents with honey combing of proximal humerus.

7. What is your differential on X-ray?

Ans. Radiologic features have *various* differentials:
- Rheumatoid arthritis
- Urate arthropathy
- Primary osteoarthritis
- Giant cell tumor of humerus
- Periarthritis (this is the most uncommon radiological differential, however, it clinically closely resembles TB—so getting an early X-ray is imperative).

8. How will you treat the patient?

Ans. This is not as complicated as in TB spine/hip. Management depends upon the stage in which the patient first presents. Patient presenting relatively early when articular surfaces are well maintained (there may be joint space narrowing) should be started on ATT with gradual mobilization of shoulder, after adequate pain relief and good response shoulder strengthening

The Shoulder

exercise should begin to prevent associated morbidity (soft tissue contractures and instability). When patient presents with destroyed (partial or complete) articular surfaces then pain relief (apart from healing obviously) is the primary goal and immobilization in spica cast in functional position should be done. If the patient fails to achieve painless joint or progresses poorly then excision of focus (debridement) and intra-articular arthrodesis in functional position will be done.

9. What is the functional position of shoulder?

Ans. *As such there are wide variations in the guidelines that are referred.* It is simplified into 30-30-30, which means 30° each of abduction, flexion, and internal rotation; or 20-30-40. It is important to understand that one should be able to provide that position where patient can feed himself well and do routine activities. "Salute position" (with wide abduction) is typically not recommended.

10. How do you judge the position of arthrodesis intra-operatively?

Ans. Abduction is judged by the position of arm in relation to body. Forward flexion is also judged so or in lateral position from the midline. For internal rotation which is supposedly the most important component (and hence should be accurate), after abduction and forward flexion, flex the elbow to 90° so that the hand is in a line between sternum and axilla, then move the hand in a range that thumb is able to reach chin.

11. What are the various methods for shoulder arthrodesis?

Ans. *Extra-articular (not preferred):* Watson-Jones, Putti, Steindler, etc.

Intra-articular:
- External fixation (Charnley and Houston)
- Internal fixation (Cofield, AO group, and Richards) combined intra-articular and extra-articular arthrodesis (Uematsu).

12. What are the problems associated with AO compression arthrodesis?

Ans. Difficulty in bending the plates and prominence of screws (so Richard used reconstruction plates).

CASE II: THE UNSTABLE SHOULDER

Diagnosis: The patient is a 28-year-old male with post-traumatic anterior shoulder instability for past 4 years. There is no associated neurological deficit and patient is able to pursue his routine activities.

1. What do you mean by shoulder instability and how do you classify it?

Ans. Shoulder instability is both a symptom and sign! Pathomechanically it can be described as inability of the head of humerus to center itself within glenoid fossa during any/some/all of the movements. This, however, is not a practical measure to judge instability, which can only be labeled by careful evaluation of patient symptomatology and examination. Various classifications have been poised to "divide" instabilities; however, they are all seemingly plagued by impracticality and imprecision. None can substitute the experienced clinicians evaluation and management.

Classification by:
- *Type:* "Dislocation" versus "subluxation"
- *Etiology:* Macrotrauma, microtrauma (repetitive) or atraumatic
- *Direction:* Anterior, posterior, inferior, superior, and multidirectional
- *Volition:* Involuntary versus voluntary
- *Comprehensive (Matsen et al.):* TUBS (traumatic, unidirectional, Bankart, surgical treatment) versus AMBRI (atraumatic, multidirectional, bilateral, rehabilitation, inferior capsular shift in some cases).

The last one is probably useful in order to group the patients, but many patients may fall in between the two groups due to mixed features making it difficult for an average surgeon.

2. What do you mean by "chronic dislocation"?

Ans. Dislocation for >6 weeks.

3. How do you recognize posterior dislocation on X-ray?

Ans. The following points help diagnosing posterior dislocations that are often missed:
- Absence of normal elliptical overlapping shadow of humerus with glenoid on routine AP view

The Shoulder

- *Vacant glenoid sign:* Most of glenoid is "vacant" of humeral head on routine AP view also known as "positive rim sign"
- *Trough sign:* Caused by reverse Hill-Sachs lesion
- *Loss of profile of humeral neck:* "Lightbulb" sign
- Void in inferior or superior glenoid fossa.

4. What defines multidirectional instability?

Ans. Simplified version would be instability in ≥2 planes in any combination (this makes it easier to fit the patient into TUBS/AMBRI).

5. What is Bankart's lesion?

Ans. Avulsion of fibrocartilaginous labrum with anterior capsule and periosteum (combined) is referred to as Bankart's lesion, when this also involves some part of glenoid bone then it is called "bony Bankart".

6. What is Hill–Sachs lesion and reverse Hill–Sachs lesion?

Ans. Impingement osseous defect (compression fracture) in the posterosuperior humeral head is called Hill-Sachs lesion (seen in anterior dislocation), when similar defect is present in anterior humerus head then it is called reverse Hill–Sachs lesion (seen in posterior dislocation).

7. What are the various risk factors for the development of recurrent shoulder instability?

Ans.

- Younger age group (75–80% in <20 years, 50% in 20–30 years)
- Posterior dislocation > anterior
- Repetitive microtrauma (athletes and overhead activities)
- Direct anterior dislocation rather than anteroinferior dislocation
- Associated bony lesions (bony Bankart, Hill-Sach, etc.)
- Poor compliance with rehabilitation program.

8. What are the various restraints for shoulder?

Ans. Importantly it is the most mobile joint of body and by virtue of compromise into stability for mobility it is also the most frequently dislocated one. The restraints have classically been divided into static and dynamic but (*it is the human nature to create and resolve confusion*) schools are divided over the concept. **Table 1** may help to give an insight that is bound to improve over time.

Table 1: Various restraints for shoulder.		
Factor	**Function**	**Abnormality**
Static stabilizers		
Congruity of humeral head to glenoid fossa (glenoids are pear shaped with surface contour and are not matching the humeral head) (head is 1.5 to 2 times larger in diameter with smaller radius of curvature, around 3 times in surface area)	<ul><li>Centering of head in concavity</li><li>Stability ratio and balance stability angle</li><li>Directional load transmission by virtue of version and conjoint movement of surfaces</li><li>"Bony cam effect" of scapular inclination</li></ul>	<ul><li>Osseous maldevelopment (dysplasia)</li><li>Osseous destruction (trauma, infection—glenoid destruction, Hill–Sachs lesion, reverse Hill–Sachs lesion)</li><li>Articular destruction (inflammation, infection, primary, posterior chondrolabral avulsion of glenoid rim)</li></ul>
Humeral head and coracoacromial arch	Concavity-compression effect	Iatrogenic (acromioplasty in rotator cuff tear), floating shoulder, coracoid avulsion
Glenoid labrum	<ul><li>Increased depth and surface area</li><li>Anchors ligaments and capsule</li></ul>	Bankart lesion (osseous, soft tissue, reverse osseous), SLAP, ALPSA (anterior labor-ligamentous periosteal sleeve avulsion), POLPSA (posterior labrocapsular periosteal sleeve avulsion), Kim lesion (concealed incomplete avulsion of posteroinferior aspect of labrum)

Contd...

Contd...

Factor	Function	Abnormality
Capsule (surface area of capsule is twice that of humeral head)	Posterior portion restrains anterior translation and vice versa	Capsular tear, plastic deformation of capsule
Negative intra-articular pressure, synovial fluid	Vacuum effect (effective atmospheric pressure), cohesive effect	Capsular rupture, defect of the rotator interval, capsular laxity, and capsular injury, arthritis and degenerative conditions with loss of synovial fluid
Coracohumeral ligament/superior glenohumeral ligament	Limits external rotation and inferior translation in adduction and posterior translation in flexion	Lesion of the rotator interval (between supraspinatus and subscapularis), rotator cleft lesions (between superior and middle glenohumeral ligament, situated deep to interval)
Middle glenohumeral ligament	Limits external rotation and inferior translation in adduction and anterior translation in midabduction (45°)	Bankart lesion and capsular injury, HAGL (humeral avulsion of glenohumeral ligaments), RHAGL (reverse HAGL)
Inferior glenohumeral ligament complex	Limits anterior, posterior, and inferior translation in abduction (45–90°)	Bankart lesion and capsular injury, HAGL, RHAGL
Posterior aspect of the capsule	Limits posterior translation in the flexed, adducted, and internally rotated shoulder	Posterior capsular laxity and injury, POLPSA

Contd...

Contd...

Factor	Function	Abnormality
Dynamic stabilizers		
Rotator cuff	Dynamic compression of the joint; steering effect	Overuse injury (fatigue) and rupture, interval/cleft injury
Biceps (long head)	Dynamic restraint to anterior and superior translation	Lesion of the superior portion of the labrum, anterior and posterior (SLAP lesion) and rupture

Typically speaking, the static and dynamic stabilizers are complementary and in any given position of shoulder both supplement each other's function. Mere congruence of glenohumeral articulation will be ineffective without ligamentous support and "dynamic" muscular "compressors". Similarly during night time when the muscles are relaxed still the rotator cuff (deemed to be dynamic stabilizer) is in enough tension to restrain the joint from dislocation thus having by itself a "static" effect.

9. How do you evaluate the patient for unstable shoulder?
Ans. I will methodically examine the patient as above to be able to decide:
- The articulation(s) involved (glenohumeral, acromioclavicular, scapulothoracic, and sternoclavicular) that are responsible for the complaints of patient
- Whether there is decentering of head
- Direction(s) of instability
- Mechanical factors responsible for decentering of head
- Dynamic factors responsible for decentering
- Age and psychological status of patient amenable for treatment
- Possibility of repairing the pathologic factor.

I will proceed with no touch examination while listening to patient's complaints and asking him to position the limb/maneuver that produces the symptoms. Then manipulative

The Shoulder

examination will be done (*Always perform the manipulative tests first on uninvolved shoulder*).

10. What else will you like to do?

Ans. I will also do an examination under anesthesia (gold standard) and radiologic investigations to look for bony articulation (CT scan) and capsuloligamentous abnormalities (MRI scan).

11. How will you look for ligamentous laxity?

Ans. Look for the following, Beighton criteria (9 sites in total, *4 are bilateral*) **(Fig. 9)**:

1. More than 10° hyperextension of the elbows.
2. Passively touch the forearm with the thumb, while flexing the wrist.
3. Passive extension of the fingers or a 90° or more extension of the fifth finger (Gorlin's sign). This is used as a "screening test".
4. Knees hyperextension greater than or equal to 10° (genu recurvatum).
5. Touching the floor with the palms of the hands when reaching down without bending the knees. This is

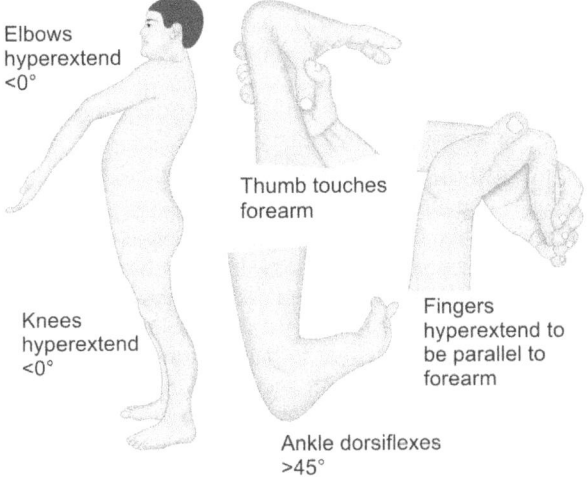

Fig. 9: Beighton criteria.

possible as a result of the hypermobility of the hips, and not of the spine as it is commonly believed.

A score of 4/9 (on Beighton score) is a major criterion in evaluating the patient on Brighton criteria.

12. What is the role of muscles as stabilizers?
Ans. The surrounding muscles are "compressors" of shoulder joint that can be produced practically in any position. They should not be classified as depressors or elevators in the perspective of shoulder stability.

13. What is the rotator cuff?
Ans. The rotator cuff is a musculotendinous structure that surrounds the shoulder joint from all sides except inferior. It is formed by four muscles that attach to the tuberosities and have the following functions:

- *Subscapularis (lesser tuberosity)*: Principle anterior compressor, chiefly in an internal rotator supplied by upper and lower subscapular nerve
- *Supraspinatus (greater tuberosity)*: Principle superior compressor, chiefly is an abductor supplied by suprascapular nerve
- *Infraspinatus (greater tuberosity)*: Principle posterior compressor, chiefly is an external rotator supplied by suprascapular nerve
- *Teres minor (greater tuberosity)*: Complements infraspinatus, supplied by axillary nerve.

14. How will you manage the patient?
Ans. I will put the patient on a supervised plan of physiotherapy for muscle balancing and strengthening exercises. The progress is judged by symptomatology. If the patient fails to improve over a prolonged program (more than 6 months) I will consider surgery for unilateral instability. Multidirectional instability (such as due to ligamentous laxity) needs to be carefully evaluated with respect to various psychological factors; the treatment options are very limited here.

Operative reconstruction is contraindicated for voluntary, habitual dislocations in a psychologically unstable patient.

15. How will you operatively manage the instability?

Ans. For a given instability there are numerous variations that have to be individually judged. A practical guide would be as follows:

- *Labral injuries producing unidirectional instability:* Bankart's repair ± capsular shift of Neer.
- *"1" + capsular injury (often anterior) (capsulolabral injury):* Bankart's repair with capsular reconstruction of Jobe's or capsular shift.
- *"1" + bony eburnation:* Bankart's repair with glenoid osteoplasty (Eden-Hybbinette or similar procedure).
- For similar posterior lesions posteroinferior glenoplasty of Metcalf can be done.
- *Loss of coracoacromial arch with anterosuperior escape of humeral head:* "Dismal injury"—reconstruction is not possible with present techniques: "Reverse shoulder arthroplasty".
- *Posterior instability due to capsuloligamentous inefficiency:* Capsular shift of Tibone.
- *Multidirectional instability:* Inferior capsular shift of Neer and Foster (or its modification) with repair of the mechanical factor if possible.
- *Hill–Sachs lesion:* Derotation osteotomy + capsular reefing "or" bone grafting of the lesion (Neer) "or" tight anterior repair (± Putti-Platt subscapularis double breasting).
- *Reverse Hill–Sachs lesion:* Modified McLaughlin procedure.
- If >40% of head involved: Shoulder arthroplasty.
- *Loss of glenoid rim*:
    - *Up to 20%:* Repair the detached labrum and capsule back to the intact glenoid cartilage to render the defect extracapsular.
    - *Up to 25%:* Reattachment of the fragment "or" Bristow-Helfet procedure if the fragment cannot be reattached.
- Reconstruction of capsuloligamentous deficiencies due to previous surgeries by tendon graft from humeral attachment.

- **Deficient tendon of subscapularis:** Hamstring tendon graft.
- **Instability associated with denervation/paralysis/irreparable detachment of muscles:** Glenohumeral arthrodesis.

16. What is the role of arthroscopic procedures?

Ans. The reconstruction of a lot of injuries to "mechanical" capsuloligamentous and labral injuries (Bankart's, SLAP, POLPSA, rotator cuff tears, capsular tears/laxity, etc.) is now possible with meticulous and advanced arthroscopic procedures. The posterior lesions are less amenable to arthroscopy and need expertise.

CASE III: DELTOID CONTRACTURE

A rare case but could be given to students appearing at centers where these cases are more epidemiologically located; else this is an important differential diagnosis for Sprengel shoulder that may come as spot case.

Diagnosis: The patient is an 18-year-old male with postinjection contracture of left deltoid. The patient is able to perform activities of daily living.

FINDINGS

History of multiple injections in the shoulder region for various reasons.

EXAMINATION

- Elbow not touching the side of body
- Drooping of shoulder
- Abnormally prominent humeral head anteriorly
- Depressed acromion
- Wasting of muscles around shoulder and loss of normal contour of shoulder
- The inferior angle of scapula is rotated towards midline
- Scoliosis with convexity to contralateral side
- There is midline deltoid depression and a tough fibrous cord is palpable that becomes prominent on adduction of arm

The Shoulder

- Increased distance of angle of acromion to vertebral border of scapula
- Limited adduction of arm (especially cross body adduction is not possible)
- *Positive Shanmugasundaram test:* Patient is unable to touch the two elbows and ulnar border of forearms when brought in front in midline in 90° flexion of elbow. Contralateral elbow has to cross midline to touch the ipsilateral elbow still ulnar border of forearms cannot completely touch each other.

1. Why do you call it contracture of deltoid?

Ans. The findings presented above suggest so.

2. What are the causes of deltoid contracture apart from injection afflicted contracture?

Ans. Other rare cause could be familial and idiopathic.

3. What drugs will cause deltoid contracture?

Ans. Commonly drugs that induce fibrosis like diclofenac injection (older nonaqueous preparations induce gross fibrosis due to irritation—remember postinjection nerve palsy) this produces continued fibrosis even days after the injection is given, tetanus toxoid injections, wrong injection of antibiotics (mostly extravasation), and repeated gentamicin injections.

4. What are your differentials and why?

Ans. The important differentials that I would keep are:
- *Sprengel shoulder (incomplete scapular descent):* Here the patient has small and elevated scapula (scapula size is comparable in deltoid contracture), low hair line, webbed neck, absent trapezius, and levator scapulae replaced by omovertebral bar that tethers scapula, cervicodorsal scoliosis, and congenital vertebral anomalies. Shoulder movements are usually full but may be restricted in abduction.
- *Klippel-Feil syndrome:* This is a syndromic association where Sprengel deformity is seen in one-third of the cases. There are associated spinal anomalies (typically unsegmented cervical vertebra fused on one side) like scoliosis, restricted movements, spina bifida, and others like cleft palate and renal anomalies.

- *Tuberculosis of upper dorsal spine*: This will have kyphotic deformity (gibbus) and with vertebral destruction there could be short scoliosis that raises scapula of other side. Shoulder joint and scapula will be normal and Shanmugasundaram test will be negative.
- *Cervicodorsal scoliosis*: This only raises the scapula on the side of convexity and no primary deltoid or scapular anomalies are seen.

5. Why only adduction is restricted in your patient, can other movements be affected?

Ans. My patient has involvement of intermediate fibers of deltoid primarily that causes restriction of adduction. If posterior deltoid fibers are involved then internal rotation will get restricted and there will be additionally external rotation contracture.

6. Why the distance of acromion angle to vertebral border of scapula increases?

Ans. Due to continued pull from contracture band of intermediate deltoid fibers the acromion gets pulled and gets lengthened.

7. Why does the shoulder droop, despite contracture it should have been up due to shortening of deltoid?

Ans. Deltoid originates within shoulder girdle so its contracture cannot lift the shoulder up. Instead due to origin from scapula and insertion into humerus the humerus gets lifted while scapular rotation externally (medial border rotated upwards) causes drooped shoulder appearance.

8. What is the cause of prominent humeral head?

Ans. The cord like contracted deltoid fibers fix the humeral length passively while the upper end of head keeps growing. Because the humerus cannot go down with lengthening it escapes upward and anteriorly making it prominent. There is anterior subluxation of humeral head that is made further prominent by inferior rotation of the glenoid.

9. How will you treat this case?

Ans. Treatment is surgical release of contracted band of fibrotic muscle. This should be followed by intense physiotherapy to maintain the lengthening.

6
The Elbow Joint

Short cases are very popular, however, long case may also be given typically to a DNB candidate—it is better to be prepared. Attempts to cover all the necessary aspects have been made in the following text.

Read times: 5-7 times for a DNB candidate, 3-4 times for a MS candidate.

EXAMINATION POINTS FOR AN ELBOW CASE

HISTORY

- *Pain*: Onset, site (bony—epicondylar, supracondylar, olecranon, radial head, and joint line; soft tissue—extensor origin, flexor origin, and bursae), duration, radiation, association with fever, and trauma.
- *Swelling*: Onset, duration, localized (laterally over soft spot "anconeus triangle" or any soft tissue site—mitotic pathology) or generalized, associated symptoms.
- *Limitation of movements*: Associated with swelling/trauma/ manipulation/immobilization/massage/fever/iatrogenic.
- *Deformity*: Congenital versus acquired, association with trauma, fever and swelling, treatment related, Charcot's arthropathy.
  Additional history: Massage, hemophilia, and manipulation attempts.

EXAMINATION

Inspection
- *Attitude*: Alignment of forearm in relation to arm (carrying angle), compare from normal, flexion deformity.

- *From front*: Flexion crease (1–2 cm above joint line, it is at the level of interepicondylar axis), swelling (epitrochlear lymph nodes, etc.), medial and lateral epicondyle, biceps tendon and lacertus fibrosus, common extensor, and flexor origin mass.
- *From lateral aspect*: Anconeus triangle and fullness over soft spot, common extensor origin, prominence of triceps tendon (elbow dislocation), olecranon process, radial head (dislocation), olecranon bursa, and biceps mass.
- *From medial aspect*: Medial epicondylar prominence, supracondylar depressions, and common flexor origins.
- *Posterior aspect (in 90° flexion)*: Olecranon process, triceps bulge, paraolecranon fossae, and three-point relationship.

Palpation

- *Superficial palpation*: Temperature and superficial tenderness
- *Deep palpation*:
    - Epicondyles, olecranon process, olecranon fossae, radial head, and capitellum (Panner's disease)
    - Myositis mass and any swelling with all characteristics (site, size, shape, surface, margins, consistency, tenderness, compressibility/reducibility, and pulsatility)
    - *Supracondylar ridges*: These palpate both medial and lateral ridges simultaneously for irregularity, thickening, discontinuity, spur, and loss of contour
    - Three-point relationship
    - Ulnar nerve (thickening, subluxation, and tenderness)
    - Joint line (for tenderness)
    - Brachial artery pulsations.

Movements

- Flexion (0–140°), extension (reversal of flexion)
- Hyperextension up to 10° is normal
- Supination (85°) and pronation (70–80°).

Measurements

- *Linear measurements*:
    - *Arm length (medial and lateral)*: Lateral length is measured from angle of acromion to lateral epicondyle, and medial

The Elbow Joint

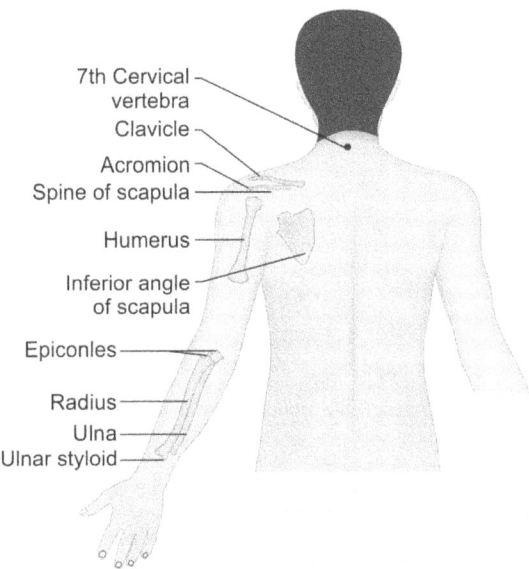

Fig. 1: Bony landmarks for upper extremity. Lengths are measured as explained in text.

length is measured from medial epicondyle to an imaginary soft tissue point on the inner aspect of arm just against the deltoid insertion **(Fig. 1)**.
- *Forearm length*: Lateral length is measured from lateral epicondyle to radial styloid process and medial length is measured from medial epicondyle to ulnar styloid process.
- *Three-point relationship measurement (in 90° flexion)*: Measurement of olecranon tip to lateral and medial epicondyles and interepicondylar distance **(Fig. 2)**.
- *Angular measurements*: Angle is formed between arm and forearm axis. [Axes are marked by joining the midpoint of lines joining the following reference points, viz. interepicondylar line at elbow, interstyloid line at wrist, and line joining deltoid insertion and a point against it (usually corresponding to tip of anterior axillary fold)] **(Figs. 3 and 4)**.

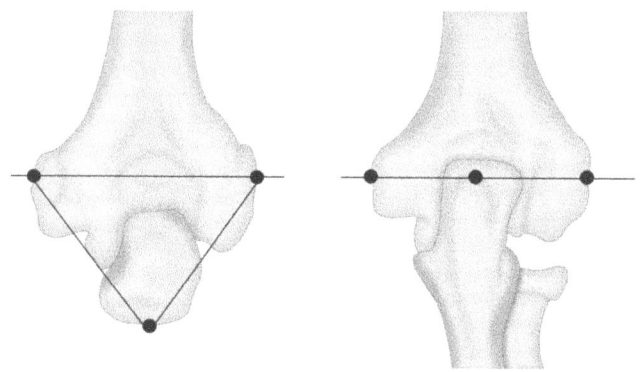

Fig. 2: Three bony point relationship around elbow in flexion and extension.

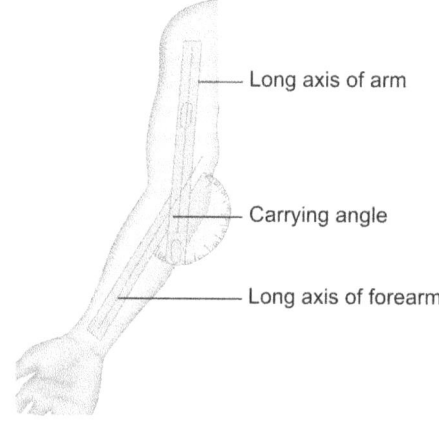

Fig. 3: Measuring carrying angle.

- *Circumferential measurements*: For wasting, measure mid-arm circumference and forearm circumference at a convenient point (usually 7 cm below medial epicondyle).

Neurological examination: Motor power of elbow flexors, extensors, supinators, pronators, biceps jerk, triceps jerk and supinator jerk, and sensory testing.

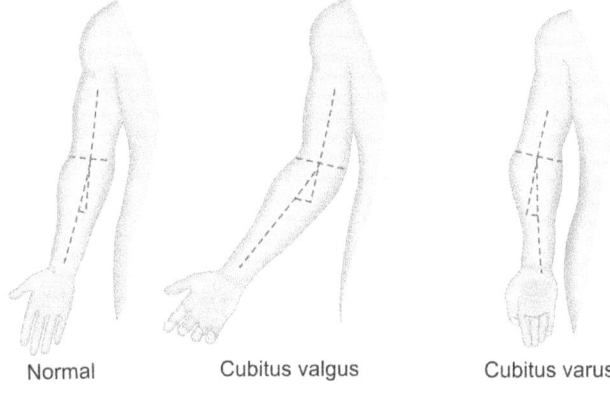

Fig. 4: Angular relationship of arm and forearm.

Special Tests

- *Varus stress test*: Test in 30° flexion to disengage olecranon
- *Valgus stress test*: Test in 30° flexion
- *Pivot shift test (for posterolateral rotator instability)*: This test is for anterior ulnar collateral ligament by applying valgus and axial compressing forces to elbow and supination torque to forearm. This maneuver produces rotator subluxation of ulnohumeral joint, which is maximum at 40° of elbow flexion.
- *Tests for lateral epicondylitis*:
    - Resisted wrist extension test
    - *Long finger extension test (Maudsley's test)*: Pain produced just distal to lateral epicondyle on resisted long finger extension in an extended upper extremity suggests lateral epicondylitis (compare from—radial tunnel syndrome)
    - Wringing test—maneuver similar to wringing clothes
    - Chair test
    - Jug test—in an attempt to lift the jug from above holding it from brim, patient feels pain in extensor origin.
    - *Cozen's test*: To an extended elbow and wrist ask the patient to make fist and passively flex the wrist in pronated forearm— produces pain at the common extensor origin **(Fig. 5)**

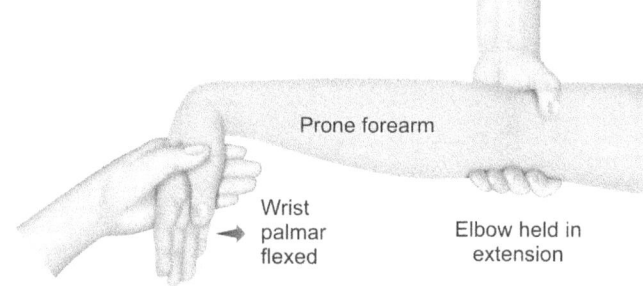

Fig. 5: Cozen's test.

- *Mill's maneuver:* With the wrist and elbow extended in supination, passively pronate forearm; this produces pain at the extensor origin
- Broom test
- Rolling-pin test
- Stir-fry test.
- *Resisted pronation*: For pronator syndrome
- *Resisted flexion and pronation*: For medial epicondylitis
- *Elbow flexion test:* For cubital tunnel syndrome
- *Long-finger extension test*: Pain produced 4 finger breadths below lateral epicondyle suggests radial tunnel syndrome.
- *Resisted elbow flexion and resisted forearm supination*: For median nerve compression at lacertus fibrosus.

Also, examine the shoulder and forearm as the compensations of elbow movements are often taken up at shoulder and the ill effects are often sustained by forearm.

1. What are the prerequisites of elbow examination?
Ans.
- Examine both elbows together.
- Examine both elbows in identical position.
- Expose whole upper limb from shoulder girdle to fingers.
- Arms lying by the side of chest is the most comfortable position for the patient.

2. What are the interpretations of three-point relationship measurements?
Ans. The olecranon, lateral, and medial epicondyle form a near-equilateral triangle in 90° flexion at elbow. In disruptions

of elbow joint, the measurements are altered and can be interpreted as below:

- *Decreased length of medial limb*: Posteromedial dislocation, medial rotation of fractured fragment
- *Decreased length of lateral limb*: Posterolateral dislocation, lateral rotation
- *Increased length of medial limb*: Fractured medial epicondyle/condyle
- *Increased length of lateral limb*: Fracture lateral condyle
- *Increased base (interepicondylar distance)*: Malunited fracture intercondylar humerus.

3. What are the fallacies of three-point relationship?

Ans.
- Displaced fracture of medial/lateral epicondyle
- Surgical intervention done leading to altered morphology and inability to palpate epicondyles
- Excision arthroplasty of elbow
- Lateral spur formation
- Ankylosed elbow in extension
- Charcot's arthropathy.

4. What is the importance of anconeus triangle?

Ans. The triangle is bounded by radial head, lateral epicondyle, and olecranon tip. The triangle directly overlies joint capsule and anconeus muscle, so this "soft spot" becomes distended early in effusions of elbow joint. Synovial biopsy from elbow joint, injections into elbow joint can be directly given by approaching this triangle. Anconeus is an important muscle in electrodiagnostic studies and can be easily approached here **(Fig. 6)**.

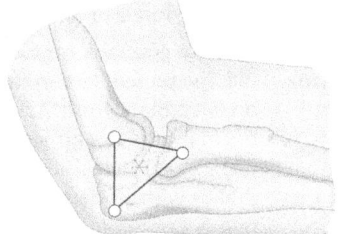

Fig. 6: Anconeus triangle.

5. How do you look for rotational deformities at elbow joint?

Ans. Internal/external rotational malalignment at elbow can be measured by measuring the external and internal rotation at shoulder in 90° abduction and while the arm is measured by the side (*the movements are to be always compared from other side*). Internal rotation deformity at elbow will restrict external rotation at shoulder and complementary increased internal rotation. This deficit or excess can be measured and is a quite accurate measure of deformity. For this measure to be effective there should be no rotational limitation at shoulder or torsional deformity of humerus and that the deformity should be unilateral. (*Remember that this measure is often only an approximation, as the dominant shoulder has an increased physiological rotation giving fallacious comparison for deformities of left elbow and masking the ipsilateral deformities.*)

Alternative method (Yamamoto et al.): Make the patient bend forward and fully internally rotate and hyperextend the shoulder (in an attempt to touch the back). Lift the hand off the back (in a normal, the hand can either be not lifted up or it is minimal). The angle made by forearm to the horizontal when compared to the opposite side gives an idea of internal rotation deformity.

6. How do you palpate for radial head?

Ans. Locate lateral epicondyle with elbow flexed to 90° then go just in front of it where a depression is first felt immediately stopped by bony silhouette of radial head. Confirm by gently rotating forearm for transmitted supination and pronation.

7. How do you look for flexion deformity of elbow?

Ans. Ask the patient to comfortably sit on chair and place his arm on flat table in front. Ask him to extend the elbow to the fullest normally the forearm touches the table completely. If forearm does not touch the table then measure the angle forearm makes with horizontal. Make sure that the interepicondylar line is horizontal to the ground before assessing the flexion deformity. (*Note: In the presence of flexion deformity, never comment on valgus deformity as even the physiological valgus varies with flexion of elbow. Similarly, however, one can say that there is varus deformity but does not attempt to quantify (measure) it when flexion deformity coexists as classically these measurements have been described in elbow extension.*)

CASE I: TUBERCULOSIS OF ELBOW JOINT

Diagnosis: The patient is a 22-year-old female with active tuberculosis of left elbow and on treatment for past 2 months with flexion deformity of 30° and further flexion of 90° (30–120°). There is restriction of pronation and supination to 0–30°.

1. Why do you call it tuberculosis of elbow?
Ans. *History:*
- Insidious onset of pain and swelling
- Prolonged symptoms with gradual progression
- Swelling (boggy) with effusion at elbow joint
- Limitation of movements over a duration
- Healing sinuses/scar
- Wasting of forearm and arm muscles
- Axillary lymphadenopathy.

2. What is your differential diagnosis?
Ans.
- Myositis ossificans
- Pigmented villonodular synovitis
- Subacute septic arthritis
- Partially/incompletely treated septic arthritis
- Mitotic pathology of muscles/synovium
- Charcot's arthropathy
- Clutton's joints.

3. What are the foci of infection for elbow joint tuberculosis?
Ans. The foci of infection are olecranon, distal humerus, radial head, and uncommonly synovial membrane.

4. What will you do to confirm diagnosis?
Ans. Anteroposterior and lateral projections of elbow joint, which reveal diffuse osteopenia, lytic foci in relevant bone, periosteal reaction, and decreased joint space. Late stages may additionally show deformation of bone ends, pathological posterior dislocation of joint, and spina ventosa of proximal ulna.

(For other diagnostic modalities, please see Chapter 2: Case I; Q9).

5. What do you mean by the term spina ventosa?

Ans. *Spina = long/short slender bone, ventosa = dilated with air.* The loculated expansile appearance resembles a dilated bone due to air. This deformity is often seen in thin long slender bone of hands and feet.

6. How will you manage the patient?

Ans. Early diseases with maintained outline of bones and somehow preserved joint space are expected to return to good function with healing of disease. I will put the patient on chemotherapy (*for regime, please see Chapter 2: Case 1; Q19*) and supervise for the response. Advanced disease with destruction of bone ends and pus collection and discharging sinuses are better managed with early excision of focus and chemotherapy with immobilization in functional position.

7. What are the other surgical options?

Ans. *Excisional arthroplasty*: For disease healed in unacceptable position or in a case of advanced arthrodesis/ankylosis, if the patient desires a mobile joint.

Arthrotomy and excision of focus: For uncertain diagnosis, nonresponders, or advanced disease.

Arthrodesis: For a heavy manual laborer.

Arthroplasty: Principles are same as discussed elsewhere (*See Chapter 10: Elbow Arthroplasty*).

8. What is the optimal position of elbow arthrodesis?

Ans. Optimal position of arthrodesis varies from patient to patient and should be determined by experimentally immobilizing the limb using plaster of Paris (POP) cast or brace. For unilateral arthrodesis, 90° flexion and mid-prone position are often acceptable. Bilateral cases may be arthrodesed in 65° for one limb in supination for personal hygiene and the other in 110° flexion in mid-prone position for ability to reach mouth, however, this is highly undesirable to do so!

CASE II: THE STIFF ELBOW AND ECTOPIC OSSIFICATION

Diagnosis: The patient is a case of post-traumatic stiff elbow with flexion contracture for past 2 years with 60° flexion deformity and further 30° range of motion.

The Elbow Joint

1. How much functional range of movements is required at elbow joint?

Ans. For activities of daily living, 100° flexion with the functional range of arc from 30–130° and 100° rotation (50° each of pronation and supination) is required.

2. How do you classify stiff elbow?

Ans. *Extrinsic causes*
- Soft tissue:
  - Capsuloligamentous
  - Muscular
- Ectopic ossification

Intrinsic causes
- Intra-articular adhesions
- Loss of articular cartilage
- Gross distortion resulting from inadequate or failed reduction.

3. What are the various causes of stiff elbow?

Ans.
- Post-traumatic:
  - Joint incongruity
  - Dislocation/subluxation
- Heterotopic ossification
- Burns
- Coronoid/olecranon/radial osteophytes
- Loose bodies
- Triceps/biceps adhesions
- Chronic infection
- Inflammatory arthritis
- Patient noncompliance
- Postsurgery.

4. How will you differentiate extrinsic from intrinsic stiff elbow?

Ans. Intrinsic stiff elbow gives a bony stop to movements while extrinsic stiffness presents with comparatively soft stop. There is associated deformity in coronal plane in intrinsic stiffness. Movements are grossly painful in intrinsic causes due to early development of arthritis. In extrinsic causes, the contracture stands out on pursuing movements. Wasting of all groups of muscles is more evident in intrinsic stiff elbow.

5. How will you manage this patient?

Ans. Evaluate with radiological investigations (X-ray and/or CT) and then categorization and management as below:
- *Acute:* Open reduction and internal fixation (ORIF), continuous passive motion, and splints (dynamic and static)
- *Subacute (<6 months)*: Splints, anti-inflammatory drugs, and close follow-up
- *Chronic (>6 months)*: X-ray ± CT scan
  - Ectopic ossification present
  - No ectopic ossification:
    - *Extrinsic causes:* Release
    - Intrinsic causes:
      - *Articular*: Soft tissue release or distraction arthroplasty for acceptable surfaces otherwise elbow arthroplasty (>50% cartilage destroyed)
      - *Impingement*: Coronoid/olecranon: Excision of bony stop.

6. What will you do for this patient?

Ans. I will put the patient on conservative regime of stretching, strengthening, and mobilization with analgesics. Then based upon the progress (if functional range of movement is not regained), I will decide surgery.

7. What surgery will you do?

Ans. I will do anterior contracture release (column procedure). Then I will reassess the movements on table, if there is restriction of flexion then I will do a posterior release also.

8. What is column procedure?

Ans. Posterolateral incision → dissection between extensor carpi ulnaris (ECU) and anconeus. Separate extensor tendon from joint capsule and LCL. Expose anterior capsule and release it as wide as possible. For posterior release, dissection

The Elbow Joint

proceeds between extensor carpi radialis longus (ECRL) and triceps and posterior capsule is released. Look for and excise the olecranon and coronoid osteophytes. Immediate continuous passive motion (CPM) is begun followed by dynamic splintage after 3 weeks and gradual weaning over 3 months.

9. What is Bhattacharya procedure?

Ans. Elbow arthrolysis procedure of Bhattacharya includes the following:
- Removal of capsular contracture
- Mobilizing brachialis and triceps from lower humerus
- Restoration of trochlear pulley
- Minimal removal of bone block without excising articular surface
- Postoperative course:
  - Instill 25 mg hydrocortisone acetate in joint with 2–5 cc of hylase
  - Compression bandage with splint in full extension
  - Second dose of hydrocortisone with 2–4 cc of lignocaine on 7th–10th day.

10. What are the contraindications of arthrolysis/soft-tissue release?

Ans. Soft-tissue release procedures should not be done in the following:
- Significant alteration of the articular contour
- Loss of cartilage >50%
- When release of one or both collateral ligaments
- Motor deficiency or spasticity.

11. What are various arthroplasty options for elbow?

Ans. The intra-articular (intrinsic) causes need the following:
- Distraction arthroplasty
- Fascial interposition arthroplasty
- Replacement arthroplasty.

12. What is distraction arthroplasty?

Ans. It keeps the injured articular surfaces distracted while simultaneously providing joint motion and protection to collateral ligaments.

Indications:
- Adjuvant to capsule release, if ligaments are damaged, or
- Significant dissection making intraoperative motion difficult, or
- >50% joint surface void of cartilage, or
- Modified joint contour.

13. What is fascial interposition arthroplasty?

Ans. It is an alternative for a poorly articulated or ankylosed joint where painless movements are desired and elbow replacement cannot be done.

Indications:
- Young patients with post-traumatic ankylosis of elbow with intact broad contour of distal humerus
- Young adult stage I and II rheumatoid arthritis with intact bone.

14. What materials can be used for interposition arthroplasty?

Ans.
- *Natural:* Fascia and fat patch
- *Synthetic*: Synthetic membranes.

15. What is ectopic ossification?

Ans. It is formation of bone at abnormal places.

Types:
- *Heterotopic ossification*: Formation of mature lamellar bone in nonosseous tissue (dystrophic process involving ligaments and capsule; can be metastatic).
- *Myositis ossificans (a misnomer)*: Benign localized reactive proliferative lesion occurring within soft tissues (muscles) that normally do not ossify.
- *Periarticular ossification*: Collection of calcium pyrophosphate crystals in soft tissue (lacks trabecular pattern).

16. What are the various causes of myositis ossificans?

Ans. The causes are classified into three types (etiological classification):
1. *Traumatic (myositis ossificans circumscripta, myosteatosis, ossifying hematoma)*: Contusions, tearing, and postoperative

The Elbow Joint

2. *Neurogenic*: Injury to neural axis
3. Myositis ossificans progressiva, which is an inherited disorder. More than 1/3rd cases are idiopathic.

17. Which muscle is commonly involved in myositis ossificans at elbow?

Ans. Brachialis muscle, others can be pronator teres and brachioradialis.

18. What are the clinical features of myositis ossificans?

Ans. Clinical features depend upon the phase in which patient is seen:
- *Acute/pseudoinflammatory phase (3rd day–3rd week)*: Pain, swelling, and ↓ROM (range of motion)
- *Subacute/pseudotumor phase (3–6 weeks)*: Painless hard mass with raised temperature locally
- Maturation (3–6 months)
- Resolution (few cases only).

19. How do you classify ectopic ossification around any joint?

Ans. Functional classification (Hasting and Graham):
- *Class I*: Radiologically evident ectopic ossification without clinical limitation
- *Class II*: Subtotal, functional, and limitation of motion:
    - *A*: In flexion and extension plane
    - *B*: In pronation and supination plane
    - *C*: In both planes
- *Class III*: Ankylosis that eliminates motion (A, B, and C as above).

20. What is the differential diagnosis of myositis ossificans?

Ans. The following are often confused with myositis ossificans:
- Deep vein thrombosis (DVT) in acute phase
- Osteogenic sarcoma
- Mesenchymal chondrosarcomas
- Synovial sarcoma
- Calcified lipoma
- Hemangiomas (phleboliths).

21. What is "zonal" phenomenon?

Ans. This applies to the functional orientation of fibroblasts to osteoblasts in all ossifying masses. Myositis ossificans matures from inside to outside. Center is less mature (higher mitotic figures and cellular atypia frequent), mature cells in periphery. "Reverse zoning" is seen in tumors. This helps to differentiate myositis from otherwise very difficult to differentiate osteoid forming tumors typically osteosarcoma histologically.

22. What are the available treatment modalities for ectopic ossification?

Ans. *Prophylaxis*:
- *Chemotherapeutic agents*:
    - *Acute phase*: Ice, compression, maintenance of ROM (CPM), support the limb, avoid massage/forceful passive mobilization.
    - *Bisphosphonates*: Merely delay the appearance of mass—not recommended now
    - *Nonsteroidal anti-inflammatory drugs (NSAIDs)*: Started on the first postoperative day and continued for 2 weeks
    - Calcitonin (doubtful efficacy)—also not recommended
    - Thalidomide (for myositis ossificans progressiva)
- *Radiation therapy*: Low-dose external beam radiation within 96 hours (20 Gy/10 fractions). Coventry (1981) recommended other regimes like 10 Gy/5 fractions, 6–8 Gy/5 fractions.
- *Excision:* Surgery.

23. What are the indications of surgery?

Ans. *Criteria for doing surgical treatment:*
- Functionally limiting joint stiffness (mechanical obstruction) or neurological or vascular complication due to mass is the only finite indication for excision. Relative indications include noncosmetic bump and if the patient demands surgery.

Prerequisites:
- Radiographic union of fracture
- Radiographic evidence of intact articulating surfaces
- Mature mass

The Elbow Joint

- Soft tissue equilibrium (do not touch a hot metabolically active mass)
- Stabilized traumatic brain injury and motivated patient.

24. How do you assess maturity of mass?

Ans. Note the following points:
- No local rise of temperature, no edema
- Normal erythrocyte sedimentation rate (ESR) and alkaline phosphatase
- Bone scintigraphy—investigation of choice (≥ 2 bone scans showing normal/decreased uptake).

In general, duration of 18 months is accepted as the sufficient time needed for maturation.

25. What is the surgical protocol?

Ans. Delayed intervention (>18 months) is recommended and has the advantage of finding a metabolically quiescent bone in a tissue in equilibrium. Also, it gives additional time for associated injuries (traumatic brain damage) to heal and stabilize.

26. How will you surgically manage ectopic ossification around elbow?

Ans. After taking care as above, I will resect the ossified mass taking care for the following:
- Incision should be selected to be able to resect all ectopic bone
- Decompress the compressed nerve
- Resection of anterior and posterior capsule
- Debride coronoid process
- Clear olecranon fossa
- Excision of terminal 1–1.5 cm of olecranon
- Correction of elbow instability
- Transposition of ulnar nerve
- Preserve collateral ligaments and annular cartilage of radial head
- Start prophylaxis.

27. What are the problems of delayed treatment?

Ans. Delay in treatment leads to:
- Progressive and advanced contracture

- Potential articular cartilage destruction
- Prolonged infirmity.

28. How will you manage old unreduced dislocation of elbow (see also case IV below for clinical features and diagnosis of elbow dislocation Q9)?

Ans. The first thing to be done is to thoroughly counsel the parents and patient about poor prognosis of treatment. Reduction can be achieved after surgery but stiffness mostly significant remains. If stiffness is not there then elbow will become grossly unstable, so it is a complex situation. The surgical procedure consists of:
- Open reduction of humeroulnar articulation—usually needs thorough debridement of intra-articular fibrosis and release of contracted ligaments. Articular surface may be grossly damaged and misshapen in long-standing cases.
- Lengthening of triceps (V→Y)
- Internal stabilization of the joint for soft tissues to heal in desired position.

CASE III: THE UNSTABLE ELBOW

EXAMINATION AND FINDINGS

- *History*:
  - Antecedent trauma
  - Overuse sports injury
  - Congenital anomalies
  - Surgery to elbow
  - Erosive arthropathy
  - Generalized ligament laxity
  - Locking/clicking with clunk when elbow supinated in extension half way through ROM
  - Assess patient's needs and demands
- Generalized joint laxity
- Arthropathy (Charcot's/syphilitic)
- *Elbow*:
  - External signs of injury/surgery
  - Tenderness over collateral ligaments

The Elbow Joint

- *Stress tests:*
  - Valgus
  - Varus:
    - Milking maneuver
    - Radiocapitellar compression test
    - Lateral pivot shift test
    - Valgus laxity in pronation
    - Valgus extension overload test
    - *Ulnar nerve*: Tinel's test.

1. What are the various restraints to elbow joint?

Ans. *Dynamic*: Anconeus, triceps, and brachialis

Static:
- Primary:
  - Ulnohumeral articulation (only stabilizes in <20° and >120° flexion)
  - Medial collateral ligament (MCL)
  - Lateral collateral ligament (LCL)
- Secondary:
  - Radial head
  - Capsule
  - Common flexor pronator and extensor origin.

Stabilizers of elbow for various stresses:

Valgus stress:
- Primary:
  - MCL:
    - *Anterior bundle:* Principle—stabilizer in 30–120° flexion
    - *Posterior bundle:* Corestraint
- Secondary:
  - Radial head
- Tertiary:
  - Flexor pronator muscle groups (FCR and FDS).

Varus stress:
- Primary:
  - LCL and annular ligament complex
- Secondary:
  - Extensor muscles with fascial bands
  - Intermuscular septa.

2. What is "fortress concept" for elbow stability?

Ans. According to O'Driscoll, the ulnohumeral articulation, lateral collateral ligament (LCL), and medial (anterior portion) collateral ligament (MCL) serve as outer "wall" and radiohumeral, common extensor and common flexor origin as inner "wall" of fortress as protection against stresses.

3. How do you classify the elbow instability?

Ans. Five criteria have been used to classify elbow instabilities **(Table 1)**.

Table 1: Criteria used to classify elbow instability.			
Articulation involved	Proximal radioulnar joint (radial head)	Ulnohumeral and radiohumeral (elbow)	Both (divergent)
Direction of displacement	• Anterior • Posterior	• Varus/valgus • Anteroposterior • Mediolateral • Posterolateral rotatory instability (PLRI)	Posterior
Degree of displacement	Subluxation	Perched	Complete
Timing	• Acute • Chronic	• Acute/chronic • Recurrent	Acute
Associated fractures	None	• Radial head • Olecranon • Coronoid	None

4. What are the various patterns of elbow instability seen?

Ans. *Valgus instability*:
- Athletic chronic overuse injuries
- Repetitive overload:
  - Intrinsic (muscular)
  - Extrinsic (external tensile overload).

Varus instability:
- Posterolateral rotatory instability (PLRI)
- Recurrent isolated radial head instability:
  - Anterior instability
  - Posterior instability.

The Elbow Joint

5. What are the various causes of elbow instability?
Ans.
- *Acquired causes*:
  - Simple dislocation
  - Fracture dislocation
  - Fractures in association with ligament injuries
  - Pure ligament injuries
  - Arthropathies
  - Hyperextension injury
  - Repetitive valgus stress
- Congenital causes
- Iatrogenic causes.

6. What is the "unified concept" of elbow instability?
Ans. The unified concept (pathomechanics) of clinical spectrum of acute and chronic elbow instability—"circle concept" (Hori's circle):
- Three sequential stages of elbow instability.
- The Hori's circle progresses from lateral to medial side.
- It may pass through soft tissue or bone or both.

7. What is the most common mechanism of injury producing unstable elbow?
Ans. Valgus strain in a supinated elbow under axial compression is the most common mechanism of injury, which is seen in fall on outstretched hand. The stresses begin laterally and pass medially "around elbow" joint anteriorly or posteriorly depending on the position and either through bone or soft tissue or both.

(*Most chronic affections of elbow affect the MCL due to peculiar disposition of elbow in valgus; however, most acute injuries affect LCL due to positional valgus stress at the time of injury!*)

8. What is the sequence of tissue injury?
Ans. The circle in progression meets three distinct stages that can arrest anywhere depending upon the severity of injuring force:
- *Stage I*: LCL disruption → posterolateral rotatory subluxation → may undergo spontaneous reduction.

- *Stage II*: Additional anterior and posterior disruption → coronoid perched over trochlea → may reduce with minimum force.
- *Stage III*: Subdivided into three parts:
  - *IIIA*: Anterior medial collateral ligament intact → stable in pronation
  - *IIIB*: Entire MCL disrupted → varus, valgus, and rotatory instability following reduction
  - *IIIC*: Entire distal humerus devoid of soft-tissue attachment → unstable even in 90° flexion in cast.

9. What are the associated fractures with this injury?

Ans. The associated fractures are coronoid, radial head, posterior capitellum, medial and/or lateral epicondyle.

10. What are your differential diagnoses?

Ans. As the patient presents with pain on activity and feeling of "not enough strength", the following serve as important differentials:
- *Anterior*: Anterior capsular tear, pronator teres syndrome, and annular ligament disruption
- *Posterior*: Traction apophysitis, triceps tendonitis/rupture, and valgus-extension overload syndrome
- *Medial*: Medial epicondylar physeal fractures, medial epicondylitis, snapping elbow syndrome, medial elbow instability, and ulnar neuritis
- *Lateral*: Panner's disease, radial head fracture, radiocapitellar overload syndrome, and PLRI.

11. How will you investigate the patient?

Ans. If the clinical examination is equivocal then manipulation under anesthesia is worth considering in a symptomatic patient after ruling out above conditions.

Radiology:
- *Plain X-rays*: To look for associated bony injury, degenerative changes, ectopic bone formation, and posteromedial osteophytes
- *Stress radiographs*: Varus and valgus stress, posterolateral stress

The Elbow Joint

- *Magnetic resonance imaging (MRI) and magnetic resonance (MR) arthrography*: Rupture of collateral ligaments and muscle groups
- *Computed tomography (CT) arthrography (86% sensitive and 97% specific)*: Undersurface tear in MCL → "T-Sign"
- *Arthroscopy*: Controversial value.

12. How will you decide treatment in this case?

Ans. I will undertake the following course (please refer to classification especially type III for a good understanding of the algorithm and the various constraints and 'circle concept'):

- Reduce and test stability clinically, if stable → splint/sling and early mobilization and muscle equilibrium and strengthening exercises
- If unstable in "1" then pronate and retest, if stable → hinged brace, forearm pronated and gradual mobilization
- If unstable in "2" then fully flex and check for up to 30° extension block, if stable → hyperflexion and pronation immobilization with 30° extension block and gradual mobilization
- If unstable in "3" then → operate!

13. How will you decide surgery?

Ans. Surgical treatment algorithm (depends much on the identified ligamentous injuries and radiological investigations):

- If all constraints can be repaired → ORIF and repair ligaments/tendons
- No to "1" but ulnohumeral articulation intact → excise unfixable radial head/replace radial head and repair ligaments/tendons
- No to "2" but ulnohumeral joint can be fixed → ORIF coronoid and or olecranon and may excise/replace radial head, repair ligaments and tendons
- No to "3" then look for "type" of coronoid fracture: For type I/II coronoid fracture → suture it, ORIF or replace/partially excise radial head and repair ligaments and tendons. For type III coronoid fracture → ORIF coronoid and apply hinged distractor.

14. What is the terrible triad of elbow injury?

Ans. It is combination of elbow dislocation and radial head and coronoid fractures.

15. How will you manage this injury?

Ans. Fundamental to management is to convert complex dislocation into simple dislocation as above.

16. What is the cause of recurrent dislocation of elbow?

Ans. Exceedingly rare, causes may be misshapen trochlear notch of ulna, lax collateral ligaments. Both congenital and post-traumatic forms are documented. Manage as above for post traumatic ones else for congenital forms → arthroplasty.

17. What is recurrent dislocation of radial head?

Ans. Disruption of annular ligament produces anterior subluxation or dislocation of radial head especially during pronation. Diagnosis is done by finding of locking/popping of elbow, decreased ROM, crepitus over radial head ± tenderness, and apprehension to hyperpronation.

18. What is your differential diagnosis?

Ans. PLRI, Monteggia fracture-dislocation, congenital dislocation of radial head, and dislocation in association with cerebral palsy.

19. How will you treat recurrent radial head instability?

Ans. Recurrent radial head instability is treated by annular ligament reconstruction (Bell–Tawse procedure) and radial head excision.

CASE IV: CUBITUS VARUS

Diagnosis: The patient is a 10-year-old male child with right side cubitus varus deformity for 7 months due to malunited supracondylar fracture of humerus with restricted flexion and pronation without any distal neurological deficit.

If there is flexion deformity then mention after diagnosis and remember that diagnosis will then not include 'cubitus varus' instead you will have to mention 'Gunstock deformity'.

The Elbow Joint

1. How do you define cubitus varus deformity?

Ans. When the forearm is deviated inwards (toward midline) with respect to arm at elbow with resulting lateral angulation *in full extension*, we call it cubitus varus. [*Note: Literally speaking any reduction of physiological valgus is also cubitus varus—although there is no true varus angulation! This further implies that even cubitus rectus is 'cubitus varus' deformity of elbow so when you do the correction of deformity then you add the normal valgus (by measuring at other elbow) to give full correction—opinions should not differ.*]

2. What is the anatomical alignment at elbow?

Ans. Forearm is aligned in a valgus of 8–15° (8–11° for males; 10–15° for females) with respect to arm in full extension with a medial angulation.

3. What if the angulation is lost?

Ans. If the alignment is neutral, we call it cubitus rectus "deformity". It is still a "deformity", as it deviates from the normal for population.

4. What is the name of this alignment of elbow?

Ans. This is called carrying angle **(Figs. 7A and B)**.

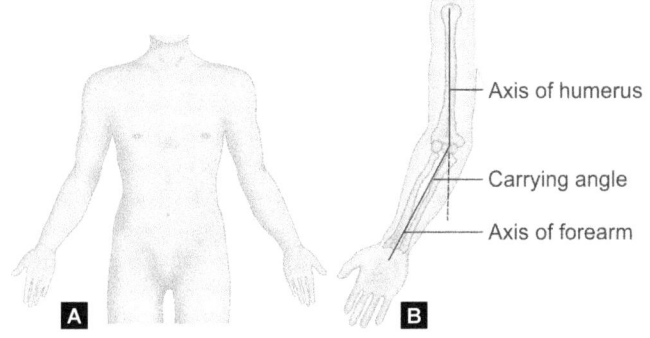

Figs. 7A and B: Carrying angle.

5. Why do you only measure it in complete extension?

Ans. The carrying angle is measured in elbow extension and supination. The carrying angle reduces in flexion and with complete flexion, the long axis of arm and forearm coincide making the angle "zero". There is no guideline that compares the reduction of carrying angle viz-a-viz elbow flexion, so measurement in any degree of flexion will be fallacious.

6. Why is the carrying angle lost in flexion?

Ans. During elbow flexion, the ulna rotates internally (minor effect) and tilts medially (major effect, due to peculiar trochlear anatomy), and this causes loss of carrying angle of elbow.

7. Why do you call it post-traumatic malunited supracondylar fracture?

Ans. There is history of trauma with relevant treatment.

On examination:
- Gunstock deformity of elbow **(Fig. 8)**, the deformity appears more like a 'gunstock' when shoulder is abducted to 90°.
- Irregularity and thickening over medial and lateral supracondylar ridges (indicate healed fracture)
- Hyperextension at elbow
- No widening at intercondylar region
- No deficiency in the region of trochlea
- Internal rotation deformity with restricted external rotation and increased internal rotation
- Maintained three-point relationship

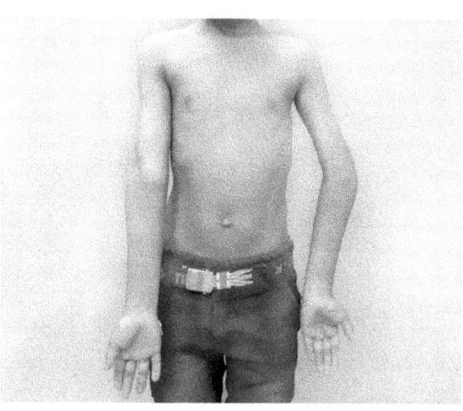

Fig. 8: Cubitus varus deformity of elbow.

The Elbow Joint

- Medial epicondyle tip is higher
- Lengthening of arm length with a normal forearm length.

8. Why the rotational deformities do not manifest?

Ans. The much more mobile shoulder joint compensates for the same so often they go unnoticed by patient or relatives.

9. Why is this not an elbow dislocation?

Ans. Though fall on outstretched hand also can produce elbow dislocation but the elbow is slightly flexed at impact (these subtle differences are never noticed by the onlookers irrespective of how good you are at history taking, so, it is only theoretical).

Clinically, following points differentiate an elbow dislocation by presence of:

- Prominent olecranon and triceps tendon insertion
- Semiflexed elbow due to dislocation
- Wasting of periarticular muscles
- The three-point bony relationship is distorted—reduced length of lateral limb of triangle—posterolateral dislocation, reduced medial limb length—posteromedial dislocation.
- Loss of movements—presents as stiff elbow
- Presence of ectopic bone as a bony hard mass that is smooth surfaced in or just above cubital fossa not tethered to skin **(Fig. 9)**.

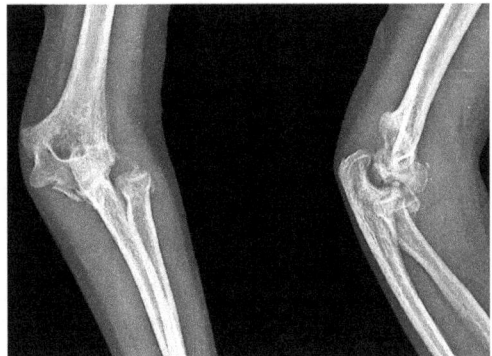

Fig. 9: Radiographs showing old unreduced elbow dislocation.

10. Is it a progressive deformity?

Ans. No, it is a static deformity *(also see Question below).*

11. What are the other causes of cubitus varus/what is your differential diagnosis (DD)?

Ans. Apart from above:
- Congenital (progressive)
- Malunited fracture lateral condyle (progressive, if due to hyperemia and overgrowth)
- Trochlear osteonecrosis (often nonprogressive)
- Malunited intercondylar fracture (static)
- Malunited medial condyle fracture (static)
- Infective damage to medial physis (progressive)
- Exostosis near to physis.

12. Why is supracondylar fracture so common and why does it occur at this site?

Ans. Young active boys in age group of 5-8 years are susceptible for this fracture more so on left side (nondominant side). Injury is commonly sustained following fall on outstretched hand (FOOSH) while flexion type may occur following direct fall on the elbow. The following reasons account for the same:
- Thin wafer of bone
- Olecranon impinges at the fossa with leverage and delivers point stress
- Soft tissues often are lax in children, which account for possible hyperextension
- The bone is actively undergoing remodeling at the site during 6–10 years of age so weakened metaphysis
- Large number of actively growing physes in vicinity account for increased vascularity at the region and resultant relative hyperemia
- Periosteal attachment to olecranon fossa (results in constant transcondylar failure); the capsule is tight anteriorly and hinges the olecranon tip against fossa.

13. What is the cause for a higher frequency of posteromedial type fracture?

Ans. The following bring the distal fragment medially:
- Pronation of forearm at fall
- Eccentric (medial) pull of biceps
- Medial column collapse
- Oblique fracture line.

14. What are the displacements of a supracondylar fracture?

Ans. Following are the displacements in a typical supracondylar fracture:
- Medial displacement (shift)
- Medial tilt
- Internal rotation
- Posterior displacement (shift)
- Posterior tilt
- Proximal migration.

15. What causes restriction of flexion in malunited supracondylar fracture?

Ans. Most commonly, malunion in extension causes restriction of flexion but there is hyperextension movement, so *per se* the arc of movement is same as that of other elbow (the joint is normal but only posteriorly tilted, so the gain in extension = loss in flexion movement). However, in some cases with extension and proximal migration of distal fragment, there is bony restriction from anterior cortex of the humerus; here, there is true restriction of flexion of elbow.

16. What neurovascular structures are particularly at risk in a supracondylar fracture?

Ans. Radial nerve in posteromedial type fracture displacement, median nerve in posterolateral type, anterior interosseous, and ulnar (flexion type: 2–3% of all supracondylar fractures are flexion type) all may be damaged (often neurapraxia and that too of mixed type is seen). Brachial artery is particularly at risk in posterolateral displacement with median nerve, which is further placed at risk by ulnar-sided tether of supratrochlear branch.

17. What are the complications of supracondylar fracture?

Ans. *Early*:
- Compartment syndrome
- *Nerve injury*: Anterior interosseous branch of median nerve is overall the most common damaged nerve in supracondylar fractures and is especially precarious in posterolateral displacement (though this is not the most common type), ulnar nerve is involved commonly in flexion type fractures, and radial nerve is commonly at risk in posteromedial displacement and is 2nd most common nerve injury.
- Vascular injury.

Late:
- Malunion
- Volkmann's ischemic contracture (VIC)
- Myositis ossificans
- Cubitus varus
- Cubitus valgus
- Tardy ulnar nerve palsy
- Chronic nerve entrapment in healed callus (Metev's sign).

18. What are the clinical signs of an irreducible fracture?

Ans. Button holing of the fragment through anterior muscles particularly brachialis, which is evident as puckering.

19. How do you classify supracondylar fracture?

Ans. Pediatric supracondylar fractures of humerus can be of flexion type or extension type. The extension type is further classified according to Gartland system **(Fig. 10)**:
- *Type I*: Undisplaced fracture
- *Type II*: Displaced with angulation but intact posterior cortex (A—angulation only, B—with rotation)
- *Type III*: Completely displaced fracture with no cortical contact (A—without rotation, B—with rotation)
  Modified Gartland system divides Type 3 into 2 subtypes:
    - IIIA: Completely displaced posteromedially
    - IIIB: Posterolateral displacement
- *Type IV*: Multidirectional instability with circumferential periosteal disruption.

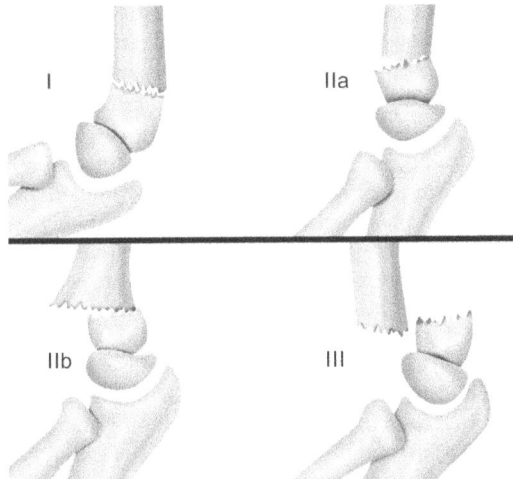

Fig. 10: Types of supracondylar fractures of elbow.

20. How do you manage the acute supracondylar fracture?

Ans. Type I fracture (Gartland's) and most of type II are managed using closed reduction and plaster slab immobilization in 90° flexion or less and pronation (in posteromedial type) or supination (in posterolaterally displaced fracture) (some people recommend skin traction or overhead skeletal olecranon screw traction). Type III fractures being unstable are managed by closed/open reduction and percutaneous pinning (posteromedial >> common than posterolateral = 3:1). Previous practice of hyperflexion is discredited now and is obsolete.

21. Why do you immobilize in flexion?

Ans. In Types I and often in Type II the posterior periosteum is spared. This acts as posterior splint, additional splinting is obtained by tightening of triceps posteriorly.

22. What precaution do you take while reducing fracture and applying slab?

Ans. One needs to keep a constant check of vascularity by keeping finger over radial pulse.

23. What configuration of cast do you use?

Ans. Above elbow, cast/slab is applied from deltoid muscle insertion to proximal palmar crease just short of knuckles and leaves the base of thumb free.

24. What if the radial pulse disappears during plastering?

Ans. Usually, the circulation is improved with reduction but if, while putting plaster, the circulation (judged by capillary filling and pulse oximeter) deteriorates then I will reduce flexion at elbow gradually till when circulation improves. If the circulation does not improve even with a plaster in less than 45° flexion after 10 minutes then vascular surgeon consult is imperative. If say the circulation is adequate but no radial pulses are palpable (pink pulseless hand), I will keep the child in close observation after plastering in adequate flexion. If then the circulation deteriorates then I will consult vascular surgeon else just the absence of radial pulses is not a criteria for judging circulation.

25. What precaution do you take while pinning the fracture?

Ans. After closed reduction, lateral pin is inserted first (in hyperflexion) followed by medial pin after bringing elbow to 80–90° flexion (it reduces risk of ulnar nerve injury). Reduction of flexion prevents subluxation of ulnar nerve.

26. How will you protect ulnar nerve?

Ans. Besides pinning the fracture medially in less flexion (or better in extension), I will push the medial soft-tissues using finger/thumb, and visualize the medial epicondyle directly through stab incision. Direct visualization is better in cases of gross swelling of elbow. Also, I will use tissue protector while inserting the medial pin.

27. How many pins and what configuration will you use?

Ans. As such two pins are adequate for most patients and though biomechanically cross-pinning is expected to provide more stability a diverging-lateral-only 2-pin configuration that engages opposite cortex also works well. The major emphasis is that the site of pin convergence should be as away from the fracture plane as possible. If stability is doubtful after two lateral only pins then third medial pin can be added with proper precautions.

The Elbow Joint

28. How do you look for adequacy of reduction?

Ans. For coronal plane alignment, a true anteroposterior (AP) view of elbow is evaluated and compared with the normal side for Baumann's angle and intact olecranon fossa **(Fig. 11)**. A crude approximation is that a change of 5° in Baumann's angle will produce a 2° cubitus varus at the malunion. Other measures are humero-ulno-wrist alignment (apparently more accurate than Baumann's angle) and metaphyseal-diaphyseal angle. For rotational alignment (axial malalignment), one should look for any deformation in the tear drop in a true lateral view and that anterior humeral line must transect capitellum (other measures like shaft-condylar angle and coronoid line can also be evaluated). Finally, sagittal plane malalignment (flexion–extension) is also looked for in a true lateral view.

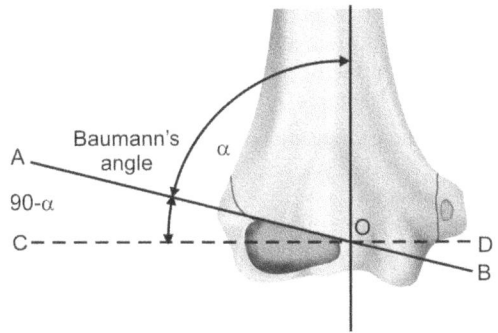

Fig. 11: Baumann's angle.

29. What is Baumann's angle?

Ans. Baumann's angle is the angle subtended between the tangent to lateral physeal line and long axis of diaphysis of humerus (normal = 64–81°; mean = 72°).

30. What is the role of traction in management of supracondylar fractures?

Ans. Though with better fixation techniques, the role of traction has reduced but in cases of severe swelling and places where facility of intraoperative imaging is unavailable, patient may

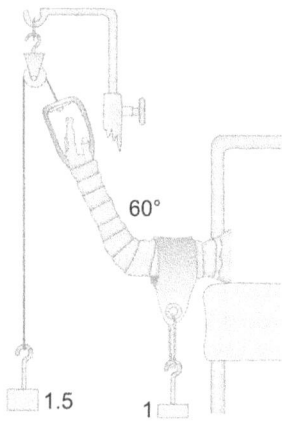

Fig. 12: Dunlop traction.

be kept in Dunlop traction (**Fig. 12**). Relative indication is in a case of open fracture with gross contamination and highly comminuted fractures.

31. What are the indications of open reduction?
Ans.
- Open fracture
- Irreducible fracture
- Associated neurovascular injury
- Flexion type fracture
- Delayed presentation (>1 week).

32. How do you look for cubitus varus deformity on a lateral view?
Ans. "Crescent sign" due to overlapping of capitellum on olecranon.

33. What are the associated deformities with cubitus varus?
Ans. Cubitus varus (medial tilt and lateral angulation) is accompanied with:
1. Internal rotation
2. Extension of distal fragment
3. Shortening
4. Medial shift

"3" and "4" are seen in severe forms only.

34. What deformities may get corrected over time?

Ans. As this deformity is not in the physiological direction of elbow, so correction, if at all, is minimal. Only extension deformity (partially) and, to a minimal extent, medial shift are corrected over time. This is the reason why this cosmetic deformity often persists.

35. Is the ulnar nerve at risk in cubitus varus deformity?

Ans. Not as commonly as in cubitus valgus but for sure there is reported tardy ulnar nerve palsy in cubitus varus deformity. This is due to medial shift of triceps, which narrows the cubital tunnel or fibrous band across the heads of flexor carpi ulnaris.

36. How will you differentiate between a lateral condyle fracture and supracondylar fracture clinically?

Ans. The points mentioned in **Table 2** must be noted to differentiate a lateral condyle fracture and supracondylar fracture clinically.

Table 2: Difference between lateral condyle fracture and supracondylar fracture.		
Findings	*Lateral condyle fracture*	*Supracondylar fracture*
Three-point relationship	Disturbed	Maintained
Arm length	Normal	May be reduced
Thickening of supra-condylar ridges	Lateral only	Both sides
Instability	To varus stress	None
Fixed flexion	Present	Absent deformity
Movements	Restrictions of rotation or flexion/extension often seen	None often (decreased external rotation at shoulder is due to bony deformity at elbow)
Hyperextension	Restricted	Often hyperextension seen
Complications	Delayed by months to years	Usually immediate and neurovascular
Long-term	Arthrosis common	Very rare

37. What is the other name of cubitus varus deformity?

Ans. Gunstock deformity (**Fig. 13**).

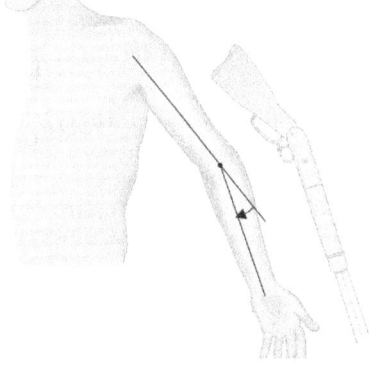

Fig. 13: Gunstock deformity.

38. Why is it called so?

Ans. The deformity resembles the loading stock of old long barrel guns.

39. What will you do for this patient?

Ans. I will confirm my diagnosis radiologically and then do a modified French osteotomy (lateral closing wedge osteotomy).

40. What radiographs will you order?

Ans. I will obtain radiographs of both elbows (preferably in a single film) in anteroposterior projection in full supination, and lateral projection (**Fig. 14**).

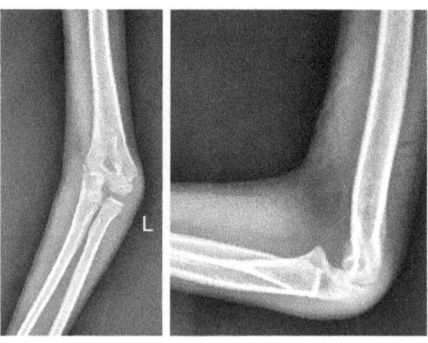

Fig. 14: Radiograph of cubitus varus deformity.

The Elbow Joint

41. Why both elbows?

Ans. To compare the degree of deformity and decide the correction needed in different planes.

42. What is the cause of fishtail deformity?

Ans. This is seen in old supracondylar fractures and is due to osteonecrosis of trochlea producing a smooth gentle curve. Trochlea is supplied by two sources. A distal fracture line disrupts the supply to lateral part of medial trochlear crista that comes through medial condyle. The other type of sharp angular wedge is seen after fracture of lateral condyle and is due to persistence of gap between lateral condylar physis ossification center and medial ossification of trochlea.

43. Who modified French osteotomy?

Ans. Bellemore modified the original osteotomy described by French **(Fig. 15)**.

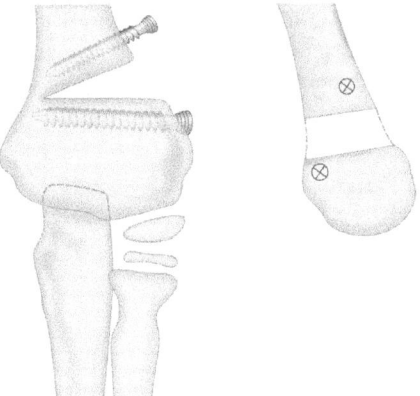

Fig. 15: Modified French osteotomy and correction of rotation.

44. What is the difference between modified and original French osteotomy?

Ans. The differences are given in **Table 3**.

Table 3: Difference between modified and original French osteotomy.	
French osteotomy	**Modified French osteotomy**
Posterior longitudinal approach	Posterolateral incision
Detach lateral half of triceps	Whole triceps (medial and lateral) detached
Ulnar nerve explored	No exploration of ulnar nerve done
Medial periosteum hinge	Medial periosteal and bony hinge, performing osteoclasis to obtain correction

45. How do you correct the rotation while doing osteotomy?
Ans. The proximal lateral screw is posterior to the coronal plane and distal slightly anterior, this disposition leads to external rotation of distal fragment when the wires are tightened.

46. What are the methods of fixing the osteotomy?
Ans. Screws and metallic suture wire, crossed thick K-wires, Steinman pin, external fixator, staples, plate, and no fixation (POP cast only).

47. What other osteotomies do you know of?
Ans. The other osteotomies are dome osteotomy (advantage of not producing shortening, less lateral bump) **(Fig. 16)**,

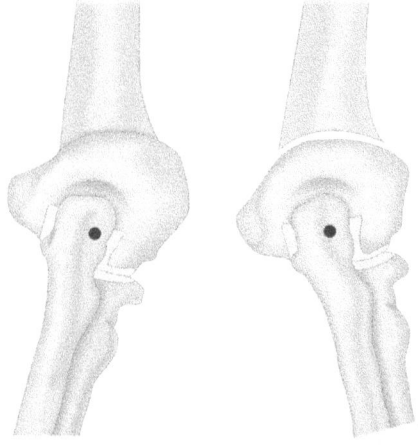

Fig. 16: Dome osteotomy for correction of cubitus varus.

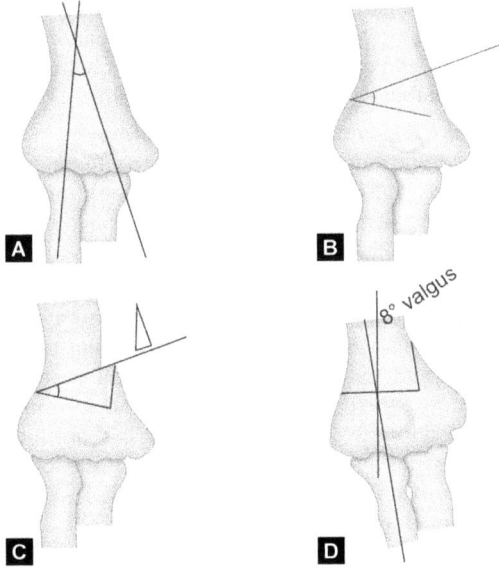

Figs. 17A to D: Step-cut osteotomy.

oblique osteotomy with derotation, three-dimensional osteotomy (Uchida et al.), step-cut osteotomy (Derosa and Graziano) **(Figs. 17A to D)**, and medial opening wedge osteotomy with bone graft (King and Secor).

48. When will you plan for osteotomy?
Ans. *Prerequisites:*
- At least 1 year following fracture (adequate duration for remodeling of bone and tissue equilibrium to regain)
- Patient demanding surgery.

49. What will you explain to the patient?
Ans. Always explain that this osteotomy is being done only for cosmetic correction and that no functional benefit must be expected out of it. Also, the lateral bump often persists after osteotomy. The complications of osteotomy should be thoroughly explained.

Cubitus varus deformity may be a risk factor for future lateral condyle fracture of humerus and development of tardy ulnar nerve palsy besides being a cosmetic unacceptability.

50. What are the complications of osteotomy?

Ans. The complications of osteotomy are stiffness, nerve injury, persistent deformity (under correction), nonunion, lazy S-deformity of elbow, etc.

51. What is Soltanpur method?

Ans. Soltanpur described a method of management of flexion type supracondylar fractures in adults and aged. Here, the condylar mass is pushed posteriorly along the axis of the forearm and the hand is rotated to full supination, while the elbow is held in flexion to correct deformities. Fixation is divided into two parts: the circular cast around the upper arm provides a firm buttress onto which the lower fragment is reduced and then the arm is immobilized in a plaster, which includes the wrist.

52. What is pseudocubitus varus deformity?

Ans. Lateral spur formation is one of the most common deformities after lateral condyle fracture due to lateral elevation of periosteum by displaced fragment. In patients with no real change in angle, the lateral prominence produces appearance of mild cubitus varus.

CASE V: CUBITUS VALGUS

Diagnosis: My patient is a 12-year-old male child with nonunion fracture lateral condyle of left humerus causing cubitus valgus deformity of elbow and is associated with tardy ulnar nerve palsy.

1. What are the causes of cubitus valgus deformity?

Ans.
- Nonunion fracture lateral condyle **(Fig. 18)**
- Malunited supracondylar fracture humerus
- Osteonecrosis of lateral trochlea
- Malunited intercondylar fracture
- Radial head fracture dislocation
- Medial epiphyseal injury and growth stimulation.

The Elbow Joint

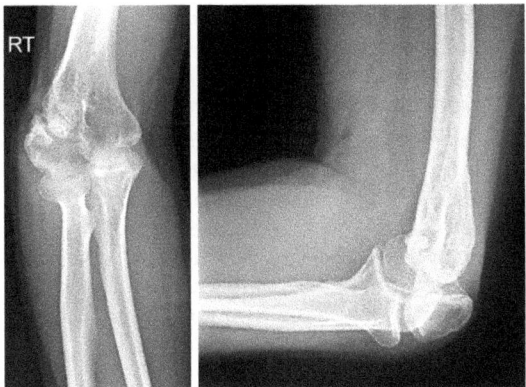

Fig. 18: Radiograph showing nonunion lateral condyle fracture.

2. Why do you call it fracture of lateral condyle?
Ans. Following points favor fractured lateral condyle:
- Disturbed three-point relationship
- Lateral supracondylar ridge thickening
- Widening of intercondylar region
- Flexion deformity (this entails you should not mention carrying angle as full extension is mandatory to measure carrying angle even though deformity is so tempting)
- Tenderness
- Abnormal mobility of lateral condyle—palpable as a mildly tender/nontender bony hard swelling situated just below the supracondylar ridge laterally that is not fixed to skin and can be moved abnormally. Usually, the movement is very slight
- Varus stress test is positive
- Ulnar nerve (may be involved as ulnar neuritis)—hypothenar muscle wasting (motor weakness comes before sensory changes).

3. When do you call lateral condylar fracture to be not united?
Ans. After 12 weeks (3 months).

4. What are the components of lateral condyle?

Ans. Lateral condyle comprises:
- Lateral trochlear crista
- Lateral condylar physis and epicondyle
- Capitellum and lateral metaphyseal region.

5. Why is nonunion common in lateral condyle fractures?

Ans. The following factors have been put forward:
- *Poor circulation to metaphyseal fragment*: Only a very small portion of lateral condyle is extra-articular and nearly all of blood supply enters from here. Damage to the same is quite common (trauma/iatrogenic) and causing nonunion and osteonecrosis
- Fragment bathed by synovial fluid
- Forces exerted by muscles arising from condylar fragment keeping it displaced
- Displaced fragment with opposition of articular cartilage to the proximal fracture surface—in this scenario, union is impossible.

6. Which type of fracture is it?

Ans. It is epiphyseal intra-articular fracture.

7. How do you classify lateral condyle fracture?

Ans. *Milch classification* **(Figs. 19A and B):**
- *Type I*: Line passing from metaphysis to capitellotrochlear groove traversing through ossification center, push-off injury (= Salter–Harris type IV)—stable, heals often with bony bar.
- *Type II*: Fracture line passing from metaphysis coursing through physis and exiting through intercristal groove (medial to lateral crista) out of ossification center, pull off injury (≡ Salter–Harris type II)—unstable type more common type.

Jacob's classification (stages of displacement) **(Fig. 20):**
- *Stage I*: Undisplaced with intact articular surface (Badelon modification—displacement <2 mm)
- *Stage II*: Complete fracture through articular surface
- *Stage III*: Fragment rotated, displaced laterally and proximally allowing translocation of olecranon and radial head.

The Elbow Joint

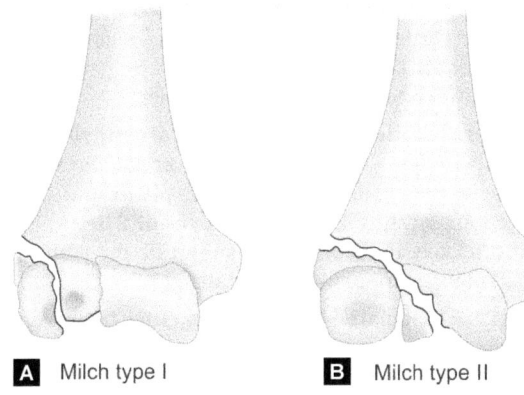

Figs. 19A and B: Milch classification of lateral condyle fracture.

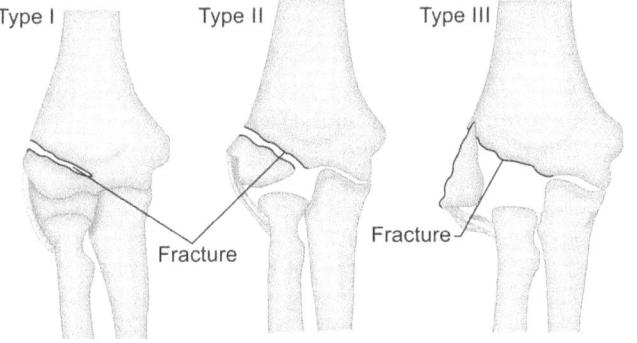

Fig. 20: Jacob's classification of lateral condyle fracture.

Finnbogason and associates (classified only minimally displaced fractures ≤2 mm):
- *Type A:* Minimal/no gap on radial/dorsal side fracture, not continuous to epiphyseal cartilage
- *Type B*: As above but fracture line continues to articular surface. Lateral fracture gap > medial
- *Type C*: As of B but fracture gap as wide medially as laterally.

8. **What muscles remain attached to lateral condyle?**
Ans. Extensor carpi radialis brevis (ECRB) (major blood supply) and extensor carpi radialis longus (ECRL), the fracture line runs between ECRL and brachioradialis.

9. **What are the displacements of lateral condyle?**
Ans. Lateral condyle is rotated both in coronal and vertical axes. There is 180° rotation in coronal plane and 90° vertical directions totaling the displacement of 270°. Milch type II is more likely to displace and subluxate the elbow, whereas type I injury is more likely to rotate.

10. **What are associated injuries to fracture lateral condyle of humerus?**
Ans. The following are the associated injuries of fracture lateral condyle of humerus:
- Elbow dislocation
- Radial head fracture
- Fracture olecranon
- Fracture medial epicondyle.

11. **What is the cause of development of cubitus valgus deformity in lateral condyle fractures?**
Ans. In type I fracture, with healing, there may be development of bony bar or arrest of lateral growth due to injury to ossification center (*see* Milch classification above). This leads to cubitus valgus deformity.

Type II fractures cannot be held securely in place with conservative methods being inherently unstable, so there is always a tendency toward lateral and proximal migration, hence, development of cubitus valgus with nonunion. Even in united fractures, there could be formation of bony bar, which tethers lateral growth.

12. **Why is the cubitus valgus of concern?**
Ans. Not all cubitus valgus deformities will concern us, but particularly the one from lateral condyle nonunion or sometimes with united fracture, if deformity is "progressive" (as in type 1). This may lead to changed elbow mechanics or neurological complications or both and thus concerns us.

The Elbow Joint

13. What are the causes of progression?

Ans.
- Nonunion with progressive lateral and proximal migration (type II)
- Damage to ossification center (type I)
- Bony bar formation (type I and II)
- Overgrowth of medial condyle (theoretical).

14. How does tardy ulnar nerve palsy develop?

Ans. Tardy (literally meaning 'tardy = slow' applied for 'late-onset' diseases) ulnar nerve palsy develops due to:
- Stretching of nerve due to medial angulation and hence resulting lengthier course
- Friction induced perineuritis, and
- Adhesions causing entrapment of the nerve in cubital tunnel.

15. What are other causes of tardy ulnar nerve palsy?

Ans. Apart from progressive cubitus valgus deformity from nonunion lateral condyle humerus fracture, the causes of tardy ulnar nerve palsy include:
- Malunited lateral humeral condyle fracture
- Displaced medial epicondyle fracture
- Elbow dislocation
- Ulnar nerve contusions
- Shallow cubital tunnel resulting in subluxating ulnar nerve
- Hypoplasia of trochlea of humerus.

16. How do you clinically diagnose ulnar nerve palsy?

Ans. Kindly *see* Chapter 7 for detailed discussion on ulnar nerve palsy and examination. Here, we will briefly describe the features.

Clinically—tingling/numbness of little finger, weak grip, and developing of claw hand. Positive card test and Froment's sign (lots of other tests described). For ulnar nerve involvement at elbow, perform flexion test; here, the wrist is fully flexed with hyperflexed elbow and position is maintained for 5–7 minutes. Compression neuropathy of ulnar nerve at elbow or neuritis, as in tardy palsy, will produce pain and/or paresthesia along the ulnar nerve distribution.

Investigation: Radiographs for bony pathology, nerve conduction velocity (NCV) localizes site of lesion.

17. Can this fracture also produce cubitus varus?
Ans. Yes, hyperemia and overgrowth of lateral part of physis in Milch type II fracture may sometimes cause cubitus varus deformity instead.

18. How will you manage this patient?
Ans. I will confirm the diagnosis by getting X-ray done in anteroposterior (AP) and lateral projections (*see* **Fig. 18** above) and also assess the displacements, condition of physis, and span of metaphyseal fragment.

19. What will you do?
Ans. I will assess the patient for surgical management in a symptomatic patient based on Flynn criteria:
- Large metaphyseal fragment
- Displacement of <1 cm from joint surface
- Open viable lateral condylar physis.

Surgical management is absolutely required for a progressive deformity, associated tardy ulnar palsy, or elbow instability. The patient should be symptomatic.

20. What surgery will you do?
Ans.
- For a patient with established nonunion (deformity <20°) having a large metaphyseal fragment, minimal migration (<1 cm upward migration from joint surface) and an open physis → open reduction (debride fibrous tissue to expose bone), *in situ fixation* in compression with a screw (cancellous/cortical), and bone grafting along with anterior transposition of ulnar nerve can be done.
- For patients with concern of cosmetic deformity (≥20°), *supracondylar corrective osteotomy (medial closing/stepcut/dome) and rigid in situ compression fixation along with transposition of ulnar nerve must suffice.*

- Patients with displaced fragments (>1 cm upward migration of the fragment from joint surface) require → translocation of fragment debriding the fracture surface and rigid fixation with bone grafting and transposition of ulnar nerve. This is particularly needed when *in situ* fixation is useless like in conditions where the articular cartilage opposes fracture surface.
- Asymptomatic nonprogressive nonunion in an adult patient with tardy ulnar nerve palsy requires transposition of ulnar nerve.

Some more clarifications over need and choice for open reduction:

Open reduction is a sort of 'extensive surgery' for this nonunion—often associated with complications chiefly stiffness that 'excels' the benefits from surgery. So, it is a better idea on table to preliminarily fix lateral condyle with K-wires and look for limitation of movements and drop open reduction, if significant limitation is produced. This is true for fragments that are moderately displaced and can be easily repositioned. For a grossly rotated fragment, it is probably better to leave it 'as it is' unless grossly symptomatic while explaining the risk of osteonecrosis to patient and guardians.

21. Why is ulnar nerve transposition always required?

Ans. Even after correction of deformity and fixation, tardy ulnar nerve palsy may still develop, so transposition must be done.

CASE VI: OLD UNREDUCED MONTEGGIA FRACTURE DISLOCATION

Diagnosis: The patient is a 9-year-old male child with 2-year-old unreduced Monteggia fracture dislocation of left forearm. There is flexion deformity at elbow of 20° with restricted extension, supination and pronation, and 'bowing' deformity of ulna with cubitus valgus deformity. (Examine nerve injury and include them, especially look for radial/posterior interosseous nerve palsy.)

1. Why do you call it old unreduced Monteggia fracture dislocation?

Ans. *Findings:*
- History of trauma (usually the mechanism is a fall on outstretched hand with maximally pronated forearm), treatment in POP cast, absence of radiograph/quack treatment, etc.
- Cubitus valgus
- Anterior ulnar bow with bony prominence anteriorly just below cubital fossa
- Radial head palpable anteriorly in elbow rather than its original location as a bony hard smooth rounded prominence that moves slightly only on attempted pronation/supination
- Restricted supination and pronation of forearm and elbow movements
- Foreshortening of forearm more over radial aspect.

2. What are your differentials?

Ans.
- Traumatic isolated radial head dislocation
- Congenital radial head dislocation
- Congenital radioulnar synostosis
- Rheumatoid arthritis (older patient)
- Recurrent radial head dislocation.

3. How do you define old-unreduced Monteggia fracture dislocation?

Ans. No strict definition, but when closed reduction is not possible then it is often called old unreduced dislocation, which is arbitrarily chosen to be 3 weeks.

4. What will you do next?

Ans. I will confirm my diagnosis on AP and lateral X-rays of elbow joint with arm and forearm including wrist joint.

5. How do you differentiate traumatic isolated radial head dislocation with congenital radial head dislocation?

Ans. The difference between traumatic isolated radial head dislocation and congenital radial head dislocation is given in **Table 4**.

The Elbow Joint

Table 4: Difference between traumatic isolated radial head dislocation and congenital radial head dislocation.

Findings	Congenital	Traumatic
Bilateral	Common	Uncommon
Trauma	Absent (may be present)	Often remembered (and necessary for clinical diagnosis)
Radial head shape in anterior dislocation	Dome shaped (rounded) without central depression	Normal
Radial head shape in posterior dislocations	Elongated and narrow head	Normal
Ulnar bow	Present (often palmar in anterior dislocation and dorsal in posterior)	Absent unless remodeling failed to occur
Capitellum	Hypoplastic or absent	Normal
Other congenital anomalies	Present	Absent

6. What are the possible complications of unreduced Monteggia fracture dislocation?

Ans.
- Tardy radial nerve palsy
- Tardy ulnar nerve palsy
- Progressive cubitus valgus
- Restriction of movements
- Functional impairment (weakness, stiffness)
- Arthrosis and pain over lateral aspect of elbow.

7. Which movement is more severely restricted in Monteggia fracture dislocations?

Ans. Supination.

8. What nerve injuries are frequently associated with this injury?

Ans. The associated injuries are posterior interosseous nerve, anterior interosseous nerve, and ulnar nerve in that order of occurrence.

9. How do you classify Monteggia fracture dislocations?

Ans. Bado classification of Monteggia lesion **(Figs. 21A to D)**:

- *Type I (60%)*: Anterior radial head dislocation with pronated bicipital tuberosity; fracture ulnar diaphysis at any level with anterior angulation (children > adults)
- *Type II (15%)*: Posterior/posterolateral radial head dislocation; fracture ulnar diaphysis with posterior angulation (exclusive to adults)
- *Type III (20%)*: Lateral/anterolateral radial head dislocation with fracture ulnar metaphysis (exclusive to children)
- *Type IV*: Anterior dislocation of radial head with fracture proximal 1/3rd radius and fracture ulna at same level.

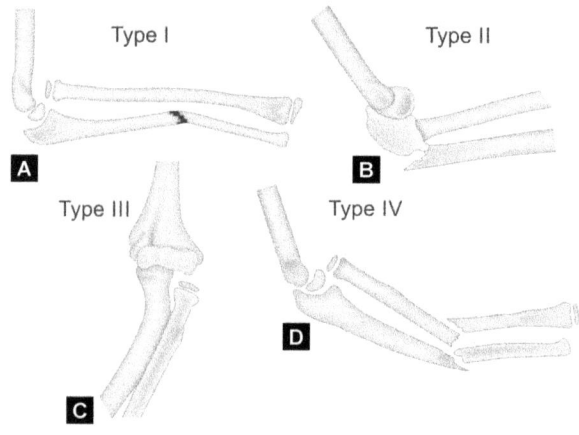

Figs. 21A to D: Bado classification.

10. What do you understand by the term Monteggia lesion?

Ans. Monteggia in 1814 described a traumatic lesion of ulna (fracture between base of olecranon and proximal third of ulna) with dislocation of radial head. Over time, various patterns of injuries with similar mechanism of production have been included into the group "Monteggia lesions" that is defined as "A group of lesion having in common a

The Elbow Joint

radio-humero-ulnar joint dislocation associated with ulnar fracture at various levels or with lesions of wrist".

11. What are Monteggia equivalents?

Ans. Type I and II only have been classically described to have equivalents.

Type I:
- Anterior dislocation of radial head (pulled elbow, nursemaid elbow, and minimal Monteggia)
- Fracture ulnar diaphysis with fracture radial head
- Fracture neck of radius
- Fracture ulnar diaphysis with fracture proximal radius (always fracture radius proximal to ulnar fracture)
- Fracture ulnar diaphysis with anterior dislocation of radial head and fracture olecranon
- Posterior dislocation of radial head with fracture ulnar diaphysis with or without fracture proximal radius
- Wrist lesions may also be found with type I Monteggia lesions or "equivalents":
  - Radioulnar dislocation
  - Slipped distal radial epiphysis
  - Fracture distal radius
  - Fracture distal radial diaphysis with sprained distal radioulnar joint (DRUJ) (Galeazzi's lesion).

Type II:
- Epiphyseal fracture of dislocated radial head of fracture radial neck.

12. How do you look for ulnar bow?

Ans. On a lateral projection radiograph, make a longitudinal line from olecranon to distal ulnar metaphysis along dorsal border. Perpendicular distance of ulna from this line of >1 mm is significant and denotes bow.

13. What will you do for this patient?

Ans. I will do open reduction of radial head with annular ligament reconstruction and ulnar lengthening/corrective osteotomy.

14. What else would you do?

Ans. I will fix the radial head using transcapitellar wire.

15. How will you do open reduction of radial head?

Ans. By using Boyd's approach, radial head and joint are exposed.

Capsule and/or annular ligament are removed, if they hinder reduction and radial head is replaced into position after inspection.

16. How will you reconstruct annular ligament?

Ans. Modified Bell-Tawse (Steel and Peterson modification) using triceps aponeurosis. A drill hole is made in ulna obliquely from medial aspect to exit from near coronoid (where original annular ligament is attached); then the tendon is passed, which does not completely encircle the radial neck. This has the advantage of avoiding notching of radial head and constriction to prevent future growth disturbance and also stabilizes it more securely with posteromedial force. Immobilize in 60° supination for 6 weeks in POP cast.

17. What other materials can be used for reconstruction of annular ligament?

Ans. *Natural*: Central/lateral slip of triceps aponeurosis, lacertus fibrosus, forearm fascia, palmaris tendon, chromic catgut ligature, and fascia lata graft

Synthetic: (Not very popular) mersilene tape.

18. What are the indications of ulnar osteotomy?

Ans. Malunited ulna with shortening or angulation needs correction for reduction and maintenance of radial head in position.

19. At what level will you do the osteotomy?

Ans. At the apex of deformity.

20. Till when can you do open reduction?

Ans. As such till 12 years of age, the results are good. However, there is no absolute contraindication for the procedure but complications like stiffness and dystrophic ossification are more common. In asymptomatic children without neurological compromise or progression of deformity masterly inactivity is the best option. However, for any of the above, one can give a fair trial of reduction. In skeletally mature patients, radial head excision can be safely done. In a skeletally immature patient, the progression of deformity and consequent nerve injury are common.

The question can have other meaning of asking time limit after injury till which reduction can be done. For this, there is again absolutely no duration limit. The only recommendation is as soon as possible (ASAP). Reductions done within 3–6 months have a good prognosis and results, however, are not disappointing for longer dislocations.

21. **What are the contraindications of doing reduction and repair?**
Ans. Deformed radial head, flattened capitellum, and valgus deformity of radial neck.

22. **What is Boyd's procedure?**
Ans. Boyd's procedure involves excision of radial head with corrective osteotomy of ulna (and fixation) and bone grafting. This is done in adult patients.

7

Wrist and Hand

EXAMINATION POINTS FOR A WRIST AND HAND CASE

The topic is difficult with respect to the examination as various specifications are to be remembered and detailed. Precision and tests are tough to learn.

Read times: 4-6 times for MS and DNB candidates.

HISTORY TAKING

In a broad division, try to first ascertain what you are dealing with—deformity/neurological condition/painful or inflammatory condition, then it will be prudent to proceed:

- *Pain*: Onset (injury/spontaneous; acute/insidious), type, location, duration, remote injury [reflex sympathetic dystrophy (RSD)], aggravating and relieving factors, activity restrictions, guarding of wrist and hand.
- *Swelling*: Onset (as above), location, duration (also whether temporary or permanent), relieving and aggravating factors, flare-ups (severity, frequency, duration), previous treatment if any, association with fever/stiffness, discoloration.
- *Deformity*: As above + abnormal contours, palm and finger alignment.
- *Loss of function*: A key factor as hand in itself is an organ, 45% of hand function is utilized for grasp, 45% for pinch (key, tip, chuck pinch), 5% for hook function, and in rest 5% hand functions as a paper weight (most primitive function).
- *Loss of power*: Any decreased strength or dexterity.
  Apart from above, it is very important to ask for history of hospitalizations and treatment (type, dose, frequency, response,

and side effects), details of trauma if present, dominant hand, effect on occupational functioning, and activities of daily living (ADL).

EXAMINATION

Inspection (keep the hand on a pillow or a firm clean support like table top having adequate contrast to render examination possible, with whole ipsilateral and contralateral upper limb exposed):

Alignment

- Normally, the hand as a whole is centered over the forearm and the middle finger (MF) forms the center that is in straight line running arbitrarily from the center of forearm. On side view, the hands and fingers in neutral alignment are in line with the forearm. Note the following common deformities conspicuous on inspection:
    - *Dorsally prominent distal radius*: "Dinner fork" deformity is common for malunited distal radius fractures
    - *Prominent ulnar head*: Distal radioulnar joint (DRUJ) disruption, rheumatoid arthritis (RA)
    - *Ulnar deviation of hand*: RA
    - *Radial deviation of hand*: Radial club hand, Madelung deformity
    - Ulnar claw hand, simian hand, wrist drop, pointing index
    - Swan neck deformity, boutonniere deformity, Z-deformity of hand and wrist—RA. Whether viewed from dorsal or volar aspect with fingers and thumb in adduction, the forearm, wrist, and hand (middle finger) should be in a straight line (axial alignment). Ulnar deviation of metacarpophalangeal (MCP) joint with radial deviation of wrist is observed in RA
    - *Contractures*: Dupuytren contracture and incarcerated trigger finger [flexion at *interphalangeal* (IP) joint]
    - Dislocation of *proximal interphalangeal joint* (PIP) joint is visible as a step off (sagittal malalignment). Rupture of extensor slip in RA produces flexion deformity of fingers at MCP joint (Vaughan-Jackson lesion).

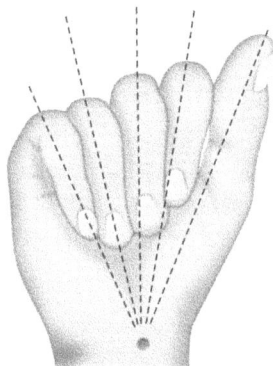

Fig. 1: On flexion of fingers, the tips point to scaphoid tuberosity.

- Rotational malalignment is judged in two ways:
  1. Ask patient to partially flex the fingers together at MCP joint—nails of index finger (IF) and those of ring finger (RF) and little finger (LF) face away from that of long finger in supinated hand **(Fig. 1)**.
  2. Ask patient to flex fully each finger in turn—the fingers should unfailingly point toward the scaphoid tuberosity.

Dorsal Aspect

- *Nails*: Vasculitic changes (local infarction—rheumatoid arthritis), splinter hemorrhage, periungual telangiectasias [systemic lupus erythematosus (SLE), scleroderma], pin-size pitting (psoriasis), hyperkeratosis, onycholysis, discoloration, ridges, anemia, dilated capillary loops over nail fold, paronychia, subungual hematoma
- *Fingers [examine from distal interphalangeal (DIP) to MCP]*: Mallet finger [avulsion of extensor digitorum communis (EDC), extensor pollicis longus (EPL) for thumb], redness, sausage shaped digits, nicotine stains, arthritis mutilans, tophi, swan neck/boutonniere deformity, Z-deformity of thumb, Bouchard nodes, Heberden nodes, Garrod pads, ulnar deviation, benediction attitude, clawing of fingers, contractures,

telangiectasia, mucous cyst, inclusion cyst, sebaceous cyst, skin and appendages [normally there are no hair from metacarpophalangeal (MP) and distal]
- *Hand:* Dropped knuckle (fracture metacarpal), foreshortening of metacarpal, fracture malunion, spina ventosa, wasting in first web space, wasting of interossei, skin and appendages, carpal bossing
- *Wrist:* Head of ulna (prominent in pronation disappears in supination), silver fork deformity, ulnar deviation, volar subluxation, volar-ulnar subluxation, cystic swelling (ganglion).

Radial Aspect

- *Thumb and first MCP joint (basilar joint):* (Skier's thumb or gamekeeper's thumb), swelling (first MCP arthritis).
- *Wrist:* Anatomical snuffbox [bound dorsally by EPL and volarly by abductor pollicis longus (APL) and extensor pollicis brevis (EPB)] for swelling.

Volar Aspect

- *Fingers and palms:* As above + pulp spaces for pits (Raynaud's phenomenon) and swelling (Felon), swelling over volar aspect of finger [giant cell tumor (GCT) tendon sheath or cystic swelling], jersey finger [avulsion of flexor digitorum profundus (FDP)], flexion arcade of fingers, palmar skin for pits and cords/nodules (Dupuytren contracture), signs of flexor tendon sheath infection [Kanavel signs—fusiform swelling extending along MP and proximal phalanx (PP) into distal palm + tenderness along volar aspect + finger held in flexed position + passive extension causes pain], thenar and mid palmar spaces for infection, thenar (median nerve—carpal tunnel, cervical spine disorders) and hypothenar (ulnar nerve lesion) wasting, both wasted—brachial neuritis, parsonage turner syndrome, or cervical myelopathy.
- *Wrist:* As above + tendon of palmaris longus (PL) (ask patient to touch the tips of thumb and LF and flex the wrist—tightens the palmar fascia and makes tendon prominent), flexor carpi radialis (FCR), flexor carpi ulnaris (FCU), compound palmar ganglion.

Ulnar Aspect

Hypothenar wasting, head of ulna (capita ulna syndrome—in RA the volar subluxation of carpals and dorsal subluxation of ulnar head accentuates the deformity with prominent head of ulna).

Palpation

Make a note of temperature.

Dorsal Aspect

- *Fingers*: For mallet finger, collateral ligaments especially for thumb, joint swelling and effusion, MCP joint for collateral ligament tenderness
- Metacarpals for deformity, tenderness, first metacarpal base for Bennett fracture
- Wrist for radial styloid, De Quervain disease (tenovaginitis of first dorsal compartment—APL, EPB), lister tubercle (2 cm ulnar to radial styloid), anatomic snuff box (for dorsal branch of radial artery, fracture scaphoid, 3-4 mm distal to it is basilar joint), second dorsal compartment [extensor carpi radialis longus (ECRL), extensor carpi radialis brevis (ECRB), intersection syndrome, ganglion is most likely to occur here], fourth dorsal compartment (EDC tendons in RA), triangular fibrocartilage complex (TFCC) just distal to ulnar styloid
- *Joint line*: The joint line dorsally is basically the dorsal lip of radius that is palpated. For this, hold the patients hand in pronation with elbows flexed with your dominant hand. The thumb of examiner's hand rests dorsally, while the IF supports distal forearm and third-fourth fingers support the hand from below. With the tips of IF and middle fingers of nondominant hand, gently palpate proximally along the metacarpal while moving the patient's hand with your dominant hand. Opening and closing gap is palpated with a firm ridge of bone along the joint line of radius.

Palmar Aspect

- As in inspection confirm the findings of felon, flexor sheath infection, midpalmar space, thenar space
- Swelling of ganglion, GCT tendon sheath, trigger finger (catching of tendon in pulley)

- Tubercle of scaphoid, hook of hamate, pisiform, pisohamate ligament and Guyon's canal, FCR, median nerve [between palmaris longus (PL) and flexor carpii radialis (FCR)], volar carpal ligament (proximal limit corresponds with the distal radial crease).

Radial Aspect

Palpate the anatomical snuff box for scaphoid tenderness and for tenderness over radial styloid region (De Quervain disease).

Movements

Wrist motion (with elbow flexed in 90°)—dorsiflexion (60–70°), palmar flexion (60–80°), radial (20°) and ulnar deviation (30–40°), pronation (90°), and supination (80–90°) **(Fig. 2)**.

Finger movements: Flexion at DIP (70–90°), PIP (110°), MCP joint (80–90°). Hyperextension at MCP joint is quite normal and is maximum at IF (up to 70°). Other method is to measure the finger-tip to transverse palmar crease distance for serial assessment and follow-up. Restricted flexion at IP joints can be due to capsular contracture/intrinsic contracture or extrinsic tightness. Perform Bunnell-Littler test to differentiate the two. Passively flex the IP joint with MCP in extension followed by MCP in flexion. Restriction due to intrinsic muscle tightness will increase the passive flexion at IP joint with MCP flexion due to relaxation of intrinsic muscles. In extrinsic tightness, the flexion decreases due to tightening of structures with MCP flexion hence restricting flexion further.

Abduction and adduction: Abduction and adduction is possible at MCP joint due to "cam effect"—the metacarpal heads are shaped like cam (larger volar articular component as compared to linear distal) so that in extension the collateral ligaments are lax allowing movement in coronal plane (this is also the reason for "James position" of immobilization). This is not possible at IP joints—bicondylar joints without a "cam". The presence of abduction and power of adduction is more important than the range of abduction! (just compare with other side).

Thumb movements: Flexion, extension, adduction, abduction, opposition.

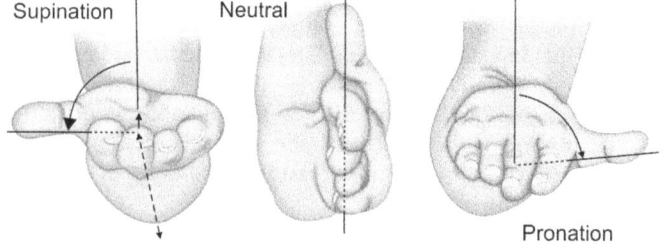

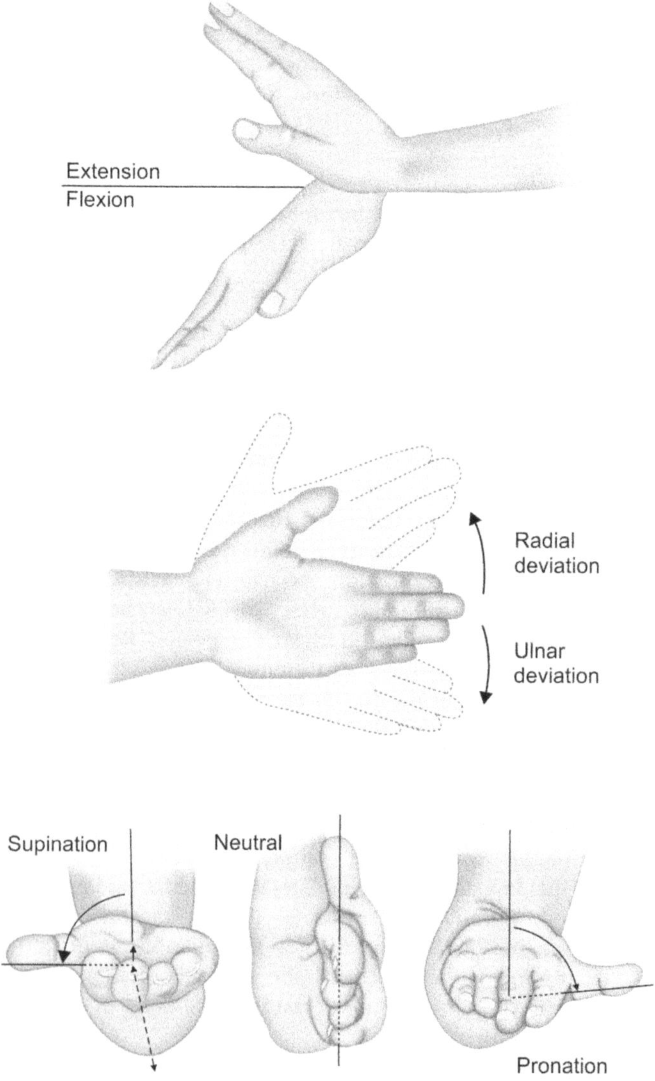

Fig. 2: Movements at wrist.

Wrist and Hand

Motor power and muscle/tendon function:
- Wrist flexors [FCR/flexor carpi ulnaris (FCU)], extensors [ECRL, ECRB, extensor carpi ulnaris (ECU)], radial deviators (FCR, ECRL, ECRB, APL), ulnar deviators (ECU, FCU)
- Finger flexors [FDP—hold PIP individually and ask patient to flex DP; flexor digitorum superficialis (FDS)—ask patient to flex the PIP while holding other three fingers in extension, this defunctionalizes the FDP as it is a single unit muscle]. This test is less reliable for IF as the FDP to IF may be separate
- Abduction (dorsal interossei) and adduction (palmar interossei) of fingers, card test
- Thumb flexion [flexor pollicis longus (FPL), flexor pollicis brevis (FPB)], radial abduction or extension (APL), palmar abduction (APB), adduction (adductor pollicis), opposition [APB, opponens pollicis (OP)], froment test (adductor pollicis).

Sensation Testing

Perform the sensory examination of hand and wrist for various nerves **(Fig. 3)** towards light test, pain, temperature, etc.

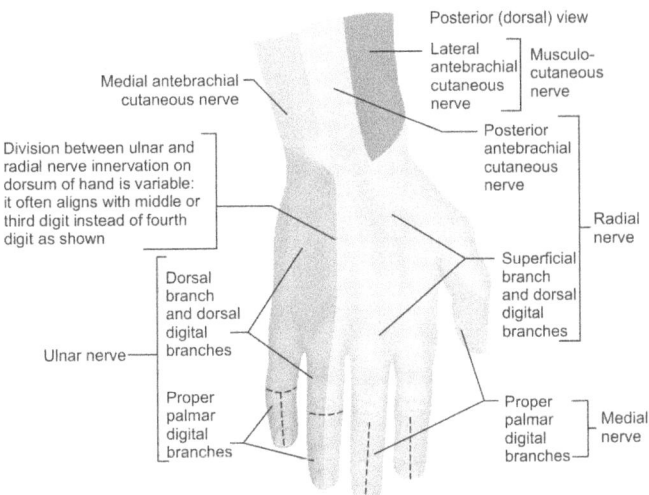

Fig. 3: Sensory distribution of various sensory nerves around hand and wrist).

Vascularity

Observe the vascularity of soft tissues. Normal hand is warm and pink. Note especially any necrotic patches or bluing of digits.

Special Tests

Percussion: Tinel test
- Carpal tunnel compression tests:
  - Tinel sign
  - *Phalen test*: Wrist flexed by gravity for 60 seconds **(Fig. 4)**
  - *Durkan median nerve compression test*: Manual pressure over median nerve at carpal tunnel for 30 seconds **(Fig. 5)**
  - *Reverse Phalen test*: Wrist and fingers extended for 2 minutes
  - *Tourniquet test*: Arm tourniquet inflated above systolic pressure for 60 seconds
  - *Hand elevation test*: Hand elevated above for 60 seconds
  - *Wrist flexion and carpal compression test*: In a supinated forearm with flexed wrist, compress the median nerve with direct pressure
  - *Closed fist test*: Tight fist for 60 seconds
- Stability testing:
  - MCP joint
  - IP joint

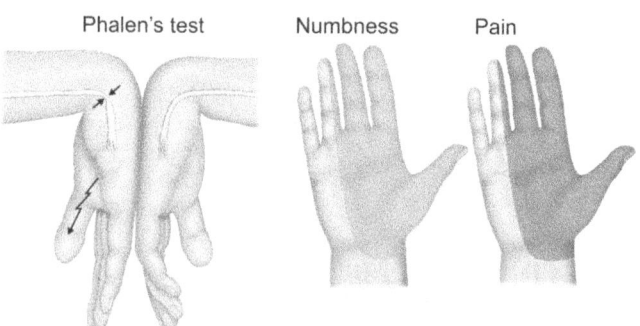

Fig. 4: Phalen test.

Wrist and Hand

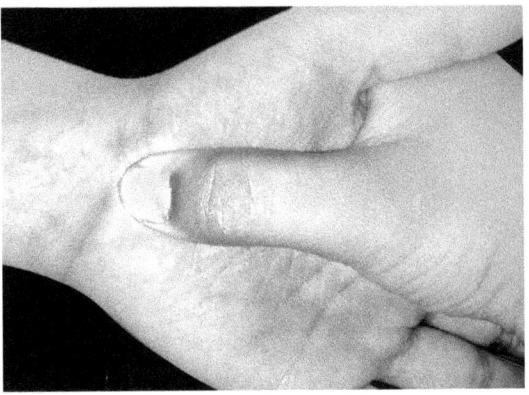

Fig. 5: Durkan test.

- Carpal instability:
  - *Scaphoid shift test of Watson*: Provocative maneuver used to examine the dynamic stability of the scaphoid and reproduce a patient's symptoms. The Watson Scaphoid Shift test provokes pain and subluxation by applying a force to the distal pole of the scaphoid while moving the wrist from ulnar to radial side **(Fig. 6)**.
  - Lunotriquetral ballottement test (Reagen test) for lunotriquetral instability (second most common instability of carpal bones)—the lunate is translated in an anterior-posterior direction while stabilizing the triquetrum by placing IF on one side and your thumb on the other. Observe of pain/crepitus/laxity **(Fig. 7)**.
  - Midcarpal instability.
- Distal radioulnar joint instability:
  - *Piano key test*: The Piano key test is also called the "stress test" or the ballottement maneuver. The examiner supports the wrist in pronation and applies force to the ulnar head. The piano key test is positive result if the ulnar head returns to its normal anatomic position when the force is removed from the ulnar head.
  - *Distal radioulnar joint grinding test*: The examiner moves the ulnarly deviated wrist in a volar-to-dorsal direction while

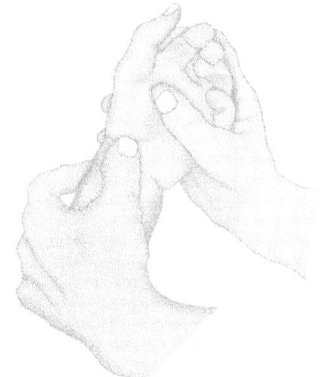

Fig. 6: Watson scaphoid shift test.

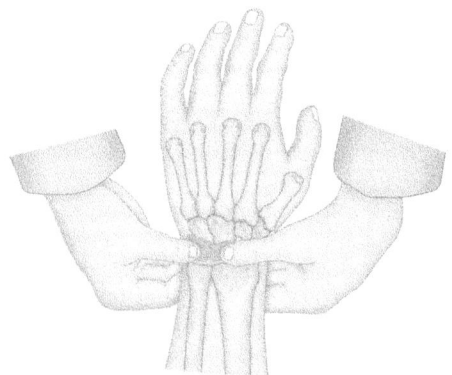

Fig. 7: Lunotriquetral ballottement.

applying an axial load across the ulnar side of the wrist to transmit load across TFCC which may cause grinding and reproduce pain.
- *Triangular fibrocartilage complex test—press test*: Observe the patient pushing himself up from seated position with the help of affected wrist. This produces ulnar side wrist pain, which indicates TFCC pathology.

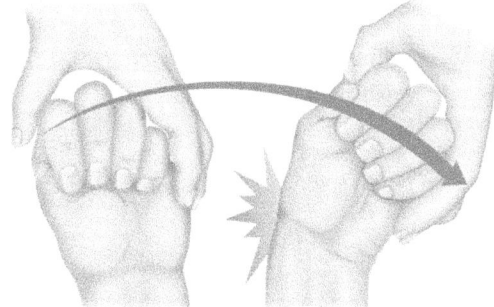

Fig. 8: Finkelstein test.

- *Grind test for basilar (trapeziometacarpal joint) joint arthritis*: Apply axially directed force along the first metacarpal holding the first MCP joint base with nondominant hand while metacarpal with dominant hand and rotate the thumb. Patient will complain of pain in basilar joint arthritis and intra-articular first metacarpal fractures (Rolando fracture).
- *Finkelstein test for De Quervain disease*: The examiner grasps the thumb and ulnar deviates the hand sharply. Pain over radial aspect of distal radius is positive test **(Fig. 8)**.
- Allen test for radial and ulnar arterial circulation.
- *Maisonneuve test*: Ask the patient to maximally dorsiflex clenched fist with forearm pronated and elbows flexed to 90°. Increased extension on pathological side indicates malunited extra-articular distal radius fracture.
- *Grip strength*: Assesses the pinch grip, key grip, chuck grip, and power grip strengths.

CASE I: PERIPHERAL NERVE INJURIES (RADIAL, MEDIAN, AND ULNAR NERVES)

This is a very important and favorite topic that is bound to come if case is present. The diagnosis is simple and straightforward to those who have practiced the case, otherwise not only examination or diagnosis but the management will also be formidable!

Read: 6–8 times (MS Orth and DNB candidates).

Diagnosis: The patient is a 28-year-old male with post-traumatic, nonrecovering, complete right high radial nerve palsy for past 9 months (with or without nonunion/united fracture of humerus).

1. What do you mean by high/low nerve (radial/median/ulnar) palsy?

Ans. *Radial nerve:*

Complete palsy (very high): Triceps paralyzed (injury in axillary region).

High: Triceps and often anconeus preserved but rest all paralyzed (injury around radial groove till it pierces septum).

Low: Brachioradialis (BR) and ECRL preserved [→ posterior interosseous nerve (PIN) palsy; ECRB in 58% cases is supplied by PIN so it may also be spared in some cases].

For ulnar and median see Chapter 7: Case II; Q 21-23.

2. Why do you call it nonrecovering?

Ans. The nearest muscle to the site of injury (BR) has not been reinnervated and the Tinel is still localized at the site of injury.

3. What function is lost in nerve (radial/median/ulnar) palsy?

Ans. *Radial:*
- Inability to extend fingers (1, 2, 3, 4, 5) (low) and wrist (low + high)
- Inability to stabilize the wrist (wrist drop) and thumb (radial abduction of thumb) (low + high)
- Loss of grip strength (accessory forearm flexion) (high)
- Accessory forearm supination (very high)
- Sensory loss (radial two-third dorsal sensation).

Ulnar (also *see Chapter 7: Case II; Q 21, 23, 29, 30*):
- Loss of grip strength (impairment of power grip > precise grasp) (high)
- Flexion of distal phalanx 4, 5 (high)
- Digital balance 4, 5 (high)
- Loss of finger function [flexion (partial), adduction, abduction] (high + low)
- Loss of thumb adduction and weakness of thumb flexion (high + low)
- Sensory loss (medial 1½ digits—low; ulnar one-third volar—high).

Wrist and Hand

Median nerve:
- Loss of thumb opposition, finger stabilization 1, 2 (low + high)
- Weakness of wrist and partial loss of finger flexion 2, 3; complete for 1 (high)
- Forearm pronation (high)
- Sensory loss (radial volar two-thirds hand).

Combined low median and ulnar nerve:
- Thumb opposition + adduction + flexion (partial)
- Finger abduction and adduction
- Finger stabilization
- Sensory loss (volar hand + dorsal ulnar 1½).

4. What is the course of radial, ulnar and median nerves?

Ans. *Radial nerve (C5-T1):* Formed in front of subscapularis from posterior cord → passes anterior to latissimus dorsi muscle → to pass through triangular space accompanied with profunda brachii artery to posterior aspect of humerus into radial groove (not spiral groove; radial groove is few mm above spiral groove) where it is separated from bone by medial head of triceps coursing obliquely laterally → pierces the lateral intermuscular septum around 122 mm above lateral epicondyle → passes into anterior compartment emerging beneath BR → deep branch (PIN) pierces supinator muscle to emerge into extensor compartment of forearm → forms cauda equina of spinner 8 cm distal to elbow joint **(Fig. 9)**.

Ulnar nerve (C8-T1, rarely C7 also): Formed from medial cord of brachial plexus → runs inferomedial to axillary artery to continue behind brachial artery over triceps muscle → passes straight to posterior aspect of medial epicondyle in "ulnar groove" between medial epicondyle and olecranon process → passes between two heads of FCU (the so-called "cubital tunnel" better called humeroulnar aponeurosis → remains deep to FCU overlying FDP muscle accompanied with ulnar artery → passes superficially; emerging beneath FCU to reach Guyon canal at wrist.

Median nerve (C6-T1): It is formed from combination of medial and lateral roots and, enters arm in close relation

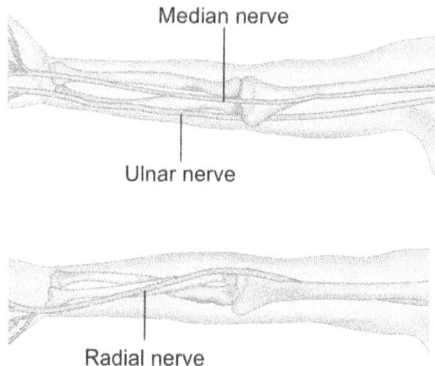

Fig. 9: Anatomy of nerves in upper limb.

to brachial artery. In the cubital fossa, nerve lies lateral to brachialis tendon and passes between two heads of pronator teres (PT) → gives anterior interosseous nerve (AIN) → continues in forearm sandwiched between FDS and FDP → emerges just proximal to wrist between FDS and FCU → passes through carpal tunnel → lies anterior and radial to FDS tendons → divides in hand into recurrent motor and sensory branches.

5. What will you do for this patient?

Ans. I will do a thorough examination of motor, sensory loss. Look for reinnervation (e.g. BR for motor recovery—radial, FCU for ulnar, etc. and advancing Tinel for nerve regeneration). I will also document the findings with electrodiagnostic studies (EDS). I will get X-rays of the arm in anteroposterior (AP) and lateral projection to look for status of fracture.

6. What are the requirements of a patient with radial nerve palsy?

Ans.
- Wrist extension
- Finger (MCP) extension
- Combination of thumb extension and abduction.

(*What is available?—motors innervated by ulnar and median nerve*)

7. What about sensory deficit?

Ans. The sensory deficit is notable but really not a disability and is partially covered up by lateral cutaneous nerve of forearm. So, it can be neglected unless there is painful neuroma.

8. How does status of fracture affect the treatment?

Ans. Osseous union should be promptly addressed to stabilize the limb and prevent additional injury to soft tissues especially nerve. In this case, I will have to prepare for bony surgery also, according to the findings. Had the duration been less (say 3 months), then I would have fixed the bone along with exploration of a nonrecovering nerve. Fracture in acceptable position with recovering nerve would have been managed with plaster of Paris (POP) immobilization otherwise surgery to fix fracture was indicated even in recovering nerve.

9. What is the role of nonoperative treatment?

Ans. *Goals:*
- Maintaining full range of motion (ROM).
- Preventing contractures particularly of first web space. It is undertaken while waiting for spontaneous nerve recovery and obviously in the interim period to surgery. Usually, a dynamic cock-up splint (external splint) is used for this purpose. However, internal splintage can also be done.

10. How will you treat this patient?

Ans. I will do tendon transfer.

11. What are the prerequisites for tendon transfer?

Ans. In order of importance:
- Correction of contractures (all joints must be supple).
- Adequate strength of the transferred tendon
    - About 85% of power is a must (Steindler)—graded as good power
    - "Omer" stated that a muscle loses at least one grade of strength after transfer, so for useful postoperative movements 4/5 power is a must.
- *Straight line of pull*: No pulley is ideal or minimum number of pulleys should be made.
- *One tendon*: One function, i.e. flex or extend.

- *Synergism*: Synergistic transfer should be preferred as much as possible; however, there are a lot of violations of this rule.
- *Expendable donor*: There should be no functional morbidity following use of a tendon.
- Tissue should be in equilibrium (tissue equilibrium— termed by Steindler)
  - Soft tissue induration should subside
  - No reaction in wounds
  - Joints are supple
  - Scars should be as soft as possible
- Pass tendon below fascial planes/sheaths and not below incision line/scar (best between subcutaneous fat and fascial sheath).
- Amplitude of transferred tendon should be as near to the original tendon for which the transfer is being done.
- Try preserving the nerve and vascular supply to muscle and vascular supply to tendon.
- Insertion of the tendon should be as close to the insertion of paralyzed tendon; at same angle, if split transfer, then keep both slips in same tension.
- Try to restore sensibility of distal organ before treatment.
- Arthrodesis/joint procedure should be done before tendon transfer.
- The disorder should be a nonprogressive one.
- Keep dissection to a minimum around the muscle to be transferred and achieve meticulous hemostasis to prevent adhesion formation.

12. What if the amplitude of transferred tendon is less than the tendon for which transfer has been contemplated?

Ans. Amplitude can be increased by two ways:
1. Converting a monoarticular muscle into bi/multiarticular, e.g. (FCU/FCR → EDC). The effective amplitude of motion is enhanced due to tenodesis effect by active volar flexion of wrist.
2. Muscle release from surrounding, e.g. BR transfer (*violates pt. 15 Q 11*).

Wrist and Hand

13. When will you do a tendon transfer?

Ans. In general, till the time a functional recovery is expected to occur, one can wait else do a tendon transfer.

Early transfer can be done if there is gap > 4 cm or there is excessive scarring/skin loss over the nerve; some may also include injection palsy and gunshot injuries in this category. Otherwise, transfer is usually done after waiting for around 1 year following injury (whether an interim repair has been attempted or not). (Remember the exact time for transfers as such vary according to the nerves involved and surgeon's preference).

14. Why do you wait for a year?

Ans. I will give adequate time for the nerve to regrow and possibly reinnervate the muscle. Neuromuscular (NM) junctions in the muscle degenerate if not reinnervated in about a year's time, so it is prudent to do tendon transfer after year as the likelihood of regaining function is meager. Moderate-to-severe atrophy of muscles is seen by 3 months, moderate-to-severe fibrosis seen by 11 months, and beyond 3 years there is fragmentation and disintegration of muscle fibers; hence, ideal reinnervation can be expected after 1–3 months, functional reinnervation up to 1 years, and no reinnervation >3 years.

15. What are the various tendon transfers for radial nerve injury?

Ans.
- JONES transfer *(violates point no. 6 Q 11)*: Classical (1916):
    - PT → ECRL and ECRB;
    - FCU → EDC III-IV;
    - FCR → EPL; EDC II, EIP (extensor indicis proprius)

    Classical (1921):
    - PT → ECRL and ECRB
    - FCU → EDC III-IV
    - FCR → EDC II, EIP, EPL, EPB, APL

    Modified JONES: PT → ECRB and rest as above
- FCR transfer (of Starr; Brand; Tsuge)
    - PT → ECRB

- FCR → EDC II-V
- PL → rerouted APL
- Boyes transfer (Superficialis transfer)
  - PT → ECRB
  - FCR → APL and EPB
  - FDS III → EDC II-V via interosseous membrane
  - FDS IV → EIP; EPL via interosseous membrane
- FCU transfer (standard transfer, this is not modified Jones transfer)
  - PT → ECRB
  - FCU → EDC
  - PL → rerouted EPL

16. Which one will you do?
Ans. *(Look for PL and ECRB power in examination).* I will do FCU transfer. *(If PL is absent, then say Boyes transfer. If the innervation to ECRB is not lost, then PT transfer is unnecessary ☺)*

17. What options are available if PL is absent?
Ans. Options in the order of preference:
- Do Boyes transfer.
- Substitute FDS III and IV for PL (Tsuge and Goldner)
- Use BR *(possible only in PIN palsy)*
- Use FCU transfer to both thumb and finger extensions *(violates pt no. 4)*.

18. What is meant by rerouted EPL?
Ans. It means that EPL is taken out of dorsal retinaculum (if the region of snuff box and junction is made between PL and EPL). This gives a combination of abduction and extension force on thumb.

19. What are the problems with standard transfer (FCU transfer)?
Ans. The main problem is of excessive radial deviation which is due to:
- Removal of the only preserved ulnar deviator (FCU) in radial nerve palsy.
- PT → ECRB transfer. ECRB is a radial deviator (albeit less than ECRL)

Wrist and Hand

- In PIN palsy, ECRL may be spared that leads to excessive radial deviation.

20. How will you avoid them?

Ans. Mainly by two methods:
1. *Planning itself*: If you are too concerned by radial deviation, then do FCR/Boyes transfer.
2. Alter the insertion of tendon by centralizing the ECRL (attach to IV metacarpal) or alternately one may attach the proximal resected end of ECU to (PT → ECRB) transfer which is not preferred as it limits total excursion.

21. What is internal splint and what is its rationale?

Ans. *Principles*:
- Should not → function in remaining hand
- Should not create deformity
- Should be phasic or capable of phasic conversion, e.g. PT → ECRB transfer described by Burkhalter for radial nerve palsy.

Indications:
- Substitute function during nerve regrowth eliminating the need of splintage.
- Helper following reinnervation → aiding power of normally innervated muscle.
- Substitute in cases where results of repair are poor or nerve irreparable.

22. Which type of nerve is radial nerve?

Ans. Radial nerve is a primary motor nerve with a small sensory component. Ulnar and median nerves are mixed nerves.

23. Does the type of nerve have any impact on outcome of repair?

Ans. Yes, primary functioning nerves whether sensory or motor have a better outcome as the chances of cross union and resultant fiber atrophy are minimum and also single modality (sensory/motor) dominant nerves have similar fibers which reform better.

24. What is Holstein Lewis fracture and what is its importance?

Ans. Spiral fracture of middle third and lower third junction of humerus with proximal spike over lateral aspect just at

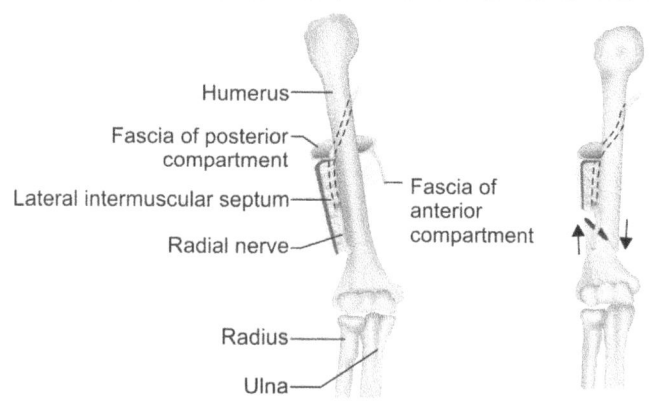

Fig. 10: Precarious location of radial nerve in vicinity of humeral shaft.

the site where radial nerve touches humerus. Commonly, radial nerve palsy was thought to be associated with fracture (**Fig. 10**).

25. What will you do for a patient who comes with fracture of humerus with radial nerve palsy?

Ans. I will wait for return of nerve function as according to Steindler formula for nerve regeneration [(1 mm = 1 day) + 30 days for motor recovery to manifest (NM junction) and nerve ends to sprout]. Usually, e.g. nerve injury is 90–120 mm above lateral condyle. Now for brachioradialis to get reinnervated that arises 20 mm above lateral condyle, it will take 70–100 days + 30 days = 4–5 months. This is the time duration one can wait (calculate as for other fractures). This is based on the premises that often the nerve injury is apraxia or axonotmesis with nerve in continuity and fair recovery is seen in over 90% cases.

26. Will you always follow this regime "or" will you always prefer to wait?

Ans. No, I will do early exploration of radial nerve for palsy associated with:
- Radial nerve injury secondary to manipulation of fracture (absolute indication)

- Open fractures
- Fractures in which satisfactory alignment is not possible by closed methods
- Fractures with associated vascular injury
- Patients with multiple trauma.

27. If you find a gap on exploration, what will you do?

Ans. I will see whether nerve ends can be coapted without tension. If not, then I will mobilize the nerve and still if not possible then I will do nerve grafting.

28. How will you assess the tension at suture site?

Ans. *Wilgis:* Take a single suture bite with 8-0 suture and if a knot cannot be tied without tension (or if it breaks) then there will be unacceptable tension at suture site (or a gap > 4 cm).

Millesi: Gap of ≥ 2.5 cm after keeping the limb in functional position indicates possibility of tension.

Elbow flexion > 90° or wrist flexion > 40° required for nerve approximation indicates tension.

Brooks: If gap cannot be closed after mobilizing the nerve, then there is bound to be tension.

29. How will you overcome nerve gap?

Ans. Following in isolation or combination are often required:
- Mobilization
- Transposition
- Limb positioning
- Resection osteotomy
- Nerve stretching and bulb suture (neuroma to glioma suture)
- Neuromatous neurotization (e.g. intercostal nerve for brachial plexus)
- Nerve grafting
- Nerve crossing (ulnar → median)
- Addition of non-neural tubes (e.g. vein segment).

30. How much mobilization can be done for a nerve?

Ans. Depends on the type of nerve but in general mobilization > 6–8 cm ↓ perfusion. (≈ 8% tension ↓ venular flow, 10–15% tension: blood flow arrest).

Practical Orthopedic Examination Made Easy

31. What are various types of nerve grafting?

Ans. The various options are:
- Trunk grafting using full-thickness segment of major nerve trunk (disadvantage—central necrosis/total graft dissolution)
- Cable graft using multiple strands of cut nerve sewn at both ends (drawback—wastes axons and ignores anatomic localization of function)
- Pedicle grafting often preferred for high combined ulnar and median nerve palsy where ulnar nerve is used as a pedicle graft to repair median nerve
- Interfascicular nerve graft (group fascicular nerve grafting)
- Individual fascicular nerve grafting—often done for paucifascicular nerve, e.g. ulnar nerve at elbow or for thin/terminal nerves, e.g. motor thenar branch of distal digital N
- Free vascularized nerve graft.

32. From where one can harvest nerve for graft?

Ans.
- *Autogenous:*
  - Lateral cutaneous nerve of thigh
  - Medial brachial and antebrachial cutaneous nerve
  - Radial sensory nerve
  - Sural nerve (up to 40 cm of graft)
  - Lateral cutaneous nerve of forearm (up to 20 cm)
  - Terminal branch of PIN (for digital nerves)
- Autologous vessels and muscle
- Allograft nerve
- Artificial conduits (veins/collagen conduits).

33. What if you find a sharp cut on exploration?

Ans. I will do nerve repair.

34. What are various types of nerve repair you know of?

Ans. *Again a tricky question, begin by speaking one of the following—if unacceptable, switch to the other group!*

Wrist and Hand

Depending on duration from injury:
- *Primary repair*: Within hours
- *Delayed primary*: Within 5–7 days
- *Secondary*: Any repair > 7 days

Depending on the technique used:
- Epineural
- Group fascicular
- Individual fascicular (funicular).

35. What do you mean by conditioning effect?

Ans. In clean sharp injuries, a delay of 2–3 weeks was often advocated on the premises that a "primed" neuron will regenerate faster at its peak metabolic activity due to "conditioning effect". Conditioning effect presupposes that axons regenerate quickly, if they have been damaged previously.

36. What is the structure of a peripheral nerve?

Ans. Epineurium has two parts—internal and external; former permeates the nerve ensheathing individual fascicles and the latter is a condensation of collagen encasing the fascicles as a group. Epineural fibrosis and scar formation after nerve injury is a function of epineurium.

Perineurium is an extension of blood-brain barrier made up of up to 10 concentric lamellae of flattened cells that are "dove-tailed". Removal of perineurium causes nerve function to fail. Up to 15% stretch, there is no injury to perineurium but it fails for stretch > 20%.

Endoneurium acts as a packing material of collagen tissue. There is no elastin. Participates in the formation of Schwann cell tube.

37. What is fascicle?

Ans. Termed funiculus by Sunderland, it is the smallest unit of nerve that can be manipulated surgically.

38. What do you understand by Wallerian degeneration?

Ans. It is the reactive change of a nerve to injury whereby distal stump is cleared of axoplasm and myelin along with regenerative changes in proximal stump. It is initiated by macrophage ingrowth stimulating Schwann cells. Schwann cell proliferation peaks around 3rd day and continues up to 2 weeks. The distal stump once cleared by Schwann cells and macrophages is left in the form of a tube that shrinks in size. Proliferating Schwann cells form "bunger's bands". The proximal stump degenerates till nearest node of Ranvier from where new sprouts grow (two to five sprouts within 6 hours). Those sprouts that establish end organ contact persist, rest all (those entangled at scar site "scar delay" and those missing their "receptive tubes") are pruned away.

39. What is topographic sensitivity?

Ans. Reinnervation of correct muscle within motor system or correct patch of skin in sensory system.

40. How do you classify nerve injuries?

Ans. *Seddon classification*:
- Neurapraxia (≡ Sunderland type I); only physiological disruption of nerve function—recovers of its own
- Axonotmesis (≡ Sunderland type II-IV); physiological disruption with partial anatomical (increasing) disruption of nerve—recovery possible (70%) but later may need surgical intervention in higher grades
- Neurotmesis (≡ Sunderland type V); complete anatomical and physiological disruption of nerve—always needs surgical intervention.

41. What is type VI nerve injury?

Ans. Combination of types I-V (added by Mackinnon)

42. What is intrinsic minus hand?

Ans. *Fingers:* Hyperextension at MCP joint + flexion at IP joints ± adduction of fingers

Thumb: Adduction and hyperextension at MCP joint + flexion at IP joint.

43. What are synergistic muscles?

Ans. Synergism is the endless repeated coordination of anatomically different groups of muscles to perform a given action, e.g. wrist extensors + finger flexors + finger adductors "or" wrist flexors + finger extensors + finger abductors.

44. What is the earliest sign of nerve recovery?

Ans. Advancing Tinel sign.

45. What is Tinel sign and what is its utility?

Ans. Paresthesia *(fornication)* experienced along the nerve distribution *(not at the percussion site)* on gentle percussion from distal to proximal over the nerve (1917, Jules Tinel)

Cause: Bare young hyperexcitable unmyelinated sprouts from injured proximal end

Seen in: Sunderland grades II-V.

Importance:
- Advancing Tinel can be used to calculate and gauge progression of recovery (spontaneous or following repair)
- Nonprogressing Tinel indicates interruption of nerve regeneration
- Static Tinel at injury site and one present distally also indicates poor prognosis
- *Advancing* Tinel seen only in grades II and III (IV and V grades show it only after repair).

Fallacies:
- Few sensory sprouts and partial regeneration may give a false positive Tinel sign.
- No estimate of motor recovery should be made from Tinel sign as it indicates sensory recovery from sensory sprouts.
- Single time estimation is also useless and needs to be regularly followed.

46. What do you mean by autonomous zone, intermediate zone, and maximal zone?

Ans. Autonomous zone is the area exclusively (no other nerve has interference in this zone) supplied by nerve in question. While clinically testing for sensory loss, a somewhat larger area is outlined that contains overlap from other nerve and this is intermediate zone. In actual, there is a still larger area that can only be tested by blocking the other nerves; however, it is clinically irrelevant as it has predominant brain representation by other nerve, this is maximal area.

47. What are the autonomous zones of radial, ulnar, and median nerves?

Ans. *Radial nerve*: Coin-shaped region over the dorsum of stretched first web space

Median nerve: Volar distal aspect of IF

Ulnar nerve: Volar ulnar aspect of distal LF.

48. What is EDS?

Ans. EDS (electrodiagnostic studies) comprises of electromyography (EMG), nerve conduction studies (NCS), and strength-duration (SD) curve. Normal muscle is electrically silent on EMG (embryonic muscle show fibrillation till ≈ 6 weeks of fetal life). Denervated muscle starts showing fibrillation potential by 18–21 days (3 weeks). If renervation occurs fibrillation potential decreases and motor unit action potential (MUAP) of low magnitude appear. Giant MUAP are seen in a partially denervated muscle which is additionally reinnervated by nearby nerve.

Normal conduction velocity is ≈ 50 m/sec (slightly more in sensory nerves), demyelization reduces speed; unmyelinated fibers have ≈ 10 m/sec of conduction velocity. Sunderland type I injury may show delay at the site of injury but otherwise NCS and EMG is normal.

49. What is strength-duration curve?

Ans. A graph plotting the intensity of electrical stimulus to the length of time it must flow to produce response.

50. What is chronaxie and rheobase?

Ans. Rheobase (Rheos = current or flow; base = foundation) is the minimal amount of stimulus strength that will produce a response when applied indefinitely (practically a few milliseconds).

Chronaxie (chronos = Time; axie=axis) is the stimulation duration that yields a response when stimulus strength is set to exactly 2 × rheobase **(Fig. 11)**.

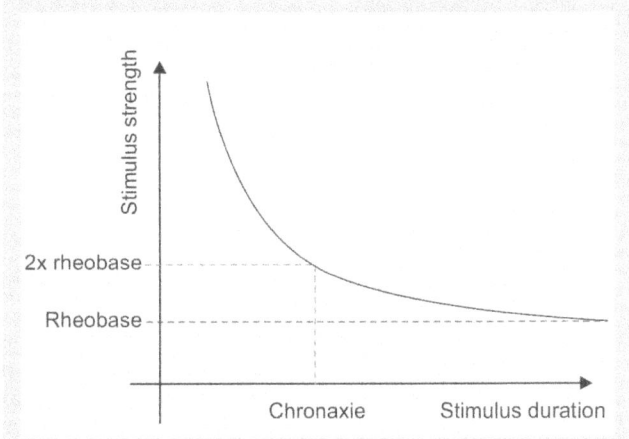

Fig. 11: Chronaxie and rheobase.

51. What is F-wave and H-reflex?

Ans. They are part of NCS (others are motor and sensory CS): F-wave—stimulation of motor nerve and recording action potential from muscle supplied by it. The stimulus travels up the nerve to spinal cord then back to limb. It measures the conduction between nerve and spinal cord (others measure conduction within limb).

H-reflex: In this case, afferent impulse travels up the sensory nerve and travels down motor nerve to produce discharge.

52. What is the importance of upward kink in SD curve?

Ans. It indicates partial denervation.

53. What do you mean by opposition of thumb?

Ans. (1) Thumb abduction → (2) MCP flexion → (3) Internal rotation and pronation → (4) Radial deviation of proximal phalanx → (5) Motion of thumb toward fingers.

54. What tendon transfer will you do for low ulnar nerve palsy?

Ans. *(Do read case II below for management of ulnar nerve palsy; it gives good guidance for understanding management of ulnar nerve lesions).*

Reconstruction system:

Requirements:
- Thumb adduction
- MCP flexion

Available:
- Wrist extensors
- FDS
- Index proprii (EIP)

Transfers:
- *Thumb adduction*: ECRB → abductor tubercle (Smith/Boyes)
- *MCP flexion with integrated IP flexion*: ECRL (Brown's 4 tailed; EF4) or FCR (if flexion contracture at wrist); tendon grafts passed volar to transverse carpal ligament attached to A2 pulley or radial band of dorsal apparatus *(see Chapter 7: Case II)*.
- *Palmar arch and adduction of LF*: Extensor digiti minimi (EDM) tendon split and ulnar half transferred to radial collateral ligament of PP or radial band of dorsal apparatus.
- *Thumb-index finger "tip pinch"*: Accessory slip of APL to first dorsal interosseous and MP joint arthrodesis. If MP joint already arthrodesed, EPB may be transferred.
- *Volar sensations*: Proximal medial digital nerve translocated to distal ulnar digital nerve.

55. What are methods for high ulnar nerve palsy?

Ans. 1, 2, 3, 4, 5 as above +:
- *Wrist flexion (ulnar side) (not frequently done)*: FCR → FCU or PL → FCU
- *DIP flexion for RF and LF*: FDP (IF and MF) → tenodesed to FDP (RF and LF).

56. What is ulnar paradox?

Ans. Normally, it is a mindset that the high are the lesions the more will be the involvement of distally innervated structures so it will produce more marked deformity(ies). But in case of ulnar nerve lesion, the primary deformity → claw hand demonstrates opposite. High ulnar nerve palsy at

Wrist and Hand

elbow damages both the long flexors and the intrinsic hand muscles. So, the pull on fingers from long flexors is lesser compared to when the ulnar nerve is involved at wrist (low lesion) where the long flexors are spared so they pull the fingers prominently in flexion. Thus, a low ulnar nerve palsy presents with marked clawing of the ulnar digits of hand while a high lesion demonstrates lesser degree of clawing which appears paradoxical as higher lesion is expected to produce a more grotesque deformity.

57. Which transfer is done to obtain opposition with adduction of thumb?

Ans. FDS (RF) transfer through pulley of volar carpal ligament (Royle Thompson); *remember that FDS transfer can be done for low ulnar nerve palsy in place of one described previously but for high ulnar nerve palsy FDP is paralyzed so this is contraindicated. It is always more comfortable not only to practice and master one technique but for exams also to remember only one method and not get confused!* Other very commonly asked transfer is littler ("muscle") transfer of abductor digiti minimi.

58. What reconstructive method will you use for combined low median and ulnar nerve palsy?

Ans. This is a severe injury with complete volar anesthesia and intrinsic palsy. Make the hand supple first and do transfers as below:
- *Finger intrinsic function*: Brand's EF4 using ECRB or Brown's EF4 using ECRL.
- *Opposition for thumb*: Do Riordan transfer (FDS through FCU pulley) or Burkhalter transfer (EIP). But it is better to remember thumb adduction as suggested in low ulnar palsy as it also works for high median and ulnar and high median and low ulnar combined palsies. Of course this does not give opposition! *(Remember—we do not have perverted memories—make it simple).*
- Sensory as above.

59. What is combined high median and ulnar nerve?

Ans. What patient loses?

- Sensation of hand
- Thumb abduction/opposition
- MP joint flexion
- Finger flexion
- Wrist flexion.

What must be replaced?
- Sensation of hand
- Thumb abduction/opposition
- MP joint flexion
- Finger flexion
- Wrist flexion.

Transfers:
Thumb adduction: ECRB → adductor tubercle
Thumb opposition → Burkhalter (EIP)
Finger flexion: ECRL → FDP and tenodesis of all fingers
Wrist flexion: ECU →FCU

But this may make extension of wrist quite weak, so one may do wrist arthrodesis that spares all wrist extensors for transfer quite safely.

60. What is Camitz transfer?
Ans. PL → APB, but done only in partial low median palsy to provide opposition (in reality a pseudo-opposition), e.g. carpal tunnel syndrome (CTS).

61. What is the cause of nerve "palsy" in postinjection nerve palsy?
Ans. As such, injection into or through nerves should not cause palsy; however, some drugs act as fibrosing agent (e.g. tetracyclines, preservatives with injectable diclofenac) that lead to "progressive" fibrosis. This constricts the nerve and cause palsy.

62. What is the treatment?
Ans. Do not wait, and if the patient presents early >3 weeks, do neurolysis (endoneurolysis). Late cases (>3 months) showing no recovery should be treated with tendon transfer. For immediate presentation, one can wait for up to no longer than 3 weeks to give benefit for recovering from possible neurapraxia due to local nerve injury or edema.

63. How do you classify fibrosis?

Ans. Millesi types (added to Sunderland classification):
- Epifascicular epineurium involved
- Interfascicular epineurium involved
- Endoneurium involved.
  Type I/II and A/B need neurolysis.

64. What are the types of neurolysis?

Ans. Epineural, perineural (interfascicular), endoneural, hemicircumferential neurolysis.

65. What are the various tests for ulnar nerve palsy?

Ans. Following are the tests in the order of importance:
- *Froment sign/Bunnel "O" sign/newspaper sign*: Paralysis of first dorsal and second palmar interosseous muscle with adductor pollicis paralysis. Patient flexes thumb as a trick/compensatory maneuver **(Fig. 12)**.
- *Card test*: To test palmar interossei (PAD = palmar-adduct; DAB = dorsal-abduct) **(Fig. 13)**.
- *Wartenberg sign*: EDM unopposed by third palmar interossei.
- *Jeanne sign*: Loss of key pinch (adductor pollicis).
- *Bouvier maneuver*: Passive block of MCP hyperextension facilitates IP extension.

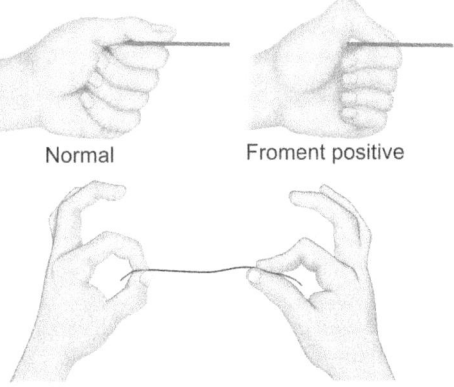

Fig. 12: Froment (upper) and Bunnel "O" sign.

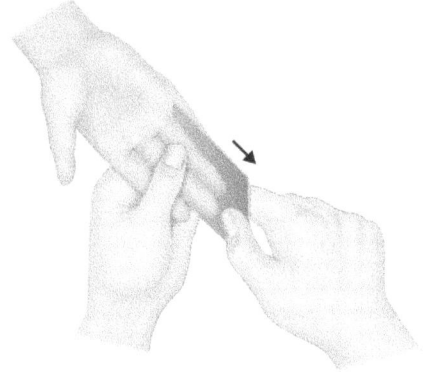

Fig. 13: Card test.

- *Duchenne sign*: Loss of MCP flexion.
- *Pitres-Testut sign*: Inability to cross fingers, e.g. IF (index finger) on MF (middle finger) tests P1D2.
- *Pitres-Testut sign 2*: Inability to make cone with extended fingers.
- *Pitres-Testut test*: Inability to radial and ulnar deviate MF.
- *Masse sign*: Wasting and loss of metacarpal arch.
- *Pollock sign*: Inability to flex DIP of RF and LF (paralysis of ulnar half of FDP).
- Look for wasting in first web space (first dorsal interosseous).
- Impairment of precision grip.
- Andre-Thomas sign.

66. What are anomalous innervations for ulnar nerve?
Ans.

- *Martin-Gruber anastomosis*: In proximal forearm between Median/AIN and ulnar nerve—additional intrinsic innervations
- *Riche-Cannieu*: Motor ulnar branch with recurrent branch of median—complete/partial intrinsic innervations
- Ulnar nerve always contains fibers from C8 and T1; additional C7 in 5–10% FCU

Wrist and Hand

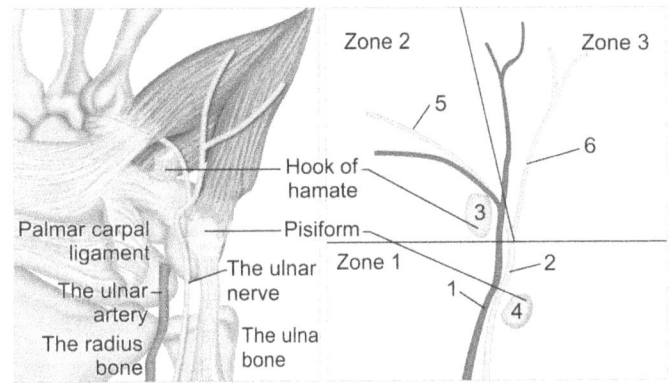

Fig. 14: Guyon canal and zones of ulnar nerve.

- *FDP innervation*: All ulnar to all median
- Dorsoulnar surface of hand may be innervated by radial nerve **(Fig. 14)**.

67. What are the boundaries of Guyon canal?

Ans.
- Wall formed proximally by pisiform and distally by hook of hamate
- Floor by transverse carpal ligament, hamate, and triquetrum bones
- Roof by pisohamate ligament.

68. Can you outline the formation of brachial plexus and its branches?

Ans. *(Learn this by heart as it may be asked anywhere and at any instance)*

Formation:

From C5–C8 nerve roots just lateral to scalene muscles, if a component of C4 received then it is termed prefixed; if from T1—postfixed. Roots → Trunks (Upper C5, 6; middle C7; lower C8, T1) → Divisions (anterior and posterior; behind clavicle) → Cords—named after their relation to axillary artery (lateral—anterior division of upper and middle trunk;

medial—anterior lower; posterior—posterior divisions of all three trunks)

Branches from the roots:
- Dorsal scapular nerve (C5) supplies rhomboids and levator scapulae and runs down deep to levator scapulae
- Nerve to subclavius (C5, 6) supplies subclavius
- Long thoracic nerve (C5, 6, 7) supplies serratus anterior.

Branches of the upper trunk (lower and middle have no branches):

Suprascapular nerve (C5, 6) supplies supraspinatus and infraspinatus

Branches of the lateral cord (L2M) (anterior divisions of upper and middle trunk).
- Lateral pectoral nerve (C6) supplies upper half of pectoralis major
- Lateral head of median nerve (C6, 7)
- Musculocutaneous nerve (C5, 6, 7) supplies coracobrachialis, biceps, and brachialis and then becomes lateral cutaneous nerve of the forearm.

Branches of the medial cord (M4U) (anterior division of lower trunk)
- Medial pectoral nerve (C7, 8) supplies the sternocostal fibers of pectoralis major
- Medial cutaneous nerve of the arm (T1)
- Medial cutaneous nerve of the forearm (C8, T1)
- Medial head of median nerve (C8 and T1) joins the lateral head and supplies most of the flexor muscles of the forearm, the three thenar muscles, and two lumbricals
- Ulnar nerve (C7, 8 and T1) supplies the ulnar forearm flexors and most of the intrinsic muscles of the hand **(Fig. 15).**

Branches of the posterior cord (ULNAR)
- Upper subscapular nerve (C6, 7) supplies subscapularis
- Lower subscapular nerve (C6, 7) supplies subscapularis (lower part) and teres major
- Nerve to latissimus dorsi [thoracodorsal nerve (C6, 7, 8)]

Wrist and Hand

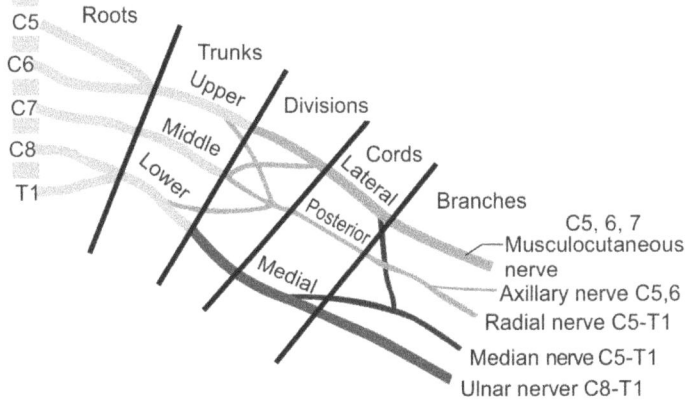

Fig. 15: Branches of the medial cord (M4U) (anterior division of lower trunk).

- Axillary nerve (C5) passes backward through the quadrilateral space in contact with the neck of the humerus and supplies deltoid and teres minor
- Radial nerve (C5, 6, 7, 8 and T1) supplies muscles of the extensor compartment of the arm and forearm leaves the axilla through the triangular space below teres major.

69. List the muscles innervated by radial, median, and ulnar nerves.

Ans. **Radial:** Arm—triceps, anconeus, radial half of brachialis, BR, ECRL, ECRB

Forearm: Supinator, EDC, ECU, EDM, APL, EPB, EPL, EIP

Median: Forearm: PT, FDP (IF, MF), FDS (I-IV), FPL, PL, pronator quadratus (PQ)

Hand: APB, FPB (partial), OP, lumbricals (I, II)

Ulnar: Forearm: FDP (RF, LF), FCU

Hand: Palmaris brevis, flexor digiti minimi, ADM, opponens digiti minimi, adductor pollicis, flexor pollicis brevis (partial), all interossei, lumbricals (III, IV).

70. What are the various tests for median nerve?

Ans. *Signs:* Pointing index, ape thumb deformity (adducted thumb)—Simian "hand", thenar wasting, sensory deficit

Tests:
- *Clasp test*: Ask patient to clasp both hands—IF remains extended
- Pen test
- Loss of opposition
- *Kiloh-Nevin sign*: Ask patient to form "O" with IF and thumb using tips; patient will extend DIP of IF and IP of thumb making peacock's eye instead.

71. What is Hilton law?

Ans. It states that a nerve passing near a joint supplied that joint.

[*It is difficult at all times to understand learn and remember all tendon transfers; as a rule, difficult aspects will not be asked (because it is rare to get hand surgeon doing good volume surgery to get as examiner) and if you pass in concepts then you may be forgiven for not knowing all the details. What you are expected to know:*

Type of palsy (high/low, complete/incomplete, recovering/nonrecovering)

Basic principles of decision making.

Examination of motor and sensory innervation and deficits—you should know how to examine: FDS and FDP separately, wrist flexors and extensors, demonstrate PL, movements of thumb and muscles especially intrinsic muscles and their nerve supply.

Additionally, you should know thoroughly the origin, course, and muscle innervation of three major nerves of upper limb.

Extensor compartments, carpal tunnel, and structures, Guyon canal may also be asked]

CASE II: LEPROSY HAND

Important but difficult case as regards the treatment part which is quite similar to peripheral nerve injuries and needs constant revision otherwise "all is volatile". Identification may be easy and barring few specific examination and characteristic points, there is nothing "special" in leprosy. Approach the case as for peripheral nerve injury that helps learning, and then grab the specific points for leprosy.

Personally, I will advise you to follow the practice in your institute for a given set of nerve involvement and not get confused in exams—remember not only does the eyes see what mind knows but also the mind knows what eyes see!

Read: 6-8 times (MS Orth and DNB candidates)

Diagnosis: The patient is a 28-year-old male with claw hand deformity of left hand due to high ulnar nerve palsy as a residual of leprosy.

FINDINGS (SEE Q1 BELOW)

1. Why do you call it Hansen disease?

Ans. *History*: Long duration → Paresthesia (ants crawling), patch (area) of numbness, glove and stocking anesthesia, paralysis, trophic ulcer, epistaxis, pedal edema. Take history of (h/o) residence in endemic area, family h/o, occupational h/o, any other disease etiology leading to thickened nerves.

Skin lesions: Macular, papular, nodules, infiltration ulcers, burns, scar

Palpate: Decreased sweating, roughness, scaling

Nerves (Cutaneous, superficial, peripheral): Test for anesthesia

Motor weakness.

Cardinal signs of Hansen (three):
1. Anesthetic lesion
2. Nerve enlargement
3. Demonstration of *Mycobacterium leprae* in lesions.

Other examination:
- *Ear lobe infiltration*: Thickening and nodularity of ear lobes
- Superciliary madarosis (loss of lateral third eyebrows) late feature of lepromatous leprosy (LL)
- Gynecomastia (testicular atrophy) late cases of LL
- Pedal edema
- Trophic changes and ulcer formation (metatarsal heads and lateral border of foot)

- V and VII cranial nerves (only cranial nerves to be involved in leprosy)
- Lymph nodes (lepromatous spectrum)
- Hepatosplenomegaly (occasional in lepromatous)

2. What nerves are commonly involved and how do you examine them?

Ans. *In the order of involvement*: Ulnar (mixed, high, low), median at wrist (then high), common peroneal at fibular neck, facial, radial (superficial at wrist and distal forearm, deep at arm), posterior tibial (clawing of toes and loss of arch), greater auricular, supraorbital

- *Supraorbital and supratrochlear*: Examine from front → run thumb/IF from midline to lateral margin of forehead); 2 cm from midline
- *Greater auricular*: Turn head to side → make sternocleidomastoid prominent → look for thickened nerve crossing the muscle → run thumb/IF above below to feel as it slips under
- *Supraclavicular*: 2 cm lateral to medial end of clavicle
- Radial nerve in radial groove (arm) and over radius (lateral aspect of forearm)
- *Ulnar nerve in cubital tunnel*: Right side with left hand and vice versa!
- Ulnar and radial cutaneous nerves over medial and lateral aspects of wrist
- *Median nerve*: Flex elbow and deep palpation of nerve at wrist between flexor tendons
- *Common peroneal nerve*: Patient sitting → flex knee and feel for nerve 2 cm below fibular head
- *Posterior tibial nerve*: 2 cm below and behind medial malleolus
- *Sural cutaneous nerve*: Between heel and lateral malleolus.

3. What is the old name of leprosy?

Ans. "Elephantiasis graecorum". In India, it has been known as "Maharog" since ages.

4. What is meant by "lepra" and "kushtha"?

Ans. Lepra = bark/scaling; Kushtha = eating away.

5. Who discovered *M. leprae* and what was his hypothesis?

Ans. Gerhard Hendric Armauer Hansen (1873) first identified it as an infectious disease rather than "older" hereditary concept.

6. Why are nerves involved and that too in a peculiar distribution?

Ans. *M. leprae* enters through naked axons in epidermis → perineural cells → endoneurium → localizes to Schwann cells → it enters nerves through endoneural blood vessels. Schwann cells are present only in peripheral nerves and the nerves are at relatively cooler regions of body, hence particularly affected (V and VII are the only cranial nerves to be involved in leprosy).

7. How does nerve damage occur?

Ans. Immune reaction to bacterial antigens is the primary cause of nerve damage. Also peripheral nerves (located in cooler areas) are common sites for trauma → localize infection; and also they pass through unyielding fibro-osseous tunnel, hence getting further traumatized following thickening. In tuberculoid spectrum, there is primary damage by caseating necrosis and in lepromatous spectrum there is slow ongoing fibrosis due to unchecked bacterial proliferation in Schwann cells with secondary ischemic damage to nerve (vasculitis).

8. What is "Jogerson Lewandoz" law?

Ans. An infection when controlled by immunological mechanisms result in granuloma formation.

9. How will you test the integrity of dermal nerves?

Ans. Pilocarpine test.

10. What is methylene blue test?

Ans. One of the tests to prove that hypopigmented patches are due to leprosy. Inject (36.5 mL) methylene blue → after around 6 days, the patches become blue and retain stain due to lipid content of lepra cells.

11. What is the differential diagnosis (D/D) of thickened nerves?

Ans. Hereditary sensory neuropathy, primary neuritic amyloidosis, Dejerine-Sotta disease, Refsum disease.

12. What is morphological index?
Ans. Percentage of viable bacilli after counting 200 bacilli.

13. What is bacteriological index?
Ans. Number of bacteria in an average microscopic field. Cochrane and Ridley scales commonly used to grade it from 1+ to 6+.

14. How do you classify leprosy?
Ans. *WHO*: Single lesion paucibacillary (SLPB), paucibacillary (PB), multibacillary (MB).

Ridley-Jopling (1962): True tuberculoid (TT), borderline tuberculoid (BT), borderline borderline (BB), borderline lepromatous (BL), lepromatous leprosy; modified in 1971 to include subpolar tuberculoid (TTs) and subpolar lepromatous (LLs) types.

(Indian Association of Leprologists (IAL) (1951 → 1953 → 1981): Tuberculoid, borderline, lepromatous, indeterminate, pure neuritic. Previous maculoanesthetic type now clubbed with tuberculoid.

National Leprosy Eradication Programme (NLEP) (clinical) classification: Nonlepromatous (N) → tuberculoid, maculo-anesthetic, pure neuritic; lepromatous (L); (N/L) → borderline and indeterminate.

Madrid (more useful):

Types: Lepromatous (macular, diffuse, infiltrative, major tuberculoid and pure neuritic), tuberculoid (macular, minor tuberculoid, major tuberculoid, pure neuritic)

Groups: Dimorphous, indeterminate (divided into macular and neuritic).

15. What are lepra reactions?
Ans. Allergic inflammatory process which is not a part of infective process either in its spread or resolution, although it may be associated one or more of these processes. The disease itself is chronic and active for a long time with bouts of exacerbating and sudden attacks of disease. They describe only an episode in major disease. These reactions are more common in lepromatous than borderline or tuberculoid spectrum.

16. What are the types of lepra reaction?

Ans. *Type I:* Observed around neural elements and skin lesions of borderline and tuberculoid types. They are likely due to bacterial antigens which are killed by therapy and get exposed to cell-mediated immunity. The reaction is typically akin to lepromin reaction with presence of epithelioid cells as the hallmark. It may be upgrading (reversal) or downgrading types. Upgrading (reversal) reaction is a BT to TT shift and downgrading one is a shift to lepromatous spectrum with new lesions having their characteristics.

Type II: [*Also called as*—erythema nodosum leprosum (ENL), Roseolar leprosy, lepra fever] seen in lepromatous spectrum with/without treatment. This reaction resembles "arthus phenomenon"—Ag-Ab complex formed at specific sites. Reaction is particularly located around medium-sized vessels **(Table 1)**.

Table 1: Types of lepra reactions.		
	Type I	*Type II*
Spectrum	BT, BB, BL	BL, LL
Lesion	Existing lesion develop erythema and edema	New modules arise in crops
Nerve damage	Frequent and severe	Not so
Systemic signs	Not common	Fever, malaise, arthralgia, lymphadenitis
Other organs	Iritis, orchitis, glomerulonephritis do not develop	Common
Course	Relapse infrequent	Common
AFB	Not seen	Broken bacteria
Investigations	Normal routine	Urine – albuminuria
Pathogenesis	Type 4 Ag-Ab reaction	Type 3 Ag-Ab reaction
Histopathology	Disorganized granuloma	Vasculitis

(BB: borderline borderline; BL: borderline lepromatous; BT: borderline tuberculoid; LL: lepromatous leprosy; AFB: acid-fast bacillus)

Type III (Lucio phenomenon, erythema necroticans): Seen in Mexican origin only, vascular lesion with diffuse infiltration, does not respond to thalidomide. Large number of organisms seen.

17. What are the types of ENL?

Ans. *Two types:* Intermittent (divided into mild and severe forms) and continuous (no reaction free period).

18. What are the bony changes in leprosy?

Ans. *Specific:* Osteitis, periostitis, bone cysts, bone resorption (longitudinal/concentric/combined).

Nonspecific: Erosions, osteomyelitis, osteopenia, septic arthritis.

Minor changes: Honey combing, pseudocyst, enlarged nutrient foramina, stippling.

19. What is reaction hand?

Ans. Subcutaneous nodules develop over dorsum of hand in type II reaction. Infiltrating edema with pain and functional incapacity is often present. If these features are associated with arthritis of IP joint → reaction hand.

20. What is frozen hand?

Ans. Subcutaneous nodules heal by leaving scar (involves palmer skin and aponeurosis) → contracture produced by fibrosis pulls up finger at MCP joint → pull in various directions produces multiforme deformities in fixed position known as frozen hand.

21. How do you define low ulnar nerve palsy?

Ans. Anatomically—distal to olecranon fossa. Clinically—involvement of intrinsic hand muscles.

22. What is high ulnar nerve palsy?

Ans. Anatomically—proximal to ulnar fossa. Clinically—involvement of ulnar half of FDP and flexor carpi ulnaris.

23. What do you understand by low and high median nerve palsy?

Ans. Low median nerve palsy typically is defined by involvement around wrist (carpal tunnel). Motor loss to OP, APB, FPB, first and second lumbrical with variable loss of palmar cutaneous sensation. High median nerve palsy in addition has motor loss to FDS, radial half of FDP, and thumb long flexor (FPL), weakness of pronation (PQ).

24. What is deformity, disability, and impairment?

Ans. *Deformity:* Alteration in form/shape/appearance of body part which is visible.

Disability: Deterioration in one's ability (capacity) which is felt by the patient. Also defined as inability (or difficulty) to carry out certain tasks.

Impairment: Anatomic, physiological, and/or psychological abnormality or loss resulting from disease/disorder that may be temporary or permanent.

25. What are the types of deformity in leprosy?

Ans. *Specific (LL/BL):* Intrinsic plus finger, twisted finger, banana finger, reaction hand, frozen hand.

Paralytic (BB/neuritic): Claw hand, wrist drop, claw toes, foot drop.

Feet: Trophic ulcer, scars and contractures, short digits.

26. What is the chemotherapy for leprosy?

Ans. Multidrug therapy (MDT).

Multibacillary: Regimen for adults: Rifampicin 600 mg (per month), dapsone 100 mg daily, clofazimine 300 mg per month and 50 mg daily. [Children (10-14 years)—half dose].

Paucibacillary: Rifampicin 600 mg monthly, dapsone 100 mg daily. SLPB: Rifampicin 600 mg, ofloxacin 400 mg, minocycline 100 mg (ROM regime).

27. How long will you continue treatment?

Ans. *Multibacillary*: Lifelong monotherapy (dapsone); MDT till skin smears negative; FDT (fixed-dose treatment) 24 pulses (in 36 months); *FDT 12 pulses in 18 months (1995).*

Paucibacillary: 6 pulses of PB—MDT. SLPB: ROM therapy.

Treatment of reactions: Steroids (types I and II); thalidomide (I); colchicines (II), *chloroquine (I and II)*, cyclosporine till subsidence of lesions and new lesion do not appear.

28. How do you diagnose and treat neuritis?

Ans. Suspect neuritis in tenderness over nerve trunk with thickening.

Swelling/redness/increased temperature.

Some functional loss in distribution.

Conservative (medical decompression): Anti-inflammatory drugs; prednisolone (60 mg/kg reduced by 10 mg every week till 3 weeks → good response, treat with 30 mg/kg till 6 months); ice packs, splint → if no improvement in 3 weeks then operate.

Operative: Indications:
- Recent onset incomplete paralysis not responding to conservative treatment
- Sudden onset complete paralysis attributed to neuritis
- Continued pain even in presence of paralysis
- Deterioration/progression of disease on conservative treatment
- Symptomatic nerve abscess.

Procedures:
- External decompression by removing constricting ligaments and/or arching tendon fibers, medial epicondylectomy for ulnar nerve
- Reduction of angulation stress: For example, anterior transposition of nerve
- *Decompression*:
  - Epineurectomy
  - Hemicircumferential neurolysis (epineurium dissected only from hemicircumference of nerve to preserve blood supply)
  - Interfascicular neurolysis.

Splinting and exercises (muscle strengthening—physiotherapy; functional re-education—occupational therapy).

29. What is claw hand?

Ans. Claw hand is deformity of hand due to functional malposition with clawing of fingers (in position of extension or hyperextension at MCP joint and flexion at IP joints) and loss of cascade (normal disposition of fingers in relaxed hand).

Wrist and Hand

It can be due to low/high ulnar nerve paralysis (partial claw hand) or due to combined ulnar and median nerve paralysis (total or complete claw hand). Other causes are soft tissue contractures, hand compartment syndrome and sequel, forearm compartment syndrome, and Volkmann ischemic contracture (VIC).

30. What is reversal of grasp or how does clawing functionally affect patient?

Ans. Major hand functions include: grasp, pinch, hook, and grip. To achieve all or any of these functions, hand must first achieve lumbrical position (MCP flexion and IP extension) followed by gradual MCP → PIP → DIP → flexion occurring in coordination. In intrinsic paralysis (intrinsic minus hand), extension at MCP occurs due dominance and DIP and PIP sequences occur before MCP flexion pushing the object away before grasping.

31. How will you assess this claw hand for treatment?

Ans. *Claw deformity* → forearm vertical on table with wrist neutral → ask patient to actively extend fingers → assess severity of deformity.

Assisted angle: Assesses extensor lag in IP joint. Patient actively extends finger with examiner stabilizing MCP joint (examiner basically replenishes lumbrical function) → if assisted angle is present, then flex MCP joint until maximum active extension of IP joint is possible. If assisted angle > 30°, then passive (static) procedures are contraindicated.

Contracture angle: Measures residual fixed flexion at IP joint. (Examiner passively extends the finger to fullest and measures the residual angle). Joint stiffness/skin/capsule contracture causing contracture angle < 30° is correctable by physiotherapy.

Flexor digitorum superficialis power: If FDS is involved, then routine procedures are contraindicated.

Flexor digitorum profundus power: If FDP to RF or LF is < grade 4 MRC, then use of FDS of these fingers is contraindicated.

Volkmann sign: If positive, then stretching by physiotherapy is required before surgery.

Hypermobility of joints: If present, then use weaker muscles for transfer to prevent later development of swan neck deformity.

32. What are the prerequisites for surgery in leprosy hand?
Ans. Determined by various factors:
- Good clinical response to antileprosy treatment
- No attacks of reaction or neuritis during previous 6 months
- No tenderness over nerve
- Deformity for at least 1 year (no possibility of spontaneous recovery)
- No joint contracture/joint damage
- Less than 10° hyperextension at PIP joint and < 15° ulnar deviation of fingers (ideally should be absent)
- Isolated contraction of muscle to be transferred must be practiced
- Compensatory abnormal movement pattern must be unlearnt and eliminated
- Supple hand

Most importantly, explain to the patient that only motor function will be restored and not sensory function.

33. How will you treat claw hand?
Ans. Primary requirement in claw hand is to provide flexion at MCP joint.

Secondary is to achieve flexion at IP joint and coordination and power.

I will get an X-ray done to look for condition of bones and joints.

Passive (Static) treatment methods to provide flexion at MCP joint (achieve only first goal and also do not address adduction of fingers).
- Zancolli anterior capsulorrhaphy of MCP joint
- Extensor diversion graft (Srinivasan)
- Palande technique (capsulorrhaphy and flexor pulley advancement)
- Extensor carpi radialis longus tenodesis.

Tendon transfer (dynamic): Even if RF and LF are involved, transfer of tendon to all four tendons must be done to provide coordinated and powerful movements:

1. *Sublimis transfer (Modified Stiles-Bunnel FF_4T phasic transfer)*: FDS of RF → four tail/slips → IF (ulnar side) and rest of fingers (radial side). Attach to dorsal lateral extensor expansion. Specific attachment provides in addition adduction of fingers. Tendon should pass anterior to MCP joint (Bunnel originally used all four FDS slips that led to intrinsic plus deformity).
2. *Zancolli Lasso:* Transfer of FDS of RF/MF to all fingers. Here, a lasso is created around A2 pulley system (modified Lasso) to provide dynamic MCP flexion (remember unassisted angle should be < 30°).
3. *Extensor to flexor four tailed (EF_4T nonphasic, Brand)*: ECRL tendon with fascia lata or palmaris or plantaris extension attached as mentioned. Brand originally described it with ECRB tendon and later modified with ECRB/ECRL.
4. Palmaris longus many tailed graft—if fingers are hypermobile. (This weaker muscle will not cause swan neck deformity).
5. Extensor indices transfer.

34. How do you ascertain adequate tension?
Ans. *Karat method*: Maintaining range of excursion between 4 and 6 cm.

Other method is to clinically pull one tendon slip that should just start excursion in nearby slip.

35. How will you address thumb function?
Ans. Adduction of thumb lost in ulnar nerve (adductor pollicis, FPB—partial) and major thenar muscle functions (APB, FPB, OP) lost in median nerve palsy (claw thumb)—so treatment required mostly in total claw hand. Aim is to provide pronation (total claw hand) and adduction (ulnar). Most commonly, FDS to RF rerouted around pisiform bone (Riordan opponensplasty) → divided into two slips → one attached to dorsum of MC (adduction) and other to dorsum

of terminal IP joint (pronation). Other transfers include lateralization of EPL tendon at wrist, APL rerouting, ECU rerouting, FPL transfer, and intermetacarpal bone block.

36. What ancillary surgeries may be required?

Ans. Web space contractures → Z-plasty (with or without skin graft or Groin).

Arthrodesis of MCP and IP joint (bone destruction and nonsalvageable joints).

Surgery for Boutonniere, Swan neck, and mallet finger deformities may be required.

37. What are the prerequisites for tendon transfers in foot?

Ans. The following must be looked for:
- No planter ulcer or septic focus
- No fixed equinovarus deformity or tarsal disorganization
- *Condition of muscles*: Powerful tibialis posterior (Grade V or at least IV+)
- No contracture of tendo Achilles
- At least 20° ankle dorsiflexion
- Conditioning of tibialis posterior muscle for voluntary contraction (training).

38. How will you manage Hansen foot drop?

Ans. Main aim is stability to have reasonable gait and stance.

I will get X-ray done to see status of bones.
- *Early foot drop*: I will do passive mobilization, splinting, physiotherapy to strengthen muscles till 1 year as spontaneous recovery is possible till that time.
- *Established foot drop*: Tibialis posterior transfer (non-phasic) → split into two → attach each into extensor digitorum longus (EDL)/extensor hallucis longus (EHL). Two routes:
  1. Circumtibial route is easier but pull is oblique.
  2. *Transinterosseous membrane*: Direct pull but more chances of adhesion.

Other method is to insert it into ligaments of foot or middle cuneiform (not preferred).

Incomplete lesions with active peronei: Do a transfer of both peronei and tibialis posterior otherwise tendency to eversion is increased.

39. How will you manage Claw-toes?

Ans. Claw-toes arise due to posterior tibial nerve palsy (Three stages: (1) Hyperextension of (metatarsophalangeal) (MTP) joint: Toe tip touches ground: Toe-tip ulcer; (2) Increased hyperextension: Toe tip off ground: Increased IP joint flexion: Toe dorsum ulcer; (3) Increased MTP hyperextension: Dorsal dislocation of toe; Toe Ball ulcer.)

- *If toes are supple*: Flexor to extensor transfer: FDL transferred to dorsum of toe and extensor tendon.
- *Stiff toes with contracture*: Shortening of toes (excision of middle phalanx) and inactivation of long flexor tendons with arthrodesis.

40. How will you manage foot ulcers?

Ans. Three types:

1. *Lepromatous*: MDT for leprosy and nitrofurazone ointment
2. *Stasis ulcer* (dorsum of foot and medial and lower third of leg): Local hygiene, antiseptic cream, dressing, elastic compression bandage and elevation, POP cast, and skin grafting
3. *Trophic ulcer* [plantar ulcer caused by prominent metatarsal heads, sensory deficit, weight bearing, increased plantar fascia tension, loss of protective function of sesamoids in flexor hallucis brevis (FHB)]:
   - *Acute (swollen hot foot with abscess):* Drainage, wash and irrigate, regular dressing, elevate limb, antibiotics
   - *Chronic:* Regular dressing with antiseptics [or MSGP (Magnesium sulfate, glycerine, proflavine) solution], POP cast, rest and immobilization (contraindicated for secondary complications—infection). Remove slough, clean, and dress to enhance granulation, split thickness skin grafting, amputation.

41. What is "Hot foot syndrome" and how will you manage it?

Ans. Acute neuropathic disintegration of foot → results from neurological deficit. Foot is hot and swollen with collapsed suspension system. It is basically acute onset Charcot foot.

42. What other deformities can be found in foot?

Ans. Cocked up toe due to unopposed extensor action (treat by extensor tenotomy); Rosette toes (bunching of toes) treated by corrective bandaging; neuropathic foot can be managed by triple arthrodesis but chances of failure are high.

43. What vaccines are available for Hansen disease?
Ans.
- Live *M. leprae*, killed *M. leprae*.
- Killed *M. leprae* with adjuvant
- Chemically modified *M. leprae*
- BCG + *M. vaccae*
- Delipified *M. leprae*
- *M. omega* (ω vaccine) [Indian Council of Medical Research (ICMR) Delhi]
- Indian Cancer Research Centre (ICRC) bacillus.

44. How do you make smears?

Ans. *Slit smears:* Incise 5 × 3 mm and scrape material from posterior auricular patch

Snip smears: Small piece of skin removed and crushed under slide.

45. What is histoid leprosy and lazarine leprosy?

Ans. Histoid leprosy is seen in LL patients with or without relapse. It has variable nodules, does not undergo ENL, absence of globi, and clears on treatment.

Lazarine leprosy (Lepra Manchada) are ulcerating lesions arising over trunk and extremity seen in BT leprosy (also seen in Lucio leprosy).

46. What is SFG index?

Ans. Solid, fragmented, and granular (SFG) index:
- 2-0-0 (all solid) (SFG index = 10)
- 0-0-2 (all fragmented) (SFG index = 0)

47. What are the characteristics of *M. leprae*?

Ans. It is an atypical (slow growing, oxidizes L-dihydroxyphenylalanine (L-DOPA) partial (weakly) acid-fast bacillus that looks like a bundle of cigars "globi" under microscope.

48. What are the stains for *M. leprae*?

Ans. Ziehl-Neelsen and Fite-Faraco stains; the latter one being better as the bacilli are acid-fast for only a particular duration of their lifetime and Fite-Faraco sort of creates acid fastness in bacilli. (Hansen originally used osmic acid).

CASE III: DUPUYTREN DISEASE

Diagnosis: The patient is a 52-year-old male with Dupuytren contracture of both hands involving the ring and LFs.

FINDINGS

- Painless nodules/cords over palmar aspect
- Garrod nodes/knuckle pads over PIP joint dorsally
- Painless flexion contracture of fingers
- Thinning of subcutaneous fat
- Adhesion of skin to contracture
- Pitting/dimpling of skin
- Lesion of plantar fascia (Ledderhose disease)
- Plastic induration of penis (Peyronie disease).

1. What is Dupuytren contracture?

Ans. It is a proliferative fibroplasia of palmar tissue predominantly involving the palmar fascia and palmodigital extension. The proliferation is seen in the form of nodules and cords that may soon after develop in secondary flexion deformity of fingers.

2. What are various risk factors for the development of this disease?

Ans. Male sex (M:F = 10:1, occurs earlier in males), Scandinavian and celtic origin, diabetes mellitus, epilepsy, alcoholism, pulmonary tuberculosis (TB), vascular insufficiency (?free radicals, ?platelet derived growth factor), cigarette smoking, and heredity (autosomal dominant with variable penetrance).

3. How do you classify Dupuytren disease?

Ans. There are three phases:
1. *Early:* Skin changes + loss of normal architecture + skin pits

2. *Intermediate:* Nodules and cords
3. *Late phase:* Above + contractures. This has four stages:
    i. Ring finger MCP joint contracture
    ii. Ring finger MCP + PIP joint contracture + LF MCP
    iii. Above + LF PIP joint and MCP joint of middle finger
    iv. Above + DIP joint hyperextension of ring or LFs or both.

4. Which finger is most commonly involved?

Ans. Ring finger (followed in order of involvement by little, middle, index, and lastly thumb).

5. What are Dupuytren nodules?

Ans. It is a firm soft-tissue mass originating in the superficial components of palmar and digital fascia which is fixed to both skin and deep fascia. They are usually well-defined and localized. In the palm, they are located adjacent to distal palmar crease while in fingers the nodules are commonly found at PIP joint or at the base of fingers. They are often painless but may become symptomatic when associated with stenosing tenosynovitis due to direct pressure on A1 pulley. Over time, they get regressed to be replaced by cord.

The dorsal side equivalents are Garrod nodes (rare) or knuckle pads which are prevalent in bilateral disease and particularly the presence of former should suggest one to search other sites for similar affection (Ledderhose and Peyronie).

6. How does the nodule form?

Ans. The earliest change is the thickening of Grapow fibers (these connect the fascia to dermis). There is hence the development of thickening of skin associated with rippling and dimpling. The local proliferation continues to form a nodule or if skin retraction occurs then a pit. (*Skin pit caused by full-thickness skin retraction is a reliable sign of early Dupuytren disease and is latter replaced by nodule or cord*) **(Fig. 16).**

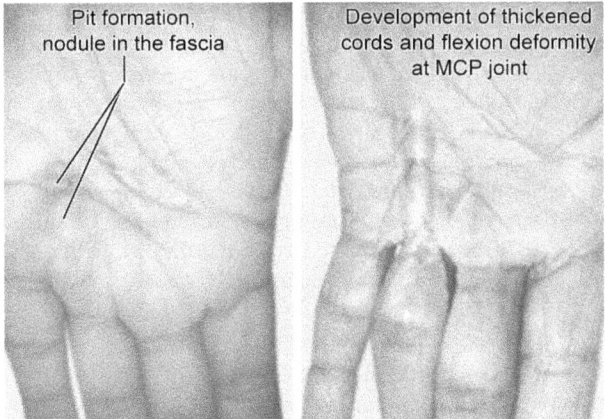

Fig. 16: Nodule formation and development into fibrous cords in later stage. (MCP: metacarpophalangeal)

7. What is the pathogenesis of cord?

Ans. Cords are often the future of nodules; however, they may arise de novo. Remember the cords or nodules are by themselves not de novo structures but often the fibroblastic proliferation in normal anatomical structures that become thickened by myofibroblastic activity and deposition of type III collagen. The cords involve the palmar, palmodigital, and digital regions and the exact distribution is complicated necessitating sound anatomical knowledge of hand; however, the important features are presented here.

For development of flexion deformity at MCP joint, the pretendinous cord is most important.

The spiral cord is the one that extends through palm to digits and has four origins; the pretendinous band, the spiral band, the lateral digital sheet, and the Grayson ligament.

Proximal interphalangeal joint contracture results from involvement of central cord, lateral cord, spiral cord, and retrovascular cord.

Distal interphalangeal joint contracture emerges from contracture of retrovascular and lateral cord.

8. What is the differential diagnosis?
Ans.
- *Non-Dupuytren disease*: Occurs in diverse ethnic groups (Dupuytren disease occurs in whites), unilateral, usually single digit, often associated with trauma, can spontaneously improve (rarely needing surgery)
- Epithelioid sarcoma
- Occupational thickening of skin and hyperkeratosis
- Localized pigmented villonodular synovitis (PVNS), palmar ganglion, inclusion cyst are differentials for large Dupuytren nodule
- Post-traumatic contracture.

9. How do you treat the patient?
Ans. General guidelines are as follows:
- Observation is limited to a patient with static disease and minimal contracture or functional compromise.
- Surgery is the keystone to treatment for majority. Typical indications are flexion deformity of > 30° at MCP joint and flexion contracture of 15° at PIP joint in the presence of a well-developed cord. The following procedures are done with their individual merits and demerits:
    - *Percutaneous fasciotomy:* Preferred for palmar cords in older patients. Higher recurrence rate; limited dissection required but greater danger to nearby tendons.
    - *Fasciectomy:* Partial, regional, limited remains the most widely done procedure. Lower recurrence rates.
    - *Segmental aponeurectomy:* Through multiple small C-shaped incisions in palm or digits, segments of diseased fascia are removed.
    - *Total fasciectomy and digital Z-plasties*: Higher complications.
    - *Dermofasciectomy:* Simultaneous excision of skin and diseased tissue. Low recurrence rates but limited to recurrent disease or treatment failures or very severe disease due to extensive dissection needed.

- *Salvage procedures:* Amputation (PIP flexion deformity > 70°, recurrent disease with exuberant scar tissue), dorsal wedge osteotomy of proximal phalanx, arthrodesis of PIP joint with partial resection of proximal phalanx, arthroplasty of PIP joint.

    Surgical release of PIP joint contracture is needed for residual deformity > 40°.

10. What are the complications of surgery?

Ans. Various complications are known, viz. neurovascular injury, hematoma, infection, stiffness, reflex sympathetic dystrophy, recurrence (true recurrence—disease at the operative site or disease extension—recurrence outside the primary surgical site), and inclusion cyst formation.

11. What can you offer to a patient unwilling for surgery?

Ans. Local agents have been tried with variable efficiency:
- Calcium-channel blockers for early disease
- Collagenase for advanced disease
- Trypsin and hyaluronidase (enzymatic fasciotomy)
- Steroid injection and local interferon injections.

12. What are the poor prognostic factors?

Ans. Male sex, family history, ulnar side lesions, alcoholism and epileptic patients, bilateral disease, etc. are associated with poor prognostic factors.

CASE IV: FLEXOR TENDON INJURY

Diagnosis: A 42-year-old male with 15 days old complete cut injury to FDS and FDP of ring and middle fingers of right hand in zone II.

FINDINGS

- Scar mark over palmar aspect of hand healed with primary/secondary intention
- Loss of finger flexion cascade
- Palpable gap at the injury site
- Palpable nodule (of retracted tendon) proximal to injury site (commonly at A2 pulley or at FDS chiasm or in palm)

- Inability to actively flex the finger at PIP and DIP *(examine both for all injured fingers)* of RF and MF
- Loss of sensation distal to the injury site (cut injury to digital nerve(s). Loss of sweat and two point discrimination.

1. Why do you say it is a cut of both FDS and FDP?

Ans. *(Also see examination of hand, motor power, and muscle/tendon function discussed earlier in this chapter).* There is complete absence of finger flexion at both PIP and DIP joints on testing active finger flexion.

2. How do you interpret the finger flexion cascade to localize tendon injury?

Ans. *(Observing flexion cascade is better than probing the wounds in many circumstances).* Allowing the wrist to drop free into extension, there is a passive tenodesis effect of long flexors that bring all four fingers into a smooth flexion cascade (arcade) with incremental flexion from IF to LF. Also, there is flexion at IP joint of thumb. Any break in this smooth transition indicates pathology (the interpretation is true for zone 1-3 injuries and some zone 4 injuries).

A finger held with slight flexion at both IP joints but with a break in cascade → FDS injury.

A finger is straighter than others but there is slight flexion at PIP joint → FDP injury *(if there is no history of cut injury, then suspect FDP avulsion; "Jersey finger"—especially for RF).*

A completely straight finger → injury to both FDP and FDS.

3. What else would you like to know from patient's history of injury that has a bearing on management?

Ans. I would specifically enquire if the finger was in flexion or extension at the time of injury.

4. What is the implication?

Ans. Injury inflicted at finger flexion suggests that the level of wound, cut FDS and cut FDP, will be different and is a favorable situation as "bunching" at repair is less likely with minimal chances of cross union and adhesions or mechanical block later during rehabilitation training.

Wrist and Hand

An injury in extension would although make it easier to find the cut structure through smaller incision, however there are higher risk of healing process and tendons becoming one scar unit.

5. What in examination would prompt you to look for possible other injuries?

Ans. Cut injury of both tendons in zone 2 will raise alarm for associated digital neurovascular injury. Cut injury at zone 3 often implicates injury to digital nerves and superficial arch injury. Cut flexor tendons except PL at zone 4 should be explored for median nerve injury. Similarly, cut injury to FCU often indicates ulnar neurovascular injury.

6. What are the zones of hand?

Ans. Verdan described five zones for flexor region of hand as shown in **Table 2** and **Figure 17**.

Table 2: Zones of hand.	
Zone	**Limits (with suggested modification)**
1	Insertion of FDP tendon at DP to insertion of FDS at MP
2	(No Man's land) Insertion of FDS at MP to A1 pulley—corresponds to distal palmar crease
3	A1 pulley to distal limit of transverse carpal ligament (only the central limited part of tendons supplied by mesotenon and attached to lumbricals are proposed to be included in this zone)
4	(Enemy territory) Underneath the transverse carpal ligament—between proximal and distal limits (synovial coverage of flexor tendons extends up to 4 cm proximal to proximal limit and some authors include this also in zone 4)
5	Muscles tendons and other structures proximal to proximal limit of carpal ligament. Extensive laceration of muscles in this region is termed "Spaghetti wrist/full house injuries"

(Remember only the classical ones unless you aspire to become a hand surgeon or encounter a hand surgeon in exams!)
(DP: distal phalanx; FDP: flexor digitorum profundus; FDS: flexor digitorum superficialis; MP: middle phalanx)

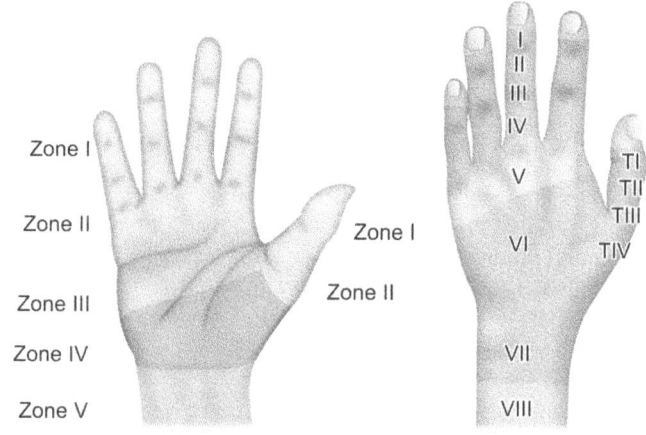

Fig. 17: Various zones for flexor and extensor tendon.

7. Why is zone 2 called "no man's land"?

Ans. Bunnell (1918) introduced the term "no man's land" for zone 2 following dismal results of primary repair and admonished surgeons to primarily remove the tendon and graft later. Problems primarily arise due to limited space fibro-osseous tunnel containing two tendons and multiple pulleys and minimal areolar tissue to allow gliding despite best of repairs. Since then with advances in suture material and techniques along with better understanding, the term should be upgraded to "some- man's land".

8. What will you do for this patient?

Ans. (Considering the wound is favorable—healed without infection/necrosis). I will ensure suppleness of joints and absence of reflex sympathetic dystrophy. I will explain the need of exploration and tendon repair with arrangements for tendon grafting and repair of digital nerve to the patient. Prognosis and need of all these procedures will be explained to the patient.

(Any injury more than 3 weeks old is a strong candidate for tendon grafting as the suture retaining strength of tendon

decreases and myostatic contractures develop precluding apposition of tendons without excessive IP flexion).

9. What care will you take during repair?

Ans. Proper exposure using midlateral incisions or Bruner incisions or both. Minimal tissue handling, avoid devascularization of tendons, avoid bunching (stuffing), strong enough repair for early mobilization, and maintaining or reconstructing pulley system.

I will expose the injury site through the transverse wound and a midlateral incision (as nerve is also involved). I will milk the tendons through the sheath using gentle pressure on palm and flexing the MP joint; else I will expose the retracted tendons in palm and pass a catheter through the digital sheath with tendons tied to the same and deliver through wound.

10. What are Bruner incisions?

Ans. Extensile zigzag incisions suitable for pure tendon injuries that keep away the scar site from repair as much as possible and do not produce function limiting wound contracture **(Fig. 18)**.

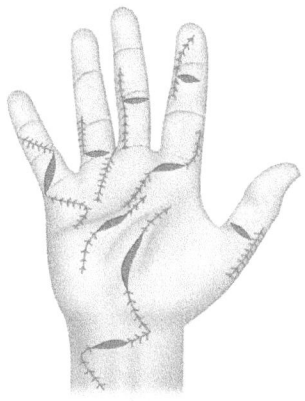

Fig. 18: Bruner incisions.

11. What should be the characteristics of suture material for repairing tendon?

Ans. The suture should have high tensile strength; have easy knotability; having minimal tissue response; not be extensible, for preventing gaping; be absorbable late after healing of tendon; and have ease of use.

12. What suture technique will you use for repair?

Ans. I will use locked cruciate core suture technique (or otherwise modified Kessler) using 4-0 ethibond along with Lin-locking epitendinous suture (or simple locked epitendinous suture) using 6-0 prolene to "tidy up" the repair.

13. What tendons will you repair?

Ans. I will repair the FDP and one slip of FDS using four-strand technique. However, if FDS is cut proximal to Camper Chiasm then I will repair both using the core suture and epitenon repair technique. If the cut in both tendons are at the same level, then only repair the FDP.

14. Why will you use the four-strand technique?

Ans. It is agreed upon that more the number of suture filaments cross the repair site the more is strength of initial repair (time-zero). However, the strength of repair is weakest at 5th day and may drop anywhere from half to one fifth of time-zero strength. Now, it is believed that some 14.7N strength is required to flex finger against moderate resistance so that three to five times this measure (around 45N) is required for the time-zero suture techniques. Most of the four-strand suture techniques easily surpass this 45N limit (especially the Becker and locked cruciate techniques—60N); also some strength is provided by epitendinous technique (10–50%). Two-strand techniques are hence weak and six and eight-strand techniques are too bulky possibly.

15. What other suture techniques you know of?

Ans. The following are various suture techniques:
- *Two-strand techniques*: Bunnell (condemned), Mason-Allen, modified Kessler

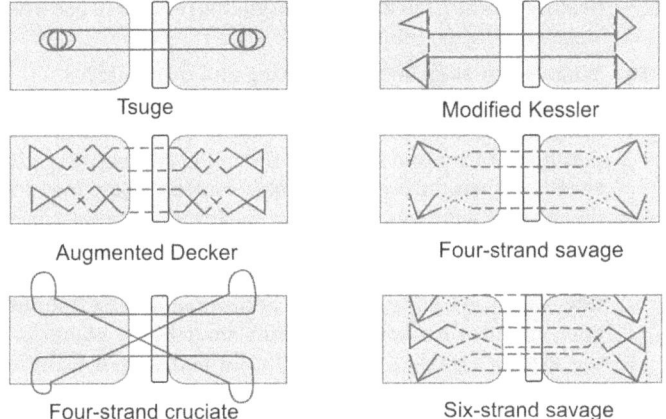

Fig. 19: Various suturing techniques for tendon repair.

- *Four-strand techniques*: Strickland, Lee, Robertson, Becker, modified Becker and Locked cruciate (McLarney)
- *Six-strand techniques*: Savage, Sandow, Lim
- *Eight-strand technique*: Silva **(Fig. 19)**

"Strands" mean the number of suture filaments actually crossing the repair site.

16. How will you protect tendon surfaces and repair?
Ans. The following should be practiced:
- Using a strong nonabsorbable suture
- Employ at least two independent sutures
- Using atraumatic technique
- Minimize exposed knots and sutures
- Minimize exposed raw surfaces of tendon
- No strangulation of blood supply to tendon ends.

17. What if repair is not possible?
Ans. There is a high chance that the repair is not possible (difficult after 2 weeks) and then I will arrange for tendon graft using PL tendon in single stage, if the peritendinous tissue is

healthy (not scarred and provide gliding) else I will use a two-stage grafting technique (less likely).

18. What is two-stage tendon grafting and rationale?

Ans. *(Ensure supple skin, sensate digit, adequate vascularity, and full passive ROM of IP joints).* If the tendon bed and peritendinous tissue are badly disrupted so that the gliding sheath for tendon is not available and/or pulley system is damaged, I will place a silicone sheath in place (as spacer) so that pseudo-sheath develops around it which will act as tendon sheath for the future graft preserving or reconstructing A2 and A4 pulley. Stage II performed at least 3 months after, requires extrasynovial grafts from PL or plantaris or toe extensor passed through the formed tunnel using rail road technique.

19. How will you manage injury to pulley?

Ans. Out of eight pulleys (five—annular and three—cruciate), A2 and A4 are the most important *(oblique pulley for thumb)* to prevent bowstringing of flexor tendon (A2 pulley) and reducing the angle of attack (A4 pulley) for flexor tendon to provide smooth flexion. Primary repair is possible only if care has been taken to deliver the tendons through L-shaped incision across the pulley. Else, a damaged pulley will be reconstructed using extensor retinaculum sheath (distal half to third) or PL tendon graft. *(It is easier to remember the important pulley locations—A2 is located in proximal half of proximal phalanx and A4 is located in middle-third of middle phalanx).*

20. How will you manage tendon injury in zone 1?

Ans. Avulsion injury of FDP—"Jersey finger" is classified into three types (Leddy and Packer):

Type I: Avulsion injury with proximal tendon stump retracted into palm. Urgent repair required as tendon degeneration (both nutrient vinculae ruptured) and myostatic contractures are highly likely. Delayed presentations (>21 days) require DIP fusion, FDP reconstruction around FDS (not through chiasm), no treatment or excision of FDP.

Type II: Tendon retracts to FDS decussation at PIP joint (commonest). Short vinculum only is ruptured. Repair to bone.

Type III: Larger piece of bone gets caught at the level of A4 pulley. Open reduction and internal fixation (ORIF) using pull-out suture or suture anchors.

Cut injury of FDP is treated depending on the length of distal stump left. If more than 0.75 cm of distal stump remains, repair the tendon under A4 pulley (modified Kessler). For small stump, either advance the tendon and attach to volar plate (*the volar plate moves with distal phalanx*) or bone. If quadriga effect is expected, then one may consider conversion to "superficialis finger" or suture the proximal tendon to distal stump and bring out the suture through fingertip as pull out sutures.

21. What is "superficialis finger"?

Ans. For small distal stump in cut FDP tendon in zone 1, the proximal stump is sutured to middle phalanx and the proximal end of distal stump is sutured to the neck of middle phalanx to prevent hyperextension deformity at DIP. The method is also used for nonreconstructible pulley in zone 2 with bowstringing of FDP.

22. What will you do for zone 4 injury?

Ans. As the space is limited, so repairs are limited to terminal digital flexors. I will repair FPL and index profundus independently while profundi to MF, RF, and LF are combined anatomically into single unit. Superficialis tendons should be repaired only if they will not come in contact with any other tendon repair. I will keep the carpal ligament open.

23. How will you manage the patient in postoperative period?

Ans. I will manage the patient with Strickland active motion protocol **(Table 3)** designed for four-strand repair with epitendinous suture (Indiana protocol). This incorporates the early active motion exercises with tenodesis motion in a Kleinert-type hinged splint.

Table 3: Management of the patient in postoperative period.					
0–3 days	0–4 weeks	4 weeks	5 weeks	6 weeks	8 weeks
Dorsal blocking splint (DBS) with wrist in 200 and MCP in 500 flexion Tenodesis splint (TS) allowing 300 wrist extension and full wrist flexion, maintaining MCP in 500 flexion	Passive DIP extension with PIP and MCP flexion (DBS) (15 repetitions/2 hours) Passive PIP extension with DIP and MCP flexion (DBS) (15 repetitions/2 hours) Tenodesis exercises within hinged splint (TS) (15 repetitions/ 2 hours)	Dorsal blocking splint removed during exercise Tenodesis exercise continue (TS)	Active IP flexion with MCP extension followed by full digital extension	Blocking exercise if active tip to distal palmar crease >3 cm	Progressive resistive exercises begin Unrestricted use of hand at 14 weeks

(DIP: distal interphalangeal; MCP: metacarpophalangeal; PIP: proximal interphalangeal)

24. What is the rationale of this program?

Ans. From the original description of Kleinert using the elastic flexion pull against active extension, various observations have modified the postoperative regime.

- Passive DIP extension with PIP and MCP flexion glides FDP away from FDS suture site.
- Passive PIP extension with DIP and MCP flexion glides both tendons away from wound.
- Combined MCP flexion and wrist extension produces the least tension on repaired site.
- Tendon loses its tensile strength in first 2 weeks and gliding function by 10 days.

- Work of flexion (resistance to tendon gliding) at 1 week is least for repairs protected for first 3 days compared to those mobilized immediately (during edema) or at 7 days.
- Interphalangeal joint flexion is critical to preventing adhesion (it is difficult to determine in Kleinert regime if flexion is really occurring at IP joints or MP joint only)
- Wrist joint with greatest moment arm for flexor tendons produces greatest tendon excursion, so tenodesis exercises have been added to active exercises.

25. What is Kleinert regime for postoperative rehabilitation of tendon repair?

Ans. The protocols for tendon repair have moved a full circle from early active mobilization in 1920s to immobilization to passive mobilization (Kleinert and Duran) to active mobilization (last two decades). Kleinert passive mobilization protocol involved the use of a protective splint with wrist and MP joints in flexion and IP joints in extension, whereby active extension was encouraged while flexion was passive using elastic rubber-band. This slowly progressed to progressive resistive exercises.

26. What is Quadriga effect?

Ans. Quadriga (Roman four-horsed chariot—single driver holding reins to four horses) syndrome was first described by Verdan in 1960. The common muscle belly of FDP to four fingers (and analogous EDS—extensor quadriga) limits independent function of flexor tendons to individual finger. Also, the muscle belly can contract effectively only if excursion of all the tendons is normal. Thus, if one of the tendon is fixed or its amplitude altered, then proportional effect will be evident in all the other slips (reduced flexion) and often produces forearm pain. Pseudoquadriga is produced by fixed contractures of IP joints.

27. How much advancement is considered critical to produce quadriga effect?

Ans. More than 1 cm advancement has been found to clinically produce quadriga effect.

28. What is lumbrical plus finger?

Ans. The term refers to extension (paradoxical) at IP joints (the action of lumbricals) on attempted flexion. This condition is seen in cases where the tendon graft is either too long or sutured in lax tension or has ruptured in attempted reconstruction for zone 2 or sometimes three injuries using tendon graft. The force in these cases is transmitted through the lumbrical muscle tendon unit instead of flexor tendon and hence paradoxical movement is produced. It is important to demonstrate full "passive" flexion before making diagnosis of lumbrical plus finger.

(Remember and do not confuse: The superficialis finger is a treatment method while lumbrical plus finger is a complication of reconstruction).

29. Why is maintaining IP joint extension and MP flexion for immobilization so stressed upon?

Ans. During immobilization, MP joints should be maintained in more than 50° flexion as the collateral and accessory collateral ligaments are lengthiest in 50–70° flexion at MP joint. In case stiffness develops, the ligaments will hence not contract and limit the flexion during rehabilitation; however, immobilization in extension will produce contracted ligaments and capsule that are difficult to stretch later by physiotherapy. This differential length (19 mm in flexion and 14–17 mm in extension) is due to differential radii of metacarpal head and eccentric volar placement (Cam effect) which places PP farthest from metacarpal epicondyle (the origin of collateral ligaments) during flexion. The effect is not seen in IP joints and prevention of flexion contracture here is priority (hence extension). Such a cast with MP joint in flexion and IP in extension is called "Clam Digger cast".

30. How do you manage partial lacerations?

Ans. Tendon lacerations of up to 90% of their thickness are stronger than completely cut repaired tendons, so a partial laceration must never be made complete. In general lacerations, up to 25% may be simply trimmed. Epitenon repair is done for lacerations involving 25–50% of tendon width. Larger lacerations are repaired as for a complete tear without disturbing the remaining intact tendon.

CASE V: CARPAL TUNNEL SYNDROME (TARDY MEDIAN PALSY)

Simple case to diagnose and present and is good to score marks. Simple and straight questions and answers.

Read times: 4–5 MS and DNB candidates.

Diagnosis: The patient is a 40-year-old female with nontraumatic incomplete right low median nerve palsy most likely due to CTS.

1. **Why do you call this CTS?**

Ans.

- *Short history:*
    - Tingling and numbness sensation in the typical median nerve distribution in the radial three and a half digits (thumb, index, long, and radial side of ring) prominent in night ("nocturnal acroparesthesia"). Variable amount of deep throbbing pain present diffusely over hand climbing to forearm or arm may be described.
    - In late cases, symptoms may progress to gritty or numb feeling in fingers, weakness of grip or pinch, and diminished finger dexterity.
    - Tinel and Phalen test (Wrist hyperflexed for 60 seconds; acceptable if Tinel positive; sensitivity 0.59, specificity 0.93) are positive.
    - On inspection of the right hand, there is thenar muscle wasting. The thumb cannot be opposed to the fingertips. Testing for APB revealed MRC power grade 3 compared to the opposite normal side with reduced muscle bulk and tone present. [In advanced cases, one may find thumb to be lying in the plane of the palm—a simian thumb (ape- thumb deformity). There may be atrophy of the pulp of the index and main fingers, dystrophic nail changes. There may be signs of ulceration or burns seen in the hand or

fingers. However, testing for FPL revealed normal power (distinguishes with high median nerve palsy.)]

2. What other differentials have you ruled out?

Ans. Also called CTS, mimics:
- Median nerve contusion
- Cervical radiculopathy (double-crush syndrome)
- Thoracic outlet syndrome
- Pronator syndrome
- Idiopathic brachioplexitis (Parsonage-Turner syndrome/ neuralgic amyotrophy)
- Intracranial neoplasm
- Multiple sclerosis
- Cervical syringomyelia
- Pancoast tumor
- Peripheral nerve tumor (schwannoma, hamartoma, etc.)
- Lower trunk brachial plexopathy
- Ulnar neuropathy
- Radial neuropathy
- Generalized neuropathy (diabetes/mononeuritis multiplex)
- Churg-Strauss syndrome.

3. What else would you like to examine?

Ans. Examination of neck to exclude any proximal abnormality (like double crush syndrome). Examine for causes of proximal median nerve compression.
- Supracondylar process of humerus (also known as ligament of Struthers)
- *Bicipital aponeurosis*: Resist elbow flexion with forearm supinated
- *Between heads of PT*: Resist forearm pronation with elbow extended/negative Phalen test at wrist
- Proximal arch of FDS (isolate long finger PIP joint flexion).

Simple test is to look for FPL weakness that identifies high median nerve palsy.

4. How do you perform Tinel test and what is the significance?

Ans. The Tinel sign is elicited by percussing in the midline from 2.5 cm proximal to 4 cm distal to the wrist crease.

Wrist and Hand

Presence of paresthesia along with a positive Phalen test has sensitivity of 0.41 and specificity of 0.9.

5. Are there any other tests you can do to identify critical median nerve compression?

Ans. *Durkan test:* Manual pressure over carpal tunnel for 30 seconds—positive if paresthesia (electric test or tingling) elicited in the median nerve distribution. More sensitive than Phalen test (acceptable if Tinel positive).

Wrist extension test (Reverse Phalen test; pray position): Active extension of wrist for 2 minutes (acceptable if Tinel is positive).

Tourniquet test (Gilliatt and Wilson): Arm tourniquet inflated above systolic pressure for 60 seconds—not significant.

Closed fist sign: Making tight fist for 60 seconds—significant only if one more sign positive.

Hand elevation test: Hand elevated above head for 60 seconds—not significant.

Ames test: To detect malingering. Make a fist and ask to press the fists together—identifies malingering if positive.

6. What are the other names for CTS?

Ans. Acroparesthesia, thenar neuritis, median neuropathy at wrist.

7. What are other clinical tests that can be performed in this case?

Ans. Hand diagram (patient marks site of pain or altered sensation on outlined hand diagram), hand volume stress test (hand volume measured by displacement, repeat after 7 minutes stress test and 10 minutes rest), static two point discrimination, moving two point discrimination, vibrometry, Semmes-Weinstein monofilaments.

8. Do you know of any invasive test?

Ans. Direct measurement of the carpal tunnel pressure by Wick method. Normal pressure inside carpal tunnel is 2.5 mm Hg. Complete intraneural flow stasis is seen at pressure above 80 mm Hg. "Critical pressure" for microvessels to cause obliteration and consequent ischemia is 40–50 mm.

In patients with CTS, the pressure has been found to be elevated to a range of 12–43 mm Hg.

9. How will you investigate this case?

Ans. I will get EDS (nerve conduction velocities and EMG):
- A distal motor latency of more than 4.2 ms and a sensory latency of more than 3.5 ms are considered abnormal.
- There is increased median-to-ulnar latency difference of the fourth finger systolic asterial pressure (> 0.5 ms).
- Electromyography may show signs of nerve damage, including increased insertional activity, positive sharp waves, and fibrillations at rest, decreased motor recruitment, and complex repetitive discharges in adductor pollicis muscle.

10. What do you achieve with EDS?

Ans. Confirm the clinical suspicion of CTS. EDS:
- Localizes the lesion
- Depicts involvement of motor, sensory fibers; defines physiologic basis (axon loss demyelination)
- Severity of lesion
- Time course of lesion (evidence of reinnervation or ongoing axonal loss).

In preoperative workup, EDS allows quantification of severity and type of lesion. Should the outcome of surgery is less than satisfactory it can be of some value in litigation.

It should not be used as a substitute for clinical examination as EDS is more sensitive and may come positive even in "clinically silent" patients.

11. Is there any role of computed tomography (CT)/ ultrasonography/magnetic resonance imaging (MRI) in carpal tunnel syndrome?

Ans. *Ultrasound* dynamic stress testing in NM ultrasound may demonstrate compression of median nerve between contracting thenar muscles ventrally and taut tendons dorsally. Mean diameter may decrease by 40%, while in normal population there is a tendency of no change or median nerve enlargement by 17%. Cross-sectional area

Wrist and Hand

of < 9.9 sq mm is taken as a cutoff for median nerve compression at pisiform level.

Computed tomography shows the bony structures clearly, but does not define the soft tissues accurately.

Magnetic resonance imaging shows high soft-tissue contrast may demonstrate space occupying lesion as a cause. Most importantly, MRI is useful in postoperative failed cases (investigation of choice) to look for real canal widening, incomplete ligament resection, scarring, or algodystrophy.

12. What is carpal tunnel and what are its boundaries?

Ans. A cylindrical, inelastic osseoligamentous space (open on both sides) bound dorsally by concave carpal arch (floor) and volarly by unyielding carpal ligament. The depth varies from 10 to 13 mm.

Carpal ligament (roof) attaches to the hook of the hamate, triquetrum, and pisiform medially, and the scaphoid, trapezium ridge, and fibro-osseous flexor carpi radialis sheath laterally.

13. What are its contents?

Ans. The most ventral (palmar) structure in the carpal tunnel is the median nerve. Lying dorsal (deep) to the median nerve in the carpal tunnel are the nine flexor tendons (four FDS, four FDP, one FPL) to the fingers and thumb. *Total of 10 structures in tunnel.*

14. What is the most common site for median nerve compression in the tunnel?

Ans. The compression has been localized to the thickest part of transverse carpal ligament (TCL) which is somewhere 1 cm distal to the proximal border of ligament. This level has been identified to be in line with hook of hamate.

15. What are the risk factors for CTS?

Ans. Certain risks factors have been identified but are not proven *causative* factors:
- Increased age (30–60 years)
- Female gender (F:M = 3)

- Obesity
- Cigarette smoking
- Vibrations associated with job tasks (rock drilling)—exertional CTS
- Repetitive movements of wrist and finger flexion
- Keyboarding (computer associated disease).

16. What are the causes of CTS?

Ans. Causes can be:
- Idiopathic
- Anatomic:
    - *Acute form* (fracture, crushing hand injury, hemorrhage, burn, median artery thrombosis, infection, pregnancy)
    - Distal radius malunion
    - *Carpal canal stenosis* (deformity congenital or acquired)
    - *Anomalous structures* (palmaris profundus, proximal origin of a lumbrical, reversed PL, anomalous branch of radial artery)
    - *Space occupying lesions* (ganglion, lipoma, fibroma, synovial sarcoma, neuroma, neurofibroma, hemangioma)
- Occupational (exertional CTS)
- Systemic
    - Pregnancy
    - Endocrinopathy (diabetes mellitus, thyroid disease, growth hormone)
    - Congestive heart failure
    - Collagen and autoimmune diseases (tenovaginitis, RA, scleroderma, gout, chondrocalcinosis, etc.)
    - Amyloidosis
    - Polyneuropathy
    - Alcoholism
    - Myeloma
    - Consequential forms (oral contraceptives, anticoagulants, lack of vitamin B6)

Wrist and Hand

- *Children's forms*
- *Congenital diseases* (mucopolysaccharidosis, mucolipidosis).

17. Carpal tunnel has tendons and nerves as contents but can you think of any muscular cause of CTS?

Ans. Yes, aberrant muscles (lumbrical, reversed PL, palmaris profundus) can decrease the volume of carpal tunnel.

18. Are there any vascular causes of CTS?

Ans. Yes, anomalous branch of radial artery, hypertrophied or aberrant median artery and vein, hemangioma, arteriovenous (A-V) malformation in the tunnel.

19. How will you manage this case?

Ans. *The following is based on general consensus.* Mild-to-moderate cases that are not rapidly advancing and are not due to acute cause (see previous in text) should be given a fair conservative trial. I will operate advanced and late cases only on an urgent basis and counsel for elective surgery to patients showing evident denervation in median nerve distribution and pronounced sensory loss particularly supported by EDS.

20. What is nonsurgical treatment for CTS?

Ans. Splinting, activity modification supplemented with oral medications are mainstay of conservative management of CTS.

Splinting: Especially at night and intermittently during day provide good relief in majority of cases, particularly those having positive Phalen test.

Oral medications: Anti-inflammatory medication ± neurotropic vitamins (B6, methylcobalamin) ± steroids ± diuretics to reduce carpal tunnel pressure.

Local adjunctive measures like ultrasonics, laser therapy, and iontophoresis have variable nondocumented effects.

21. What is the role of corticosteroid injections?

Ans. Steroid injections provide rapid relief but there is no documented benefit after 3 months over oral steroids and over long-term when compared to splinting and non-steroidal anti-inflammatory drugs (NSAIDs). There is no concrete information as to type, dose or location of injection. They may be of help in patients with symptoms less than 1 year, normal two-point discrimination, no thenar atrophy, less than 1–2 msec prolongation of sensory motor latencies, and no denervation potentials (mild or moderate cases). Failure to improve with steroid injections is a poor prognostic factor and even surgical release may not be helpful in these cases.

22. What are the poor prognostic factors where conservative treatment often fails?

Ans. Age older than 50 years, duration of symptoms longer than 10 months, constant paresthesia, stenosing flexor tenosynovitis, and a positive Phalen test result in less than 30 seconds.

23. What are surgical approaches to CTS?

Ans.
- Open carpal tunnel release:
  - Wrist-palm incision (Milford, Taleisnik, Phalen, etc.)
  - Double incision technique by Wilson
  - Palm only incision (Lee et al.)
  - Minimal open release (Bromley et al.)
- Endoscopic technique (single portal technique of Agee and double incision technique of Chow).

24. What are the complications of open release?

Ans. Iatrogenic nerve injury (palmar or motor cutaneous branch), injury to thenar branch (commonly aberrant), scar tenderness, pillar pain (most common complication following release due to laceration of palmar cutaneous branch), weakened grip strength, injury to superficial palmar arch and recurrence.

25. What are the contraindications for endoscopic release?

Ans. Wrist stiffness, proliferative synovitis, and space occupying lesions.

26. What is the role of internal neurolysis during open release?

Ans. Once popular, this has been absolutely abandoned and is counterproductive.

27. What are common causes of failed release and persistent symptoms or recurrent CTS?

Ans. Incomplete ligament release, fibrosis/painful scar, tendon adhesions to nerve, missed double-crush syndrome, recurrent tenosynovitis. Others are reformation of the flexor retinaculum, scarring in the carpal tunnel, median or palmar cutaneous neuroma, palmar cutaneous nerve entrapment.

28. How will you manage failed CTS?

Ans. A very difficult problem even for experts. Re-evaluate with EDS studies; MRI is a must. At revision surgery, neurolysis of median nerve with fat or muscle transfer and vein wrapping are some of the methods described to improve results.

CASE VI: MALUNITED DISTAL RADIUS FRACTURE

This is a very common case to see in our subcontinent. Not a frequent examination case, but in regions or places where large number of DNB students appear for examinations, the case may be kept. It is a fact that not many surgeons expertise in treatment of malunited distal radius fractures so the questions will be more directed to treatment of distal radius fractures rather.

Read: 6–8 times to grab the different concepts.

Diagnosis: This is a 56-year-old female with a malunited distal radius fracture for 8 months duration. There is 1 cm of radial shortening and reduced grip strength. [Look also for complex regional pain syndrome (CRPS) and mention if present]

Findings of a typical malunited Colles fracture.
- Inspection
  - Dinner fork deformity
  - Shortening of forearm

- Mannus rectus or valgus
- Swelling at wrist
- Prominent ulnar head.
- Palpation (above +)
    - Distal radial swelling
    - Irregular distal radius
    - Tenderness at carpal region or dorsal wrist joint line (late cases due to degenerative changes) or wrist instability
    - Wrist widening.
- Movements
    - Reduced palmar flexion, ulnar deviation, and combination of other movement loss depending on stiffness and wrist instability
    - Reduced forearm movements [supination (significant) and pronation (less prominent)
- Maisonneuve test may be positive
- Reduced grip strength
- Shortening of radius
- Wrist widening (measurements).

1. What type of malunion is this, would you like to be more specific?

Ans. This appears to be extra-articular malunion but I would need radiographs to confirm absence (or presence) of intra-articular extension of original fracture. Dorsal malunions are further classified as type I [correctable dorsal intercalated segment instability (DISI)] or type II (fixed DISI).

2. What other malunions you know of?

Ans. Apart from intra-articular and extra-articular malunions, can also be subgrouped as volar (Smith) or dorsally (Colles) displaced malunions with shortening.

3. What would you like to do for this patient?

Ans. Firstly, I would like to get radiographs to primarily evaluate the fracture. I will order standard AP, lateral, and one clenched fist X-ray of wrist (to look for carpal instability).

Wrist and Hand

4. What else can you expect to see on X-rays?

Ans. Reflex sympathetic dystrophy (algodystrophy) changes, associated ulnar styloid fracture.

5. What are the consequences of malunion that concern patient?

Ans. Intra-articular malunions produce irregular cartilage surface (late degenerative changes). Extra-articular malunions alter intracarpal, radiocarpal (RC), and DRUJ mechanics. Grip strength is reduced. TFCC strain may produce constant ulnar pain on activity. Altered loading patterns and premature osteoarthritis are quite possible.

6. How do you define malunion of distal radius on radiographs?

Ans. There is no constant definition. Agreed values are as follows: RC malunion—RC joint step-off of > 1 mm. Dorsal malunion—10° of extension and more (greater than 20° from normal). There is still more disagreement on malunion in coronal plane (<10° of radial inclination is considered significant), acceptable distal radius shortening (loss of 5 mm or more of radial height is considered significant), acceptable displacement of DRUJ surface, and malunion of ulna. (*It is all dependent on onlooker; in view of an experienced surgeon, a displacement is a displacement and malunion if united! - really a bookish definition, but I am sorry*). Any malunion associated with RC subluxation is a significant malunion and needs corrective action.

7. What is the incidence of malunion?

Ans. Most common complication following distal radius fracture. Around 23-25% radiological malunion is seen. Clinically, symptomatic malunion is very low somewhere around 5-7% following various treatment methods.

8. What are the values for various parameters of distal radius?

Ans. Radial inclination = 17-25° (22° average)
Palmar/volar tilt/inclination = 2-20° (11° average)

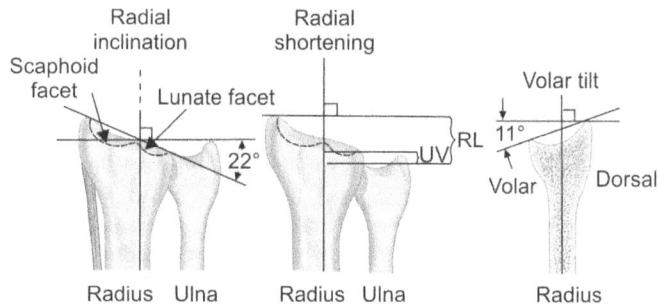

Fig. 20: Understanding various radiological parameters for distal radius.

Radial length/height (from distal radius lunate fossa to radial styloid) = 9.9–17.3 mm (mean of 11 mm), < 9 mm is significant **(Fig. 20)**

Ulnar variance (from distal radius lunate fossa to ulnar articular surface) = –2.3 to ± 4.6 mm (average 0.9 mm), on a zero rotation view.

9. **What is the most concerning aspect of distal radius malunion?**

Ans. Dorsal tilt disables most of the mechanics around distal radius that concerns all patients; additionally for a manual laborer, radial shortening is of additional concern as it weakens the grip strength (and alters the TFCC/DRUJ biomechanics). For intra-articular malunion, development of wrist arthritis is a big concern (some 91% patients develop arthritis having step-off >2 mm while only 11% develop arthritis if the step-off is <2 mm), and should be managed with priority.

- Dorsal tilt of 10–20° alters midcarpal stability (Fernandez)
- Dorsal tilt of 20–30° increases forces on the radial articular cartilage that may produce degenerative changes (Fernandez)
- Radial tilt of 20–30° severely limits function (Fourrier)

Wrist and Hand

Table 4: Graham and Hastings criteria of treatment.

Group	Radial measurements	Radio-ulnar length	DRUJ reducible by radial osteotomy	Acceptable DRUJ articular surfaces	Reconstruction indicated
I	Unacceptable	Unacceptable	Yes	Yes	Distal radial osteotomy
II	Acceptable	Unacceptable	Not applicable	Yes	Ulnar shortening
III	Unacceptable	Unacceptable	No	Yes	Distal radial osteotomy and ulnar shortening
IV	Unacceptable	Unacceptable	No	No	Distal radial osteotomy and distal ulnar shortening

(DRUJ: distal radioulnar joint)

10. How will you treat this patient?

Ans. I will clinically assess the symptoms and functional loss and decide the treatment based on Graham and Hastings criteria **(Table 4)**. If the malunion is asymptomatic and nonconcerning to the patient (i.e. not functionally limiting the patient's activities), then I will just advice patient to continue mobilization of the joint and improve muscle strength.

11. How will you manage dorsal tilt?

Ans. I will do an osteotomy [at the or as close to deformity center of rotation and angulation (CORA)] from dorsal approach and do tricortical iliac bone grafting under fluoroscopy control to reproduce the distal radius anatomy (as compared to the normal side). Similarly for other malunions, wedge-shaped grafts in different lengths and stabilized using volar or dorsal-locked plates (as the case may be) are used—nothing very special **(Fig. 21)**.

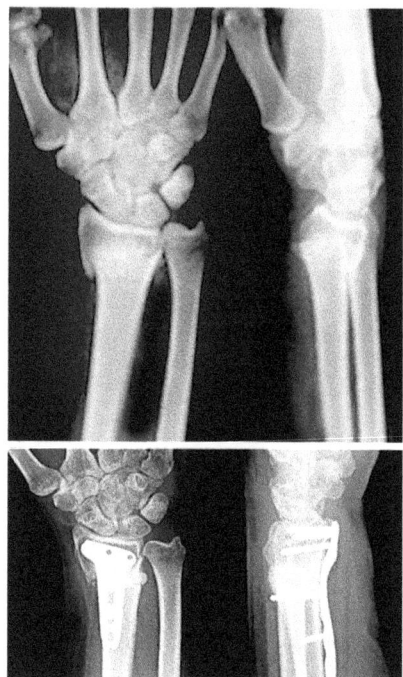

Fig. 21: Correction of dorsal tilt and radial height.

12. How will you manage intra-articular malunion?

Ans. I will get a CT scan of the distal radius malunion and plan surgery accordingly. In general, the simple intra-articular malunions and malunions with dorsal subluxations are better dealt with dorsal approach; while, volar RC subluxation with malunion is better treated with volar approach. There is a trend to avoid incising the volar stouter capsule for good functional outcome and also familiarity of intra-articular reduction through dorsal approach (die-punch reduction) makes this approach preferable. DRUJ and TFCC need specific management on a case-to-case basis.

13. What is the timing of osteotomy?

Ans. As such, early (8 weeks following injury) for developing fracture collapse and late (> 40 weeks) osteotomies have both been described and studied; there could be a favor for early procedure as this prevents development of joint contracture and had reduced disability period.

14. What are the contraindications of radial osteotomy?

Ans. Presence of significant RC or intercarpal arthritis will preclude deriving any significant benefit from deformity correction. Osteoporosis is a relative contraindication.

15. What else will you assess?

Ans. After a radius corrective osteotomy, the ulnar side should be paid attention to along with DRUJ. Usually, a well done radial osteotomy corrects DRUJ but in various cases there remains positive ulna variance or DRUJ instability. In these cases, ulnar side procedure is needed (this is also preoperatively guided by the Graham and Hastings criteria discussed previously). If DRUJ is unstable or there is DRUJ arthrosis, then Sauve-Kapandji type procedure is good **(Fig. 22)**. If there is positive ulna variance, then ulna osteoplasty is

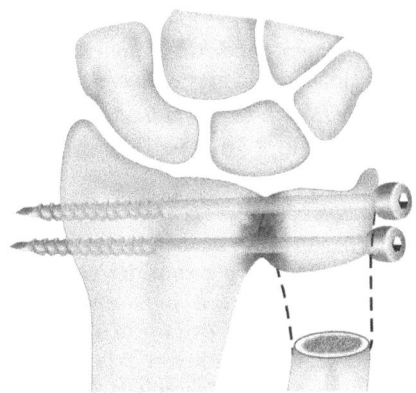

Fig. 22: Sauve-Kapandji procedure.

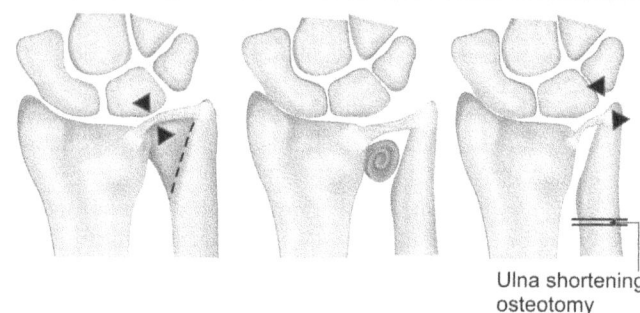

Fig. 23: Bower hemiresection interposition arthroplasty.

done to reduce ulnar length. This can be achieved in three ways:
1. Intra-articular arthroscopic method (Wafer procedure)
2. Extra-articular complete ulnar head excision—Darrach procedure (likely to produce DRUJ instability)
3. Partial distal ulnar excision—(Bower hemiresection or Watson matched resection) **(Fig. 23)**.

16. What various named fractures do you know?

Ans. *Colles (pronounced as "collis"—English literature) fracture (Pouteau fracture—French)*: Dorsal displacement and tilt, volar displacement and tilt, impaction, and supination. Fracture of ulnar styloid may or may not be a component.

Smith fracture (Smith-Goyrand fracture): Reverse of Colles.

Barton fracture: Intra-articular *shear* fracture of *dorsal* rim of radius with RC subluxation.

Reverse Barton fracture (volar Barton fracture; Smith-Goyrand II): Fracture of *volar* rim of radius with RC subluxation (many people consider volar Barton as Barton fracture—this is incorrect; it is reverse Barton fracture. Also, Smith fracture I is extra-articular fracture with volar displacement and Smith fracture II is intra-articular fracture with volar subluxation as described).

Chauffeur fracture: Radial styloid fracture.

Hutchinson fracture: Radial styloid fracture ± scapholunate disruption.

Moore fracture: Distal radius fracture with ulnar dislocation and entrapment of ulnar styloid fracture under annular ligament.

Die-punch fracture: Fracture through lunate fossa (depressed fracture).

17. **What is Colles fracture?**
Ans. As typically described by Colles, extra-articular fracture occurring at the corticocancellous junction of distal radius some one and a half inch above (around 4 cm) the carpal surface, more so a transverse fracture throwing the carpus dorsally with dorsal displacement and angulation at the fracture site.

18. **What are the complications of Colles fracture?**
Ans. The following are the common complications of Colles fracture:
- Early complication:
    - Median nerve injury (acute CTS), rarely ulnar nerve injury
    - Plaster cast-related problems—neurovascular compromise
    - Loss of reduction
- Late complications:
    - *Malunion*: Most common significant complication
    - *Nonunion*: Uncommon but can be seen
    - *Stiffness*: Commonly seen of wrist and finger joints, elbow stiffness if above elbow cast used
    - Carpal tunnel syndrome
    - Reflex sympathetic dystrophy (CRPS type 1)
    - *Rupture of EPL tendon*: This may result from even a trivial injury and is not the result of direct tendon injury but possibly occurs from vascular injury to the tendon where its watershed zone falls near the fracture line of Colles fracture. Friction across malunited Colles is another common cause.

- DRUJ instability and injury (TFCC tear)
- Ulnar styloid nonunion.

19. How do you identify CRPS type 1?

Ans. Complex regional pain syndrome type 1 is a sympathetic disorder that can result from trauma or closed manipulation of fracture or from surgical treatment. It commonly presents with hyperalgesia (sensitivity to even moving air), allodynia, discoloration (red/dusky limb), hyperhidrosis, stiffness of nearly all joints in the region, weakness, and trophic changes of skin in late cases—loss of hair, smooth shiny skin, nail changes. Radiologically, there is significant osteopenia of all bones in the region.

20. How do you classify distal radius fractures?

Ans. There are a lot of classifications but the preferred are Melone, universal, and AO (remember any one of the classifications), Fernandez and Frykman are of historical significance only.

Melone classification (my personal preference): Based on distal radius, "four parts" divided into (1) radial styloid, (2 and 3) dorsal medial and dorsal lateral parts (of lunate fossa) and (4) radial shaft.

- *Type I*: Stable, undisplaced, and minimally comminuted (Colles equivalent)
- *Type II*: Comminuted, stable displacement of medial complex
  - Posterior displacement—die—punch fracture: moderate-to-severe displacement
  - Displaced fracture involving radioscaphoid joint—involves more than simple radial styloid
- *Type IIb (irreducible)*: "double die-punch" fracture (irreducible injury)
  - Dorsal medial component fragmentation—persistent RC incongruity > 2 mm
  - Requires open reduction ± bone grafting for restoration of articular congruity

- *Type III*: Die-punch or lunate load fracture (depressed fracture)
  - Involves additional fracture from shaft of radius that projects into flexor compartment (volar spike)
- *Type IV*: Transverse split of articular surfaces, wide separation with rotational displacement
  - Open reduction and internal fixation with plating ± bone grafting.

21. What is Kapandji method of fixation of distal radius?

Ans. Intrafocal "double basket like" pinning typically described for extra-articular fractures. The k-wires pass through the fracture site (interfocal) and act to buttress the distal fragment in position resisting the displacing forces.

22. What is the role of external fixator for fixation of distal radius?

Ans. Typically indicated for open fractures for wound management. It has been used for distraction (ligamentotaxis) reduction of severely comminuted fractures to maintain alignment. The role of spanning external fixators has reduced now with the introduction of locked plates (internal fixator) and anatomic reduction. Nonspanning dynamic fixators have come into vogue for ease of application, minimally invasive surgery, and no implant remaining in the body after removal at fracture union.

8

The Spine

Spine cases are considered formidable and are sometimes simple and sometimes tricky. It is best to prepare thoroughly these cases as there is high probability of faltering in examinations for limited exposure and differing concepts that are undergoing rapid and extensive change—I am not sure if concepts would change while this chapter is in writing!

Read times: 7-9 times for MS and DNB candidates, I am afraid that topic could not be more simplified, as much of classical and recent developments have to be mingled.

EXAMINATION OF SPINE

HISTORY TAKING

- Pain (*try to search for 'pain generators' and whether it is referred from other site, give particular attention to 'red flag signs'*):
  - *Onset (acute/insidious)*: Acute in post-traumatic, jerk, pyogenic infection (diskitis), and tubercular infection; while insidious onset in mechanical low back pain, spondylitis, facet joints, and vascular structures, metastasis (unless precipitated by trauma), primary bone tumors, and hemangioma.
  - *Site:* Axial pain (localized pain) at all spinal levels often results from "mechanical" (non-neurogenic) structures like musculotendinous structures, zygapophyseal joints, vertebrae, and annulus fibrosus, while radiating pain is due to the involvement of neurological structures that

may be related to disk herniation, degenerative process, neuroforaminal stenosis or other space-occupying lesions, intrinsic diseases of cord/nerve root (herpes zoster).

- *Nature*: Throbbing acute unbearable pain results from acute pyogenic infections, traumatic/pathological fracture (barring osteoporotic fracture), and severe constant pain may result from cauda equina syndrome, advanced tubercular infection, acute cervical/dorsal/lumbar strain.

  Dull constant aching pain is often the result of mechanical problems originating as above.

- *Radiation*: The radiated (from other site) and radiating (to other site) pains both are noticed. Pain from lumbar or cervical regions often radiates as "lightening sensation" in the limbs, while dorsal segments radiate in "band-like" fashion. The general rule for radiating pain (from neurological structures) is simple and constant in that "it is the spinal level of pathology and not the exact structure involved that determines the radiation pattern". Axially radiated pain from various sites that require mention include aorta, carotid arteries, costovertebral and costotransverse articulations, pancreas, lung, pleura, gallbladder, stomach and proximal duodenum, diaphragm, kidneys, ureter, and pelvic organs in female. Affections other than spine may also present with radiating pain and include lower trunk brachial plexopathies, neuropathies, heart, and pericardium to upper limb and sacroiliac joint, sacrum (stress fracture), ilia, and hip joints.

- *Diffuse/localized*: Localized pain often results from focal injury to mechanical structures whereas diffuse pain is often radiated.

- *Aggravating and relieving factors*: Rotation and extension were classically attributed to zygapophyseal joints. Forward flexion is painful in diskogenic pain. Excursion as such is painful in inflammatory conditions of spine. Neuroforaminal stenosis causes neurogenic claudication that comes up after exertion and is relieved by forward flexion/sitting. Whereas sitting and getting up from seated position is often painful in

diskogenic pain, sleeping with knees and hips flexed often relieves pain.
- *Trauma:* Note the following—energy dissipated from impact, direct/indirect (like lifting heavy weight, seat belt injuries)
- *Deformity:* Onset, duration, sudden increase (collapse in pathological fractures), association with pain and fever (tuberculosis), and stiffness (ankylosing spondylitis)
- Loss of power/weakness and balance.

Other history: Genitourinary complaints, gynecological complaints and all pertinent symptoms/findings as above, Marfan's syndrome, ankylosing spondylitis, and vascular claudication.

Past medical history: Diabetes mellitus, tuberculosis, hypertension, hematological disorder, pulmonary disorder, treatment for osteoporosis, neurological disorder (like epilepsy, Parkinsonism), and HIV status (preoperative workup).

Personal history: Smoking, alcohol, and drug addiction.

EXAMINATION

Inspection

- *Attitude and deformity:* "military attitude", levels of shoulder, forward bending (scoliosis, kyphosis, and ankylosing spondylitis) **(Fig. 1)**, side bending (list).

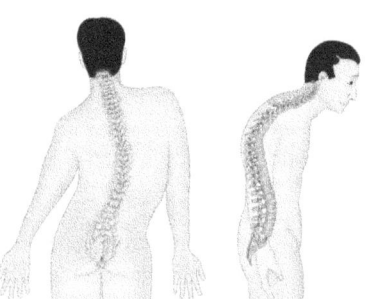

Fig. 1: Scoliosis (left) and kyphosis (right) deformity of spine.

- *From side*:
  - Kyphotic deformities (normal thoracic kyphosis is 21–33° measured by Cobb's method) **(Fig. 2)**:
    - *Knuckle*: Due to single vertebra
    - *Gibbus*: 2–3 vertebrae
    - Short angular/rounded kyphosis (>3 vertebra): small segment of spine involved from 4–8 vertebrae
    - *Rounded kyphosis*: Ankylosing spondylitis, senile osteoporosis, Scheuermann's disease, and osteomalacia.
    - *Loss or partial reduction of kyphosis*: Early tuberculosis with "boarding" due to spasm, flat back syndrome, iatrogenic (postscoliosis correction).
  - Lordosis of spine (average lumbar lordosis is 40–60°, cervical lordosis = 20–40°, thoracic kyphosis = 20–45°):
    - Increased lordosis:
      - Females
      - Obese
      - Spondylolisthesis
      - Fixed flexion deformities at hip
      - Compensatory to increased thoracic kyphosis
      - Constitutional.

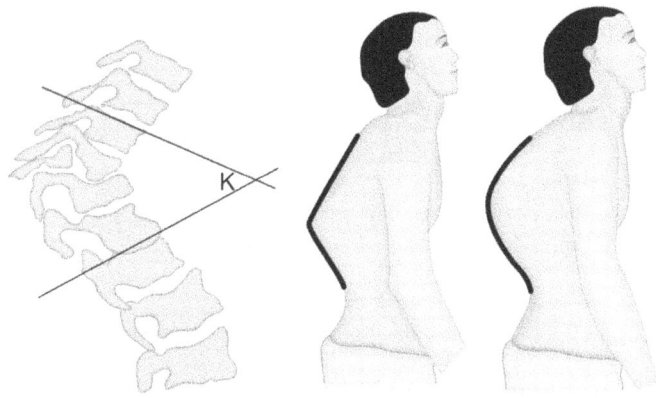

Fig. 2: Knuckle (left), gibbus (middle), rounded kyphus (right).

- Reduced lordosis (flattening/reversal):
  - "Sniffing position" of cervical spine where face of patient is thrust out anteriorly due to flexion at cervicothoracic junction but extension at upper segments (ankylosing spondylitis).
  - PIVD (prolapsed intervertebral disk)
  - Infection
  - *Lumbar flatback*: Osteoporotic/traumatic anterior wedging, advanced degeneration of disk, and long thoracolumbar spinal fusion
  - Ankylosing spondylitis.

- *From back*:
  - *Position of head (centrally aligned over pelvis)*: Plumb line—drop a plumb line from occiput "inion" and for a straight spine, it should pass between the clefts of buttocks.
  - Hair line
  - Webbing of neck/short neck
  - Position of shoulders
  - Comparative position of scapular spine
  - Scapular angles
  - Step-off deformity (spondylolisthesis) **(Fig. 3)**
  - Kyphotic and lordotic deformities (as tested above—its better only to mention them as 'confirm of above findings' rather than stressing them much as most examiners do not like these to be examined from behind!)
  - *List*: "A list is an abrupt planar shift (no definite curvature) of the spine above a certain point to one side in coronal plane"—usually seen in lumbar region.
  - Iliac crest
  - Posterior-superior iliac spine (dimple of venus)
  - Lateral body margin
  - Skin for:
    - Lumbar lipoma, hair patch **(Fig. 4)**
    - Port wine stain (of spina bifida/meningomyelocele)
    - *Café au lait* spots
    - Nodular skin swelling (neurofibromatosis)
    - Dermal hemangioma

The Spine

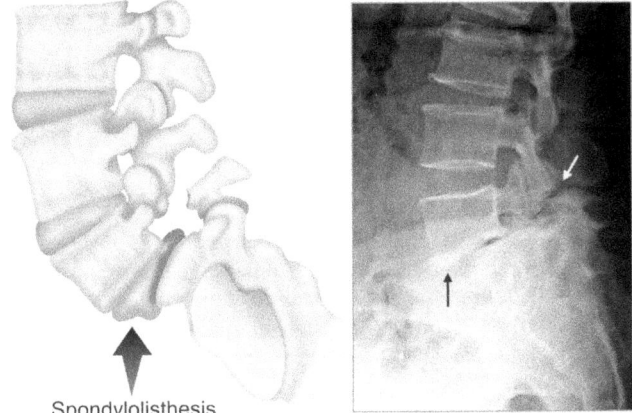

Fig. 3: Spondylolisthesis of L5 over S1.

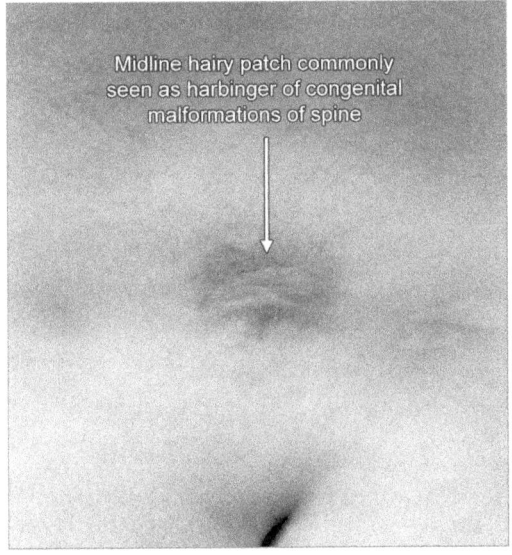

Fig. 4: Midline hairy patch.

- Scars
- Sinuses
- Paravertebral spasm
- Swelling:
  - Meningomyelocele
  - Paravertebral abscess
  - Hernia
- Scoliosis:
  - Sidedness (right/left sided convexity)
  - Forward bending for making it more prominent (Adam's test) and looking for flexibility, site of primary curve by noting the site of rotation and "razor-back" deformity
  - Lateral bending to look for possible correction and hence flexibility **(Fig. 5)**
  - Compensatory curves (note rotation is localized only to the primary curves and rest all other curves are better termed compensatory unless there are two primary curves in an unusual case!).

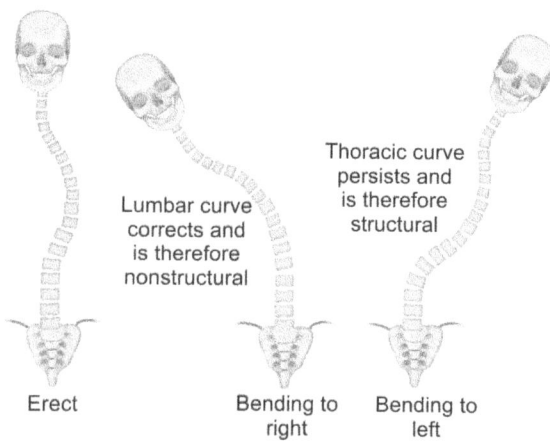

Fig. 5: Lateral bending of spine to look for compensatory (flexible curves) and differentiate from structural curves.

- *From front*:
  - Head seated squarely over shoulders and chin positioned over sternal notch
  - Hyoid bone
  - Thyroid cartilage
  - Sternocleidomastoid muscle
  - *Sternum*: Pectus excavatum and pectus carinatum
  - Umbilicus.
- *Gait*: Shuffling gait (posterior cord syndrome), slapping foot gait (high stepping gait), broad-based gait (halting gait), Alderman's gait, festinating gait, antalgic gait, etc. (*See Chapter 10*)
  - Heel walking—to test ankle dorsiflexors (L5 root).
  - Toe walking—to test ankle plantar flexors (S1 root).

Palpation

Confirm the findings of inspection:
- Local temperature.
- Tenderness:
  - Direct pressure (superficial tenderness often indicates affections of skin); for deep tenderness, give direct pressure over spinous process
  - *Twist (rotator) tenderness*: Push the spinous process to either side in an attempt to rotate the vertebra
  - *Thrust tenderness*: By gently "thrusting" the spine with a closed fist.
- Palpation of all spinous processes from inion (note C2, C7, T1, and T12) above to coccyx below to identify defect (spina bifida), thickening/deformity (congenital, affections of posterior elements in mitotic pathology), iatrogenic defect (laminectomy) and alignment (normally straight) and abnormal prominence of spinous processes (upper spinous process becomes prominent in all anterior wedging conditions that distract open the spine from behind like traumatic/osteoporotic/tubercular anterior wedging and retrolisthesis, while the lower spinous process is made prominent by forward subluxation of spine as in fracture dislocations and spondylolisthesis).
- Kyphotic and lordotic deformities as examined above.

- *Soft tissue and paraspinal gutters*: Interspinous region for supraspinous ligament and sites for Pott's abscess.
- From front, palpate the carotid tubercle (tubercle of Chassaignac), sternal notch, and deformities.

Percussion
- Spinous process
- Costotransverse joints.

Movements
- *Flexion:* Cervical spine—chin to chest, lumbar spine—forward bending [measured by the final position of trunk in relation to vertical plane or distance of fingers from floor (normal = 90° or <10 cm finger floor distance)]
- *Extension:* Cervical spine—looking roof, lumbar spine—backward bending (normally 20-30°), often limited in patients with facet arthropathy and in foraminal narrowing as extension further narrows the foramina.
- Lateral rotation to right and left side for cervical spine (normal = 80°)
- Lateral bending (thoracic spine)—floor-fingertip distance
- For flexion and extension of thoracic spine, which is minimal, make the patient sit on a wooden straight back chair and ask to bend forward and backwards. More accurate measurement can be made by direct measurement (vide below)
- Rotation in sitting position (for lumbar spine)—measure angle between plane of shoulder to pelvis.

Measurements
- Mark two points from T1 to S1 and a point at L1. Measure and ask patient to bend forward, increase of T1-L1 by >8 cm and L1 to S1 by more than 8-10 cm is normal.
- *Modified Schober's test*: Mark two points—one point 10 cm above and the other 5 cm below lumbosacral junction. Measure the distance before and after forward flexion. At least there must be an increase of >5 cm otherwise it is pathological.
- *Chest expansion*: Abnormal is <2.5 cm than the average normal value for age and sex (measure at the level of the

4th intercostal space). Up to 65 years of age, normal value for males is 5.5–7 cm and for females 4–5.5 cm. >65 years of age, the normal value for males is 3–4 cm and for females 2.5–4 cm. *You can safely refer to 5.0 cm as the normal for most healthy adults.*
- Iliocostal distance (from front)
- Iliooccipital distance (from back).

Neurological Examination

- *Cervical spine*: Lateral rotators (right by left sternocleidomastoid and vice-versa), forward flexors [both sterno-cleido-mastoid muscle (SCM) together], extensors (posterior intrinsic muscles and trapezius), and lateral benders (scalene)
- *Beevor's sign (for lower thoracic nerve roots)*: Patient performs a quarter squat with hands behind head. Watch the movement of naval up/down or to any side, which indicates involvement of lower abdominal musculature (below T9)
- Examination of limb muscles (in distribution, myotomes):
  - Bulk
  - Tone
  - Power
  - Coordination
  - Balance
  - Involuntary movements (chorea, athetosis, dystonia, tics, myokymia, hemiballismus, asterixis, and myoclonus)
- *Sensory examinations*:
  - Fine touch and sharp-dull discrimination
  - Crude touch and stereognosis
  - Two-point discrimination
  - Pressure
  - Temperature (cold and hot)
  - Vibration sense
  - Positional sense (proprioception)
- *Vasomotor examination*: Starch-iodine test and Guttman's test
- *Reflexes*:
  - Superficial [upper motor neuron (UMN)-dependent reflexes]:
    - Trapezius reflex (C3-C4)
    - Deltoid reflex (C5-C6)
    - Scapular reflex (C5-T1)

- Abdominal muscle reflexes (T7-L1)
- Cremasteric (T12, L1)
- Anal wink reflex (S2-S4)—used to determine end of spinal shock
- Bulbocavernosus (S2-S4)
- *Plantar reflex (Babinski sign)*: This is a pathological reflex and appears only in UMN lesions
- Throckmorton's reflex (percuss the dorsum of foot in MTP joint region—great toe extension with flexion of other's is normal).

- Deep [lower motor neuron (LMN) local reflexes with inhibition from UMN]: It is lost in LMN lesions and becomes hyperactive in UMN lesions (*a cervical level is UMN for lumbar levels!*)—
  - Biceps (C5-C6)
  - Triceps (C6-C7)
  - Brachioradialis (C6-C7)
  - Inversion of radial jerk (C5-C6)
  - Knee (L2-L3-L4)
  - Ankle (S1-S2)
  - Medial hamstring (L5)
  - Tibialis posterior (L5)

- Ankle clonus and patellar clonus (due to loss from UMN inhibition).

Special Tests

Nerve root tension signs:

- *Lhermitte's sign (technically a symptom)*: Electric shock-like sensation radiating into limbs. If the sensation comes with cervical spine flexion then cervical pathologies are more evident and if it comes with trunk flexion then it indicates thoracic cord lesion. The sign was first described for multiple sclerosis.
- *Spurling's maneuver*: Extension and rotation of cervical spine produce radicular pain, it is pseudoradicular, if the pain radiates to occiput or scapula or limbs but not below elbow.
- Upper limb tension test 1 (ULTT1) for C5, C6, and C7 and is considered median nerve dominant
- ULTT2 stretches C6 and C7, two variants—median and radial nerve dominant

- ULTT3 stretches C8 and T1—ulnar nerve dominant
- Axial cervical spine compression test
- Straight leg raising test (SLRT) (passive) **(Fig. 6)**
- *Crossed SLRT (well leg SLRT, Fajersztajn test)*: Extremely sensitive for L4-5 and L5-S1 disk.
- *Lasegue's test (Bragard's test)* **(Fig. 7)** *(does not increase the discomfort to hamstrings as in SLRT)*: Stop at the hip flexion where pain is induced and dorsiflexion ankle and foot → radicular pain exacerbated, strengthens the diagnosis of sciatica.
- *Modified Lasegue's test (Kernig's maneuver)*: Raising the leg with knee flexed and slowly extending knee.
- *Bowstring sign of McNab*: Perform SLRT → stop at the hip flexion where pain is produced → flex knee to 90° → press the sciatic nerve in popliteal fossa → strengthens the impression of sciatica

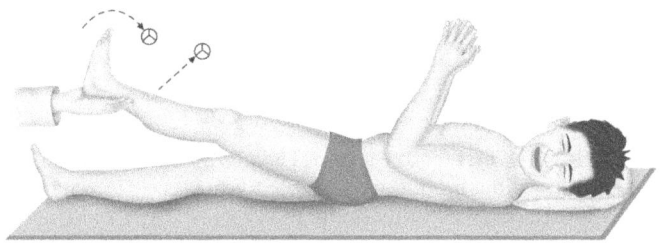

Fig. 6: Straight leg raising test (SLRT).

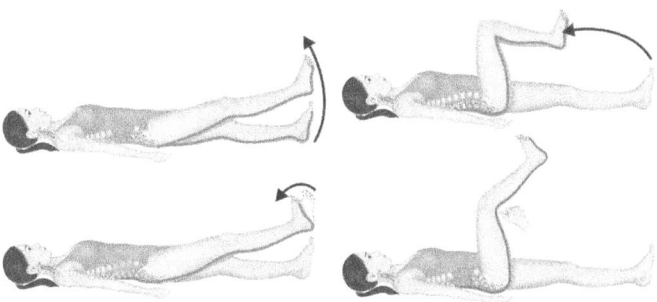

Fig. 7: Lasegue's (left) and modified Lasegue's (right) test.

- Cram test (similar to Lasegue's test) → flex hip of a supine patient then extend the knee. Reproduction of pain indicates positive test.
- *Slump test*: Patient seated → flex dorsal spine with extended cervical spine → flex cervical spine also → ask patient to straighten one leg → ask patient to dorsiflex the foot. Pain at any point means positive.
- *Femoral nerve stretch test (reverse SLRT)*: For L2-L4-prone patient → lift the thigh keeping buttocks stable
- *Single-leg hyperextension test for spondylolysis*: Ask patient to stand with one leg extended than other (straddle position) → ask patient to lean backwards → pain produced on the affected side
- Tests to increase the intrathecal pressure:
  - Valsalva maneuver
  - *Milgram's test*: Maintain active SLRT for 30 seconds once in >30° and <30° hip flexion. If positive in <30° hip flexion then it indicates prolapsed intervertebral disc (PIVD)
  - *Naffziger's test*: Jugular compression in seated position → pain in lumbar region suggests intrathecal space-occupying lesion in lumbar region.

1. How do you localize a spinal level from examination?

Ans. The findings mentioned in **Table 1** are classical for a particular level along with other findings.

Table 1: Localization of spinal level by sensory-motor examination and pertinent reflex involvement.

Level	Sensory findings	Motor deficit	Reflex involved
C4	Lateral neck region	Trapezius	Trapezius reflex
C5	Middle deltoid region in arm ('regimental badge area')—*axillary nerve*	Deltoid, biceps (partial)	Biceps reflex, deltoid reflex
C6	Dorsum of first web space (thumb); lateral forearm—*musculocutaneous nerve*	Biceps brachii, wrist extensors	Brachioradialis (supinator) reflex, inversion of radial reflex, biceps (weakness)

Contd...

Contd...

Level	Sensory findings	Motor deficit	Reflex involved
C7	Long finger	Wrist flexors, long finger extensors, triceps	Triceps jerk, scapular reflex
C8	Little finger, ulnar aspect of palm—*ulnar nerve*	Long finger flexors, hand intrinsic	Scapular reflex
T1	Medial aspect of elbow and lower arm—*medial brachial cutaneous nerve*	Intrinsic muscles of hand typically interossei	
T2	Medial upper arm and adjacent chest		
T4	Nipple		
T10	Umbilicus	Flexion of trunk (Beevor's sign)	Abdominal reflex
L1	Anterior proximal thigh at groin fold (inguinal ligament)—*ilioinguinal nerve*	Iliopsoas	Cremasteric reflex
L2	Mid-thigh (pocket region)—*lateral, anterior, and medial femoral cutaneous nerves of thigh*	Iliopsoas	
L3	Lower thigh and medial aspect of patella—*obturator nerve*	Quadriceps	Patellar tendon reflex (partial)
L4	Medial aspect of leg and ankle—*saphenous nerve*	Tibialis anterior	Patellar tendon reflex
L5	Lateral and anterolateral aspect of leg, dorsum first web space (medial plantar nerve and lateral cutaneous nerve of calf)	EHL, EDL, gluteus medius	Tibialis posterior reflex, medial hamstring reflex

Contd...

Contd...

Level	Sensory findings	Motor deficit	Reflex involved
S1	Lateral aspect of foot over plantar aspect, posterior calf—*lateral plantar nerve*	Gastrosoleus, peronei, gluteus maximus	Tendon Achilles reflex, plantar reflex
S2	Posterior thigh region, proximal calf	Lax external sphincter in rectal examination	
S3-5	Perianal area	-Do-	Anal reflex, bulbocavernosus reflex

(EDL: extensor digitorum longus; EHL: extensor hallucis longus)

2. How do you test for plantar reflex and what is its interpretation?

Ans. (*Explain the procedure to the patient*). Stroke the lateral aspect of foot from heel upwards making a "J" at the region of metatarsal heads. Normally, there is a progressive sequence of:
- Toe flexion
- Ankle dorsiflexion
- Inversion of foot.

This denotes intact innervation up to L5-S1 level. Mute plantar response can occur in a normal individual and in spinal shock. The pathological appearance of a different sequence is a Babinski reflex (extensor plantar response), which is characterized by:
- Extension of great toe
- Fanning out of other toes
- Ankle dorsiflexion
- Knee flexion followed by ipsilateral hip flexion
- Contralateral hip and knee extension (withdrawal reflex).

This dramatic sequence can be overridden in a conscious patient and only first few stages are seen in a typical UMN lesion.

The Spine

3. What are the other ways of eliciting this reflex?

Ans.
- Squeezing the heel cord (Gordon's sign)
- Squeezing the calf
- Pressing firmly the medial border of leg/tibial crest (Oppenheim's sign)
- Stroking lateral malleolus.

4. What other pathological reflexes appear in a UMN lesion?

Ans.
- Hoffmann's sign [palmar flexion of thumb (and observing a pincer movement between thumb and index finger) on rapidly tapping the distal phalanx of middle finger from palmar aspect] **(Fig. 8)**
- *Inverted radial reflex*: Tapping the distal brachioradialis tendon produces a hypoactive brachioradialis reflex with hyperactive finger flexion **(Fig. 9)**.
- *Tromner sign*: Similar to Hoffmann's reflex but here the middle finger is elevated and distal phalanx is flicked toward palm.
- *Crossed adductor's sign*: Ipsilateral patellar reflex causes contralateral thigh adductors to contract.
- *Chaddock's sign*: Abduct little toe and release it to slap against other toes or flick third and fourth toe down rapidly to look for great toe dorsiflexion.

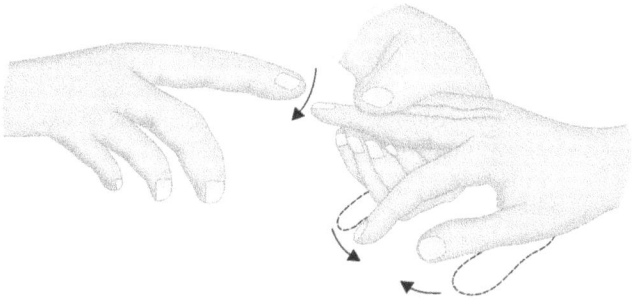

Fig. 8: Hoffmann's sign.

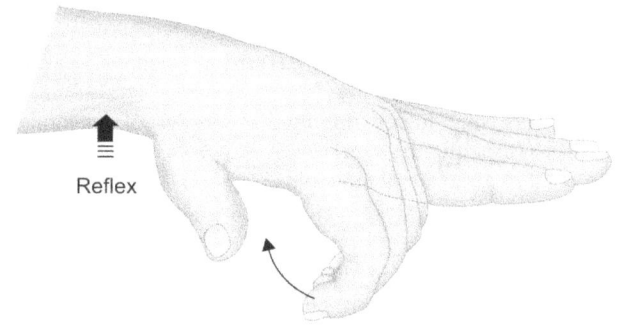

Fig. 9: Inverted radial reflex.

- Clonus!
  (*Note that they may be present in a patient with brisk reflexes and may not necessarily indicate pathology; however, asymmetry is of significance.*)

5. What is the bladder dysfunction associated with spinal cord injury?

Ans. The following should help to explain the mechanism of two different cord bladder functioning. First, there are two differently innervated muscles in bladder control. One is the bladder motor (detrusor), which is under local spinal control S2-4, whereby any stimulus that arises due to bladder filling leads to contraction of bladder and emptying. The other one is the innervation of sphincters, which is inhibited (relaxed) by local reflex (S2-4) and stimulated by sympathetic system (L1-2). Now, secondly, there is a higher control, which has an inhibitory influence on local reflex (S2-4).

Now, if local reflex is released from all upper inhibitions (as happens in UMN lesion), the bladder becomes an "*automatic bladder*", which will contract as soon as it fills up and there will be detrusor hypertrophy due to hyperactive local reflex (S2-4). If this local reflex is lost (as will happen in S2-4 lesions like cauda equina syndrome—LMN lesion), the bladder will not be able to contract due to its lost motor supply and also the sympathetic (L1-L2) reflex is still activating the sphincters that additionally prevent emptying. This type of bladder keeps filling till the capacity is exceeded when the urine dribbles due to exceeded competency of sphincters—"atonic bladder". With time, however, intramural reflexes develop whence with overfilling the bladder may contract due to direct detrusor stimulation—the so-called "autonomous bladder". (*Remember the aphorism—the one who is released from higher control becomes "automatic", while the one who gains self-control due to loss of virtually everything becomes 'autonomous'.*)

6. How do you predict the level of cord involvement with the vertebral (spinal) level?

Ans. Table 2 shows the rule of thumb for an adult to predict the level of cord involvement with the vertebral (spinal) level.

Table 2: The level of cord involvement with the vertebral (spinal) level.	
Vertebral level	*Cord level*
C1-C7	Add one to know corresponding cord level
T1-6	Add two
T7-9	Add three
T10	L1 and L2
T11	L3 and L4
T12	L5 and S1
L1 (cord ends at lower border of L1)	Rest sacral and coccygeal segment
Below L1	Cauda equina

7. What is clonus?

Ans. It is a pathological hyperreflexia of normal deep tendon reflexes produced due to release of the normal reflex from higher control. Sustained clonus (>5 beats of clonus) is significant and represents UMN lesion. Ill-sustained clonus can occur in an otherwise normal individual.

8. What do you do to make reflexes more prominent, if they are not elicited by normal maneuver?

Ans. I will do Jendrassik's maneuver by asking patient to either clench his teeth tight or pulling the interdigitated fingers of both hands apart to enhance the reflexes.

9. How do you differentiate between rigidity versus spasticity?

Ans. Both represent types of hypertonia. *Rigidity* is pathologically due to *extrapyramidal* affection. It can be of cogwheel type (jerky or intermittent regular resistance to motion) or lead pipe type (present throughout the range of motion). *Spasticity* is more of practical concern in the context of spine examination and is due to affection of *pyramidal system* (corticospinal pathway). It is classically a UMN lesion and is of clasp-knife type whereby resistance is offered only to the initial part of movement and disappears on persisting with the same. A hysterical hypertonia classically increases with the effort applied.

10. What is central cord syndrome?

Ans. Central cord syndrome occurs in the cervical level often due to hyperextension injuries or in an elderly due to stenotic cervical canal.

The upper limb is more severely affected with initial affection of pain and temperature and later involvement of upper limb motor function and lower limb with progression. The syndrome may also be produced by central canal syrinx or sometimes intraspinal tumors.

11. What is anterior cord syndrome?

Ans. It is due to involvement of ventral portion of cord (interruption of ascending spinothalamic tracts and descending motor tracts. It is characterized by:
- Loss of pain and temperature sensation
- Loss of motor control below the affected level
- Preservation of proprioception and crude touch

12. What is Brown-Sequard syndrome?

Ans. Hemisection injury of spinal cord:
- Ipsilateral motor loss below the level
- Loss of reflexes at the level
- Contralateral loss of pain and temperature one to three levels below the level of lesion
- Ipsilateral loss of proprioception and position sensation and crude touch
- Band of hyperesthesia at the level.

CASE I: SPINAL TUBERCULOSIS (POTT'S DISEASE)

CLINICAL FINDINGS

- *Pain and stiffness of spine*: Pain may be referred to arms, intercostal neuralgia in cervical and thoracic regions. In thoracolumbar region, "girdle pain" or epigastric pain may be indicated.
- Paravertebral spasm and "boarding"
- Kyphotic deformity
- Tenderness (deep thrust and rotational)
- Night cries
- Abscess formation and paraspinal swelling
- *Constitutional symptoms*: Evening rise of temperature, night sweats, anorexia, weight loss, asthenia, tachycardia, and anemia
- *Gait*: Upper thoracic disease—"military attitude"; lower thoracic and upper lumbar disease, "Alderman's gait"
- Paralysis.

In heroin addicts, a distinct syndrome has been reported having acute toxic reaction with fever, back pain, weight loss, night sweats, and rapidly developing neurological deficits.

1. What are your differential diagnoses?

Ans. Apart from spinal tuberculosis:
- Pyogenic osteomyelitis and diskitis
- Metastasis from primary tumor elsewhere (older age group)
- Primary tumor of spine (younger people—think of lymphoma, as such anything is possible like multiple myeloma, giant cell tumor (GCT), and aneurysmal bone cyst (ABC)]

- Actinomycosis of spine
- Brucellosis, *Salmonella typhi*, *Vibrio cholerae* pyogenic diskitis (as differential diagnosis for paradiskal type)
- Eosinophilic granuloma (Calve's disease)
- Hemangioma
- Early thoracic disease has the following differentials:
  - Rickets
  - Scoliosis
  - Osteochondroses (Scheuermann's disease)
  - Schmorl's disease.
- Isolated ivory vertebra:
  - Lymphoma, Paget's disease, and osteoblastic metastasis.

2. How does the organism reach vertebral column?

Ans. Associated active infection is seen in <10% cases (*most commonly—pulmonary and urogenital; uncommon—cutaneous or lymphadenopathy*). The infection reaches spine mainly via:
- Arterial vascular channels
- Batson's perivertebral venous plexus.

Other uncommon routes are direct spread from mesentery or cisterna chyli and direct implantation.

3. Why is Pott's disease most common in dorsolumbar (DL) region?

Ans. More than 50% cases are seen in DL region due to:
- Greater extent of movements
- Degree of weight-bearing and hence microfractures
- Larger area of spongy cancellous bone
- Proximity to kidney and cisterna chyli.

In decreasing order of involvement: DL region → lumbar → upper dorsal → cervical → sacral

Children have higher incidence of cervical spine TB.

4. What are various types of tubercular involvement of spine?

Ans.
- *Paradiskal involvement*: Infection spreads through epiphyseal arteries → disk and adjacent vertebral bodies. This type is more common in lumbar lesions and is overall the most common type.

The Spine

- *Complete lesions*: Destruction of one/two vertebral bodies, more in children under 10 years → prone to late-onset paraplegia
- *Central lesions*: Infection spreads through Batson's plexus/posterior vertebral artery. Concentric collapse of body. Minimal diskal involvement or paravertebral shadows. This type is more common in dorsal spine.
- *Anterior lesions*: Infection under anterior longitudinal ligament. Collapse and diskal involvement are late.
- *Posterior lesions (appendiceal/apophyseal spinal TB)*: Single pedicle involvement (Winking owl appearance), spinous process involvement (Beakless owl). Increased chances of neurological deficit due to proximity to spinal canal and often delayed diagnosis (in lumbar appendiceal TB, neurological deficit is late to appear due to ample space in canal).
- *Skip lesions*: Lesions separated by 2–3 normal vertebral levels
- *Spinal tumor syndrome*: Lesion starts at posterior margin with cord compression by ensuing granulation tissue.
- True tuberculosis arthritis at occipito-atlanto-axial joint.

5. Why do you see bony ankylosis in spine with healing whereas fibrous ankylosis in hip joint?

Ans. Hip joint is a synovial joint with hypertrophied synovial membrane and granulation tissue (pannus) that intervenes the apposition of cancellous bony surfaces, also the cartilage destruction is often not complete thus with healing disease there is fibrous ankylosis. In spinal TB, there is apposition of large cancellous surfaces preceded by destruction of intervening disk; this is aided by paraspinal spasm and weight transmission acting as compression devices. (*In fact, absence of bony fusion and fibrous pseudoarthrosis are "at risk" factors for late recurrence of disease.*)

6. What are the differences in childhood and adult spinal TB?

Ans. The differences between childhood and spinal TB are:
- Average vertebral loss in children is nearly twice that of adults.
- Collapse is rapid and severe in children due to flexibility.

- There is constant increase in deformity in children due to growth even after healing of disease.
- Children are more prone to late onset paraplegia.

7. Is there a method to predict the future deformity?

Ans. The deformity at 5 years (follow-up) can be predicted with a fair level of accuracy by calculation of pretreatment vertebral body loss according to the following formula:

$$Y = a + b \times X$$

Y = Final deformity (in degrees) at 5 years follow-up, X = pretreatment vertebral body loss, $a = 5.5$ and $b = 30.5$ are constants.

[Other methods can be read from Chapter 94 of the book Essential Orthopedics: Principles and Practice, 2nd edition (Varshney MK, Jaypee publishers)]

8. What are the various types of collapse in spinal TB?

Ans. Various types of collapse in TB spine are:
- Telescopic—along the long axis (more common in lumbar spine)
- Flexion—in the sagittal plane of one spinal segment on other (dorsal spine).

9. Why does the collapse so happen?

Ans. Weight is transmitted through articular processes (anterior ones) located posteriorly in cervical and lumbar spine (from where the line of weight-bearing passes), whereas in dorsal spine, the line of weight-bearing passes anteriorly through body (anterior column) so flexion collapse occurs.

10. What is cold abscess?

Ans. Cold abscess consists of TB debris, disintegrated bone lamellae, serum, caseous material, granulation tissue, bone marrow, and TB bacilli.

11. Where does all cold abscess track into?

Ans.

Cervical lesions:
- Retropharyngeal abscess—collection behind prevertebral fascia
- Spread lateral to posterior triangle of neck and present at posterior border of sternocleidomastoid muscle

The Spine

- Mediastinum:
  - Mediastinitis (may be life-threatening)
- Axilla/cubital fossa (along brachial plexus).

Dorsal lesions:
- Paravertebral abscess (*upper dorsal spine—squaring of mediastinum; mid-dorsal spine—fusiform swelling*)
- Extrapleural space
- Intrapleural space—empyema thoracis
- Along intercostal nerves and vessels.

Lumbar lesions:
- Psoas abscess
- Petit's triangle/lumbar triangle
- Scarpa's triangle
- Posterior aspect of thigh/popliteal region.

12. What are the radiological findings of spinal tuberculosis?

Ans. Osteopenia, decreased disk space, and loss of paradiskal margins are the earliest and most common findings.

Severe thoracic disease may show up as "bird's nest appearance" due to crowding of ribs and "eggs" as destroyed vertebral bodies.

In anterior lesions, erosion of anterior part of vertebral body without much change in disk space shows up as "aneurysmal phenomenon" akin to erosion by aortic aneurysm.

In heroin addicts, the features may be atypical including ivory vertebra **(Fig. 10)**.

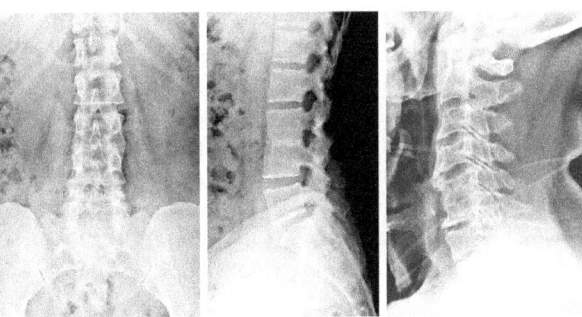

Fig. 10: Radiology of tuberculosis (TB) spine.

13. What other imaging modalities you know of?

Ans. Magnetic resonance imaging (MRI) is the imaging modality of choice as both osseous and soft-tissue details are evident. Intervertebral disk height is often preserved in TB, whereas they are destroyed quite early in pyogenic infection. Also in gadolinium-enhanced images, the abscess shows peripheral enhancement, whereas granulation tissue solid mass enhances *in toto*. The role of computed tomography scan (cannot differentiate granulation tissue from abscess) and scintigraphic (neither sensitive nor specific) scanning have lost ground to MRI.

14. How do you classify Pott's spine?

Ans. Clinicoradiological classification of tubercular spondylitis (Kumar, 1988):

I. *Predestructive*: Straightening of curves, paraspinal spasm, marrow edema (MRI); <3 months

II. *Early destructive*: Disk space, paradiskal erosion (K <10°), marrow edema + osseous break, marginal erosions or cavitations; 2–4 months

III. *Mild angular kyphos*: 2–3 vertebrae involved (K: 10–30°); 3–9 months

IV. *Moderate kyphosis*: >3 vertebrae involved (K: 30–60°); 6–24 months

V. *Severe kyphosis*: >3 vertebrae involved (K >60°); >2 years

Stage III and further all have vertebral body destruction and collapse + appreciable kyphosis.

15. How do you classify Pott's paraplegia?

Ans. Remember, Pott's paraplegia is more common in dorsal and cervicodorsal lesions, as the spinal canal is narrower and there is propensity toward kyphosis and retropulsion. In the lumbar lesions, it is less common as the canal is wider and cord ends at lower border of L1.

Girdlestone and Griffith's classification:

- Early onset paraplegia—develops within 2 years of disease onset.
- Late onset paraplegia—develops after 2 years of onset.

Hodgson's classification (etiological):
- Paraplegia due to extrinsic causes, viz. abscess, sequestrate, diskal fibrosis, pathological subluxation/dislocation of vertebrae, and transverse ridge of bone anteriorly
- Paraplegia due to intrinsic causes, viz. meningitis/meningomyelitis, inflammatory thrombosis, etc.

Seddon's classification:
- Paraplegia of active disease
- Paraplegia of healed disease.

16. What are the causes of Pott's paraplegia?

Ans. Active disease (good prognosis):
- Compressive pathology:
  - Inflammatory edema
  - Granulation tissue and caseous tissue with sequestrated material
- Infective vasculitis
- Spinal tumor syndrome
- Pathological dislocation of spine
- Direct infiltration of bacilli into cord with ensuing inflammatory process.

Healed disease (mechanical pathology with guarded prognosis—treatment surgical):
- Stretching of cord over bony ridge at apex of deformity (internal gibbus)
- Progressive constriction of cord due to epidural fibrosis.

17. How do you stage/grade paraplegia?

Ans. Kumar's clinical staging:
- *Stage 1*: Patient unaware, examination reveals extensor plantar response or ankle clonus (sustained)
- *Stage 2*: Patient has incoordination and reports weakness but manages to walk with support
- *Stage 3*: Patient confined to bed "paraplegia in extension" and variable sensory blunting (<50%)
- *Stage 4*: "Paraplegia in flexion" with sphincters involved, some also include flaccid paraplegia in this stage, sensory involvement >50%.

  (*Incoordination is the earliest symptom and clonus is the earliest sign.*)

18. What is the cause of paraplegia in extension?

Ans. During progression of disease, it is a stage when there is differential involvement of fibers in cord (predominantly related to the types of fibers) whereby the inhibitory pathways to local reflexes are lost but motor power and intrinsic tone of muscles are still there so these produce a "spastic" state and the antigravity muscles predominate producing paraplegia in extension and brisk reflexes with clonus.

19. What is the cause of flaccid paraplegia?

Ans. It is the end-stage in evolution of disease whereby all motor control and muscle tone are lost due to severe compression and possibly arachnoiditis.

20. How will you manage the patient?

Ans. After confirming diagnosis, I will manage the patient on middle path regimen and start antitubercular therapy (ATT) with brace stabilization and continue close supervision to assess and look for surgical indications. If the progression is good the course is followed.

21. What is middle path regimen?

Ans. In short, it can be stated as "drugs for all and surgery for failure"; *the above protocol described comes under middle path regimen.* This includes symptomatic supervised closely observed conservative treatment with expectation of improvement and includes rest, ATT, gradual mobilization, aspiration of large abscesses and collections to reduce discomfort, management of sinuses, and close observation with clinicoradiological progress.

22. What ATT course do you give?

Ans. *Please see Chapter 2: Case I*

23. Why DOTS is not preferred?

Ans. DOTS (directly observed treatment in supervision) is often not possible for orthopedic patients, as they are often unable to visit the center regularly due to disability! Also, uncomplicated musculoskeletal tuberculosis is classified as class 1 in WHO regime that can be given intermittently. *Do learn WHO regime from standard pharmacological texts.*

The Spine

24. Is there any condition when you will not give ATT during perioperative period?

Ans. There is only one condition where ATT is not required in perioperative period—late onset paraplegia from progressive deformity in a patient with healed inactive disease.

25. What are the indications for surgery in Pott's paraplegia/paresis?

Ans. Indications for patients on middle path regimen:
- No neurological recovery even after 4 weeks of chemotherapy
- Development of neurological complications during chemotherapy
- Recurrence of neurological complications during chemotherapy
- Worsening of neurological complications during chemotherapy
- Advanced cases of neurological involvement (stage 4)
- Rapidly advancing paresis, which is advancing daily
- *Common indications (whether or not neurological complications present)*: Patients with prevertebral cervical abscess and difficulty in deglutition, dorsal spine involvement with spasmodic respiration, older patients in whom one would like to avoid complications of prolonged recumbency.

26. What are the indications of surgery in a patient who does not have neurological complications?

Ans.
- Failure of clinical improvement after 6-10 weeks of ATT (modified from original middle path regimen that observes for 3-6 months—most examiners observe for up to 3 months)
- Recurrence of disease
- Primary drug resistance or history of irregular chemotherapy
- *To prevent deformity*:
  - *Adult*: Vertebral body loss >1 in dorsal and DL regions and >1.5 in lumbar region

- Children who present with a kyphus >30° before start of treatment
- *Rare indications*:
    - To establish diagnosis (only when CT-guided biopsy inconclusive)
    - In patients with persistent sinuses and abscess
    - Tuberculosis of cervical spine with paravertebral abscess causing difficulty in deglutition and respiration.

27. Why do you perform surgery?
Ans. Surgery is performed to:
- Drain abscess
- Debride sequestrated bone
- Decompress spinal cord
- Stabilize the spine for prevention or correction of deformity.

(*Basically, this is a play question! Option "1" and "2" achieve "3" and "4" has often to be added to "2" in multisegment involvement,* this question estimates whether you are aware of surgical procedures and their role.)

A combination of all is often required.

28. If there is no improvement for a patient on middle path regimen then what will you do?
Ans. This is an indication for surgical decompression.

29. How will you decompress?
Ans. *Choose one of the options as below*:
1. Abscess drainage around spine/pelvis
2. Abscess drainage + limited debridement
3. Radical debridement of disease focus and anterior arthrodesis + bone grafting
4. Above + posterior fusion to prevent progression of deformity.

It is fair to choose option "1" for limited disease, viz. single level perispinal collection without any neurological complications or any evidence of instability but better to choose option "3" for adult patients and option "4" for children for ≥2 level disease where operative procedure is planned.

Option "2" is not very much favored and most spine surgeons agree to the conclusions of working party on tuberculosis of spine in Medical Research Council trial that Hong Kong procedure of radical debridement and anterior strut grafting is superior.

Nowadays, option "1" is practiced as a minimally invasive guided procedure like ultrasound-guided pigtail drainage of abscess that is quite satisfactory for limited disease.

30. How will you manage disease and drain abscess at various locations?

Ans. *Common routes are mentioned with special situations in subtabs*:

- *Cervical spine*: Avoid rupturing into septic pharynx, so evacuate by neck (extraoral); except in emergency when direct posterior pharyngeal wall incision may be given:
    - 1st and 2nd cervical vertebrae → approached transorally with or without supplementary occiput to C2 fusion
    - 3rd–7th cervical vertebrae → standard anterior approach between carotid sheath and esophagus (anterior triangle), or through posterior triangle.
- *Thoracic region*: Do costotransversectomy (for abscess drainage only) additional decompression of anterior spinal canal would need extrapleural anterolateral decompression (ALD).
    - Cervicothoracic region → sternum splitting approach "or" anterior approach
    - If anterior arthrodesis is also required then use transpleural approach instead of costotransversectomy.
    - Lateral rachiotomy (modified costotransversectomy) is reserved for late-onset paraplegia with large kyphotic deformity where lateral exposure of dura is required.
- *Lumbar region*: Direct drainage along lateral border of sacrospinalis between last rib and rest of ilium:

- Dorsolumbar junction → left-sided abdominothoracic approach through bed of 11th rib
- Lumbosacral junction → extraperitoneal route/paramedian transperitoneal route.

31. What is Hong Kong procedure?

Ans. This is a radical debridement of spine with anterior strut grafting whereby spine is approached anteriorly. The sequestrated and caseous material is removed up to bleeding bone up and below and back to posterior longitudinal ligament (*the decompression should go back to dura mater in cases of neurologic deficit when spinal cord decompression is necessary*). Angular deformity, if present, is corrected with the strut graft.

32. What are the choices for strut graft?

Ans. In terms of preference:
- Full thickness iliac crest
- Vascularized rib graft
- Rib strut graft
- Vascularized fibula
- Fibular cortical strut graft.

33. What is anterolateral decompression?

Ans. Position the patient in right lateral position (avoids venous congestion and excessive bleeding, lung and mediastinal contents fall anteriorly). Semicircular (Convex laterally) incision centered at the pathological site spanning a distance 5–6 cm proximally and distally and apex of incision 9–10 cm laterally is placed (Capner incision). Skin with fascia is lifted to minimize bleeding. 2–4 ribs are identified and traced up to transverse process. Ribs are cut some 8–9 cm from transverse and lifted up and removed. Transverse process is removed from their base completing costotransversectomy (Menard procedure). For ALD, identify the intercostal nerves and vessels laterally, tracing them medially guides the pedicles, which are then removed along with diseased vertebral bodies over posterolateral aspect, hence, decompressing anterolateral part of spinal canal (*the question may be asked*

The Spine

in the form like—what structures are removed in ALD?). Some 3-6 cm of anterolateral canal should be exposed for proper decompression *completeness of which is judged by the reappearance of evident cord pulsations and passing a small red rubber catheter up and below the spinal canal for adequate space*. In younger children, posterior fusion on the other side can be done.

34. What is the role of laminectomy?

Ans. Now condemned, as it is ineffective in decompressing the anterior part of cord (*which is the most common site of compression*) and, in addition, it renders the spinal segment unstable (unless circumduction fusion done simultaneously). It can be considered, however, only for limited cases in patients in whom the lesion is posterior (appendiceal TB) or those with spinal tumor syndrome (posterior epidural tuberculoma).

35. Is it recommended to use instrumentation in spinal tubercular "infection"?

Ans. Anterior surgery alone is often ineffective and *posterior instrumentation is often additionally* required as a staged procedure or in single sitting, which is now an established modality. Also, posterior fusion alone without instrumentation or anterior surgery is considered as a poor planning, as it does not control progressive kyphosis. Implant-associated infections are related to altered local environment and bacterial thriving around implants due to relative inadequacy and ineffectiveness of host defenses and antibiotics, respectively. Biofilm formation plays a significant role in evading defense mechanisms and safeguarding bacteria from chemotherapy. *Mycobacterium tuberculosis* has limited tendency to adhere or produce biofilms, so risk of persistent infection is smaller. This has led to now an increasingly popular use of anterior instrumentation.

36. What are the indications for anterior instrumentation?

Ans. Often the graft failure occurs, if they are used for disease that spans *more than two disk levels*. In these cases, the option is either to use simultaneous anterior instrumentation or a two-staged surgery. In the two-staged surgery where first a posterior instrumented fusion is done followed by anterior debridement and fusion, the first stage prevents loss of correction.

37. How will you manage dorsal spine TB?

Ans. Mehta and Bhojraj have proposed a system for *surgical* management of dorsal spine TB (based on type of involvement):
- *Group A:* Paradiskal/central involvement without deformity—transpleural debridement with fusion (no instrumentation)
- *Group B*: "A" + deformity — above + posterior instrumentation
- *Group C*: "A" but too ill to undergo transpleural surgery — transpedicular decompression and posterior instrumentation
- Group D: Posterior involvement only — posterior decompression only.

38. What are the factors that affect the surgical outcome?

Ans. *Good outcome can be expected in*:
- Minimal destruction and small graft required for maintenance
- Good intraoperative correction
- Involvement of lower lumbar segments.

Poor outcome is more common in:
- No perioperative chemotherapy
- Poor nutrition
- Vertebral body loss >2
- Junctional lesions
- Marked preoperative kyphosis
- Frank instability
- Postdebridement defects requiring grafts spanning >2 disk spaces.

39. How does graft failure occur?

Ans. There are four types:
- Displacement
- Fracture

- Absorption
- Subsidence.

40. Why is deformity, especially kyphosis, of concern?
Ans. There is:
- Foreshortening of trunk
- Short stature
- Cosmetic problems
- Reduced pulmonary function
- Secondary cardiac and respiratory problems
- Progression leads to internal cord stretching and late onset paraplegia.

41. What is K-angle?
Ans. K-angle (short for kyphosis angle) is a measure of present kyphotic deformity. There are two methods to measure the same, one along the posterior border of vertebrae (Dickson 1967) and the other by dropping tangents to end plates of upper and lower end vertebrae. Angle >60° indicates severe deformity and requires surgical correction or anterior transposition of cord.

42. What are the risk factors for severe increase in deformity?
Ans. The following are associated with increase in deformity:
- Patients <10 years of age at onset
- Initial kyphosis >30°
- Vertebral body loss >1.5
- Involvement >3 vertebral bodies
- Evidence of instability in X-ray
- Computed tomography showing involvement of both anterior and posterior structures
- Children who have no/partial fusion.

43. What are "spine at risk" signs?
Ans. There are four "spine at risk" signs **(Fig. 11)** (given by Dr Rajasekaran):
1. Facet dislocation
2. Retropulsion sign
3. Lateral translation sign
4. Topple sign.

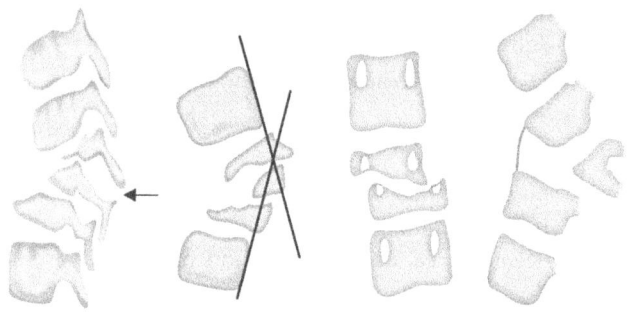

Fig. 11: The four "spine at risk" signs.

(*Score = maximum of 4, minimum of 0; score >2 is associated with higher increase in final deformity.*)

44. Can you classify deformity progression in children?

Ans. Three main types of deformity progression are seen in children during growth spurt **(Figs. 12 and 13)**:

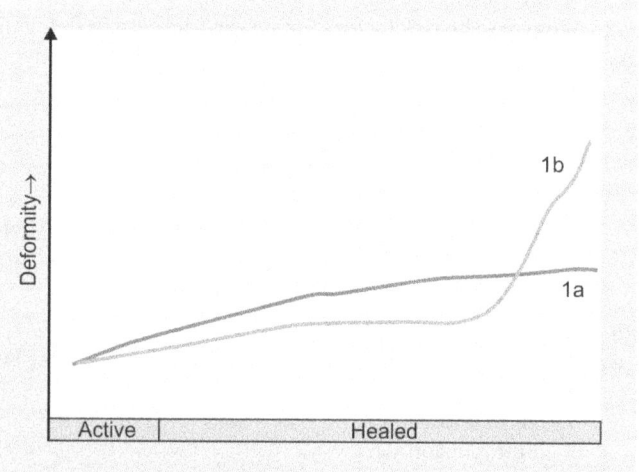

Fig. 12: Type 1 deformity progression.

The Spine

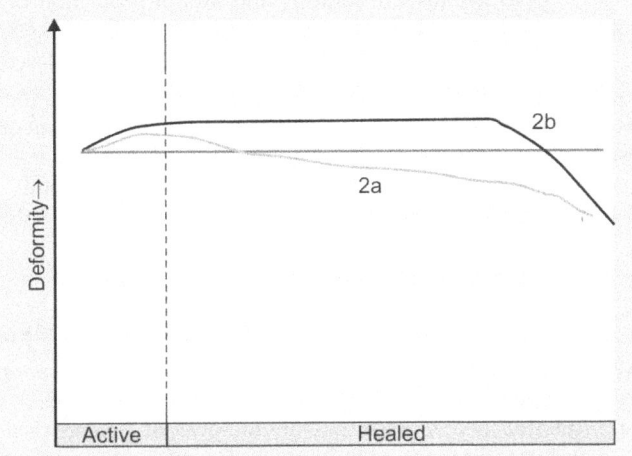

Fig. 13: Type 2 deformity progression.

1. It is a continued deformity throughout entire growth period.
   - Deformity increases continually after active period
   - There is a lag period of 3–6 years
2. It shows beneficial effects during growth with a decrease in deformity.
   - Immediately after growth period
   - After a lag period of 3–6 years.
3. In this type, no major change in deformity.

45. Does level of spine involved, have a bearing on deformity progression?

Ans. Yes
- Dorsal level has higher deformity at presentation that progresses fast and the articular facets are horizontal, so there are early subluxation and dislocation.
- Dorsolumbar junctional disease has worst prognosis because of inherent instability at the transitional zone

from kyphosis to lordosis and loss of protection of rib cage.
- *Lumbar has best prognosis*: There is often telescopic collapse due to narrowness of pedicles.

46. What factors are associated with poor recovery of cord?

Ans.
- Inactive disease with poor mechanical compression
- Complete paralysis
- Paralysis for >1 year
- Presence of severe kyphosis
- Older age and poor nutrition
- Presence of myelomalacia and syringomyelia on MRI.

47. What surgery will you do for healed disease with paraplegia?

Ans. Anterior decompression with removal of healed disease and stabilization with bone graft with/without anterior instrumentation

48. What are the indications of surgery to prevent deformity in spinal tuberculosis?

Ans.
- Loss of 0.75 vertebral levels in dorsal/dorsolumbar region and loss of 1.0 in lumbar region
- Children with >"2" spine at risk signs.

49. How will you manage severe kyphotic deformity?

Ans. For patients without neurological complications, manage as per Q27. For paraplegics with severe kyphotic deformity, do anterior transposition of cord using extrapleural anterolateral approach. A more aggressive and probably better method is to stabilize spine posteriorly followed by anterior debridement and bone grafting in healed disease using transthoracic approach. For healed disease anterior debridement followed by posterior instrumentation and anterior fusion using titanium cages filled with bone grafts is used.

50. How will you manage craniovertebral lesions?

Ans. Behari et al. classified patients into four grades depending up on presentation and respective treatment:

- *Grade I*: Neck pain only and no pyramidal signs—treat with brace immobilization and medical therapy only
- *Grade II*: Independent patient but minor disability—treat as above
- *Grade III*: Partial disability requiring assistance with activities of daily living—anterior decompression followed by posterior fusion
- *Grade IV*: Severe disability with respiratory compromise—treat as for grade III.

51. What are the advantages of costotransversectomy?

Ans. The advantages of costotransversectomy are:
- It attacks the main cause of paraplegia
- Drainage is away from cord
- It does not weaken spine
- No great operative risk.

This does not decompress the anterior compressive pathology that requires ALD.

CASE II: LUMBAR DISK DISEASE (PROLAPSED INTERVERTEBRAL DISK DISEASE)

1. What is the cause of pain in PIVD?

Ans. The following have been pointed variously as cause of pain:
- Irritation of nerve root due to:
  - Compression (?—pure compression produces only motor and sensory changes without pain so inflammation should coexist, *dorsal root ganglion* is very sensitive to compression and vibratory forces and may be an important pain generator)
  - Stretching
  - Friction
  - Occlusion of vasa nervorum (by inflammatory emboli/thrombi/vasculitis)
  - Degeneration of nerve fibers (due to relative ischemia—'cry of dying nerves')
  - Combination of above (*this has been deliberately added here if you are exhausted of etiology then you*

can "extend" your viva with this universal option—
beware this can offend an ostentatious examiner)
- Persistent pain due to facet joint arthropathy ('vertebrogenic pain' from zygapophyseal joints, the capsule and synovial folds possess pain fibers)
- Engorgement of extradural veins
- Tearing of annulus fibrosus containing sensory nerve endings ('sinuvertebral' nerve) present in outer thirds of annulus
- Biological factors (now considered much important):
  - Neurochemical changes due to localized or systemic inflammatory changes against extruded nucleus.

2. What fibers are responsible for mediation of pain?

Ans. Small, myelinated (A-delta) fibers, and unmyelinated C fibers.

3. What are various types of disk herniations?

Ans. Pathological staging (Eismont and Currier) clarifies the variously used terms **(Fig. 14)**:
- Dehydration, desiccation with early degeneration of disk material (the "degenerative disk disease")

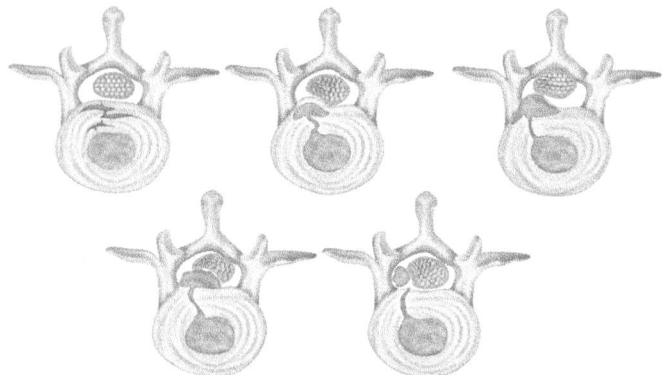

Fig. 14: Various types of disk herniations—disk bulge (top left), prolapse (top middle), subligamentous extrusion (top right), noncontained disk sequestration (bottom left), migrated disk (bottom right).

- Prolapsed of nucleus pulposus (circumferential symmetric disk extension around the vertebral border) within annulus fibrosus ('Disk Bulge'). (Contained herniation)
- Disk "protrusion" consists of focal or asymmetric extension of disk beyond vertebral border. (Contained herniation)
- "Extruded" disk material through annulus but is in continuity with the remaining nucleus but not through posterior longitudinal ligament ('disk extrusion'). (Contained herniation)
- "Sequestrated" disk material through both annulus and posterior longitudinal ligament, which is not continuous with the disk material ('disk sequestration'). (Uncontained herniation)
- "Migrated" disk identifies disk material displaced from the site of extrusion (may or may not be sequestrated).

  To this is added "intermittent disk herniation of 'Falconer' or 'concealed disk' of Dandy"—this is not obvious in position of flexion on table but can be reproduced by hyperextension of spine.

  Contained herniations mean that disk is still subligamentous. "3" and "4" may present as a firm ridge with herniation across the canal.

4. What are the various sites of disk herniation?

Ans. Topographically, disk herniation can be:
- Central zone
- Lateral recess—includes the colloquial variably used terms like "paracentral", "posterolateral", and "juxtacentral"
- Foraminal
- Extraforaminal zone

"3" and "4" are commonly indicated in the term "far lateral disk herniations".

5. What do you mean by the term sciatica?

Ans. Sciatica is the common term for "referred pain" to lower limb and can occur in other lumbar spine disorders.

6. What are your differentials?

Ans. The following must be considered:
- Inflammatory disorders:
  - Infections
  - Ankylosing spondylitis
- Vertebral tumors—both primary and metastatic
- *Nerve tumors*: Ependymoma, meningioma, and neurinoma (most likely to resemble PIVD—pain increases on coughing)
- Spondylolisthesis
- Radiculitis
- Spinal stenosis, foraminal stenosis/lateral recess syndrome
- Piriformis syndrome
- Gynecological/genitourinary condition.

7. Why is the symptomatology more often episodic spanning months to years of symptom-free intervals sometimes?

Ans. There can be regression in symptoms due to:
- Degeneration of compressed nerve fibers
- Adjustment of nerve root in displaced position
- Diminution of swelling of herniation
- Disappearance of edema of nerve root
- Disappearance of central excitatory state
- Spontaneous resolution of inflammation.

8. Are there any features that help you to judge the site of prolapsed disk?

Ans. The following features can serve as "localizing signs" and help to distinguish the various herniations:

Central disk:
- Asymmetric muscle weakness and wasting in legs
- Radicular sensory loss over sacrum, perineum, and back of leg
- Impotence, urinary frequency, and/or retention

Peripheral disk herniation:
- Segmental root pain

- Corresponding segmental muscle weakness and wasting
- Absent segmental reflexes
- Late development of sphincter disturbance and bilateral signs.

9. What do you understand by "axillary" and "shoulder" presentation of disk?

Ans. These describe the presentation of herniated material in relation to nerve root. Axillary presentation means that disk material is inferomedial to the nerve root whereas "shoulder" presentation is understandably superolateral to the nerve root **(Fig. 15)**.

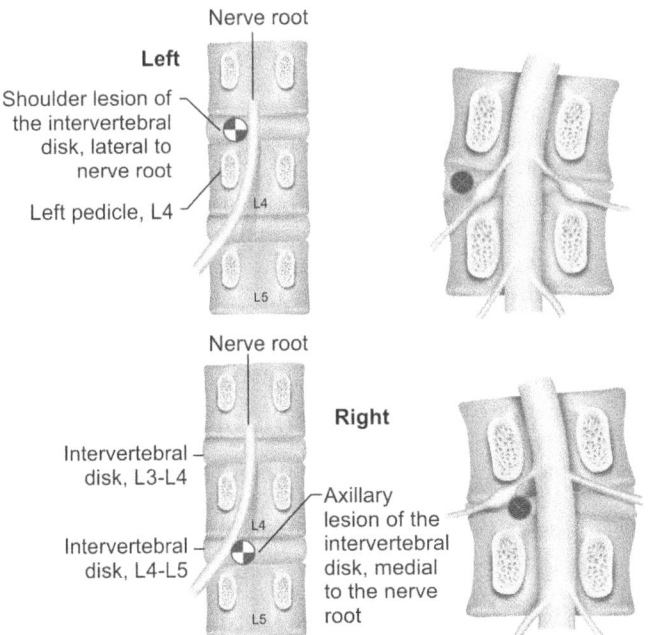

Fig. 15: Shoulder (left) and axillary (right) presentation of disk prolapse.

10. **What is its significance?**
Ans. (*It is in the very human nature to flee away from irritating factors.*) The body tries to "take away" and reduce stretching of the nerve "over" the "irritating disk" by adjusting the body posture and giving some respite. This is done by "tilting" toward the affected side in axillary presentation and away from the affected side in shoulder presentation. This presents as the typical list observed in PIVD.

11. **What are the red flag signs and their importance?**
Ans. Red flag signs in patient history should alert one for an early MRI, these include:
    - Constitutional symptoms like fever, chills, sweats, weight loss, and anorexia
    - History of significant trauma
    - History of malignancy
    - Osteoporosis
    - Age >50 years and <18 years
    - Severe or progressive neurological deficit and multiroot deficits
    - Ongoing infection
    - History of immunosuppression.

12. **What are the various presentations of back pain?**
Ans. Fairbank and Hall classification:
    - *Type I*: "Simple" or "nonspecific" back pain—acute attack, no obvious reason, radiates up to buttocks; never below knee, worse with sitting better with activity. All right with activity. Treatment is activity.
    - *Type II*: "Chronic back pain"—chronic persisting signs and symptoms, insidious onset, pain may progress from back → buttocks → thigh → legs depending on severity, so-called "thermometer pain". Tends not to respond to physiotherapy.
    - *Type III*: "Neurogenic claudication"—walking-related back pain, intolerant of walking or standing straight
    - *Type IV*: "Unclassifiable"—tumor, infection, and psychogenic back pain.

The Spine

13. How will you differentiate between neurogenic and vascular claudication?

Ans. The following features favor neurogenic claudication:
- Patient feels pain with weakness in legs so that they may fall, but in vascular claudication, it is often a cramp or tightness that progresses to pure pain.
- Patient has a variable walking distance and has no relation to speed of walking; whereas in vascular claudication, the walking distance constantly decreases and appears early with brisk walking.
- Symptoms appear proximally (back → buttock → leg) and progress distally in neurogenic claudication, whereas they are reverse (leg) in vascular claudication.
- Patient or spouse often notes a flexed posture after some walking in neurogenic claudication, whereas limp often occurs early in vascular one.
- Easier to walk uphill (due to inherent flexion of spine while going up) in neurogenic.
- Riding a bicycle is not painful in neurogenic claudication.
- Often not possible to "walk through" the pain (as can be done in vascular claudication).
- Longer duration of recovery from pain in neurogenic claudication—5–30 minutes (1–3 minutes in vascular).
- Taking simply a flexed posture reduces the pain and gives respite in neurogenic claudication but patient has to sit and take rest in vascular claudication.

14. How do you localize a segmental lesion?

Ans. It can be localized based on the clinical finding of positive stretch testing and corresponding involvement in respective sclerotome, myotome, and deep and/or superficial reflexes.

15. What are the findings for lumbar fourth segment involvement?

Ans. The following findings support lumbar fourth nerve root involvement:
- Positive sciatic nerve stretch test
- Weakness of tibialis anterior and/or knee extension (quadriceps muscle)

- Sensory loss over medial leg and ankle
- There may be weakness of patellar tendon reflex
- Patient is unable to walk over heel (or in weakness with power >3/5, there would be fanning of toes with loss of arch).

16. What are the findings in fifth lumbar root involvement?

Ans. Following would be seen apart from positive stretch testing:
- Weakness of extensor hallucis longus (EHL), extensor digitorum longus (EDL), knee flexion (hamstrings), tensor fascia lata (TFL), and gluteus medius (hip abduction)
- Sensory loss over lateral and anterolateral leg and dorsum of foot (typically in the first web space—deep peroneal nerve territory)
- Weakness or mute posterior tibialis reflex and medial hamstring reflex
- Positive Trendelenburg sign (variable)
- Trendelenburg gait (variable).

17. When do you call sciatic stretch test to be positive?

Ans. Firstly, the stretch test should be performed passively (passive SLRT). The nerve is stretched only during 35-70° range of movement in SLRT (*a typical L5 or S1 nerve is deformed by 2-6 mm in SLRT*). In the first 35°, the slack in the nerve is taken up and beyond 70°, the deformation of sciatic nerve occurs beyond spine and is not sensitive for radicular pathology. So, a stretch test for being positive should elicit pain during this range. Sometimes with intense acute inflammatory reaction, it may not at all be possible to lift the leg. This can be taken as positive with other findings but should prompt for an urgent search for pathology. A mere feeling of "posterior stretch" is NOT a positive SLRT and is common between 70° and 90° range (*not all of us are athletes*).

18. What is the interpretation of cross-leg SLRT?

Ans. Cross-leg SLRT (well leg SLRT) is quite specific and sensitive for prolapsed symptomatic disk. This test is positive due to micromotion of ipsilateral (affected side) nerve root on performing the test in asymptomatic limb. This test signifies that the disk is central or there is a large lateral recess herniation, and it is more specific for a "free" disk fragment.

19. What does the segment testing indicate with respect to level of herniation?

Ans. A herniated disk produces radiculopathy in nerve root that crosses the disk at that level. For example in L4-L5 disk herniation, L5 nerve root lies in the lateral recess that presents with the radicular signs. This is due to the peculiar disposition of nerve roots in the spinal canal. Understand the following thoroughly. Nerve root leaves the *cauda equina* ("cord") one level "above" its exiting foramen (so, L5 nerve root that will exit the L5-S1 foramen beneath L5 pedicle will leave the cauda equina "cord" at L4 vertebral body). From here, it descends obliquely in the lateral recess crossing the lower body of L4 and L4-L5 disk and turns outwards beneath the pedicle of L5 before ever coming in vicinity of L5-S1 disk. This topography of nerve root distribution explains that for a given level of disk herniation, the affected nerve root will be the lower nerve root. Hence, L4-L5 disk herniation will affect L5 nerve root as the L4 nerve root has already exited before ever coming in vicinity of L4-L5 disk and S1 nerve is still in cauda equina that will separate from it at middle of L5 vertebral body, which lies below disk.

Caution: This holds true only for a typical moderate-sized posterolateral (lateral recess) disk herniation.

Various factors modify the radicular presentation as below and now should be understood after grasping the above said:

- *Size of disk*: A large sequestrated disk can affect the nerve against it and any nerve root in vicinity (so in above example, L5, S1, and sometimes L4 may be affected)
- *Presentation of disk*: Axillary disk tends to displace down and medially, so a sequestrated fragment can involve the classical nerve root at the level and one level below (in above example L5 and S1). Similarly, a shoulder

presentation can involve in addition nerve root of one level above (but is quite uncommon)
- Far lateral disk herniations (foraminal and extraforaminal) may spare the classical nerve root but involve the exiting nerve (so in above example, L4 will be involved).

20. What is cauda equina syndrome?

Ans. As a disk herniation can involve a nerve root, so also it can involve cauda equina, if the herniation is central! The weakest part of annulus fibrosus is posterolateral and then posterocentral. L4-L5 disk is the usual culprit. Clinical diagnosis rests on several components of central disk herniation, viz.:
- Pain radiating along the back of thighs and legs (often symmetrical)
- Numbness in buttocks, back of legs, and sole
- Perineal sensory deficit, decreased rectal tone
- Paralysis in L5 and S1 supplied muscles of foot and TFL and gluteus medius
- Loss of tibialis posterior, medial hamstring and ankle (gastrosoleus) reflex
- Trendelenburg sign and gait
- Bowel or bladder or both incontinence (they travel centrally in cauda equina) with post-void residue of >50–100 mL.
- Babinski's reflex would be mute.

Such a case is most unlikely as this is a surgical emergency!

21. What will you do for patient?

Ans. After clinically examining the patient, I would confirm my diagnosis using radiological and neurological investigations.

22. What radiological investigations would you order?

Ans. I will get an AP and lateral projection X-rays of lumbosacral spine after preparing patient.

23. What will you see on X-ray?

Ans. I will observe the following:
- Physiological spine curves

The Spine

- Reduction of suspected or other disk space ("*vacuum phenomenon*" is quite characteristic for PIVD in conjunction with clinical findings)
- Auxiliary findings of canal stenosis, osteophytes, and facet joint arthropathy
- Osteopenia ("red flag" sign)
- Spondylolisthesis.

24. What else would you like to do?

Ans. I will get MRI study of L-S spine done. If I find osteopenia or suspected inflammatory process, I will order for gadolinium-enhanced study.

25. If MRI scan shows a large disk with other disks, what will you do?

Ans. The anatomical level should be ideally correlated with neurological level, so I will order electrodiagnostic studies (EMG-NCV) for the same.

26. What do you want to look for in EDS?

Ans. Confirmation of:
- Radiculopathy (whether single level or multiple)
- Evidence of denervation/reinnervation (partial/complete)
- Associated myopathy, if present.

And at last, whether this corresponds to the anatomical level determined above. Often in piriformis syndrome where there is entrapment of sciatic nerve in piriformis muscle rather than spine, the clinical tests and radiological investigations are inconclusive and electrodiagnostic studies may reveal the etiology.

27. After establishing diagnosis, how will you proceed?

Ans. I will discuss the results of investigations with the patient and explain various treatment options then decide accordingly.

28. What is the role of conservative treatment?

Ans. If a symptomatic patient with Fairbank type "2", "3", "4" opts for conservative treatment or the patient is in type "1" category then the following modalities are used in conjunction:
- *Rest*: Often not indicated for more than 2-3 days. It is just to tide over the acute painful stage and make patient feel

comfortable. Advise patient to rest with a pillow beneath knee. Prolonged recumbency potentiates prolonged disability and continued or augmented pain.
- *Lifestyle changes*: Tobacco cessation, limited alcohol intake, and weight management
- *Physical training*: Toning back muscles and stretching tight muscles and strengthening exercises for weak muscles, Pilates (incorporates Zen meditation and yoga)
- Ultrasound massage, microwave or shortwave diathermy, and electrical stimulation trans-cutaneous electrical nerve stimulation (TENS)
- Acupuncture, osteopathic manipulation, magnets, and intradiskal electrothermal annuloplasty (IDET)
- *Pharmacological treatment*: Analgesics and muscle relaxants with or without night sedation.
- Adjunctive pharmacological treatment for osteoporosis, facet joint arthropathy (disease-modifying agents for osteoarthritis), etc. (TNF-α inhibitors and systemic steroids are *not* approved for this condition), membrane stabilizers, antidepressants, etc.

29. If a patient does not progress after a fair duration of above treatment but is still not willing for surgical treatment, what else can you do?

Ans. I will opt for semi-invasive procedures like epidural injection or chemonucleolysis.

30. What is the philosophy and indications of epidural injection?

Ans. Considering altered "biological" environment and inflammation as an important cause of pain, extradural deposition of steroids is a good proposal. The indications are as follows:
- Patient with acute signs and symptoms:
  - Painful SLR/femoral nerve stretch test
  - Sciatic scoliosis
  - Appropriate neurological deficit
- Patient with acute on chronic attacks with long symptom-free intervals

- Patient with acute on chronic symptoms with a different level of disk pathology (e.g. after previous surgery).

Complications could be headache, sciatic pain during treatment, and transitory muscle weakness.

31. What is chemonucleolysis?

Ans. It is an alternative form of treatment for PIVD as well as formal discectomy/percutaneous nucleotomy. Enzymatic digestion of proteoglycans reduces the water-holding capacity of nucleus pulposus, which shrinks. Effect takes 4–8 days. Chymopapain (heat labile cysteine protease from carica papaya) or chymodiactin (less heat labile, easier production) is used.

Indications:
- Single level disk/prolapsed disk
- Failed response to adequate conservative treatment
- Classical history and MRI documented disk.

Contraindications:
- Known sensitivity
- Cauda equina syndrome
- Pregnancy
- Previous surgery at the level
- Sequestrated or free disk fragment
- Demonstrated spinal/lateral recess stenosis
- Ongoing litigation.

32. What are the indications of operative treatment?

Ans. *Indications*:
- Progressing neurological deficit
- Cauda equina syndrome
- Severe peripheral neurological deficit, viz. foot drop
- Failure of conservative treatment to relieve pain and neurological signs and symptoms
- Severe persistent pain and disability for more than 1 year.

Prerequisites:
- Compressive pathology concordant with patients signs and symptoms

- Motivated patient with a strong will to return to work
- No pending/ongoing litigations
- No psychological issues.

33. What are the various options available for surgical removal of disk?

Ans.
- Spinal fusion
- Options (for radiculopathy and nerve root compression–decompression and discectomy):
  - Standard open discectomy:
    - Laminectomy
    - Laminotomy
    - Fenestration
  - Microdiscectomy (using microscope)
  - Endoscopic discectomy
  - Percutaneous automated discectomy.

I will prefer option 1b (for larger disk with displaced nerve root) otherwise 2 (microdiscectomy) due to shorter hospital stay and faster return to work.

- Intervertebral disk replacement.

34. Are there any factors that determine a favorable result? (Reverse for unfavorable result)

Ans. Presence of only radicular symptoms, positive tension signs, no back pain, noninvolvement of workmen compensation act, higher socioeconomic status, and minimal psychosocial stressors.

35. What are the signs of complete discectomy?

Ans. There is no absolute answer as to how much disk to remove. Fragments that are loose and easily reached should be removed to minimize recurrence. Aggressive end-plate curettage should be avoided. The goal of the surgery is not complete discectomy but removal of enough material to relieve symptoms and prevent recurrence. After removal of disk, the inflamed nerve root may be erythematous but should move freely and easily with a very gentle retraction. Congestion of epidural vessel is reversed. This is the time to methodically inspect the epidural space medially around the root, anterior to the sac, distally to the level of the inferior pedicle, as well as proximally for other possible fragments.

36. What will you do if there are no further fragments but the root is not free?

Ans. Consider a foraminotomy.

37. What is the usual amount of disk material removed in discectomy?

Ans. Around 5 g in open discectomy but varies markedly with the level of operation and surgical technique (average 1–7 g).

38. What are the indications for fusion?

Ans. Posterior fusion can be done after laminectomy or facetectomy during disk removal. The indications are as follows:
- Associated listhesis
- Congenital malformation
- Advanced intervertebral arthrosis
- Instability due to bone removal
- Need to return for heavy manual work.

McNab's indications for fusion:
- Less than 50 years old with normal disk height and root entrapment associated with changes in posterior facet joint necessitating joint excision
- Progressive history of backache-associated severe sciatic pain and nerve root irritation where mechanical instability is deemed to be the more important cause
- Recurrent episodes of low back pain in otherwise emotionally stable patients.

39. What are the various methods for fusion?

Ans. The basic principle for performing fusion is to prevent further segmental motion, which is thought to be an important pain generator (posterior spinal segments or disk itself—anterior pain generator). The various methods to achieve this are briefed below:
- Posterolateral intertransverse process fusion ± instrumentation—most common procedure but leaves the disk behind

- Posterior lumbar interbody fusion (PLIF) ± instrumentation—requires instrumentation as potentially destabilizes the segment for immediate postoperative period
- Transforaminal lumbar interbody fusion (TLIF) ± instrumentation—approach to disk more lateral than PLIF, near total disk excision so more solid fusion than PLIF
- Anterior lumbar interbody fusion—anterior approach, which is somewhat better tolerated but does not reliably decompress posterior neural elements and is relatively unstable as it depends only on compressive graft fit
- Circumferential (anterior and posterior) fusion—combines anterior lumbar interbody fusion (ALIF) and PLIF, but more extensive.

40. What are the causes of failure of open discectomy?

Ans. The following may account for failure:
- Removal of lamina >25% or predisposes to facet fracture
- Recurrent/persistent disk herniation
- Epidural fibrosis
- Arachnoiditis
- Lumbar canal stenosis
- Wrong level and wrong side
- Emotionally unstable patient/patient requiring Workman's compensation.

41. What is percutaneous nucleotomy or percutaneous automated discectomy?

Ans. It is also known as percutaneous aspiration discectomy.

Indications:
- Herniation within disk—incapacitating or radicular leg pains made worse by standing or sitting and eased by lying down
- Failure of conservative treatment for >6 weeks
- Myelographic/MRI evidence of subannular disk herniation consistent with patient's symptoms and signs
- At least two of the following:
    - Weakness of plantar flexors/extensors
    - Wasting of above muscles

The Spine

- Lost/diminished reflexes
- Sensory deficit in specific distribution.

42. What are the complications of discectomy?

Ans. Complications of discectomy are:

- Recurrent symptoms/failed back syndrome, e.g. due to wrong level, recurrent herniations (same or different level)
- Dural tear and cerebrospinal fluid (CSF) leak—require resurgery
- Nerve root injury
- Infection (diskitis)
- Arachnoiditis
- Epidural fibrosis
- Epidural hematoma
- Cauda equina syndrome
- Iatrogenic instability.

(Additionally, one may read the steps of discectomy for a more extensive viva session!)

CASE III: SCOLIOSIS

FINDINGS

History

- Insidious onset deformity of spine first noted accidentally
- Gradually progressive deformity
- Painless deformity (there may be associated general weakness).

Examination

- Features of any of the following:
  - Polio
  - Neurofibromatosis
  - Von Recklinghausen's disease
  - Down's syndrome
  - Marfan's syndrome
  - Hurler's syndrome
  - Meningomyelocele/spina bifida occulta

- Osteogenesis imperfecta
- Charcot-Marie-Tooth disease
- Friedreich's ataxia
- *Or none*: Idiopathic variety
- Raised shoulder on the convex side in thoracic curves (affected side), on concave side in lumbar curves
- Scapula rotated outwards and forwards with elevation on convex side
- Thoracic/thoracolumbar/lumbar curve with convexity to right/left side
- Forward protrusion of chest wall on affected side
- Increased flank creases on opposite (concave side)
- Higher anterior superior iliac spine (ASIS) and posterior superior iliac spine (PSIS) on concave side
- *Adam's anterior bending test*: More prominence of structural curve on convex side with hump (rib hump in thoracic and thoracolumbar curves), partial/complete correction of compensatory curves or nonstructural scoliosis
- Spinous processes turned into concave side
- Plumb line to judge balance of curve
- *Flexibility testing (flexible/Rigid curve)*:
  - Forward bending
  - Pushing the curve from convex side and noting the correction
  - Lifting the patient up from head
- *Measuring the*:
  - Distance of plumb line from center (midline)
  - Iliocostal distance reduced on concave side
  - Ilioccipital distance reduced on the side of decompensation (under correction)—often to the side of convexity
  - Wasting in limbs
  - Limb length inequality
- Neurological examination of limbs
- Limb length measurements
- Hip examination for fixed deformities and a quick look at knee and foot/ankle deformities
- Ober's test
- Gait pattern.

The Spine

It is imperative to note the following:

- *Family history of Charcot-Marie-Tooth disease, Friedreich ataxia, Marfan's syndrome, and neurofibromatosis (they will not tell if you do not ask!)*
- *Age of parents (Down syndrome)*
- *Growth and developmental history (to judge further curve progression—"time left"):*
  - *Secondary sexual characteristics*
  - *Menarche*
  - *Milestone achievement*
- *Symptoms for spinal pathology (possible neuromuscular cause):*
  - *Gait*
  - *Coordination*
  - *Bowel and bladder function and specifically late onset bed-wetting.*
- *Midline defects (possible neuromuscular scoliosis):*
  - *Hairy patch*
  - *Swelling/mass*
  - *Port-wine patch (Naevi)/Café au lait spots*
  - *Skin dimples*
- *Congenital malformations (possible congenital scoliosis):*
  - *Skull deformities*
  - *Cleft lip/palate*
  - *Mandibular hypoplasia/small chin*
  - *Tapering/small ears*
  - *Malformations of limbs*
  - *Transverse/longitudinal defects*
- *Always note the nonstructural causes of scoliosis—tumor, infection, herniated disk (these often are painful while the structural scoliosis only produces mild discomfort and not characteristic pain pattern).*

This schema should make you answer the following questions quite reasonably.

Diagnosis: The patient is a 12-year-old female with right-sided thoracic structural scoliosis with lumbar compensatory scoliosis. There is no clinical evidence of midline spinal defects or neuromuscular affection and the limb lengths are equal. There is no evidence of associated congenital defects.

1. How do you define scoliosis?

Ans. It is lateral curvature of spine of >10° with associated rotation of vertebrae.

2. What are good prognostic signs in scoliosis?

Ans.
- Male sex (although overall males predominate but females are likely to have large curves)
- Late onset (>10 years) idiopathic scoliosis
- Gradual progression (or static curves)
- Single lumbar/thoracolumbar curve.

3. Why do you call thoracic curve as structural and lumbar curve as compensatory and why not other way around?

Ans. The Adam's forward bending test reveals rotation that is accentuated on forward flexion. The rib hump becomes more prominent. While the lumbar curve partially corrects and does not show any rotational component on forward flexion.

4. What is the basis of Adam's test?

Ans. Technically, spine is an asymmetrical cylinder with long anterior and short posterior distance. With forward flexion, the anterior distance is "cramped" and posterior distance "open" up, if the spine is straight. It is imperative to the fact that unless there is advanced anterior wedging of vertebrae, which is uncommon, the scoliosis *is actually a lordotic deformity* most prominent at the apex. Forward flexion compresses the lordosis and buckles out the lordosis to side making rotation more prominent **(Fig. 16)**.

In a rotational deformity where the anterior part of spine (vertebral body) has rotated away from their anatomical location, the "fixed" deformities would get accentuated by virtue of the technically "posterior line" now getting compressed and throwing rotated vertebral bodies further into disarray. While the compensatory curves by virtue of being flexible realign to reproduce the normal biomechanics and hence "reduce".

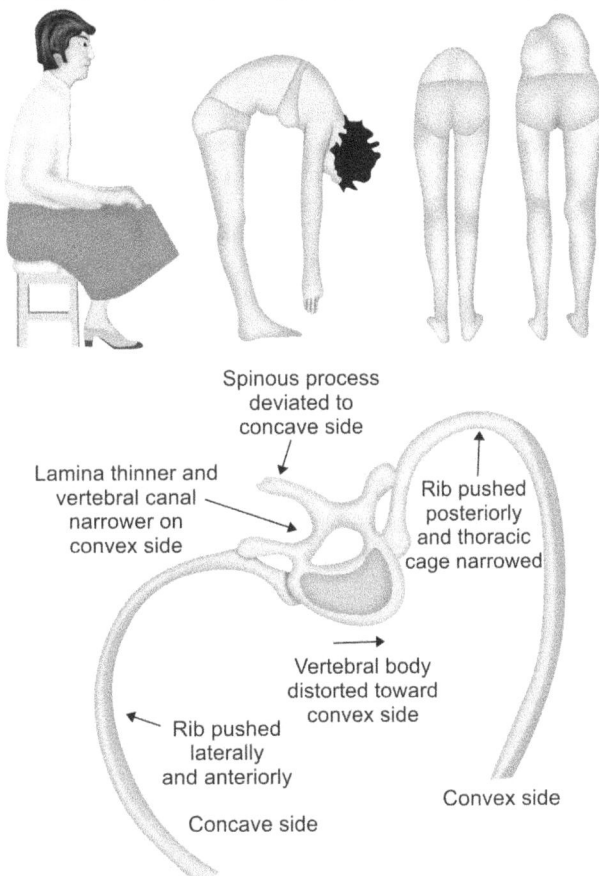

Fig. 16: Adam's test.

5. What are the interpretations of Adam's test?
Ans. Adam's test tells the following:
- Site of primary curve
- Flexibility of spine

- By virtue of accentuation of curve, the test also tells us the "future" of ongoing process in terms of expected outcome.

6. What do you understand by the term "postural" scoliosis, "compensatory" scoliosis, and "structural" scoliosis "or" is postural scoliosis same as compensatory scoliosis?

Ans. *Postural scoliosis*: A curve that corrects totally on bending forward/lying down/traction or other maneuvers. Clinically, there is no rotation of vertebrae (*this defies the definition of "scoliosis"; however, there is supposedly no other better term! Please also read 'list in examination'*), there is no structural change.

"Compensatory" scoliosis/curve (secondary curve/minor curve): Curve developed as a compensatory measure to "structural" or pathological defect elsewhere **(Fig. 17)**. There may be rotation but it is *not fixed* (except otherwise in 'intermediate idiopathic scoliosis' where the compensatory curve also shows clinical rotation, this type is fortunately

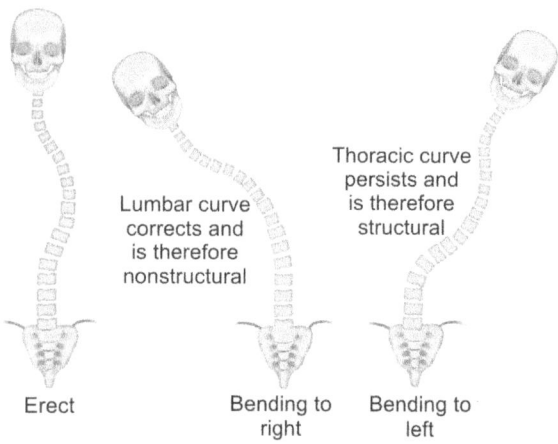

Fig. 17: Lateral bending of spine to look for compensatory (flexible curves) and differentiate from structural curves.

uncommon). The curve and rotation disappear, if the primary "defect" elsewhere is corrected.

"Structural scoliosis": The structural defect lies in the curve, which shows *fixed rotation* of vertebra and spinous process (and ribs). This rotation is persistent on clinical examination and needs intervention to correct.

"Postural and compensatory" are etiological terms and are not technically subset of each other, so always choose the correct word!

7. What are the characteristics of a compensatory curve due to limb-length inequality?

Ans. This type of curve begins at lumbosacral junction and is convex to the short side. There is no compensatory curve between the curve and pelvis; this differentiates it from all other curves except congenital forms that may extend to sacrum.

8. Is it possible to have a step-off "offset" head on thorax, which is compensated well over pelvis?

Ans. Yes, in high thoracic curves with cervical compensation, the head is dragged by cervical spine to one side and appears as an offset but may be well compensated over pelvis.

9. How do you determine the flexibility of curve?

Ans. By various distraction and manipulative tests:
- Forward bending "Adam's test"
- Lifting the patient up from head
- Lateral bending
- Pushing the curve from convex side.

10. What are the findings that can point the etiology to paralytic curve?

Ans. The following are the common findings in a paralytic curve [due to post-polio residual paralysis (PPRP)]:
- High thoracic curves (may also be seen in congenital scoliosis, rarely in neurofibromatosis and virtually never in idiopathic scoliosis)
- Collapse of ribs on convex side in contrast to the often present forward thrusting chest in idiopathic variety

- Almost certain progression
- Appearance within 1-2 years of disease process
- Muscle charting then reveals other findings (PPRP patient have normal sensory examination).

11. What are the characteristics of neuromuscular curves?

Ans. Common features of neuromuscular curves include:
- Large curves early in life
- Stiff curves due to secondary contractures
- Progressive curves that progress even out of rapid growth period
- Long "C" curves
- Sagittal plane deformity
- Presence of pelvic obliquity.

12. Is it necessary for the shoulder to always remain up on the convex side?

Ans. No, in cervicothoracic curves, shoulders may remain at the same level. More importantly in idiopathic scoliosis with double thoracic curve, the shoulder on the convex side is lower than the other side! This has been called *Signe d'épulae* (the sign of shoulder).

13. What are the interpretations of superficial abdominal reflex?

Ans. An absent reflex may not be abnormal but an asymmetric reflex demands further comprehensive evaluation by advanced radiological investigations to rule out spinal pathologies most prominently syringomyelia.

14. How will you further evaluate the patient?

Ans. I will get radiographs of the whole spine in AP and lateral projections with lateral AP right and left bending films and "hump view" to characterize the curve. Additionally, I will obtain the AP view of pelvis and optional radiographs of left hand and wrist to estimate bone age.

15. What information will you get from X-rays?

Ans. The following information can be retrieved:
- Etiology:

- Congenital—failure of formation (type I deformity) like:
  - Segmented hemivertebra
  - Semi-segmented hemivertebra
  - Incarcerated hemivertebra
  - Nonsegmented hemivertebra
- Congenital—failure of segmentation (type II deformity) like:
  - Formation of bar (partial failure)—anterior, posterior, lateral, and mixed
  - Block vertebra (complete failure)
- Congenital failure of formation and segmentation (type III deformity)
- Paralytic curve—high curves with sloping and collapsed ribs on convex side
- Neurofibromatosis—short, sharp, and stiff (rigid) curves
- Idiopathic

- Site of primary curve (regional classification) and classification into types (King's or SRS)
- Severity (magnitude) of deformity
- Compensatory curves
- Rotation (Moe and Nash method, etc.)
- Prognostication [rib vertebra angle difference (RVAD) **(Fig. 18)**]

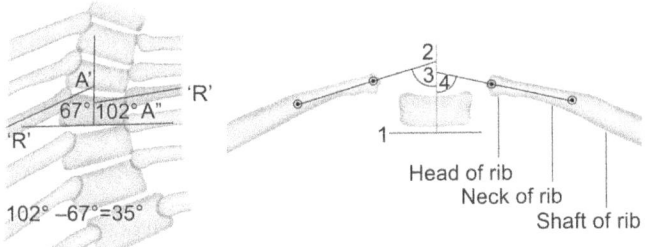

Fig. 18: Rib vertebra angle difference (RVAD).

- Compensation
- Flexibility and amount of correction possible (bending films).

16. What information is obtained from bending films?
Ans.
- Determine the curve type—i.e. structural curves
- Determination of flexibility of curves—by calculation the flexibility index of curves
- Determine the fusion level in lumbar spine
  - The distal extent can be estimated by the flexibility of disk below the chosen distal fusion vertebra
  - Centering the distal planned fusion vertebra over sacrum.

17. What is flexibility index?
Ans. Flexibility index = [Cobb's angle on standard PA film – Cobb's angle on a bend film]/Cobb's angle on standard PA film × 100

18. How do you classify curve?
Ans. Regional classification of primary curves is based on the location of "apical vertebra":
- Thoracic curve—2nd thoracic vertebra to T11-T12 disk at apex
- Thoracolumbar curve—12th thoracic or 1st lumbar vertebra at apex
- Thoracolumbar—lumbar main curve: L1-L2 disk to 4th lumbar vertebra at apex
- Cervicothoracic curve—C7 or T1 at the apex
- Lumbosacral curve—L4-5 disk to S1

Sometimes, it is difficult to identify a single vertebra at apex when instead disk is found—then term "apical disk" is used.

19. What is apical vertebra and what are its characteristics?
Ans. Apical vertebra is the vertebra situated at the apex of curve and its location determines the regional type of curve (see above):
- It is situated farthest from midline.
- It is the most rotated vertebra.

The Spine

- It is the least tilted vertebra into the curve.
- Lordosis is maximal at the apical vertebra.
- It is at the center of primary curve (often but not necessarily).

20. What are end vertebrae?

Ans. These determine the extent of primary curve on AP projection:
- These are the vertebrae "most tilted" into the curve.
- These are the last vertebrae in the curve to show rotation (least rotated vertebrae).
- They are surrounded by disk spaces that are either parallel (neutral disk) or the subsequent disk shows opening into concavity.
- The pedicle width is equal on both the sides.

These vertebrae are helpful for measuring the magnitude of deformity and determine the level till which fusion is to be achieved during surgery. Any one of the above findings is sufficient to define an end vertebra.

21. What is then a neutral vertebra?

Ans. This is specifically in relation to a double primary curve where a single vertebra marks the junction of two curves. This vertebra is surrounded by disks that open into the convexity of their respective curves and there is no neutral disk.

22. How do you measure the magnitude of deformity?

Ans. After identifying end vertebrae and apical vertebra, magnitude of scoliosis can be measured by three popular methods:
1. *Cobb's method*: (Simpler and more reproducible of the two)—draw parallel lines from the upper border of upper end vertebra and from lower border of the lower end vertebra and drop perpendiculars from a convenient point of these lines to intersect at a comfortable location. Measure the angle formed at intersection **(Fig. 19)**.
2. *Ferguson's method*: Mark the center of end vertebrae and the apical vertebra. Join the centers and measure the angle at intersection **(Fig. 20)**.

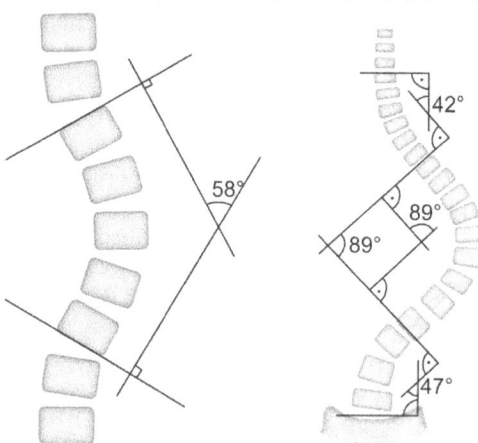

Fig. 19: Cobb's method for measuring curve.

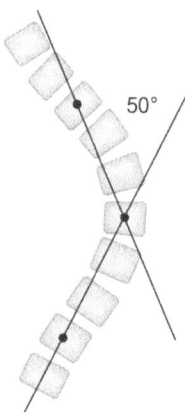

Fig. 20: Ferguson method.

3. *Whittle and Evans protractor method (Oxford Cobbometer)*: This is principally based on Cobb's method but directly yields the measure and obviates the need to draw lines.

The Spine

23. What is the criticism of Cobb's method?

Ans. The following are the criticisms against Cobb's method:
- Firstly (and the one difficult to understand), it is a nonlinear expression of the curve size and progressively underestimates the true magnitude of deformity. Understandably, the rotational deformity (3D) in transverse plane is the true deformity in scoliosis that secondarily produces a lateral curve (*remember the aphorism—'rotation + lordosis' = lateral curvature*). This means that measurement of rotation and its change will vary linearly with the true change in deformity (*extremely sorry to introduce unavoidable mathematical terms*). Arguably hence measurement of deformity in coronal plane (AP radiograph) will not give "true" picture. Thus, Cobb's angle measurement will not truly determine the corresponding deformity change (hence nonlinear) and should not be used as a population measure. This also precludes its expression in "percentage change" of deformity; it will be a logarithmic equation.
- Interobserver variation of up to 5° has been observed. This is of concern as curve progression by 5° over a given period above a certain deformity is often taken as a measure of curve progression!

(*All above are theoretical, most of the prognostication, classification, and management guidelines run on Cobb's angle measurement. Nothing in prejudice but changing this practice would mean like redefining chemistry with subatomic particles other than proton, neutron, and electron!*)

24. What are the methods to measure rotation of vertebrae?

Ans. The rotation on AP projection is noted when the pedicle shows progressive "eclipse".
- Nash and Moe—measuring pedicle distance from sides of vertebral body, grade "0" when they are equidistant and grade "4" when pedicle is past the center **(Fig. 21)**.
- Perdriolle templates.

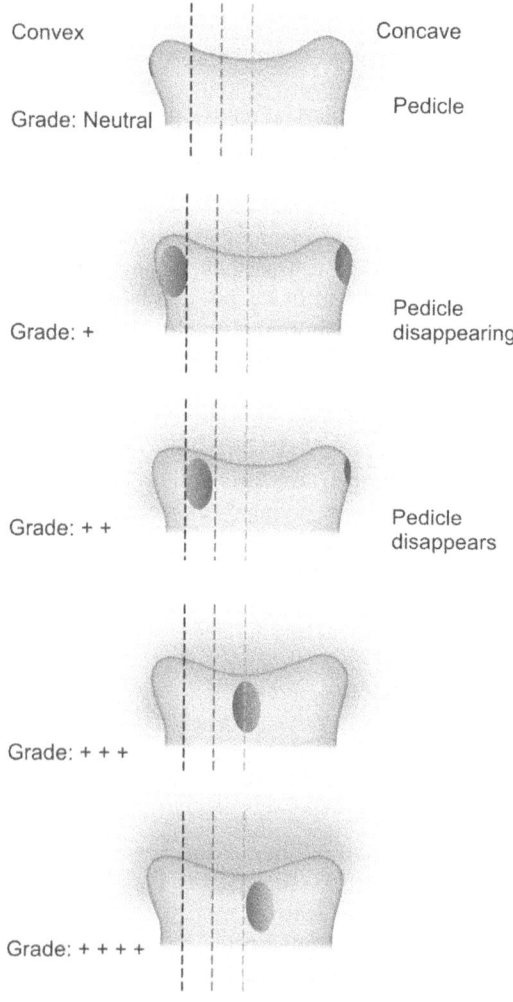

Fig. 21: Nash and Moe method.

25. What is RVAD (rib-vertebral angle distance)?

Ans. It is a method to prognosticate idiopathic thoracic curves in infancy described by Mehta. The measurement is done at the apical vertebra—draw lines along the neck of ribs adjoining apical vertebra and measure the angle they subtend with vertical line drawn at the center of vertebra. The angles measured on two sides are subtracted and if the difference (RVAD) is >20°; the curve is likely to progress.

26. How do you assess the maturity in terms of bone age?

Ans. Bone age indirectly and roughly determines the time remaining for the curve to progress so that what will be the ultimate outcome. Various methods in terms of popularity are as follows:

- *Risser sign* **(Fig. 22)**: Divide the iliac apophysis into four equal regions and grading is done according to the extent of ossification from anterior to posterior with Risser IV indicating complete capping of apophysis and corresponds to completion of vertebral end plate growth and static curve (Risser '0' = no ossification of apophysis,

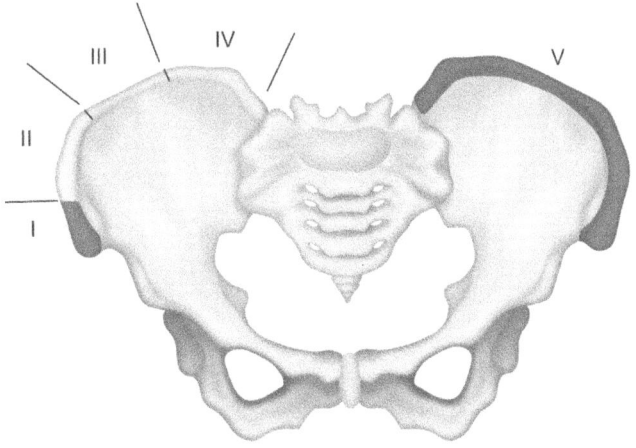

Fig. 22: Risser sign.

'5' = fusion of apophysis to ilium). (*Some growth of curve still can occur, Risser IV is not a full stop!*)
- Triradiate cartilage (open—immature)
- TW3 and particularly digital skeletal age (DSA) are considered more reliable if at all one would like to assess skeletal age by radiological methods.
- TW2 (Tanner and Whitehouse second)—comparing the standard film of AP projection of left hand and wrist against the standards referred.
- TW1—various anthropometric measures
- Vertebral ring apophysis ossification (Bick et al.).

Other measures like chronological age and menarche are unreliable. Height velocity in turn is a somewhat reliable method.

27. How do you classify curves in idiopathic scoliosis?

Ans. King and Moe types for thoracic curves (**Fig. 23**):

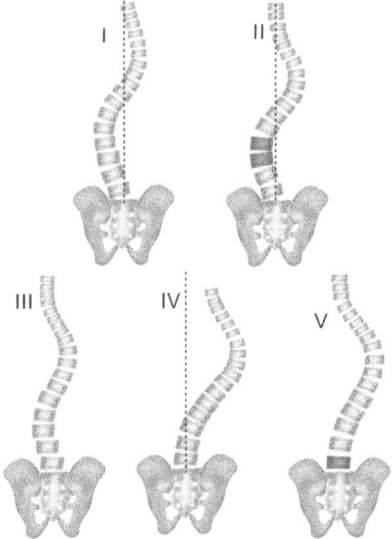

Fig. 23: King and Moe classification.

The Spine

- *Type I*: Lumbar >thoracic (or equal) with lumbar curve less flexible
- *Type II*: Thoracic >lumbar (or equal) with thoracic curve less flexible and lumbar curve crossing midline
- *Type III*: Thoracic >lumbar with very flexible lumbar curve that does not cross midline
- *Type IV*: Single thoracic curve and L4 tilted into the curve with L5 balanced over pelvis
- *Type V*: Double structural thoracic curve.

Coonard expanded King's classification to include lumbar, thoracolumbar, and triple curve patterns giving nine types. Lenke et al. classification (2001) is more comprehensive, adding sagittal alignment to the classification, and utilizes three components of spine to produce classification, viz. the six curve types, lumbar modifier, and thoracic *kyphosis* modifier.

28. How do you look for sagittal alignment and what is its importance?

Ans. On a lateral radiograph, drop a plumb line from center of C7 vertebral body. The line normally is anterior to the thoracic curve, posterior curve, and passes through the posterior corner of S1 (*sagittal vertebral axis*). Sagittal vertical axis (SVA) is said to be present, if the line passes plumb line is anterior to the anterior aspect of S1 and negative SVA exists when it is posterior to anterior body of S1. Generally, the lumbar lordosis is 20–30° more than thoracic kyphosis for maintaining sagittal balance, which should be taken care for while correcting the curves.

29. How do you prognosticate and differentiate infantile, juvenile, and adolescent idiopathic scoliosis?

Ans. Prognostication and differentiation of infantile, juvenile, and adolescent idiopathic scoliosis are discussed in **Table 3**.

Table 3: Prognostication and differentiation of infantile, juvenile, and adolescent idiopathic scoliosis.

	Infantile	Juvenile	Adolescent
Age at presentation (definition)	Up to 3 years	4–9 years	10–20 years
Frequency	Moderate	Infrequent	Commonest form (>50%)
Side dominance	Left thoracic, left:right = 2:1	Right:left = 6:1	Right:left = 8:1
Associations	Developmental disorders like DDH and congenial deficiencies like heart disease often found	Often none (look for hypermobile joints)	None Moderate (around ¼th of curves progress)
Risk of curve progression	<6 month low, >1 year—high, most of curves <6 month of age resolve (90%)	High (progression during growth spurts)	Quite effective for curves <30°
Bracing	May delay progression of curve but they ultimately progress	Reduce rate of progression but often fail (the early the onset, the poorer is outcome)	Posterior fusion ± instrumentation (preferred) <11 years—add anterior fusion
Surgical management	<8 years—instrumentation only 8–11 years—anterior + posterior fusion with/without instrumentation >11 years and closed triradiate cartilage—posterior fusion (± instrumentation)	<8 years—instrumentation only 8–11 years—anterior + posterior fusion with/without instrumentation >11 years and closed triradiate cartilage—posterior fusion (± instrumentation)	—

The Spine

30. How do you manage the patient conservatively?

Ans. Conservative treatment is a supervised treatment planning that is decided on the following points for idiopathic scoliosis:
- Type of bracing
- Duration of bracing
- Curve magnitude and progression
- Skeletal maturity.

The following serve as guidelines for bracing:
- Patient with Risser sign <II with curve progression >5° and magnitude up to 20°
- Patient with Risser sign <II with curve magnitude >20°
- Patient with Risser sign II or more with curve magnitude >30°.

The following may be kept on observation:
- Patient with Risser sign >II and curve magnitude <30°
- Patient with Risser <II with a nonprogressive curve up to 20°.

Bracing is done for 20–22 hours in a day. CTLSO (cervicothoracolumbosacral orthosis; Milwaukee brace) or TLSO (thoracolumbosacral orthosis; Boston or Miami brace) are often used with former preferred for upper thoracic curves. The threshold of surgery for upper thoracic (apex above T7) curves is kept lower.

31. What are the general operative guidelines for idiopathic scoliosis?

Ans. The surgery for scoliosis has evolved over time:
- Classical posterior fusion and POP cast gave way to Harrington's rod instrumentation, which utilized the principle of distraction and compression for correction.
- Luque (1970s) then introduced "segmental" instrumentation utilizing sublaminar wires. This system utilized translation and derotation for achieving correction in contrast to Harrington's instrumentation.
- The system of segmental instrumentation was expanded with the introduction of "hook and rod" constructs (mid 80s).

- This further expanded with introduction of pedicular screws in 1990s. Now, pedicular screws for all levels are there that give excellent stabilization and early rehabilitation.

What has remained constant over the years is the necessity to obtain a solid fusion of spine irrespective of the instrumentation used.

Indications:
- Inability to control a curve with bracing
- Curve >50° (some say >40° for immature spine and >50° for mature spine).

Principles:
- Selective fusion of primary curve is the rule while allowing compensatory curves to spontaneously correct.
- Always include the end vertebrae in fusion.
- Use anterior procedure in immature patients (infantile and juvenile) to prevent crank shaft phenomenon.

Type I curve: This requires fusion of both thoracic and lumbar curves (T4-L3/4) with multisegment construct using translation and derotation technique for correction. Screw and rod construct can also be effectively used.

Type II curve: Fusion of thoracic curve alone with careful derotation at apical vertebra. This is probably done better with the use of all-screw rod construct and translating the spine in addition to rotating the rod. Failing to achieve apical derotation locks the lumbar spine and keeps it from decompensating.

Type III and IV: Fuse the primary curve up to end vertebrae.

Type V: Both the curves should be fused. There is a tendency of upper curve to correct when major curve is fused. Guidelines by Lenke (upper curve >30° that corrects <20°, grade ≥I rotation at apical vertebra, T1 tilt into concavity, elevation of shoulder on convex side of upper curve) may help the surgeon to decide necessity of upper curve fusion.

As regards the need of anterior instrumentation (fusion often done from proximal to distal end vertebrae), types II-IV can be effectively managed with anterior procedure taking special care for preventing future kyphotic collapse by combining posterior procedure in immature spine (see **Table 3** above). For type I curve, combined approach is generally reserved for curves >80°. For lumbar and thoracolumbar curves, maintenance of lordosis is an important aspect that can be done by using titanium cage with bone grafts anteriorly and/or rigid rod systems.

Last is the consideration of thoracoplasty to reduce the "rib hump" that remains often uncorrected after scoliosis surgery. Posterior rib resection by either sectioning medial portion of ribs (the razor ridge) only, or by sectioning and suturing the remaining portion of rib to medial border; both seem to be effective.

32. What is crankshaft phenomenon?

Ans. In cases of immature spine with significant growth potential if only posterior fusion is done then due to continued growth of anterior portion, the spine rotates over posterior fused portion as axis (like a crankshaft) and the deformity increases. Risk factors are young age at surgery and significant curve remaining at the time of arthrodesis.

33. How will you manage congenital scoliosis?

Ans. The issue of conservative versus operative is not as confusing for congenital scoliosis as conservative management hardly has any role. The real issue is regarding what type of surgical procedure to use and obviously when? (*Question should not have been put in answer but this question is very much required to proceed!*)

As opposed to idiopathic scoliosis, an early surgical procedure is desirable in congenital scoliosis.

Principles:

- Operate early to prevent structural changes in spine (problem of height gain is immaterial as without intervention there is only abnormal 'width' gain rather than height)
- Surgical means of correction vary with nature of anomaly, location, curve size and flexibility, and age of child.

The following serve as general guidelines:
- Posterior fusion—reserved for small curves with limited remaining growth potential for anterior elements (to avoid crankshaft)
- *Combined anterior and posterior fusion*: Deformity with a large growth potential
- *Convex hemiepiphysiodesis*: Prerequisites—
  - ≤6 vertebrae involved
  - Curve <70°
  - Age <6 years
  - Absence of pathological congenital kyphosis or lordosis.
- Hemivertebra excision—reserved for children with unacceptable deformity, fixed lateral translation of curve and hemivertebra located at the apex of curve (safest being lumbar and lumbosacral spine)
- Use of instrumentation for large curves in children >5 years. Intraspinal anomalies and rigid curves are contraindications for its use.

34. What are different types of growing rod used for surgical treatment of scoliosis?

Ans. There are 3 systems of growing rod—single growing rod, dual growing rods, and the vertical expandable titanium prosthetic rib implant. Each system has its advantages and disadvantages.

The current expandable spinal implant systems appear more effective in controlling progressive scoliosis, allowing for spinal growth and improving lung development. All have a moderate complication rate, especially rod breakage and hook displacement.

35. What is principle behind growing rod?

Ans. Most operations addressing spinal deformity in the young child actually arrest growth. This may have unfavorable effects on the growth of the thorax, lungs, and the size of the trunk. The growing rods theoretically allow for continued but controlled growth of the spine. One or two rods span the curve percutaneously (minimally invasive). The rods attach to the spine at the top and bottom of the curve with hooks or screws. The curve can usually be corrected 50% at the time of the first operation. The child is then followed every 6 months to have the spine "lengthened" (differential distraction) about 1 cm to allow the child's growth. Often, the rods are kept longer than usual, so lengthenings are less invasive than the initial procedure and only involve opening through one incision. Children have to wear a brace to protect the instrumentation. When the spine has grown and correction is acceptable, remove instrumentation and perform a formal spinal fusion operation.

36. What are the complications of growing rod?

Ans. The complications of growing rod are hook displacement, pedical screw loosening, and rod breakage.

37. What is Shilla procedure?

Ans. The Shilla procedure uses the same ideas as growing rods, but does not require multiple lengthening procedures. The apex of the curve is fused and special screws are used at the top and bottom of the spine. These screws can slide along the rods as the child grows.

38. What is Shilla?

Ans. Shilla is the name of hotel where McCarthy the originator for system was staying and got this idea.

39. What is the role of bracing in congenital scoliosis?

Ans. Practically none. During observation of long flexible curves, bracing can be applied but these are uncommon.

40. What are the problems with bracing?

Ans. Compliance, have to wear until skeletal maturity, stressful for family/patient, lung function affected, compensatory curves can increase, some progress even after wearing brace.

9

Miscellaneous Short Cases

CASE I: CHRONIC OSTEOMYELITIS

Very important and typical case, aims to score candidate's knowledge of infection and approach toward management with respect to bone (just making diagnosis will not suffice as it is quite straightforward).

Read times: 3–5 times (MS orth and DNB candidates).

Diagnosis: The patient is a 31-year-old M/F with 3-year-old chronic osteomyelitis of R/L tibia with deformity (angulation and/or shortening; with or without pathological fracture). There is associated stiffness of knee joint.

COMMON FINDINGS

History

Bone pain, past history of trauma/surgery/swelling or discharge. History of discharging bone pieces is virtually pathognomonic.

Inspection

- Sinus fixed to bone or healed puckered scar
- Exposed necrotic bone
- Soft tissue (contractures).

Palpation

- Bony tenderness
- Fixed sinus or scar

Miscellaneous Short Cases

- Deformity
- Irregular thickened bone
- Irregular surface
- Surgical hardware.

Nearby Joints

Look for stiffness that is common due to treatment and reactive changes.

Nearby Soft Tissue

Often there are skin and soft tissue changes due to recurrent cellulitis, etc.

1. Why do you call it as chronic osteomyelitis and how do you define chronic osteomyelitis?

Ans. Characteristic history and examination as given. Also note in history classic "Walenkamp" phenomenon—classic history of cyclical pain increasing to severe and deep tense pain subsiding with pus breakage and temporary healing. Chronic osteomyelitis is by definition "bone infection predicated on preexisting osteonecrosis", and there is no relation of preceding time duration; it is chronic in literal terms that infection persists for long. Osteonecrosis usually takes around 3 months to establish (and separation of sequestrum from parent bone) hence most texts refer this time duration, however, strictly speaking this may not be acceptable to majority.

2. Who first coined the term osteomyelitis?

Ans. Nelaton (1834) popularized the use of term "osteomyelitis" probably first instigated by Reynaud in 17th century.

3. How do you differentiate a tubercular sinus from pyogenic sinus?

Ans. The following points help one differentiate the two:
- Tubercular sinus has bluish margins and is undermined.
- There is serous discharge unless there is superadded infection or extravagant infection.
- Anesthesia or paresthesia in the skin surrounding the sinus.

4. How do you clinically differentiate cellulitis from osteomyelitis?

Ans. Cellulitis has peau d'orange appearance of skin with features of lymphangitis and bleb formation. Osteomyelitis has given (see examination) features.

5. What will you do next?

Ans. Radiograph of involved extremity and adjacent joints in both anteroposterior (AP) and lateral projections to confirm diagnosis and plan treatment.

6. What do you see on X-ray and does this confirm your diagnosis?

Ans.
- Sequestrum;
- Involucrum formation;
- Ill-defined bone destruction with areas of remodeling and local irregular cortical thickening;
- Loss of corticomedullary differentiation;
- Focal cortical defects → cloacae; and
- Soft tissue scars.

The features confirm my diagnosis of chronic osteomyelitis.

7. What is the differential diagnosis for chronic osteomyelitis?

Ans.
- *Tumor*: Ewing's sarcoma, eosinophilic granulomas, lymphoma, osteoid osteoma, intraosseous ganglion and osteosarcoma.
- *Trauma*: Stress fracture.
- *Osteonecrosis*: Especially of hip, knee [femoral condyles—with corticosteroid therapy or human immunodeficiency virus (HIV) infection].
- *Miscellaneous*: Fibrous dysplasia, Paget's disease, cellulitis, hemophilia, Gaucher's disease (pseudo-osteitis), Caffey's disease (infants), hypervitaminosis A, chronic cutaneous and subcutaneous infections (deep mycotic infections).

8. What is sequestrum and what is its importance?

Ans. Separated microscopic or macroscopic necrotic fragment of usually cortical bone (which appears radiodense) surrounded by infected granulation tissue and pus (radiolucent) from viable parent bone (parent bone is important as otherwise a bone graft used to treat infected nonunion or to fill Brodie's abscess cavity may also be called sequestrum!).

Diagnostic importance: Necessary to make diagnosis of chronic osteomyelitis.

Biological importance: It serves as a focus for continuing infection leading to recurrent bouts of acute and chronic osteomyelitis.

(It takes approximately 2-3 months for sequestrum to isolate and separate. Sequestrum may be absent in children less than 12 months of age—whole bone becomes a sequestrum as periosteum is loosely attached, also small sequestra may be absorbed overtime)

9. Why is the sequestrum dense on X-ray?
Ans.
- *Avascular*: Decrease in resorption of bone (unable to take part in remodeling).
- Surrounded by radiolucent granulation tissue and pus enhancing the contrast.
- Hyperemia of surrounding bone due to inflammation making it relatively osteopenic.

10. What are different types of sequestra?
Ans. *According to shape*:
- *Pencil like*: Infants.
- *Cylindrical or tubular*: Infants (**Fig. 1**).
- *Ring*: External fixator.
- *Conical*: Amputation stump.
- *Annular*: Amputation stump.
- *Coralliform*: Perthes.

Consistency:
- *Coke like*: Tuberculosis.
- *Feathery*: Syphilis.
- *Sand like*: Tubercular osteomyelitis in metaphysis.

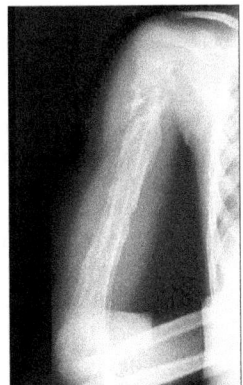

Fig. 1: Sequestration of whole humerus in a child.

Colored:
- *Black*: Amputation stump and long exposure of necrotic bone to air while also attached to parent bone (formation of ferrous sulfide), fungal infection.
- *Green*: Pseudomonal osteomyelitis.

Miscellaneous:
- *Muscle*: Volkmann's ischemic contracture.

11. What are the gross characteristics of sequestra and how will you recognize them during surgery?

Ans. Ivory white brittle piece of bone with smooth (pus facing) and rough (granulation tissue) surfaces lying free from parent bone in the cavity. Does not show any punctuate capillary bleeding (paprika sign). Sinks in water and has a dull note to percussion. It has a closed Haversian canal on histopathology.

12. What is involucrum and its importance?

Ans. Immature, subperiosteal, reactive, living new bone formation around a dead bone.

Biological importance: It walls off abscess; it surrounds and can merge with parent bone or become perforated with holes "cloacae" through which pus and granulation tissue may pout or pus discharges.

Treatment related importance: Only if three walls of sequestrum are seen fully on two perpendicular views should sequestrectomy be undertaken otherwise a pathological fracture will result and it will get converted into infected nonunion.

(It takes 10 days for new bone to be radiologically visible after subperiosteal deposition.)

Physiological and pathological variants (D/D of involucrum) include:
- 50% infants less than 6 months age: B/L symmetrical thin layer along diaphysis of femur, radius, humerus;
- Hypervitaminosis A; and
- Metastatic leukemia.
- Neuroblastoma.

13. What is the common site of osteomyelitis and why?

Ans. Metaphysis of bone is most commonly involved in hematogenous osteomyelitis:

- Hair pin bend arrangement of arterioles (Hobo).
- Relatively less phagocytosis [↓ reticuloendothelial system activity, (Hobo1921)].
- Sluggish flow (Treuta).
- Tortuous blood vessels and skimming of bacteria.
- Dead (apoptotic) and degenerating cartilage cells from physeal plate serving as medium for bacterial growth (Duthie and Barker 1955).
- Microfractures and local hematoma common in young active children (Morrissy).

14. What are the causes for diaphyseal osteomyelitis?
Ans.

- Long-standing osteomyelitis in children (grows out to diaphysis);
- Posttraumatic osteomyelitis;
- Implant related osteomyelitis;
- Tubercular osteomyelitis;
- Drug abusers (heroin addicts—pseudomonas);
- Immunocompromised (fungal); and
- Salmonella osteomyelitis (often bilateral and may be symmetrical).

15. In what forms of osteomyelitis will you not see a periosteal reaction?
Ans. Human immunodeficiency virus associated osteomyelitis, tubercular osteomyelitis (some cases), long standing resolving osteomyelitis that began in childhood.

16. What is the cause of chronicity of infection?
Ans.

- Presence of unabsorbed and retained sequestra serving as a constant source of infection.
- Unobliterated cavities (dead spaces alive with bacteria!).
- "Microbiological shift" (change of aerobic cocci to gram-negative or anaerobes).
- Multiple types of bacteria "mixed infection" and antimicrobial resistance.

17. How will you decide management?

Ans. Work-up to confirm osteomyelitis and individualize management and classify host (Cierny-Mader classification; see below).

Blood investigations include hemogram with erythrocyte sedimentation rate (ESR), liver function test (LFT), renal function test (RFT), blood sugar [BS; fasting (F) and postprandial (PP)], albumin, prealbumin, transferrin (for judging nutritional status of patient).

Advanced imaging for localizing lesion and treatment planning.

Anatomic type
- *Stage 1*: Medullary osteomyelitis (endosteal)
- *Stage 2*: Superficial osteomyelitis (surface only)
- *Stage 3*: Localized osteomyelitis (full thickness cortical involvement and cavitation)
- *Stage 4*: Diffuse osteomyelitis (that are mechanically unstable)

Physiologic class
- *A host*: Healthy
- *B host*:
  - *Bs*: Systemic compromise
  - *Bl*: Local compromise
  - *Bls*: Local and systemic compromise
- *C host*: Treatment worse than the disease

Factors affecting immune surveillance, metabolism, and local vascularity
- *Systemic factors (Bs)*: Malnutrition, renal or hepatic failure, diabetes mellitus, chronic hypoxia, immune disease, extremes of age, immunosuppression or immunodeficiency.
- *Local factors (Bl)*: Chronic lymphedema, venous stasis, major vessel compromise, arteritis, extensive scarring, radiation fibrosis, small-vessel disease, neuropathy, tobacco abuse.

Miscellaneous Short Cases

Young children are included as super A1+++ hosts.

As such it is a redundant classification for practical purposes and treatment guidelines based on this classification are hard to find.

18. How will you manage this patient?

Ans. After investigation and work-up with confirmation of diagnosis I will do sequestrectomy and saucerization of the containing or parent bone (also *see* Q30).

19. How will you perform?

Ans. Explain the procedure to patient. Under anesthesia, position and clean and prepare the patient. Methylene blue dye is injected through the sinus tract to clinically mark (live tissue stains grey and dead one blue) the various tracts and culprit sequestrum. No attempt is made to cut through sinus tracts and they are removed in toto with careful dissection. There is often a bone defect at the site of pus discharge which if adequate is used to remove the sequestrum otherwise defect is elongated in oblong fashion with rongeur or multiple drill holes and completing window. This is followed by removal of sequestrum and granulation tissue. There moved material is sent for histopathology, staining, culture, and antibiotic sensitivity. Eburnated necrotic bone is removed till healthy bone is encountered taking care not to risk parent bone's strength. In the end an oblong saucer-shaped cavity with smoothened edges is aimed for. Thorough inspection is done to search any additional sequestra and lavage is done. Cavity management and wound closure over drain is performed.

20. What are the prerequisites of surgery (sequestrectomy and saucerization) for chronic osteomyelitis?

Ans. *Absolute*:

Radiological: Well-formed involucrum surrounding the discretely visible sequestrum adequately at least two-thirds diameter of bone (three intact walls on two views ensure three-fourths intact walls).

Clinically: Symptomatic patient with pus discharge or chronic unrelieved disabling pain due to osteomyelitis *per se* and type A/B host.

Ethical: Salvageable limb and patient willing for prolonged and multiple treatments.

Relative: Stopping antibiotic treatment at least one week prior to surgery (otherwise cultures will be misleading).

21. What is leukergy?
Ans. Agglomeration of white blood cells (WBCs) in peripheral venous blood seen in association with burns, polycythemia rubra vera, ischemic heart disease, etc. Otremisky, et al. (1993) used it to diagnose and monitor early sepsis.

22. What is the role of technetium-99 (^{99}Tc) bone scintigraphy?
Ans. It serves as a screening tool only ($\approx 10\%$ specificity).

Phase I: Arterial (flow) phase.

Phase II: Venous phase.

Phase III: Focal bone uptake.

Phase I + Phase II: Positive (+ve) with negative (-ve) phase III → soft tissue infection.

All phases +ve: True skeletal infection (false +ves—postsurgical, implants).

[*Teaching note*: Gallium-67 (^{67}Ga) scintigraphy provides the best way to detect vertebral osteomyelitis radiographically, Indium-111 (^{111}In) labeled leukocyte imaging is the test of choice for osteomyelitis elsewhere in body].

23. What is leukocyte imaging (Indium-111 labeled)?
Ans. Increased specificity (over ^{67}Ga scanning) which can be further increased if used in conjunction with sulfur colloid scans that delineate areas of normal bone activity whereas leukocyte scan highlights the involved regions. "Incongruence" of ^{111}In labeled leukocyte scans and sulfur colloid scans are highly suggestive of infection.

24. What is the role of magnetic resonance imaging (MRI) and computed tomography (CT) scans?
Ans. Magnetic resonance imaging (contrast enhanced) has very high specificity and sensitivity and a negative MRI effectively rules out infection. CT scans may be done to plan surgery.

25. What is the role of sinogram?
Ans. Most important investigation to do before surgery. It demonstrates sinus tracts and their source and hence most important guide to surgery **(Fig. 2)**.

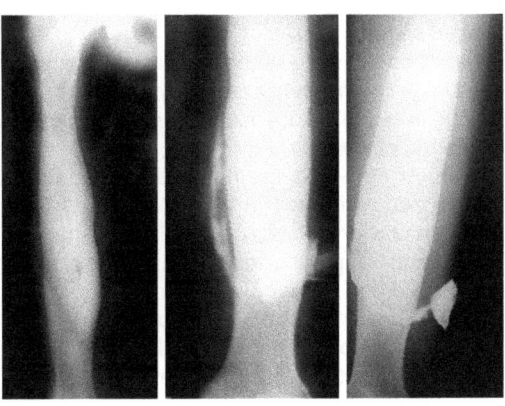

Fig. 2: Sinogram.

26. When can we see septic arthritis secondary to osteomyelitis?
Ans. In infants less than 6 months (Trueta) when there is physiological connection between epiphyseal and metaphyseal vasculature through physeal plate **(Fig. 3)**.

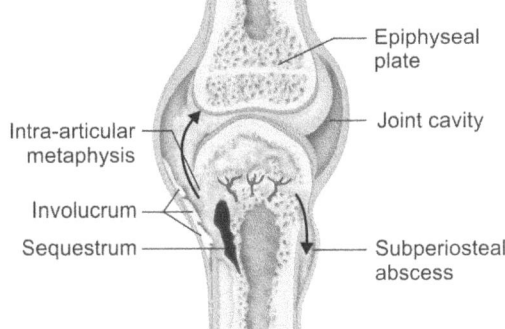

Fig. 3: Spread of osteomyelitis to produce septic arthritis.

Practical Orthopedic Examination Made Easy

In intra-articular location of metaphysis—proximal humerus, neck of femur, proximal radius, distal fibula in adults.

27. What were the various modalities of treatment in preantibiotic era?

Ans. "Rest and Poultice" method—till discharge of sequestrum occurred spontaneously.

Carrel and Dakin—acute clinical sterilization of wounds using Dakin's solution in a closed system.

W Howes (1874) advocated use of sequestrectomy and granulation of wound.

Winnett Orr—laid the fundamental principles of wide drainage and rest between World War I and II [immobilize fracture in plaster of Paris (POP) in best position → thorough debridement → pack wound with vaseline gauze → keep immobilized and do not disturb wound till granulation and healing → repeat if complications occur].

Use of maggots—Connors used it in American civil war and Baer and Eastman during World War I.

28. What are the causes of knee stiffness in osteomyelitis of femur?

Ans.
- Quadriceps tethering or sinus;
- Sympathetic effusion;
- Patellofemoral and tibiofemoral adhesions;
- Quadriceps contracture (multiple surgery);
- Cast immobilization; and
- Reflex sympathetic dystrophy.

29. What is Klemm's triad?

Ans. Determines the outcome in osteomyelitis:
- Vitality and stability of bone;
- Virulence and antibiotic sensitivity of bone; and
- Condition of soft tissue envelope.

30. Outline the principles for treatment of chronic osteomyelitis?

Ans. Treatment for osteomyelitis is initiated along the following path:

Miscellaneous Short Cases

- *Thorough debridement of necrotic tissue and bone*: Sinus tract, necrotic bone, infected granulation tissue, sequestra, eburnated bone is removed and saucerization done for providing wide window.
- Stabilization of bone.
- Obtaining intraoperative cultures.
- Dead space management.
- Soft tissue coverage.
- Limb reconstruction.
- Systemic antibiotic treatment.

31. What do you mean by saucerization?

Ans. Like the saucer has a shallow base similarly the bone cavity is converted into open roof shallow base cavity to drain the exudates outside bone compartment. This is achieved by making a cavity in length at least as large as the infected cavity with 5 mm margin around (or 10-15% larger than the sequestrum length). There should be no undermining and cavity should have smooth borders. It is better to make an oblong cavity else there are increased chances of fracture with a rectangular or square cavity with sharp corners.

32. How do you assess adequacy of necrotic bone removal?

Ans.
- *Dead bone removed till "Paprika sign"*: Punctuate bleeding from Haversian system → healthy bone (not reliable—tourniquet).
- "Laser Doppler" intraoperative—cumbersome.

33. What is pulsed lavage?

Ans. Irrigation with 10-14 L of normal saline using fluid pressure 50-70 pounds/sq. in. and 800 pulses/min. There is no indication for adding antibiotics or emulsifying agents.

34. How do you manage dead spaces following wound excision?

Ans. Healing by secondary intention is discouraged as scar formed is itself relatively avascular and frequently breaks down.

- *Antibiotic beads*:
  - *Nonbiodegradable*: Polymethylmethacrylate (PMMA) beads impregnated with (gentamycin, vancomycin, tobramycin, clindamycin, cefazolin). Local concentration of up to 200 times that of systemic is achieved. Short-term (10 days), long-term up to 80 days and permanent placements are described. Beads need removal as granulation tissue may make removal difficult later. Beads contain 2.4–3.6 g tobramycin per 40 g cement and 1–4 g vancomycin per 40 g cement. Beads are placed from deepest to most superficial. Open wound treatment and suction—irrigation methods are incompatible with this treatment.
  - *Biodegradable beads*: Calcium hydroxyappatite (up to 12 weeks), poly (D,L-lactide)—initial burst followed by sustained release, polygly-colic and polylactic acid beads.
- Local muscle, myocutaneous flap, free flap, composite flap, etc.
- Cancellous bone graft (Papineau).

35. What are the disadvantages of antibiotic impregnated beads?

Ans.

- Require second surgery for removal;
- Local immune compromise;
- Local minimal inhibitory concentration (MIC) active only for 2–4 weeks; and
- Act as substrate for bacteria in long term—glycocalyx formation.

36. What is bead pouch technique?

Ans. Often used nowadays as an interim measure between wound excision and definitive skin coverage. The cavity is filled with antibiotic impregnated beads completely and covered by sterile transparent or lucent adhesive covering to prevent secondary wound infection. It has the advantage that no dressings are required during this period **(Fig. 4)**.

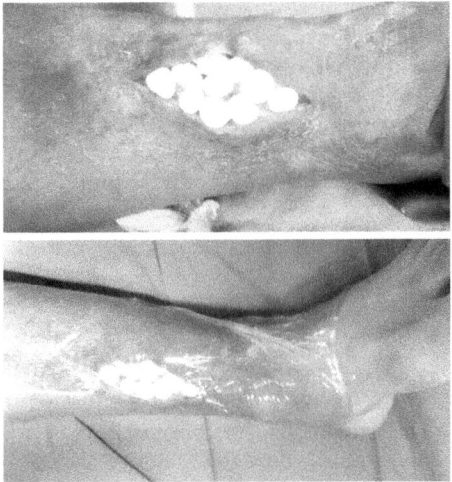

Fig. 4: Bead pouch technique.

37. **What is glycocalyx?**
Ans. It is now applied as a general term to extracellular polysaccharide material and probably glycerol techoic acid of bacteria aka "the sweet husk of cell" that is the main constituent of biofilm. It specifically protects bacteria from phagocytosis, recognition, helps cling to inert implant material and form biofilms that may contain numerous colonies of bacteria safely hidden from host immunity, e.g. *Streptococcus epidermidis*. Biofilms stimulate release of prostaglandin E receptor 2 (PGE2) from monocyte that inhibits T-lymphocyte proliferation, B-lymphocyte blastogenesis and immunoglobulin production; also it interferes with white cell chemotaxis and degranulation. For this reason implants have to be removed for complete eradication of infection.

38. **What is quorum sensing?**
Ans. "Quorum sensing" is a communication between the sessile form of pathogenic organisms. The organisms communicate with each other through lactone containing molecules that

help them gain increasing resistance against the administered antibiotics while also helping them sense the invasion by immune cells. It has been seen that these sessile organisms are also able to target the neutrophils through toxins that kill them directly and once the immunity around the region falls these bacteria change to planktonic forms enabling them to migrate to other places and colonize the nearby or distant regions.

39. What are Morrey and Peterson's criteria for acute osteomyelitis?

Ans. They determine the likelihood of having osteomyelitis (acute).

Definite: Pathogen isolated from bone or adjacent soft tissue or there is histologic evidence of osteomyelitis.

Probable: A blood culture is positive in the setting of clinical and radiographic features of osteomyelitis.

Likely: Typical clinical settings and definite radiographic evidence of osteomyelitis are present and there is a response to antibiotic therapy.

40. How do you diagnose acute osteomyelitis?

Ans. Peltola and Vahvanen's criteria (diagnosis requires two of the following four criteria):
- Purulent material on aspiration of the affected bone.
- Positive findings of bone tissue or blood culture.
- Localized classic physical findings:
  - Bony tenderness; and
  - Overlying soft tissue edema, erythema.
- Positive radiological imaging.

41. What are the differences of osteomyelitis affecting different age groups?

Ans. *See* **Table 1**.

Table 1: Differences of osteomyelitis affecting different age groups.

Feature	Infancy	Childhood	Adult
Source	Umbilical cord/ hematogenous	Hematogenous	Direct inoculation

Contd...

Contd...

Feature	Infancy	Childhood	Adult
Location	Epimetaphyseal, intra-articular	Metaphyseal	Metadiaphyseal
Constitutional symptoms	Failure to thrive	Marked symptoms of inflammation	Moderate
Local temperature	Raised little, pseudoparalysis	Raised	Moderate
Adjacent joint	Septic arthritis common	Less frequent	Uncommon, affected in intra-articular metaphysis or long-standing infections with pus tracking under periosteum and perichondrium
Periosteum	Perforated by pus	Extensively lifted by pus	Locally lifted by pus
Sequestrum formation	Less	Very frequent and usually one or two	Small and multiple
Chronicity	Less chances	More	May persist for life
Deformity	Shortening	Shortening, angulation, lengthening!	No effect or shortening in bone loss

42. What are the complications of chronic osteomyelitis?

Ans.

- Recurrences and relapses;
- Limb length discrepancy **(Fig. 5)**;
- Pathological fractures;
- Septic arthritis;
- Septicemia;
- Joint stiffness;
- Soft tissue abscess formation and cellulitis;
- Soft tissue contractures;
- Amyloidosis; and
- Squamous cell carcinoma of the sinus tract.

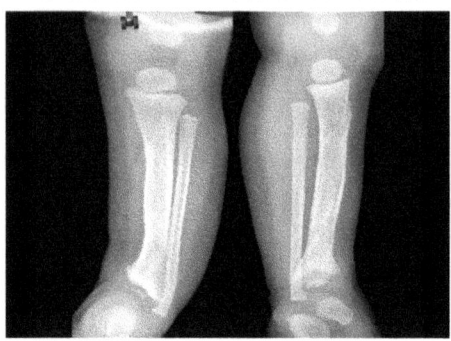

Fig. 5: Limb length discrepancy due to osteomyelitis tibia.

43. What is Garre's osteomyelitis?

Ans. This is a chronic form of disease (sclerosing nonsuppurative osteomyelitis of Garre) characterized by symmetrical thickening of bone and irregularity but with conspicuous absence of abscess and sequestra (remember Brodie's has abscess but no sequestra). Children and young adults are often affected. Low-grade anaerobic infection could be the cause. Guttering the bone or drilling multiple holes may alleviate pain. Should be differentiated from Paget's and osteoid osteoma.

44. Is there any classification method that provides estimated rehabilitation time for patient?

Ans. Yes, May's classification (**Table 2**).

\multicolumn{3}{c}{Table 2: May's classification.}		
Type	**Description**	**Rehabilitation time**
I	Intact tibia and fibula	6–12 weeks
II	Intact tibia and fibula but needs bone graft for structural support (i.e. cavitary defect and not a circumferential defect)	3–6 months
III	Tibial defect ≤ 6 cm long and intact fibula	6–12 months
IV	Tibial defect > 6 cm with intact fibula	12–18 months
V	Tibial defect > 6 cm with unstable fibula	> 18 months

CASE II: NONUNION OF LONG BONES

NONUNION, PSEUDOARTHROSIS AND MALUNION

With the exception of nonunion of fracture neck femur and pseudoarthrosis of spine in ankylosing spondylitis (Anderson's lesion) these are given as short cases. Malunions are uncommonly kept for MS exam but may very well be given in DNB exams. Again malunions around hip are given more often as long case, if at all.

Read times: 3–5 times (MS and DNB candidates).

Diagnosis: The patient is a 26-year-old male with nonunion of fracture R/L lower third both bones (if fibula is also involved) leg for one year. There is posteromedial angulation at middle and distal third junction with 2 cm shortening of leg and 20° external rotation of distal fragment. There is restricted dorsiflexion at ankle.

Common Findings

Inspection

- Scar, discoloration (due to plaster treatment), sinus(es) —infection
- Deformity (angular/rotational)
- Shortening
- Bayoneting of fragments
- Swelling (hypertrophic)
- Wasting.

Palpation

- Temperature
- Tenderness (deep palpation and palpate with nail of your thumb)
- Palpable defect (palpate with nail of thumb running from above down)
- Abnormal mobility (check in two planes)
- Crepitus
- Loss of transmitted movements (rotate the distal part)
- Telescopy and distraction of fragments (lax nonunions and pseudoarthrosis)
- Prominence or absence of other bone (fibula) and its status

Movements

Check for range of motion (ROM) of nearby joints as stiffness due to previous treatment is common.

Neurovascular status distally

Both iliac crests and legs for bone graft.

1. How do you define nonunion, delayed union, slow union, and pseudoarthrosis?

Ans. *Nonunion*: Simply, when a fracture fails to unite permanently of its own. Comprehensively "nonunion of fracture is said to exist when the fracture shows clinically, radiologically and biologically no signs for progression of healing after giving adequate time [US Food and Drug Administration (FDA) considers this as 9 months with failure of progression for three consecutive months) for the type and site of fracture which will not unite unless some fundamental alteration in the line of management is undertaken" (quite vague and demands speculation for future events). According to Brinker nonunion is a fracture that according to treating physician will not heal unless some intervention is required. This is a permanent end situation.

Delayed union: Fracture is said to have gone into delayed union when healing has not advanced at the average rate for the location and type of fracture. This is a "temporary" phase (fracture still shows progress toward healing) and will progress to permanency of union or sometimes nonunion.

Slow union: Here the fracture takes longer than usual to unite but passes through the stages of healing without departure from normal both clinically and radiologically. The ultimate outcome is union. Some people differentiate between slow union as being slow to start with from delayed union where fracture struggles in later stages of healing.

Pseudoarthrosis: This is a distinct nonunion characterized by hypermobility at the fracture site with cleft formation between ends and lined by pseudocapsule. The cavity is usually fluid-filled.

2. What are the causes of nonunion?

Ans. *Local factors:*

Fracture related:
- Open
- Infected
- Comminuted
- Segmental
- Fractures of irradiated bone
- Intra-articular fractures

Treatment related:
- Inadequate immobilization (most common)
- Inadequate reduction
- Inadequate fixation
- Inadequate blood supply
- Inadequate soft tissue cover
- Interposition of soft tissue
- Inadequate apposition "distraction"

Systemic:
- Age (elderly)
- Malnutrition (albumin < 3.4 g/dL; lymphocyte count < 1,500/mm^3)
- Corticosteroid therapy
- Immunosuppressive treatment
- Systemic (hepatic, renal) disease
- Metabolic bone disease
- Anticoagulants
- Burns
- Smoking
- Alcohol
- Radiation.

3. How do you classify nonunion?

Ans. *Infected nonunion:*

Umiarov's classification:

Type I: Normotrophic without shortening.

Type II: Hypertrophic with shortening.

Type III: Atrophic with shortening.

Type IV: Atrophic with bone and soft tissue defect usually with shortening.

May's classification for tibia (see Chapter 9: Case I; actually it is a classification for osteomyelitis of tibia, however type III, IV, V include nonunion).
Type III: Tibial defect 6 cm or less with intact fibula.
Type IV: Tibial defect more than 6 cm, intact fibula.
Type V: Defect more than 6 cm with no usable fibula.

Noninfected nonunion:

Weber and Cech (**Fig. 6**; modified Muller and "Judet and Judet" classification systems).

Hypervascular nonunion:
- "*Elephant foot*": Inadequate fixation or immobilization, premature weight bearing.
- "*Horse hoof*": Moderately unstable fixation.
- "*Oligotrophic*": Inadequate apposition, displaced fracture.

Avascular nonunion:
- *Torsion wedge*: Intermediate fragment healed to one main fragment of bone but not to other.
- *Comminuted (necrotic)*: Has one or more necrotic fragments.
- *Defect (gap)*: Loss of intermediate fragment.

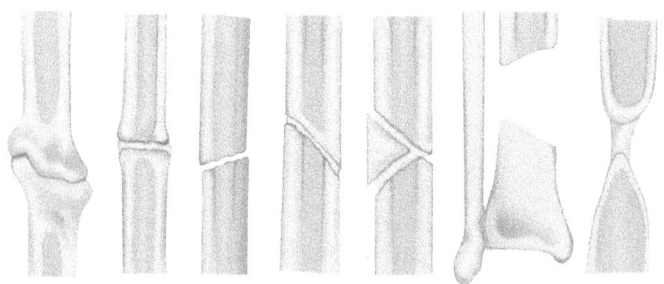

Fig. 6: Weber and Cech classification.

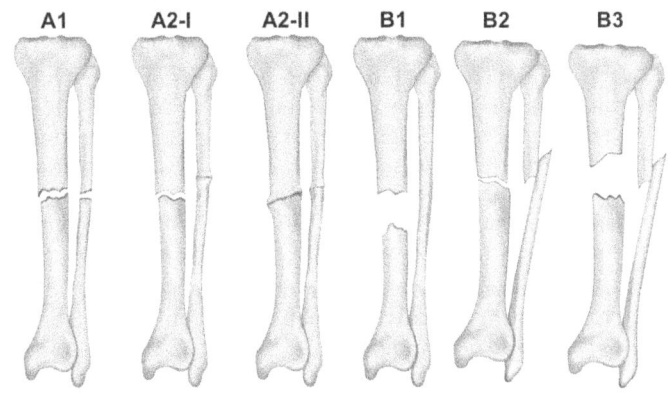

Fig. 7: Paley's classification.

- *Atrophic*: Ends porotic and atrophic usually loss of blood supply.

Paley's classification for tibial nonunion (Fig. 7; clinical and radiological):
- Type A (<1 cm bone loss)
  - *A1*: Mobile deformity
  - *A2*: Fixed deformity
    - *A2-1*: Stiff nonunion without deformity
    - *A2-2*: Stiff nonunion with fixed deformity
- Type B (>1 cm bone loss)
  - *B1*: Bony defect no shortening
  - *B2*: Shortening but no defect
  - *B3*: Both (shortening with defect).

4. What is the basis of Weber and Cech classification?

Ans. Viability of bone ends determined by strontium uptake.

5. How do you clinically determine that this is a nonunion and not delayed union or pseudarthrosis?

Ans. Presence of painless abnormal mobility at the site in two perpendicular planes is deemed pathognomonic of nonunion. Other findings are:
- Crepitus;
- Telescopy of fragments (lax nonunion);

- Loss of transmitted movements; and
- Palpable gap or defect in avascular nonunions.

Patient is unable to bear weight if it is in lower limb. In delayed union there is residual pain at fracture site and tenderness on manipulation of the fracture with abnormal mobility usually in one plane. Abnormal mobility if at all present is not gross. Pseudarthrosis is characterized by gross abnormal mobility typically in all directions and crepitus is often absent as the ends are covered by fibrocartilage.

6. Is it necessary that a nonunion has to be painless?

Ans. No, following are the causes of painful nonunion:
- Infected nonunion.
- Interposition of soft tissue especially viable muscle and nerves.
- Nonunions of intra-articular fractures.
- Bayonet nonunions impinging surrounding tissues with adventitial bursa formation and bursitis.

7. How do you clinically differentiate a stiff from a lax nonunion?

Ans. Stiff nonunions have arc of motion less than or equal to 7° (classically < 1 cm defect) that is not adequately bridged by fibrocartilage to resist movements grossly. Often only micromotion can be elicited; even the patient may bear weight partially in such cases. They are also called nonmobile nonunions (or short fibrous nonunions). Lax nonunions (arc of motion > 7°) on the contrary are inadequately supported by connective tissue and demonstrate the classical signs of nonunion. These are also called long nonunions or mobile nonunions.

[Intra-articular short fibrous nonunions (fibrous ankylosis) are often painful and the concept of painless nonunion does not apply to them].

8. Do all nonunions demonstrate abnormal mobility (or can you tell me something about nonmobile nonunions)?

Ans. Not necessarily. As above stiff nonunions typically hypertrophic ones may not at all demonstrate abnormal mobility, also some site specific nonunions like in diaphyseal tibial nonunion where fibula is intact mobility may be masked at least in mediolateral plane. Some metaphyseal tibial and femoral nonunions also ingeniously mask abnormal mobility only on the sheer basis of proximity to mobile joint—judgment testifies the surgeon's clinical competence.

(In these cases give the clinical diagnosis as malunion if deformity is present but there is no tenderness or if tenderness is present then—uniting fracture when time frame from injury is short or delayed union if time period is long. If there is no deformity/tenderness/abnormal mobility then case will not be kept in exam and better search for something else or you are grossly missing something!).

9. What are the common sites of occurrence of nonunions?

Ans. Typical sites include—fracture femoral neck, fracture of carpal scaphoid, fracture neck of talus, fracture lateral condyle humerus, fracture capitellum, fractures of distal third shaft of tibia.

10. What are the causes of nonunion for fracture shaft of tibia?

Ans. Distal third of tibia is poorly surrounded by muscles so that segmental periosteal blood supply (derived from anterior tibial artery) is limited.

Secondly these fractures are often open and caused by high velocity injury further compromising the blood supply.

Surgical intervention is an added risk factor for jeopardizing the blood supply.

Lastly in middle-third fractures of tibial shaft the endosteal blood supply derived from posterior tibial artery that supplies 90% of cortex is most severely affected.

11. How do you clinically identify infected nonunion?

Ans. Following are the features of infected nonunion (infected nonunions fall into Cierny-Mader type IV osteomyelitis):
- Painful nonunion [painless if there is significant gap (>1 cm) filled with mature fibrous tissue].
- Raised local temperature.
- Discharging sinus.
- Scar healed by secondary intention with "puckering".

- Tethered skin.
- Irregularity of bone on either side (representing osteomyelitis).

[It is not always that you get an active infection with nonunion, more often than not it is a quiescent infection. Healing of infection in bone is virtually equivalent to reversing virginity of a girl. So if active infection is not seen then make diagnosis of "infected nonunion with quiescent infection"—there is no term like quiescent infected nonunion. Similarly healed infected nonunion (which means that nonunion has healed which was infected) should also not be used ideally speaking. Also healing of infection cannot be clinically "detected". Single plane mobility with tenderness at fracture site and lesser duration of fracture would be clinically diagnosed as "delayed union"].

12. What will you do next?
Ans. Radiograph of involved extremity (to confirm diagnosis) with adjacent joints.

13. Does this confirm your diagnosis?
Ans. Yes or No!

Describe the location, type of nonunion along with condition of bones and ancillary findings of infection and soft tissue. Comment on joints, status of hardware and deformities.

Delayed union:
- Slight resorption of bone ends with "Wooly" appearance (No evidence of sclerosis or very slight).
- Medullary canal is open at both ends.
- Fracture line is clearly visible.
- External and internal callus are minimal.

Nonunion:
- Marked sclerosis of ends with rounding off appearance.
- Medullary canal closed **(Fig. 8)**.
- Diffuse osteoporosis of both fragments.
- Fracture gap persists and widened due to unsuccessful bridging.
- Proximal end convex and distal end concave (pseudoarthrosis).

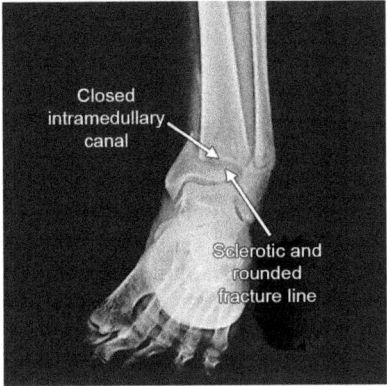

Fig. 8: Radiograph of tibia nonunion.

14. How does infection affect fracture healing?
Ans. Infection is not an etiological factor for nonunion, i.e. it does not cause nonunion; fractures are known to unite in the presence of infection. However, active ongoing uncontrollable infection is a predisposing factor for nonunion of fracture. Various mechanisms are responsible to this effect:
- Dissection of pus through planes and periosteum—devascularizing the ends.
- Fragmentation and dissolution of fracture hematoma.
- Inflammatory mediators that promote fibrous tissue formation.
- If fixation was done then implant failure occurs destabilizing the fragments.
- Increased catabolic response at fracture ends than anabolic activity (this also causes porotic ends).

15. How does nonunion develop?
Ans. The inherent tendency of fracture is to heal and to this end there is a fine interplay of innumerable factors that also have a reserve capacity, i.e. some deviations are tolerated but not constant and gross distractions from normal process.

Quality of bone, vascularity, protection, and stress are some of important mechanical and biological factors that can be modulated to produce positive effect. Response to stress is as follows:

- *Intermittent compressive hydrostatic stress (pressure)*: Chondrogenesis
- *Intermittent strain*: Fibrogenesis
- Low levels of mechanical stimuli (micromotion)
    - *Good vascularity*: Ossification (osteogenesis)
    - *Poor vascularity*: Chondrogenesis

    Type of healing also depends on type of stabilization (Q: What are the various types of callus response with your chosen mode of treatment?):
- *Cast (closed treatment)*: Periosteal bridging callus and interfragmentary enchondral ossification.
- *Compression plate*: Primary cortical healing (cutting cone type).
- *Intramedullary healing*: Early—periosteal bridging callus and late—medullary callus.
- *External fixator*: Depends on rigidity.
    - *Less rigid*: Periosteal bridging callus.
    - *More rigid*: Primary cortical healing.
- *Inadequate immobilization with*:
    - *Adequate blood supply*: Hypertrophic nonunion (failed endochondral ossification).
    - *Poor blood supply*: Atrophic (avascular) non-union.
- *Inadequate reduction with displacement at fracture site*: Oligotrophic nonunion.

16. What are the principles of treating nonunion?

Ans. Following are some of the principles of managing nonunion:
- Infected and noninfected nonunions can both be managed with compression distraction method commonly provided with Ilizarov method.
- For infected nonunion with active infection and discharging pus initially thorough debridement should be done followed by second stage stabilization ± bone grafting when the infection settles.

Miscellaneous Short Cases

- For infected nonunion with quiescent infection single stage debridement with Ilizarov fixation ± bone grafting may suffice.
- Hypervascular nonunion:
    - Long bone nonunion (femur, tibia, humerus) that has been treated with nailing can be very well managed with exchange nailing using a larger diameter nail.
    - If the cause of nonunion is torsional instability following nailing, then it is advisable to use augmentative or auxiliary unicortical plate fixation (preferably locked plate) ± bone grafting (usually not necessary as it is a mechanical failure).
    - *Plate fixation and bone grafting*: For femoral metaphyseal nonunions, if site permits the application of locked distal femoral plates with bone grafting is preferred for distal nonunions. For proximal femoral nonunion, proximal femoral nail with bone grafting is a better option.
    - If the site of nonunion is too near the joint, then hinge prosthetic replacement could be an option in less active population.

17. What are the various types of bone grafts?

Ans. Bone grafts or bone transplants are natural bone tissues obtained to provide either structural stability (cortical) or stimulate osteogenesis (cancellous) or both (usually). (Bone graft substitutes are synthetic or semisynthetic derivatives that have various effects on bone healing.)

Vascularized: Fibula (free vascularize or double-barrel fibula transfer, centralization of fibula, reversed flow vascularized pedicle), iliac crest, greater trochanter, coracoid process (with muscle), rib.

Nonvascular graft:

Cortical: Fibula, tibia, autoclaved diaphyseal grafts.

Cancellous: Iliac crest mulberry grafts, tibial condyles, femoral condyles, olecranon, excised head of femur, posterior superior iliac spine, malleoli.

Corticocancellous: Tibial upper metaphysis, tricortical iliac graft.

Mesh cage bone graft technique: Metallic cage (slightly smaller than adjacent bone) filled with cancellous bone chips and demineralized bone matrix.

Grafts may also be classified as autograft, syngraft (isograft—from identical twin), allograft (homograft), xeno (hetero) graft or according to shape, composition and method of application [onlay (single or dual of Boyd)], inlay, intercalary, peg (neck femur, epiphysiodesis), H-graft, chip, shell, osteoperiosteal, pedicle, sliding and intramedullary (augments stability, improves screw purchase, added potential for intramedullary healing between host bone and graft, e.g. humeral nonunion).

18. What is the mechanism by which grafts enhance healing?

Ans. Biological properties of bone grafts are osteoinduction (process that supports the mitogenesis of undifferentiated mesenchymal cells, leading to the formation of osteoprogenitor cells that form new bone), osteoconduction (property of a matrix that supports the attachment of bone-forming cells for subsequent bone formation) and osteogenesis (combination of above to form bone). Osteogenic property is defined as propensity to generate bone from bone forming cells.

19. How do grafts heal?

Ans. *Cancellous (osteoinduction more prominent than osteoconduction)*: By a process called "creeping substitution" (Phemister) whereby capillaries invade the tissue followed by granulation tissue and macrophages that resorb the bone while simultaneously also the process of osteogenesis is going on over the scaffold of graft.

Cortical (mainly serves as structural graft, osteoconduction prominent): Process is somewhat similar but slow resorption occurs along Haversian canals and then regeneration occurs. This may take years to complete depending on size and vascularity.

Miscellaneous Short Cases

20. What grafting options are available for infected nonunion?

Ans.
- Papineau open bone grafting (three-stage technique; Rhinelander, Higs, Roy-Camille, etc. also described similar techniques):
  - Debridement (usually multiple at 5–7 days interval) with intramedullary stabilization.
  - *Grafting*: Once granulation tissue appears use "match-stick" cancellous grafts 3–6 cm × 3 mm × 4 mm in overlapping circular fashion with or without saline irrigation and wound packing.
  - *Skin cover*: Either spontaneous or various flaps or graft for coverage.
- Mini-Papineau.
- Posterolateral bone grafting of tibia (Harmon's method, especially if anterior skin is unhealthy).
- Phemister bone grafting.
- *Friedlander technique*: Thorough debridement plus stabilization and closure followed by open bone grafting.
- Ilizarov method with or without bone grafting.
- Huntington's two-stage tibialization of fibula for infected gap nonunion (quiescent infection).

21. What is Phemister bone grafting and modified Phemister grafting?

Ans. DB Phemister (1947) devised a technique for treating delayed unions and established nonunion of tibia (even infected ones) by placing "subperiosteal" "cortical" bone grafts (onlay) across fracture site. The fracture site was not opened. Modification (Charnley and Forbes) included placing "corticocancellous" grafts "subcortically" by raising "osteoperiosteal" flaps. Charnley additionally used "Shingling" (raising osteoperiosteal flaps of bone longitudinally across fracture site) originally devised by Naughton Dunn (1939). Later, process of "Petalling" ("fish-scaling" originally described by Uhtoff) was also combined to above; Forbes actually analyzed the results of Charnley method and also used petalling in combination. Petalling has the effect of creating artificial ensheathing callus at ends which is connected by process of shingling.

Philosophy of Phemister grafting:
- Fibrous union should not be broken down by refreshing or resection as it disturbs the ongoing healing process and increases instability.
- Nonunion heals if induced to do so.
- Rigid immobilization is unnecessary.
- Can be used in presence of recent sepsis provided graft is inserted through normal tissues away from fracture site.

22. What are the various modalities of enhancing fracture healing?

Ans.

- Autogenous (vascular/nonvascularized) bone grafting.
- Bone marrow injection (app. 20 mL of marrow harvested from iliac crest or greater trochanter for nonunions less than 5 mm).
- Stem cell injection (100–150 mL bone marrow centrifuged to produce 2–4 mL aspirate containing multipotent marrow cells and osteogenic stromal cells).
- Platelet rich plasma and related peripheral blood concentrates.
- *Electrical*: What can be modulated?
    - Piezoelectric effect of Yasuda.
    - Bioelectric or steady state potentials (Friedenberg and Brighton).

    How?
    - *Constant direct current stimulation (invasive percutaneous electrodes)*: Stimulates inflammatory like response—stage I of fracture healing.
    - *"Capacity coupled generators" (alternating current)*: Affects cyclic adenosine monophosphate (cAMP); collagen synthesis and calcification during repair.
    - *PEMF (pulsed electromagnetic field, time varying inductive coupling)*: Calcification of fibrocartilage (not fibrous tissue).

Miscellaneous Short Cases

- Ultrasound.
- External shockwave treatment.
- Bone morphogenic proteins:
    - BMP-2 (rhBMP-2; 1.5 mg/kg in collagen sponge);
    - BMP-7 [rhBMP-7 aka OP-1(osteogenic protein-1)]; and
    - BMP-14 (GDF-5/MP-52).

23. What are bone graft substitutes?

Ans. *Osteoinductive*:
- Allograft bone.
- Demineralized bone matrix [contains Type-I collagen, noncollagen protein and osteoinductive growth factors like transforming growth factor (TGF)-superfamily, bone morphogenetic protein (BMP), growth and differentiation factor (GDF)].
- Purified human BMP.
- OP-1 device
- INFUSE [rhBMP-2/ACS (absorbable collagen sponge)].

Osteoconductive:
- $CaPO_4$: Available as powder, ceramics (coralline, synthetic, etc. prepared by *sintering* (heating to temperature > 1000°C) cements and composite.
- $CaSO_4$.
- Allograft [stored at (–60°C); tested for HIV, hepatitis B virus (HBV), hepatitis C virus (HCV), syphilis—India; additionally for human T-cell leukemia-lymphoma virus (HTLV-I) and II and cytomegalovirus (CMV)—US, sterilized by γ-irradiation or ethylene oxide].

Hydroxyapatite:
- Bioactive glass (beads of silica, calcium oxide, disodium oxide and pyrophosphate).

Osteogenic and osteopromotive:
- Selective cellular retention (Cellect).
- Bone marrow aspirate injection or implantation.
- Platelet-rich plasma and blood concentrates.
- Stem cells.

24. What is distraction osteogenesis?

Ans. Actually it is distraction histogenesis. This is based on the philosophy of tissue generation under tension—"A living tissue (capable of regenerating) when put under steady traction can be lengthened to any extent in the line of tension vector by virtue of increased metabolism and vascularity". For bones the principles of compression and distraction osteogenesis both apply. Additionally, Ilizarov method can be used to its best by "accordion maneuver" and "trampoline effect" to enhance union.

- *Small segment nonunions (short stiff nonunions)*: Can be crushed by pressure effect in compression and then growth of fibrocartilage ensues which slowly ossifies due to trampoline effect if patient is bearing weight.
- Diseased or malunited segments can be removed for relatively longer nonunions and if the resulting gap less than 4 cm then acute docking in compression followed by lengthening can be done.
- For long and atrophic nonunions where the gap will be more than 4 cm; it is better to hold out the extremity to its length and do bone transport (internal/external/combined, as there is risk of kinking neurovascular bundle) in various modes:
    - Monofocal;
    - Bifocal; and
    - Trifocal.

25. What is corticotomy?

Ans. Best defined as "an open, subperiosteal, low-energy partial osteotomy of bone cortex, followed by manual osteoclasis of the remainder of cortical circumference maximally preserving the periosteum, endosteum and bone marrow with its blood supply as well as the muscle and soft tissue surrounding the bone". The term "compactotomy" is specifically used for diaphyseal corticotomy. Torsional corticotomy usually requires "external rotation" to prevent stretching radial and peroneal nerves.

26. What are various types of corticotomy?

Ans.
- *Transverse*: Lengthening, correction of deformity, bone transport.
- *Longitudinal*: To widen bone (overcoming defect in one of two bones improve shape of a thin atrophic limb).
- *Splinter*: Splints off a piece of bone with attached periosteum, soft tissue and skin—bridging nonunion, eliminate partial bony defects.
- *S-shaped corticotomy*: Chronic osteomyelitis.
- Complete.
- *Partial*: To correct bow in bones, e.g. osteogenesis imperfecta.

27. Where in bone will you do corticotomy?

Ans. Should be done at the center of rotation of angulation (CORA; apex of deformity) if done to correct deformities. For lengthening and other purposes metaphyseal location is best suited:
- Regenerate is of best quality.
- The nutrient artery has already branched and it is easier to preserve the same.
- Lastly the origins and insertions of muscles are adapted for extremity growth (that takes place at ends of bone)—so lengthening at ends of bone is more physiological.

Center of rotation of angulation basically is a locus from where all deformities in that plane can be addressed. Coexistence of various types of deformities (e.g. angular, translational, rotational, etc.) at various sites makes assessment of CORA more difficult and then multiple CORAs exist. For uniplanar angular deformity correction of deformity along the bisector of deformity (CORA) corrects the deformity completely. Calculation of CORA is a bit complicated but it should be sufficient to remember that there are two methods for doing so. First one is trigonometric which is more accurate; the other one is graphical method which is more of approximation.

28. What is the physiological effect of distraction osteogenesis "or" tell us some nonorthopedic uses of distraction osteogenesis?

Ans. There is increase in blood supply of limb by 330% so it can be used for treatment of peripheral vascular disease and trophic ulcer.

29. What are the complications of corticotomy?

Ans. Damage to vascularity, displacement after corticotomy, incomplete corticotomy, premature consolidation.

30. How do you assess regenerate?

Ans. Radiologically:
- No defects or shark bite lesions on three sides (if present—accordion maneuver).
- Complete ossification of radiolucent central growth zone.
- Uniform radiographic density that is half way between density of adjacent bones.

31. How do you reduce pin site infection?

Ans.
- Proper care.
- Proper tension
- Using special pins:
  - Titanium pins (900% less chances of infection, steel pins inhibit respiratory burst of granulocytes).
  - Hydroxyapatite (HA)-coated pins.
  - Silver coated pins (antimicrobial action of silver ions).

32. What is the rate of distraction and when do you start it?

Ans. Distraction at corticotomy site is done at the rate of 1 mm/day in equally divided intervals usually four (each 0.25 mm). Ideal will be to use motorized continuous motion distracters. Rate of distraction can be increased (up to 2 mm/day) in children or oblique corticotomy whereas it should be reduced in older age groups/diaphyseal corticotomy/poor bone quality. Distraction is started (latency) usually on fourth or fifth day former one being favored for children, oblique

Miscellaneous Short Cases

corticotomy. Waiting for an additional day or two (≈ 7 days) may be required for high energy, diaphyseal, comminuted corticotomy or accidental osteotomy, osteopenic or sclerotic bone and fragments rotated more than 30° for rotational osteoclasis.

33. What are the various types of bone transport?

Ans.
- *External bone transport*: Combined bone loss replacement (up to 5–7 cm) with correction of deformities and limb lengthening [can be monofocal (single corticotomy) or bifocal (dual site corticotomy and movement in opposite directions toward each other)].
- *Internal bone transport using olive or hooked wires*: For defects 7–10 cm and larger.
- *Combined bone transport*: For larger defects due to major bone loss combined with limb deformities, deep soft tissue scars and local blood supply insufficiency.

34. What are advantages and disadvantages of your technique?

Ans. External bone transport is easier and can simultaneously correct deformity and shortening but produces more skin scarring and is inadequate for major bone loss. Internal bone transport is better for larger bone defects and easier for patient as fewer wires are involved but it is difficult to apply and does not have enough "compression effect" at docking site.

35. For fracture of legs, which has better prognosis as regards union—a fracture of both bones or fracture of tibia only?

Ans. Fracture of both bones as nonfractured fibula quite often produces distraction at fracture tibia and prevents apposition of displaced fracture tibia. Even in simple fractures of both bones, fibula may unite early and become load sharing reducing axial loading of tibia. Partial fibulectomy may allow closer apposition of tibia and with weight bearing union could be enhanced.

36. How do you decide the treatment for nonunions?

Ans. Treatment options are decided on the basis of type of nonunion, location (epi-/meta-/diaphysis), age, bone quality, functional demands, movements at nearby joints, secondary changes in soft tissue, infection, prior treatments and presence of deformity and shortening. Most hypervascular nonunions will heal if adequately stabilized in optimum position combined with bone grafting. Sometimes biological enhancements (bone marrow, stem cells, electrical, etc.) may alone be used if fracture is acceptably aligned. Deformity correction may be done acutely with open methods if deformity is not grotesque (<4 cm shortening; <10-15° angulation). For larger deformities gradual correction would be a better option. Infected nonunions require specialized modalities (see above). Avascular nonunions often require diligent measures and planning for achieving union along with adjuncts.

(*You should be a part surgeon, part detective, and part historian. History has a way of repeating itself, without a clear understanding and appreciation of why previous treatments have failed; the learning "curve" becomes a "circle")

37. How much shortening is acceptable for treating nonunions of various bones?
Ans. *Shaft humerus*: 4-5 cm.

Both bones forearm: Up to 4 cm (proximal third of radius and distal 5-8 cm of ulna are dispensable and can be sacrificed for defects in these regions). Ideology is that elbow joint is primarily formed by proximal ulna and wrist joint by distal radius—this holds true for creating single bone forearm in complicated lesions.

Lower limb bones: Less than 3 cm (up to 1.5 inch of deformity can be hidden without producing ankle equinus).

38. How do you treat epiphyseal (intra-articular) nonunions?
Ans. These are usually oligotrophic type. Interfragmentary screw (e.g. cannulated lag screw) with arthroscopic intra-articular setting of bone and arthrolysis if required is most recommended. This may be followed by neutralization plating.

39. What is SCONE?
Ans. Slow compression over nail using external fixator.

Miscellaneous Short Cases

40. What is dynamization?

Ans. Supporting efforts at healing by providing or producing micromotion at fracture site—generally recommended for delayed unions.

Nails: Remove the screw that is farthest from nonunion (advantage—minimally invasive with immediate return to weight bearing, disadvantage—axial and rotational instability).

External fixator: This is both therapeutic (axial loading—further bony union) and diagnostic (↑ pain at fracture site suggests fracture has still not united). Achieved by removal/loosening/exchange/farther shifting of external struts spanning nonunion.

41. What principles underlie enhancing healing by exchange nailing?

Ans. Improves local mechanical environment (two ways) and local biological environment (two ways).

Mechanical advantages:
- *Larger diameter nail (usually 2-4 mm larger)*: Stronger and more stiff construct.
- *Widening and lengthening of isthmic portion of medullary canal*: Increase in stability due to increase in cortical contact area.

Biological advantages:
- *Reamings*: Local bone graft.
- *Reaming*: Decrease in medullary blood flow → dramatic increase in periosteal blood flow and periosteal bone formation.

Exchange nailing is applicable for both viable and nonviable nonunion. Preferred if circumferential bone loss less than 30% (failure rate high if defect >2 cm and/or >50% circumferential bone loss).

(*Additional information*: "Ultrasound adjuncts" have not been found useful for nonunions with intramedullary nail *in situ*).

42. What is the role of synostosis and amputation for managing nonunions?

Ans. Synostosis entails creation of bony continuity between paired bones above and below nonunion site functionally creating one bone extremity, e.g. single bone forearm. *Amputation; least preferred and is indicated for*:

- Frail, elderly unfit patient with infected nonunion.
- Unreconstructable neurologic function which precludes restoration of purposeful limb function.
- Patient wishes to discontinue medical and surgical treatment.
- When ultimately all viable reconstructive methods have failed and left over plans will produce less satisfactory function than with amputation.
- When reconstruction is impossible.

43. What are various types of callus response?

Ans. Callus is like sex—it is natural, it unites two ends, and it requires a bit of movement.

Primary callus response:

- Begins to form after two weeks of injury.
- Derived from *cambium layer* of periosteum and exuberant *external callus* beneath the intact periosteum.
- Spread from fracture end.
- Undergoes involution and does not cause bone union.
- Independent of environmental and hormonal influences.

External bridging callus:

- Under the control of hormonal and mechanical factors.
- Paracrine hormonal influences principally determine the blood supply.
- Inhibited by rigid fixation.
- Seen in cast immobilization and interlocking nails.

Late medullary callus:

- Seen in combination with external bridging callus.
- Dependent on medullary vascularity and independent of environment.
- Not inhibited by rigid fixation.

- Seen with plate fixation.

  [*Teaching note*: Sources of osteoprogenitor cells:
  - *DOPC*: Previously determined osteoprogenitor cells—present in the inner layer of periosteum (cambium and marrow).
  - *IOPC*: Inducible osteoprogenitor cells derived from undifferentiated soft tissue cells].

CASE III: PSEUDOARTHROSIS OF TIBIA

Diagnosis: The patient is a 6-year-old M/F with anterolateral angulation of left tibia at lower-third middle-third junction **(Fig. 9)** for 4 years. There is 1 cm true shortening of leg and wasting of 2 cm over calf muscles and patient is walking with short limb gait. There is associated right sided scoliosis of dorsal spine and café-au-lait spots over trunk.

COMMON FINDINGS

Inspection

- Anterolateral angulation of leg
- Foot deformity (type VI)
- Ankle valgus curly toes

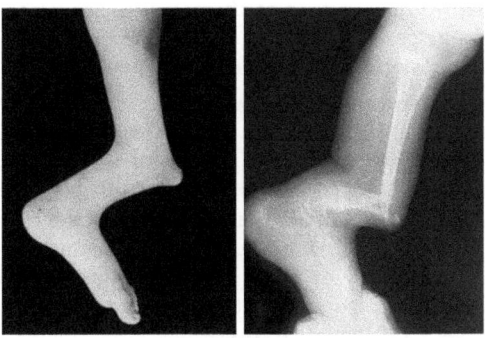

Fig. 9: Clinical and radiographic picture of congenital pseudarthrosis of tibia.

- Signs of neurofibromatosis
- Deformities in other limbs (fibrous dysplasia).

Palpation

- Thinning of tibia at angulation
- Tenderness
- Abnormal mobility (pathological fracture)
- Fibula and its status
- Wasting
- Constriction bands
- Contracted and prominent tendo-Achilles.

Associated Findings

- Other limb deformities
- Previous surgical procedures, etc.

1. What is your etiological diagnosis?

Ans. I would like to give differential diagnosis of congenital pseudarthrosis of tibia with neurofibromatosis (see below), congenital longitudinal deficiency of tibia (paraxial tibial hemimelia), congenital longitudinal fibular deficiency (paraxial fibular hemimelia), fibrous dysplasia, nonunion of tibia (if previous surgical procedures have been done and trauma +), rickets, postosteomyelitic pathological fracture, fibrous dysplasia.

2. What would you do to confirm your diagnosis?

Ans. I would get X-rays of leg with knee and ankle joints in anteroposterior (AP) and lateral projections.

3. What do you see on X-rays?

Ans. There is a pathology involving lower-third and middle-third junction of tibia with area of sclerosis or lucency (cyst formation). There is thinning of tibia or hour glass constriction and fibula is also dysplastic (you may find frank nonunion at the site). This suggests the diagnosis of congenital pseudoarthrosis of tibia (first described by Hatzoecher 1708, Barbar associated with neurofibromatosis; incidence = 0.005%, 1:190,000 live births).

4. When you do not see pseudarthrosis of tibia then why do you call it congenital pseudarthrosis of tibia?

Ans. Congenital pseudarthrosis of tibia is a misnomer, it is often neither congenital nor is there a primary or true pseudarthrosis. The nonunion (pseudarthrosis) develops usually after birth due to congenital "defect" in tibia. The defect lies in bone, periosteum, surrounding tissue and possibly nerve or vascular supply (likened to hamartoma) weakening the bone.

5. What are the diseases most commonly associated with congenital pseudoarthrosis of tibia?

Ans. Neurofibromatosis and fibrous dysplasia.

6. How do you look for pseudarthrosis and what is its impact on congenital pseudarthrosis of tibia?

Ans. Crawford criteria for neurofibromatosis (at least two of the following):
- Multiple café-au-lait spots (>5 mm and at least 5 mm).
- Positive family history.
- Definitive biopsy.
- Characteristic bony lesions such as congenital pseudoarthrosis of tibia; short sharply angulated, stiff (3S) scoliosis of spine.
- Fibroma molluscum (subcutaneous nodules) is not present until adolescence but they are typical of chronic disease.

The neurofibromatosis does not have any effect on the type of treatment or prognosis of disease.

7. How do you differentiate between skin lesions of neurofibromatosis and those of fibrous dysplasia?

Ans. The café-au-lait spots of congenital pseudarthrosis of tibia have smooth edge (coast of California) however, in fibrous dysplasia the lesions have appearance of coast of Maine (irregular edge).

8. How do you classify congenital pseudarthrosis of tibia?

Ans. Various classifications; Crawford, Boyd's, Anderson system **(Table 3)**.

Table 3: Classification of congenital pseudarthrosis of tibia.

Boyd	Description	Anderson equivalent
I	Patients born with anterior bowing and tibial defect	
II	Anterior bowing + hourglass contracture (fracture by 2 years) associated with neurofibromatosis (worse prognosis)	Dysplastic type
III	Bone cyst	Cystic type
IV	Sclerotic segment of tibia (no narrowing), usually develops stress type fracture—nonunion	Late/sclerotic type
V	Also have dysplastic fibula	Fibular type
VI	Intraosseous neurofibroma/Schwannoma (rarest type) Foot deformity [congenital talipes equinovarus (CTEV)/Streeter's band associated]	Clubfoot/congenital band type

9. What is conservative treatment for congenital pseudoarthrosis of tibia?

Ans. Done for patients without fracture or pseudarthrosis (prep-seudarthrosis). Total contact plastic clamshell orthosis, ankle-foot orthosis (AFO; prior to walking), knee-ankle-foot orthosis (KAFO; infant starting to walk). Worn indefinitely full-time; if fracture does not occur tibial bowing usually gradually improves and reformation of medullary canal often requires up to 5–10 years. If there is sufficient straightening of tibia, medullary canal is reformed and adequate cortical thickness then orthosis may be discontinued. Explain to parents that this is not a permanent remedy and may be of little use; ultimately surgery including amputation may be needed.

10. What are goals of surgical treatment and what are various modalities available?

Ans. *Goals:*
- Union at fracture site

Miscellaneous Short Cases

- Maintaining union
- Obtaining acceptable limb length.

Treatment options:

- McFarland type posterior bypass graft from opposite tibia (this is prophylactic grafting done in imminent fracture cases, inadequate bone structure, child whose activity cannot be controlled).
- EyreBrook's delayed bone grafting (older the patient with presentation greater are the chances of success).
- *Boyd's dual onlay cortical bone grafting with bicortical screw fixation (bone of parents/allograft)*: Early success but much ultimate failure.
- *Farmar's cross-legged vascularized pedicle bone grafting from opposite tibia*: Problematic as it is cumbersome and potential for infecting uninvolved tibia.
- *Sofield Miller's double proximal and distal osteotomy followed by reversal of tibial shaft with intramedullary nailing*: Reversing healthy bone to involved site may stimulate osteogenesis.
- Intramedullary nailing with iliac crest bone graft (Charnley).
- *Intramedullary bone graft with vascularized fibula and iliac crest*: Transfixes ankle and subtalar joint (retrograde insertion of rod).
- Microvascular fibular graft (contralateral), rib, iliac crest with excision of tibial pseudarthrosis.
- Electric current stimulation of osteogenesis.
- *Ilizarov method*: Compression, compression plus tibial lengthening, compression followed by distraction, distraction alone for hypertrophic nonunion.
- Amputation (McCarthy); Boyd/Symes type to produce end bearing stump:
  - Failed three surgical attempts
  - Shortening > 5 cm
  - Deformed foot

- Prolonged hospitalization
- Pseudarthrosis < 2.5 cm from ankle joint.

11. What are the complications of treatment?

Ans.
- Refracture;
- Limb length discrepancy;
- Ankle and subtalar stiffness;
- Progressive anterior angulation;
- Ankle valgus; and
- Donor site morbidity.

CASE IV: AMPUTATION STUMP

Simple case, having good chances to be put up in DNB exam. Very commonly performed surgery so practical aspects must not be of concern. Some theoretical aspects of course need polishing.

Read times: 2–3 times (DNB candidates), MS orth may get a short question instead.

Diagnosis: The patient is a 37-year-old male with healed, mature below knee amputation (BKA) stump of right leg done 15 cm from knee joint line with skewed flaps. The patient is using below knee prosthesis for mobilization for last 3 years.

If you know the reason for doing amputation—include in diagnosis.

FINDINGS

- Conical amputation stump covered with soft tissue (muscle and skin).
- No protruding or impinging bony ends.
- Healed incision line without sinus/discharge/excoriation/erythema/ulcers/keloid formation.
- There are no callosities.
- Vascularity of the stump is fair.

1. How do you define amputation?

Ans. Amputation is a procedure where a body part is removed through one or more bones (cf—disarticulation where it is removed from joint).

Miscellaneous Short Cases

2. What are the indications for doing amputation?

Ans. Amputation is philosophically required for:
- *Dead*: Complete irreversible loss of vascular supply to limb.
- *Dying*: For example, PVD, tumor, burns.
- *Deadly (dangerous)*: Necrotizing fasciitis, gas gangrene, etc.
- *Damn nuisance (damn useless limb or damn painful limb)*: Trauma/chronic osteomyelitis, nerve injury, trophic ulceration or neuropathic disorder, congenital, complete irreparable brachial plexus injury, etc.

3. What are the goals of amputation?

Ans.
- Ablation of diseased tissue;
- Reconstruction;
- Optimize patient function and reduce morbidity (palliation); and
- Provide a physiological end organ.

4. Why do you call flaps skewed?

Ans. The scar line is anterior from midline in coronal plane having long posterior flap.

5. What are various methods of configuring of flaps?

Ans. *Principles*:
- Use defined flaps in elective amputation with apex of flaps just distal to planned level of bony resection.
- Use any available flaps in trauma aiming to preserve length.
- Tailor flaps at least as long as diameter of the stump.
- Thick flaps without undermining or undue dissection.
- Flaps should not adhere to bone.
- No dog ears or unnecessary folds.

Options:
- *Equal anterior and posterior flaps*: Suits most amputations.
- Equal medial and lateral flaps [Scandinavian flaps—especially for peripheral vascular disease (PVD)].
- Long posterior flap (skewed flap)—commonly done in BKA and PVD.

6. What is the ideal length for amputation stumps at various places?

Ans. Amputation level is not primarily decided by ideal length at least now with the advent of modern prosthesis. The most distal level that will heal without complications and provide a functional stump should be chosen.

- Above the knee amputation (AKA):
  - 12 cm from medial joint line or 18 cm below greater trochanter tip.
- Below the knee amputation:
  - Ideal level is at musculotendinous junction of gastrocnemius. Ideal length would be 15 cm from medial knee joint line (stumps < 12 cm are less efficient and <6 cm do not function as below the knee stump); minimum working length is 9 cm.
  - Rule of thumb—allow 2.5 cm (1 inch) for every 30 cm (12 inch) height otherwise preoperatively flex the knee at right angle and if the residual tibia extends at least three finger breadth beyond insertion of medial hamstring tendons then patient can be fitted for below-knee prosthesis.
- Above the elbow (A/E) amputation:
  - 20 cm from acromion.
- Below the elbow (B/E) amputation:
  - 18 cm from tip of olecranon.

7. How do you determine adequacy of vascularity of flaps?

Ans. *Clinically*: Skin temperature, level of dependent rubor, feel pulses (the level till pulses can be felt will support the skin adequately even distally some 5–8 cm can survive by collateral circulation).

Investigations:

- *Doppler*: Inaccurate in elderly patients (calcified vessels)—ankle brachial pressure index more than 0.45 provided 90% chances of healing.
- *Toe systolic blood pressure (BP)*: 55 mm Hg is minimum required for distal healing.
- *Transcutaneous PO_2*: Minimum 35 mm Hg for healing.

Miscellaneous Short Cases

- Arteriogram or digital subtraction angiography.
- Skin blood flow (^{133}Xe clearance), thermography, thallium scanning, etc. largely research tools.
- Intraoperatively adequate bleeding form flaps and oozing from muscles (remember to deflate tourniquet).

8. How will you assess the patient for amputation (or what precautions will you take before proceeding with amputation)?

Ans. Tissue perfusion as above.

Immune competence and nutritional status of patient for adequate healing: Serum albumin at least 3 g/dL, hemoglobin level at least 10 g/dL, lymphocyte count more than 1,500/mL.

Systemic: Control diabetes, optimize renal, cardiac, and liver functions.

Psychological: Early plan for return to function, preoperative counseling, rehabilitation assessment.

Preoperative pain control: Coordination with experts in pain management.

9. What intraoperative precautions will you take for tailoring an ideal stump?

Ans. Planning flaps as mentioned.

Muscles divide some 5 cm distal to level of bone resection, stabilize muscle mass to prevent sensation of instability during prosthetic fitting and ambulation.

Nerves: Divide cleanly with sharp knife after gentle traction and allow to retract at least 1 inch. Large nerves should be ligated for they contain vessels, e.g. sciatic nerve.

Vessels: Large arteries and veins should be doubly ligated to secure hemostasis. In general hematoma formation should be prevented by meticulous hemostasis.

- *Bone*: Plan a level as this is often the reference point (apart from flaps). No sharp ends or margins, bevel the end to give desired shape and should not impinge or come in direct contact (and adhere) with skin flaps.

- *Closure*: There should be no tension at margins, interrupted monofilament sutures to give good scar.
- *Drains*: If infected or hematoma expected.
- *Dressing*: Compression soft dressing or molding dressing reinforced by POP cast or slab.
- Prevent contractures.

10. What do you mean by muscle stabilization?

Ans. Muscles must be so secured that they do not wiggle under the effect of prosthetic fitting during mobilization as it gives a sensation of constant discomfort.

Methods:
- *Myodesis (preferred)*: Here the muscle or tendon is attached to bone by drill holes. Should not be done for ischemic limb (↑ chances of wound breakdown). It effectively counterbalances the antagonists, provides good strength and minimizes atrophy, maximizing residual limb function, prevents contractures.
- *Myoplasty*: Here the muscle is sutured to periosteum or fascia of opposing group (antagonists) for counterbalancing action.

11. How will you prevent contractures?

Ans. The following are the various methods to prevent contractures:
- Make the patient lie prone;
- Muscle setting exercises;
- Myodesis;
- Early mobilization and pain control (prevents spasm); and
- Immediate postoperative prosthetic fitting.

12. What are the complications of amputation surgery?

Ans. *Early*:
- Wound hematoma.
- Flap breakdown, infection (especially in diabetics), clostridial infection secondary to perineal contamination.
- Joint contracture.
- Wound pain, phantom sensation, phantom pain.

Late:
- Joint contracture, instability.
- Pain due to pressure of ill-fitting socket, phantom pain, neuroma.
- Stump edema due to venoconstriction, unstable—too much soft tissue left failure to perform myodesis.
- Skin verrucous hyperplasia, skin maceration, fungal infection or intertrigo, blisters, abrasion, atrophy, callosities, follicular hyperkeratosis, sycosis barbae, allergic reactions to material of cup or liner.
- Bone spur formation—due to periosteal bone formation—avoid periosteal stripping osteoporosis, fracture.
- Cosmesis sitting asymmetry, bulbous stump, e.g. symes in females, severely scarred stump.

13. Why do you prefer distal amputation?

Ans. More acceptable, ethically preserves as much normal tissue as possible, less energy expenditure and higher compliance.

Energy expenditure depends upon:
- Length of residual limb (amputation level), unilateral or bilateral **(Table 4)**.
- Reason for amputation.
- Aerobic capacity and cardiopulmonary efficiency, patient age and fitness.
- *Speed of gait*: Walking speed decreases with more prox amputation, gait symmetry.
- Weight of prosthesis and weight concentration.

Table 4: Energy expenditure and level of amputation.

Level of amputation	Beyond baseline (energy consumption)
Long BKA	10% +
Medium BKA	25% +
Short BKA	40% +
Average AKA	65% +
Hip disarticulation	100% +

14. What is the timing of prosthetic fitting?

Ans.
- *Immediate* [immediate postoperative prosthesis (IPOP)] *(See Chapter 10: Prosthetics and Orthotics).*
- *Prompt* (7-10 days): With evidence of stump healing ("preparatory prosthesis").
- *Early* (≈ 3 weeks): After the stump has healed.
- *Late*: After the stump has fully matured—less chances of wound breakdown.

Stump modulation occurs for up to 6 months postoperatively; therefore, the patient should be assessed regularly. Usually a new socket has to be given after 2-3 months. The patient should be explained thoroughly that repeated visits in the early period are essential and normal.

15. What do you understand by preprosthetic care?

Ans. *Postoperative or preprosthetic care*: This phase includes the time period during which the amputation stump undergoes maturation.

Goals of preprosthetic care:
- Promotes wound healing;
- Reduces postsurgical edema;
- Molding of residual limb;
- Preventing flexion contractures;
- Maintain muscle strength in the affected limb;
- Maintain muscle strength in the unaffected limb; and
- Maintain body symmetry.

16. What is pylon prosthesis?

Ans. Pylon or endoskeletal (means—structure of "prosthesis", do not confuse with osteointegrated prosthesis) prosthesis with adjustments began to appear in 1960 for use as temporary limbs. Ultimate concept being an adjustable endoskeletal structure that could be carried in to definitive prosthesis, the pylon being covered with resilient foam shaped to match the contralateral leg. Basic technique involves fitting plaster socket on operating table that incorporates an aluminum fitting to which pylon can be attached bearing an artificial

foot. Patient is made to touch down the prosthesis within 24 hours and can bear weight in ensuing days. The benefits are as follows (not all are accepted by community without controversy at large):
- Control of postoperative edema;
- Reduction of postoperative pain;
- Improved wound healing;
- Early gait training and walking;
- Reduced hospital stay;
- More rapid stump maturation;
- Earlier fitting of definitive prosthesis;
- Psychological benefit to patient "waking up with arm or leg";
- Prevents contractures; and
- More frequent sparing of knee joint when amputation is done for PVD.

Difficulties:
- Cast loosening with edema subsidence;
- Pistoning effect can increase edema and wound breakdown;
- Heaviness of cast, impedes walking; and
- Muscle atrophy.

17. What are the advantages of through knee amputation?

Ans. *Advantages*:
- Large end bearing surfaces of distal femur are preserved;
- Long lever arm controlled by strong muscles is created; and
- The prosthesis used on the stump is stable.

18. What is inactive residual extremity syndrome and how do you manage it?

Ans. Some patients in spite of being treated with well-performed amputation experience persistent residual extremity pain, swelling, a sense of instability and inability to tolerate extended prosthetic ambulation. Extremity hence undergoes atrophy and becomes a passive participant in mobilization. This symptom complex is known as inactive residual extremity syndrome. The Ertl osteomyoplastic lower extremity amputation reconstruction is described to treat such patients for transtibial and transfemoral amputations.

Technique: Osteoperiosteal flaps are raised from end stump of bone and bone further resected → the osteoperiosteal flaps are closed over medullary canal sealing it off (osteoplasty) → superimposed myoplasty attaching antagonizing muscle groups is performed → skin is contoured to underlying myoplasty.

19. What is phantom limb sensation and phantom limb pain?
Ans. Phantom limb sensation is the feeling that amputated limb is still present sometimes in contorted positions. In early days the sensation is often accompanied with pain that can be managed with analgesics. It is later replaced by intermittent paresthesia and still further by mere awareness of absent limb. Some patients experience *"jacitation"*—distressing phantom limb pain with involuntary jerking of stump. This is resistant to treatment and is more likely to be present in patients with chronic pain and sepsis before amputation. Cause is not known but "trigger points" may be identified in some; other proposed mechanisms include absence of normal afferent barrage (C-fiber atrophy) especially at night, hypersensitive axonal sprouts from cut nerve ends, changes in spinal cord physiology (altered peptide concentrations, etc.), extrapolation by brain of limb location.

CASE V: EXAMINATION OF SWELLING

Examination of a bony swelling is not only interesting but a vast topic, viva of which can proceed in any direction sometimes to the weirdest of extents. Only the most basic aspects of it are presented here that are must for candidate to learn and without which only an exceptional examiner would forgive. The details of various tumor types are better learnt from standard textbook(s).

Read times: 2–4 times for MS and DNB candidates; better judge it from your capability.

Diagnosis: The patient is a 17-year-old male with solitary, nontender benign looking swelling over upper leg. The swelling is fixed to tibia,

Miscellaneous Short Cases

around 6 × 4 cm, spherical, bony hard, smooth, nonlobulated with defined edges. The swelling is nonfluctuant, noncompressible or reducible, nonpulsatile and does not transilluminate. The overlying skin (and muscle) is not fixed (rather tethered) to the swelling.

Look for solitary or multiple lesions, type of bone (long/flat), site affected (metaphysis/diaphysis/epiphysis).

1. Why do you call it a benign swelling?

Ans. Brief history suggests that swelling appeared insidiously followed by pain and that the swelling has progressed from the size of a lemon to pear in last 6 years.

On inspection:
- The skin is not stretched or shiny smooth.
- There are no dilated veins.
- There is no discoloration.
- There are no secondary skin changes (inflammation, ulcer formation or fungation, loss of skin appendages).

On palpation:
- Local temperature not raised.
- Nontender swelling.
- Well-defined edge (margins are for ulcer).
- Smooth surface.
- Not tethered to skin or surrounding soft tissue.
- No pain on bearing weight or movements.
- No evidence of pathological fracture (not a very consistent finding for differentiating a benign from a malignant swelling—better drop it!).

2. How do you determine that the swelling is fixed to or emanating from bone?

Ans. The swelling is continuous with bone when I palpate the edges of the swelling. There is no intervening tissue between bone and swelling. The swelling congruently moves with the movements of bone. The swelling arises from beneath the muscles which overlie it.

3. What else would you like to examine?

Ans.
- Sessile or pedunculated.
- Deformity in the bone secondary to the swelling.

- ROM of nearby joints.
- Lymphadenopathy.

4. How will you differentiate that the swelling is below the muscle or above it?

Ans. Ask the patient to tense the muscles overlying the swelling by appropriate resistive maneuver, e.g. pressing the knee down for an anteriorly located lower thigh swelling. Observe the following:
- Movement of the swelling in the direction of muscle fibers and perpendicular to it.
- Prominence of swelling.

If the swelling becomes more prominent on tensing the muscle, it indicates that the swelling overlies the muscle otherwise disappearance of swelling suggests that it is deep to the muscles. A swelling arising from the muscle itself shows variable change depending upon where it lies within muscle fibers and the support for swelling increases if it lies in the superficial fibers making it more prominent and vice versa. Now here the assessment of mobility takes an important role.

The mobility of a swelling that overlies the muscle is not changed while that of a swelling arising from muscle is lost when movement is attempted in the direction of fibers or perpendicular to a taught muscle (swelling that underlies the muscle often disappears unless it is large and bony or stony hard).

5. How do you determine if a swelling is soft/firm/hard on clinical examination?

Ans. A *stony hard* swelling is not indentable offering some friction or a "gritty feeling" to the examining hand. *Bony or woody hard* swelling is also not indentable but is smooth or lobulated. *Rubbery swelling* is hard to firm or firm like touching the nose tip. A swelling that is soft and squashable offering some resilience is "*spongy*". Swelling feeling like your ear lobe (spongy and squashable) is a "*soft*" swelling.

Bony swelling may have some typical surface characteristics like "crackling egg-shell consistency" of a giant cell tumor (GCT), variable consistency (firm on surface to bony hard at

Miscellaneous Short Cases

pedicle) for an osteochondroma. Swelling may be indentable like a "ping pong" ball in aneurysmal bone cyst (ABC).

6. What is your differential diagnosis?

Ans. Benign bone tumors like osteochondroma, osteoma, GCT, osteoid osteoma, chondromyxoid fibroma, osteoblastoma, ABC.

Learn and remember the tumor distribution as per diaphyseal location, metaphyseal location, epiphyseal location, which may be asked for enumeration—it is always better to develop your own list. A brief list is presented here:

- *Epiphyseal lesions*: Chondroblastoma, chondrosarcoma, giant cell tumor.
- *Metaphyseal lesions*: Any lesion.
- *Diaphyseal lesions*: Ewing's sarcoma, osteoblastoma, lymphoma, adamantinoma, fibrous dysplasia, eosinophilic granuloma.
- *Flat bones*: Ewing's sarcoma, metastasis, myeloma, chondrosarcoma.
- *Vertebral body*: GCT, metastasis, Ewing's sarcoma, eosinophilic granuloma.
- *Posterior elements of vertebra*: ABC, osteoid osteoma, osteoblastoma.

7. How do you stage benign bony swellings?

Ans. In Enneking classification the benign bone tumors are classified according to activity of the tumor:

- *Latent*: Remains static or heals spontaneously like nonossifying fibroma.
- *Active*: Progressive growth limited by natural barriers like ABC.
- *Aggressive*: Progressive growth, invasive, not limited by natural barriers like GCT.

8. What is Enneking classification of bone tumors?

Ans. Enneking classified the malignant and benign bone tumors **(Table 5)**.

Enneking classification of malignant bone tumors is based on a combination of parameters [grade of tumor (G1: low-grade, G2: high-grade), compartment involved (T) and metastasis (M)].

Table 5: Enneking classification of malignant bone tumor.

Stage	Grade	Site	Metastasis
IA	G1	T1	M0
IB	G1	T2	M0
IIA	G2	T1	M0
IIB	G2	T2	M0
III	G1/G2	T1/T2	M1

Table 6: Staging of bone sarcoma by AJCC.

Stage	Grade	Primary tumor	Metastasis in regional lymph nodes	Distant metastasis
IA	G1/G2	T1a/b	N0	M0
IB	G1/G2	T2a	N0	M0
IIA	G1/G2	T2b	N0	M0
IIB	G3/G4	T1a/b	N0	M0
IIC	G3/G4	T2a	N0	M0
III	G3/G4	T2b	N0	M0
IV	Any G	Any T	N1	M0
IV	Any G	Any T	Any N	M1

Compartment is defined as a natural barrier to tumor extension like bone, fascia, synovial tissue, periosteum or cartilage. The tumor may be intracompartmental (T1) or extracompartmental (T2).

Stage I is a low-grade tumor while II is high-grade one. Substage "B" means an extracompartmental tumor and stage III is a metastatic tumor.

American Joint Committee Classification (AJCC) for staging of bone sarcomas is more comprehensive as follows **(Table 6)**:

G1: well-differentiated, G2: moderately differentiated, G3: poorly differentiated, G4: undifferentiated. T1: tumor 8 cm or less in greatest dimension, T2: tumor more than 8 cm in greatest dimension (a: superficial tumor, b: deep tumor). N0: no regional lymph node metastasis, N1: regional lymph node metastasis.

9. What is the stage of tumor when it presents with an extraosseous component?

Ans. Often stage IIB.

10. What will you do next?

Ans. I will get an X-ray of the involved region in at least two perpendicular planes.

11. What will you see on an X-ray?

Ans. Specifically I will look for parent bone and changes (site, extent, cortical breach, etc.), tumor mass, destruction pattern, periosteal reaction and tumor mineralization patterns (osteoid, chondroid, reactive bone mineralization).

12. What are the various types of periosteal reactions?

Ans. Takes 10 days to three weeks to appear:
- *Type I*: Solid periosteal reaction **(Fig. 10)**.
    - *Shell formation*: Simultaneous bone removal of bone from endosteal surface with surface deposition of bone. Thickness depends on the balance between the two.

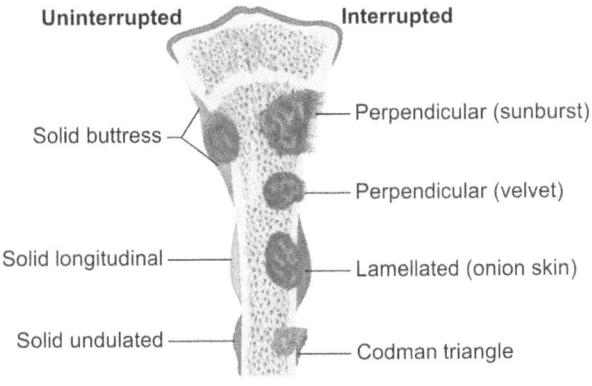

Fig. 10: Various types of periosteal reactions.

- *Smooth shells*: Associated with benign tumors.
- *Lobulated shells*: Due to focal variation in growth rate.
- *Ridged shell*: Trabeculated, septated or soap-bevel reaction. This is due to uneven destruction. Seen in nonossifying fibroma, GCT, ABC, enchondroma and some malignant tumors like chondro/fibrosarcoma, plasmacytoma and metastasis from thyroid, melanoma, renal.

- *Type II*: Continuous periosteal reaction with cortical persistence.
  - *Solid periosteal reaction*: Multiple layers of bone deposition due to chronic stimulation of bone by a relatively slow growing bony lesion, e.g. osteoid osteoma, subacute osteomyelitis. It is referred to as cortical thickening or hyperostosis.
  - *Single lamellar reaction*: Single layer of new bone in the form of a uniform radiodense line considered hallmark of benign process, e.g. histiocytosis X, osteoid osteoma, fractures.
    - Dense undulating periosteal reactions are a variant seen with low-grade osteomyelitis, osteoarthropathy associated with paraneoplastic lesions or varicose veins, periosteitis.
  - *Lamellated reactions*: Seen with active bone-destroying lesions like acute osteomyelitis, Ewing's sarcoma, and osteosarcoma.
  - *Parallel speculated reaction*: "Hair-on-end appearance" seen with more rapidly destroying malignant process due to bone formation along the radial neovascularization.

- *Type III*: Interrupted periosteal reactions seen with aggressive tumors reaching subperiosteal location after cortical breach.
  - *Buttress*: Solid bone formation at cortical margins of a slowly but constantly growing lesion.
  - *Codman angle*: Represents the buttress lesion in an aggressive neoplasm. First described by Ribbert was elaborated upon by Codman in 1926. It can be seen

in any lesion that aggressively lifts the periosteum like acute osteomyelitis, ABC, osteoma, osteosarcoma, chondrosarcoma. They result from subperiosteal bleeding and bone formation and are themselves free from tumor.
- *Type IV*: Complex periosteal reactions.
  - *Divergent speculated pattern aka sunburst pattern*: Combination of reactive bone formation and malignant bone formation, it contains areas of reactive and sarcoma bone with intervening areas of cellular tumor and tumor products. It is highly suggestive of osteosarcoma but can also be seen in osteoblastic active metastasis and hemangioma.

13. **What are the various types of bone destructions?**

Ans. Bone destruction has to be analyzed on the following grounds before grouping them:
- Pattern of bone destruction and configuration of marginal interface.
- Cortical breach.
- Presence of sclerotic rim.
- Expansion of parent bone.

Type I: Geographic bone destruction:
- *Geographic lesion with sclerotic margin*: Seen in nonossifying fibroma, unicameral bone cyst, chondroblastoma, fibrous dysplasia.
- *Geographic lesions without sclerotic margins*: GCT.
- *Geographic lesions with ill-defined margins*: Seen in GCT, fibrosarcoma, and chondrosarcoma. Aggressive benign neoplasms such as enchondroma, chondroblastoma, desmoplastic fibroma.

Type II: *Moth-eaten destruction (regional invasion)*: Multiple scattered holes that vary in size interspersed with apparently preserved bone. This pattern is seen in Ewing's sarcoma, primary lymphoma, chondrosarcoma, fibrosarcoma, and osteosarcoma, sometimes acute osteomyelitis.

Type III: *Permeative destruction*: Poorly demarcated with indistinct margins. Can be seen in numerous destructive processes not limited only to neoplastic (round cell tumors, angiosarcoma, high-grade chondrosarcoma, etc.), mechanical, inflammatory (acute osteomyelitis), and metabolic lesions of bone.

14. What else would you like to do and why?

Ans. I would get detailed radiological investigations to determine and plan management:
- *Bone scan*:
    - Intramedullary extent of tumor—classically the bone was cut 6 cm proximal to the lesion demarcated by scintigraphy.
    - Polyostotic disease.
    - Metastasis.
    - Biological activity of tumor.
- *CT scan*: Bony extent and margins of tumor and cortical breach.
- *MRI*:
    - Medullary extent.
    - Soft tissue component and extent.
    - Involvement of vital structures.
- *Angiography*:
    - Tumor blood supply.
    - Embolization to reduce intraoperative bleeding.
    - Relationship of major vessels to tumor.
    - Feasibility of intra-arterial chemotherapy.

15. Which bone tumor metastasizes to bones?

Ans. Osteosarcoma.

16. What will you do for this patient?

Ans. Management planning is done only after characterization of the tumor that includes doing a bone biopsy before proceeding any further.

17. What are the principles of bone biopsy?

Ans.
- Should be done at the conclusion of staging (to avoid radiological artifacts).
- Avoid sampling error, take multiple samples from the lesion (this is necessary for sarcomas but single specimens may suffice for carcinomas).

Miscellaneous Short Cases

- The biopsy tract should be incorporated into the planned surgical incision.
- Biopsy should be done from the representative tissue.
- Biopsy tract should be the shortest way to tumor.
- Should not violate more than one compartment.
- Should not be done from intermuscular planes.
- Should be remote from the main neurovascular bundle.
- Try not to violate the cortex and take sample from the extracortical bone tissue (to prevent weakening the bone by creating a stress riser defect).
- Bone window should not have any sharp corners (avoiding stress risers)—prefer an oblong window.
- Avoid transverse incisions (prefer longitudinal incisions).
- Do a sharp dissection, close with a subcuticular stitch.
- Obtain meticulous hemostasis (to avoid hematoma formation); a drain if absolutely needed must be placed in the line of incision, or through the wound.
- For an incisional biopsy take tumor tissue, reactive tissue, pseudocapsule, capsule.
- Biopsy should be ideally done by the surgeon going to finally operate the patient.

18. What are the various types of biopsy?

Ans.
- Fine needle aspiration cytology (FNAC; not very useful for sarcomas).
- Core or trephine biopsy using a 14-gauge needle (usually recommended for most bone tumors).
- Incisional biopsy (for failed core biopsy, vascular bone tumors, ABC).
- Excisional biopsy (usually done for small lesions <2–3 mm in longest diameter).

19. What surgery will you do for this patient and what are the various advantages and disadvantages of the resection procedures?

Ans. Four types of excision based on the relationship of dissection plane to the tumor and pseudocapsule **(Fig. 11)**.

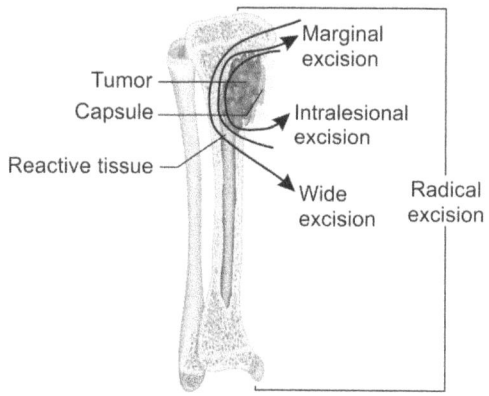

Fig. 11: Types of bone tumor excision.

- *Intralesional excision*: Performed within the tumor mass and removes only a portion of tissue, the pseudocapsule and macroscopic tumor are often left behind.
- *Marginal excision*: Dissection plane passes through the pseudocapsule, may leave microscopic tissue behind.
- *Wide (en-bloc) excision*: Removal of tumor tissue, pseudocapsule, and a cuff of normal tissue (some >1 cm) peripheral to the tumor tissue in all directions. This is often the desired procedure for a sarcoma but the normal tissue is a matter of controversy.
- *Radical excision*: Removal of tumor and entire containing compartment, taking care of skip metastasis 1, 2 done for benign lesions or for palliative procedures in metastases. 3, 4 for curative malignant lesion. Amputation can be 2, 3, and 4 depending upon the plane through which it passes.

20. What is the difference between a "satellite" lesion and a "skip" lesion?

Ans. "Skip lesions" are present in the same anatomical compartment; they are "not" in continuity with the main tumor mass that forms outside the pseudocapsule.

Miscellaneous Short Cases

"Satellite lesions", in turn, are formed within the pseudo-capsule and are in continuity with the main tumor mass.

21. What is three-strike rule?

Ans. The four key components are:
- Bone;
- Nerves;
- Vessels; and
- Soft tissue envelop.

If any of the three key components are involved then limb salvage is not worth considering "three-strike rule".

22. What are the types of chemotherapy?

Ans.
- *Adjuvant chemotherapy*: Given after surgical procedure for control of residual tumor and metastasis or micrometastasis.
- *Neoadjuvant chemotherapy*: Given before the surgical procedure and after it ("Sandwich technique") often for a limb salvage procedure. It is aimed to:
  - Chemotherapeutic drugs start acting immediately helping control micrometastasis.
  - Reduce the stage of tumor (at least 90% kill is desired, if <90% then change agents—there is no evidence of increased survival in those that do not respond to initial or deemed most effective agents).
  - Determine the response of tumor to chemotherapy (sort of "sensitivity testing" for drugs).
  - Reduce mass and vascularity of tumor.
  - Buy time for surgical intervention and prosthetic design.
- *Definitive chemotherapy*: For tumors that are highly chemosensitive (Ewing's sarcoma).
- *Palliative*: For tumors that cannot be resected.

23. What is the role of radiotherapy?

Ans. Adjuvant radiotherapy had been largely replaced with chemotherapy. Use of megavoltage and orthovoltage radiation to control micrometastasis and tumor volume reduction has now but immensely helped the limb salvage procedures. It can be given in neoadjuvant or adjuvant modes. Radiotherapy acts by rupture of chemical bonds of complex molecules, generation of highly reactive free radicals and hydrolysis, direct deoxyribonucleic acid (DNA) damage and strand breakage and lastly to damage to vascularity which is quite prominent in sarcomas. The damage is more pronounced in rapidly dividing cells (high turnover) but success is dependent on the rate of recovery of surrounding normal tissue.

Dosage is measured in terms of Rad (radiation absorbed dose) which is a measure of the energy imparted to the matter by ionizing radiation per unit mass (1 Rad—0.01 J/kg). Grays (Gr) = 1 joule of energy absorbed by a mass of 1 kg tissue (= 100 Rad). Radiation is given in daily fractionated doses resulting in repair of normal tissues but exponential kill of tumor tissue. Multisite radiation (multiaxial radiation) protects the normal tissue from excessive radiation but the total energy delivered to the tumor is high often in the form of "limit movement" (large amount of energy delivered in packets over few seconds). Tumors that are amenable to radiotherapy are few and include Ewing's sarcoma, osteosarcoma, and myeloma.

24. What is the most common soft tissue tumor in children?
Ans. Hemangioma.

25. What is the most common soft tissue tumor in adults?
Ans. Lipoma.

26. What is the most common malignant soft tissue tumor in children and adults?
Ans. It is rhabdomyosarcoma for children and malignant fibrous histiocytoma for adults.

27. What is the most common primary benign and malignant bone tumor?
Ans. Osteochondroma and osteosarcoma.

28. What is the most common bone tumor of hand?
Ans. Enchondroma.

29. What is the most common secondary benign bone tumor?
Ans. Aneurysmal bone cyst.

Miscellaneous Short Cases

30. What is the most common secondary malignancy of bone?

Ans. In the order—malignant fibrous histiocytoma, osteosarcoma, and fibrosarcoma.

31. What is the most common sarcoma of foot and ankle?

Ans. Synovial sarcoma.

32. What is the most common sarcoma of hand?

Ans. Epithelioid sarcoma.

33. What are the common anterior spinal tumors?

Ans. Giant cell tumor, hemangioma, eosinophilic granuloma, metastasis, chordoma, multiple myeloma.

34. What tumors do you find in posterior spinal elements?

Ans. Aneurysmal bone cyst, osteoid osteoma, osteoblastoma.

35. Can you tell characteristic immunostains for some tumors?

Ans. Lymphoma (+CD20), Ewing's sarcoma (+CD99), chordoma (keratin, S100), adamantinoma (keratin).

36. Is genetics associated with bone tumors or they are developmental?

Ans. Yes, it is only a fact of matter that we have not identified all. Some common ones are:
- Ewing's sarcoma t(11;22)(q24;q12); and
- Synovial sarcoma t(X:18).

37. What are the various osteosarcoma variants?

Ans. 11 variants (first three are forms of osteosarcoma):
- Osteosarcoma of jaw
- Multicentric osteosarcoma
- Secondary osteosarcoma

Variants of primary osteosarcoma:
- Conventional
- Low-grade intramedullary
- Low-grade superficial (parosteal and periosteal)
- High-grade intramedullary
- High-grade superficial
- Small cell variant
- Chondroblastic variant

- Giant cell rich osteosarcoma
- Osteoblastic
- Fibroblastic
- Telangiectatic.

CASE VI: VOLKMANN'S ISCHEMIC CONTRACTURE AND COMPARTMENT SYNDROME

Often considered as a difficult case needing specialized review and guidance. The case is moderately important and is a good choice for examiners. Diagnosis is often clear and emphasis is on examination and identifying other lesions (nerve injuries) and approach to treatment. The viva can quickly jump to compartment syndrome and its management so kindly be thorough with the details of compartment syndrome—*I recommend reading from Chapter 16 of the book Essential Orthopedics: Principles and Practice, 2nd edition for comprehensiveness.*

Read times: 4-6 times (MS orth and DNB candidates).

Diagnosis: The patient is a 14-year-old male with posttraumatic (if etiology known then mention it viz supracondylar fracture humerus, both bone forearm fracture, etc.) moderate Volkmann's ischemic contracture (VIC) of left forearm of 7 months duration with median nerve involvement. There is associated metacarpophalangeal/interphalangeal (MCP/IP) joint contracture of 2-4th digits of hand.

FINDINGS

- Wrist flexion.
- Volkmann's sign positive.
- Pronated forearm, wasting.
- Flexed elbow.
- Cord-like induration on the flexor side, extensors affected or spared.
- MCP joints flexed or extended and IP joints flexed or extended.
- Paresthesia or anesthesia in the hand and fingers (related to the involved nerve).
- Flexed and adducted thumb.
- Claw hand.

Miscellaneous Short Cases

- Deformity and trophic changes due to ulnar and median nerve involvement.
- Additionally, there would be signs of causative injury (deformity in forearm bones, supracondylar region of humerus deformity, etc.).

1. Why do you call it Volkmann's ischemic contracture (VIC)?

Ans. History of trauma followed by swelling and functional loss. There is treatment with POP cast that produced increasing pain not abated by analgesics. Slowly developing contracture. Wasting and fibrosis of muscles, involvement of skin with scar (contracted). Typical posture of hand and attitude of limb. Volkmann's sign positive and other findings as above.

2. What is Volkmann's sign and what is its significance?

Ans. Inability to actively extend fingers (at IP and/or MCP joints) without flexing wrist "and" passive extension of fingers possible only with wrist flexion (or conversely wrist flexion with passive finger extension). It differentiates the deformity due to nerve palsy and those due to intrinsic muscle contracture of long flexors. Also it can differentiate between intrinsic minus hand from long flexor contracture **(Fig. 12)**.

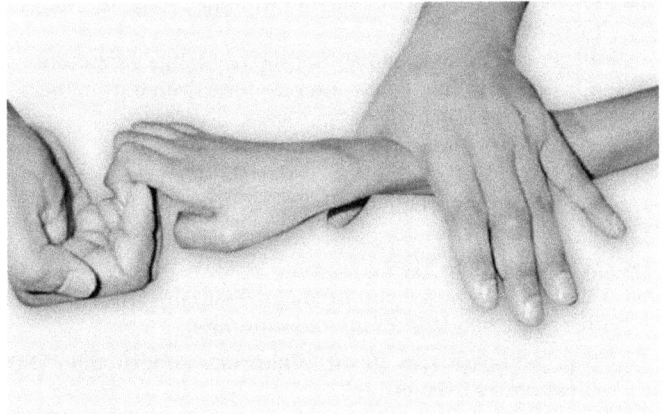

Fig. 12: Volkmann's sign.

(One may wonder why the Volkmann's sign is not described in a supposedly simpler way—"finger flexion with passive wrist extension", the explanation is—try on yourself and you will appreciate that it is a normal finding—the tenodesis effect).

3. What is the pathogenesis of Volkmann's sign?
Ans. The sign is due to "constant length phenomenon" of the fibrotic muscles that lose their elasticity and produce fixed length. Because the flexor group is predominantly affected so on passive extension the flexion at wrist and fingers is the prominent finding.

4. Do you see any other condition that produces "constant length phenomenon"?
Ans. Constant length phenomenon may be seen with tethering of tendons in callus or in scar tissue. In leg, tendon of flexor hallucis longus (FHL) may get incarcerated in the callus of healing distal one-third tibia fracture or in surgical scar ("check-rein deformity"). At wrist deep cut injury may incarcerate flexor tendons in the healing tissue of the surgical wound.

5. What is your differential diagnosis?
Ans. Cases are usually very evident but some milder versions may be confused with:
- Post-traumatic hematoma and resulting contracture.
- Osteomyelitis and muscle involvement either by intervention or disease process.
- Hemangioma of forearm muscles.
- Pseudo-VIC [tethering of muscle often flexor digitorum profundus (FDP) to healing fracture].
- Burns.

6. Who described VIC?
Ans. Richard Von Volkmann of Halle, Germany (1881) resulting from tight bandage for injured extremity.

7. How will you test flexor digitorum superficialis (FDS) contracture in isolation?
Ans. Flex FDP to fullest to relax it completely then stretch FDS.

8. What is Seddon's ellipsoid?

Ans. Seddon described ischemic zone of injury usually following brachial artery injury that acquires ellipsoid shape which is in general different from conical ischemic zones observed in lung and liver ischemia. The long axis of the ellipse runs usually around anterior interosseous artery with center just above mid-forearm. Nerve at the center is the one most affected in VIC; which is often median nerve whereas ulnar nerve often is at periphery and is variably involved. FDP and flexor pollicis longus (FPL) lying on either side of vessel are the most severely affected muscles. Necrotic muscle is colloquially termed "muscle sequestrum".

9. How do you classify VIC?

Ans.

- *Seddon*:
  - *Grade I*: Ischemia.
  - *Grade II*: Ischemic contracture.
  - *Grade III*: Ischemic contracture with nerve involvement.
- *Zancolli*:
  - *Type I*: Contracture involving forearm muscles with normal intrinsic muscles.
  - *Type II*: Contracture involving forearm muscles with paralysis of intrinsic muscles.
  - *Type III*: Contracture involving forearm muscles with contracture of the intrinsic muscles.
  - *Type IV*: Combined type.
- *Tsuge (types)*:
  - *Mild (aka localized VIC)*: Further subdivided into proximal [pronator teres (PT) chiefly involved] or distal (pronator quadratus) or middle-third (FDP) involvement. No or mild nerve involvement, e.g. ulnar nerve in proximal type. Often presents with involvement of ring finger/middle finger but in advanced cases there may also be involvement of index finger/little finger.

- *Moderate*: Deep muscles (FDP, FPL) + superficial muscles (FDS, wrist flexors, PT) + involvement of thumb and nerve involvement.
- *Severe*: Moderate + extensors (often partial) and skin involvement + severe contractures and joint stiffness.

10. Why is median nerve more commonly involved?

Ans. Median nerve is often entrapped at the center of ischemic ellipsoid and contracting cicatrix in later stages hence it suffers maximum damage. Ulnar nerve situated at periphery of the zone is variably involved depending on the severity of disease and involvement. Radial nerve is involved only in extensive disease process spilling on to extensor region.

11. What muscles are most commonly involved?

Ans. *Deep muscles*: FDP (partial or complete) and FPL are the first ones to be involved; then depending on the severity of involvement FDS, PT, flexors of the wrist, pronator quadratus, extensors in that order may be affected.

12. What assessment will you do before surgery?

Ans. Muscle groups involved and spared (for tendon transfer), nerve involvement, skin involvement (there may not be enough initial space available for free vascularized transfer due to skin contracture). Then we stage the disease and decide treatment.

13. When can you do surgery?

Ans. Ideal is to wait for at least 3 months [Seddon; for necrotic region to segregate and spontaneous recovery of muscle and nerves stops (some say 6 months)] and should be done within a year (Tsuge) to produce good results. Deformity is said to be established if the interval from injury is more than 6 months (the trend now is changing to perform surgery as soon as feasible without waiting or delaying to preserve maximal function).

14. How will you treat this case?

Ans. I will get an X-ray done to look for the status of bones (malunion/crossunion/nonunion) as they also require treatment. Then I will do initial physiotherapy and stretching to reduce stiffness and improve contractures and do muscle slide operation with neurolysis.

15. What are the various modalities of management?

Ans. Treatment is devised according to the stage of presentation (this staging is not the stage of disease progression or severity—the Tsuge classification).

- *Acute stage (up to 24 hours)*: Treat like compartment syndrome.
- *Subacute or delayed stage (from 24 hours to 3-6 months)*: Presenting as edema and induration of forearm with paresthesia or anesthesia and motor weakness or loss. The deformities are progressing during this stage. It is an opportunity to improve sensations and motor function and prevent stiffness and deformity. Mobilization and supervised physiotherapy (dynamic splinting, stretching) is undertaken. Surgery is indicated if there is neurological impairment, failure of conservative treatment or radiological (MRI) evidence of fibrosis. Neurolysis and displacement of nerve from contracting cicatrix to subcutaneous plane, excision of scar is done. If nerve damage is severe then excision followed by grafting may be attempted.
- *Established VIC (Tsuge classification of disease severity)*:
  - *Mild type*:
    - *Stretching and physiotherapy*: If muscle mass is available.
    - Tendon transfer or lengthening when there is loss of muscle mass by Z-Plasty (of involved FDS, FDP, FPL tendons) or FDS to FDP transfer (Parkes; by attaching cut distal end of FDS to cut proximal end of FDP "motorization of FDP").
    - The other way of transfer is to transfer extensor tendon to flexor. For involvement of multiple tendon units prefer muscle sliding operation (Page's operation) or less favorably proximal row corpectomy.

- *Moderate type (classic type)*: Initial stretching followed by:
  - Muscle sliding operation (of Max page) with neurolysis (preferred for preserved muscle mass).
  - When there is no useful finger flexion left or there is proximal skin problem then branchioradialis/extensor carpi radialis longus (BR/ECRL) transfer to flexors (FPL and FDP respectively) and complete release of contracture and neurolysis is the usual option. Other options are proximal row carpectomy or forearm shortening by 2-3 cm (Garre's operation).

    Severe type: Preferred treatment includes early excision of all necrotic tissue with complete neurolysis of ulnar and median nerves to give them fair chance to recover (at least 3 months). This can be followed by tendon transfer as above or if no tendons are available then Gracilis (muscle after expanding skin with tissue expanders) or lattissimus dorsi or medial gastrocnemius (myocutaneous) free innervated muscle graft. Carpectomy (Griffiths) and wrist arthrodesis are other uncommonly performed operations in isolation.

In old cases with no available motor, severe contracture and nonsalvageable nerve injury; a combined procedure of flexor tenodesis with intermetacarpal fusion with thumb in opposition can be done. Nonsalvageable (damn useless) limb can even be amputated.

Thumb function needs to be addressed in moderate and severe types: Release of first web space contracture followed by reconstruction of motor function by use of extensors or by intermetacarpal fusion with thumb in opposition.

(Always begin answer by "stretching and physiotherapy to correct contractures and stiffness" then better choose appropriate surgery as above, those underlined are now standard).

16. Why is tendon lengthening not preferred?

Ans. Lengthened tendons often fail to function due to recontracture and adherence to skin and each other. Further it is ineffective for paralyzed muscles.

17. What is muscle slide operation?

Ans. It is the distal slide (by 3 cm) of flexor pronator mass subperiosteally from common flexor origin and interosseous membrane protecting carefully the ulnar nerve and anterior interosseous nerve, artery, and vein. Flexor carpi ulnaris (FCU) may need to be elevated till the level of wrist. This is followed by anterior transposition of ulnar nerve. The muscles are dissected in the order (ulnar nerve → FCU → PT → FDP → PT (distal origin) → Palmaris longus (PL) and FCR → FDS → FCU at interosseous membrane). Advantages are—simple surgery, can be completed in one operation and secondary tendon transfers are possible after this procedure.

18. What are the disadvantages of muscle slide operation?

Ans.
- Ineffective for paralyzed muscle.
- Some scar tissue is left behind.
- There is a risk of recurrence of contracture with growth of the bone.
- There is a decrease in strength of grip especially inflexion of the distal interphalangeal (DIP) joint.
- All flexor muscles are treated alike irrespective of the severity of damage.

19. What is the most common cause of VIC?

Ans. Long bone fractures either as a primary cause or secondarily due to ill-supervised or ignored treatment. Fracture both bones of leg is the most common cause of compartment syndrome (not of proximal tibial metaphyseal fracture). In the upper limb forearm VIC is most common following fracture of both bone forearm and its management related complication frequently tight cast; fracture supracondylar humerus in children is the second most common cause.

20. What are the various compartments in forearm?
Ans. There are four compartments:
1. Superficial volar (FDS, FCR, FCU, PL);
2. Deep volar [FDP, FPL, pronator quadratus (PQ)];
3. Dorsal; and
4. Mobile wad of Henry [brachioradialis, ECRL, extensor carpi radialis brevis (ECRB)].

21. Can you name some eponyms with the name Volkmann?
Ans. Richard von Volkmann:
- Volkmann's ischemic contracture
- Volkmann's deformity (congenital talar subluxation or dislocation)
- Volkmann's splint (for fracture of lower extremity)
- Volkmann's triangle (posterolateral corner of tibia)
- Volkmann's spoon (sharp spoon to curette away carious bone or other diseased bone)
- Volkmann's cheilitis (lower lip swelling, ulceration, crusting, and mucus gland hyperplasia)

Alfred Wilhelm Volkmann (Father of Volkmann RV):
- Volkmann's canals in bone.

(Kindly read in detail the management according to Zancolli's classification from Chapter 106 of the book Essential Orthopedics: Principles and Practice, 2nd edition)

CASE VII: TORTICOLLIS
[TORTUS (L.): TWISTED; COLLUM (L.): NECK]

1. What is your diagnosis?
Ans. My case is a patient of congenital muscular torticollis (CMT) of right side in a male child of one and a half years. There is associated congenital talipes equinovarus (CTEV) of right foot.

2. Why do you say that this is torticollis and how do you determine the side?
Ans. *On inspection*:
- There is contracture of right side sternocleidomastoid muscle.

- The head and neck are tilted toward involved side.
- Ear of the ipsilateral side is touching the shoulder.
- The chin is lifted toward the left side (child seems to be looking in the direction opposite to the side which is involved).

On palpation:
- There is tightness and thickening of the sternocleidomastoid muscle of right side.

Also examine for identifying the etiology of torticollis (*See* Q4 and 5).

3. What is the cause of congenital muscular torticollis?

Ans. The CMT is caused by fibromatosis within the sternocleidomastoid muscle. It may involve the muscle diffusely, but more often it is localized near the clavicular attachment of the muscle. Various hypothesis preferred are:
- Malposition of the fetus in utero (resulting in intrauterine or perinatal compartment syndrome of sternocleidomastoid muscle more common toward right side).
- Birth trauma (with resultant hematoma formation followed by muscular contracture—pseudotumor formation).
- Infection.
- Vascular injury (and fibrosis of muscle).

4. What are the other musculoskeletal disorders that you will look for?

Ans. Developmental dysplasia of hip (associated in 7–20% of CMT), metatarsus adductus, talipes equinovarus.

5. What are the other possible causes of torticollis in a child?

Ans. *Pediatric local etiology:*
- Congenital causes, such as pseudotumor of infancy, hypertrophy or absence of cervical musculature, spina bifida, hemivertebrae, and Arnold-Chiari syndrome.
- Otolaryngologic causes, such as vestibular dysfunction, otitis media, cervical adenitis, pharyngitis, retropharyngeal abscess, and mastoiditis.
- Esophageal reflux.
- Syrinx with spinal cord tumor.

- Traumatic causes, such as birth trauma, cervical fracture or dislocation (atlantoaxial rotator subluxation), and clavicular fractures.
- Juvenile rheumatoid arthritis.

Pediatric compensatory etiology:
- Strabismus with fourth cranial nerve paresis.
- Congenital nystagmus.
- Posterior fossa tumor.

Pediatric central etiology: Dystonias include torsion dystonia, drug-induced dystonia, and cerebral palsy.

6. How will you treat a case of CMT?

Ans. Evolution of CMT takes around 12-24 months so any surgical intervention should be deferred until evolution of fibromatosis is complete.

In infancy stretching of the sternocleidomastoid by manipulation should be done.
- Manual—by parents.
- Plaster casts.

Surgical intervention can be done after the age of 2 years and the options are:
- Unipolar or bipolar release of sternocleidomastoid muscle.
- Selective denervation.
- Dorsal cord stimulation.

Postoperatively immobilization in corrected position by plaster casts, hard cervical collar or head halter traction for 3-6 weeks is done depending on the tolerance of child. Physical therapy including manual stretching of the neck to maintain the overcorrected position is then immediately begun. Manual stretching should be continued 3-5 times daily for 3-6 months.

7. What are the complications of surgery?

Ans. Complications include injury to spinal accessory nerve or nearby vasculature including the jugular veins and carotid artery. Other complications include neck muscle atrophy,

Miscellaneous Short Cases

loss of muscle control, instability, variable numbness or sensory loss, pain, and neck deformity.

8. What are the features in a child presenting late?

Ans. In a delayed presentation there are fixed anatomical changes that are hard to reverse. These include:
- Facial asymmetry;
- Elevation of ipsilateral shoulder; and
- Frontal-occipital diameter of the skull may become less than normal.

9. What precaution will you take before treating a child presenting with delayed presentation?

Ans. One should clearly explain to the parents that the fixed anatomical structures will or may not reverse in spite of the corrective surgery and the surgery only cosmetically corrects the deformity. One should also not be aggressive as the chances of complications are much higher due to secondary contracture and shortening of neurovascular structures.

10. Why do you then do the surgical correction?

Ans. For a neglected case the primary indication for doing surgery is cosmetic correction of unsightly "wryneck" that has immense psychological implications for a school going child. Also without surgery the deformities become fixed and may even progress. However, the above should be clearly followed and borne in mind.

10
Miscellaneous Topics

GAIT

Gait analysis is an important part of examination for lower limb and spine evaluation and no candidate would be spared if he does not possess the requisite knowledge of the same. The topic is difficult and needs lots of practice and guidance for proper presentable knowledge.

Read times: 5–7 times (MS Orth and DNB candidates).

1. **What do you understand by gait?**
Ans. Gait is a dynamic posture allowing bipedal unassisted mobility by virtue of sound interplay between coordination and balance primarily of the lower limb and pelvis. Gait involves complex neuromuscular coordination of the lumbar spine, pelvis, hips, and those structures distal to them. Any dysfunction in the lower limb will become observable during gait.

2. **What do you understand by walking, running, and jumping?**
Ans. *Walking*: Bipedal unsupported gait pattern where at any time at least one foot is in contact with the ground.

   Running: Gait pattern where at least at some point of time feet are in air and one foot touches the ground in alternation.

   Jumping (both feet): Where at any point of time either both feet are touching the ground or are in the air. In single foot jump the other foot never comes in contact with ground.

3. What are the prerequisites for gait evaluation?

Ans. The following needs to be closely conformed to:
- Gait should be observed in all three planes with and without shoes (bare foot).
- Patient should be covering the private parts only during the gait examination.
- Observe gait while the patient walks along walkway of 1.1 m wide and 6 m long.

4. What is gait cycle?

Ans. It consists of two distinct phases—the swing phase and the stance phase with their subphases **(Fig. 1)**.
1. Swing phase (40% of the gait cycle—remember body tries to preserve energy)
    - Acceleration phase
    - Midswing phase
    - Deceleration phase
2. Stance phase (60% of the gait cycle—*even while walking we rest more*; actually balance is more important than speed. So as a corollary one is more "unstable" while running).
    - Heel strike
    - Foot flat
    - Midstance

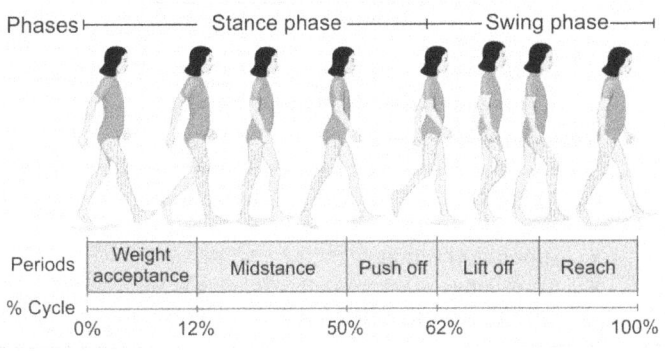

Fig. 1: Gait cycle.

- Heel off (Push off)
- Toe off

Two periods of double support:
1. Immediately after the initiation of stance phase
2. Just before the end of stance phase.

5. What are the various dysfunctions that can influence the gait?

Ans.

- Neurological (may involve dysfunction of one or a combination of the following parts of the CNS and/or PNS):
    - *Motor:* CVA and cerebral palsy
    - *Sensory:* Tabes dorsalis and blindness
    - *Cerebellum:* Friedreich's ataxia
    - *Basal ganglia:* Parkinson's disease
- Systemic disease:
    - *Joint disease:* Rheumatoid arthritis, osteoarthritis, and JRA
    - *Crystal arthropathies:* Gout
    - *Muscle disease:* Duchenne's muscular dystrophy and dermatomyositis
    - *Bone disease:* Rickets, osteomalacia, and Paget's disease
- Structural:
    - *Limb length inequality:* DDH, polio, femoral/tibial fracture
    - *Alignment disorder:* Coxa valga/vara, genu varum/valgum, and tibial/femoral torsion.

6. How to describe gait?

Ans. Observe the following anatomical and functional features during gait (observe from front, back, and side):
- Head position
- Shoulder position
- Arm swing
- Trunk position/rotation
- Base
- Pelvic tilt
- Limb motion

Miscellaneous Topics

- Thigh segment
- Patellar position/rotation
- Knee position
- Tibial position/rotation
- Ankle
- Calcaneal position
- Navicular position
- Midtarsal joint
- Metatarsals
- Toe position
- Foot position/shape
- Propulsion
- Swing phase.

The patient is walking with a bipedal unsupported gait having equal smooth alternating and rhythmic stance and swing phases with a normal base. The patient walks with a steady head in coronal plane centered over the shoulders. The shoulders are at same height. There is no trunk sway or rotation. Arm swing is equal and alternate on both sides. There is no pelvis drop on either side and the limbs move in coordination alternately during swing phase. During stance phase the patellar and knee heights are equal and there is no pelvic drop. The foot on both sides maintains its arch and stance phase progresses smoothly through heel strike, foot flat, midstance, heel off, and toe off. This patient has a normal gait.

[First mention bipedal or single limb or three/four point gait commenting type of support used. Then comment on the two phases of gait, their length, smoothness, coordination, alternation, and any abnormality. Then one may differ and would describe the pathological features first (like short stance phase with ipsilateral shoulder dip and trunk sway, etc. for antalgic gait) and then describe the other normal findings. Otherwise one may describe the features observed during swing and stance phases sequentially—both are correct and choice is yours. *Always remember to conclude with your diagnosis of type of gait*].

7. What do you understand by base of gait?

Ans. The distance between medial borders of both feet (normally 2–4 inches).

8. What is "double support" during gait cycle?

Ans. This is also known as "double leg stance". During gait cycle the body is supported on both feet for a brief period that extends from somewhere between push off and toe off on one foot and between heel strike and foot-flat on contralateral side. This comprises some 10% of gait cycle.

9. What is cadence and its importance?

Ans. Number of steps taken in one minute (normal 90–120/min). The period of double support is inversely proportional to cadence.

10. Can you comment on some common types of gait and their mechanism?

Ans. The various types of gait observed are [see also (Chapter 3)]:

- *Trendelenburg's gait (abduction lurch gait)*: It may be unilateral or bilateral. It depends upon the abductor lever arm (*See Chapter 2: Examination points for hip case, Q 33*) any abnormality of which leads to Trendelenburg's gait. When present unilaterally, the patient lurches on the affected side and the pelvis drops on the opposite hip. Bilateral Trendelenburg's gait is also known as *waddling gait*.
- *Short limb gait*: The patient lurches to the affected side and the pelvis drops to the same side (different from Trendelenburg gait in which the pelvis drops to the opposite side). If the shortening is less than 4 cm, it is compensated by the hyperextension at the knee and equinus at the ankle. Typical short limb gait is seen only when the shortening is more than 4 cm.
- *Antalgic gait*: Patient walks with shortened stance phase (avoids taking weight on the same limb). Any condition leading to pain in the lower limb (from hip to foot) leads to antalgic gait.
- *Stumbling gait*: Gait of bilateral CTEV.

Miscellaneous Topics

- *Waddling gait or duck walk gait*: It is wide base gait with increased lumbar lordosis, the patient sways to the same side after putting weight on the limb. Seen commonly in pregnancy, bilateral DDH, osteomalacia, and myopathies.
- *Knock knee gait*: While walking the knees point to each other and cross each other and the feet are kept apart. Typical in-toeing gait except the position of the knees on flexion are crossed or near to each other.
- *Quadriceps gait or "hand to knee gait" or "five fingers quadriceps gait"*: In cases of weakness of the quadriceps (PPRP—quadriceps are the most common muscles affected in the polio) the patient walks by supporting his knee with his hand during the extension to bear weight. The typical gait is produced to stabilize the knee. The patient does this typical action externally or by putting his hand through the pocket.
- *Gluteus maximus gait or "extension lurch gait"*: The gait is rarely seen these days as the most common cause was the weakness of the gluteus maximus due to PPRP. The patient lurches backward during walking.
- *Gluteus medius gait*: The gait is similar to the Trendelenburg's gait as the abductor forces of the hip are affected.
- *Stiff hip gait*: The patient walks by moving his whole pelvis along with the affected side (swaying to opposite side to clear ground); there is no or minimal movement at the affected hip.
- *Stiff knee gait*: The patient lifts his pelvis during the swing phase of the gait cycle to get the ground clearance.
- *High stepping gait or Russian march gait*: The gait is seen in cases of foot drop; patient lifts the affected limb higher and puts the forefoot first over the ground while entering into the stance phase. (Remember—normal gait cycle starts with heel strike).
- *Scissors gait*: This pattern of gait is seen in cases of weakness with spasticity (weakness is more than the spasticity) of the both lower limbs (CVA, cerebral palsy,

early stages of lathyrism, etc.). One leg crosses directly over the other with each step as the blades of the scissors **(Fig. 2)**. This is also called as the circumduction gate.

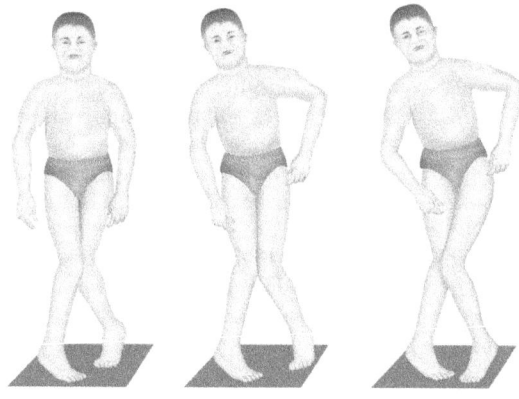

Fig. 2: Scissors gait.

- *Hemicircumduction gate*: The patient moves his limb while dragging his body along with the limb in hemicircle **(Fig. 3)**. The pattern is seen in cases of hemiparesis (CVA and cerebral palsy).

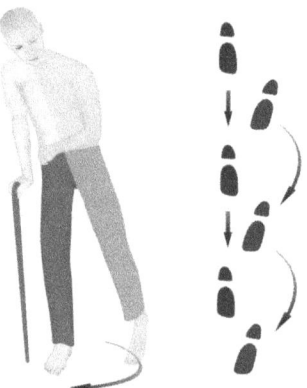

Fig. 3: Circumduction gait.

Miscellaneous Topics

- *Stamping gait*: It is seen in cases of loss of proprioception (sensory ataxia, tabes dorsalis, vitamin B_{12} deficiency, and alcoholism). The patient walks as he has no idea where his foot is leading to thumping noise over the ground due to sudden striking of the foot. The pattern can be imagined as descending the stairs in complete darkness.
- *Short shuffling gait or festinating gait*: Difficulty in starting and stopping the gait cycle with forward stooping posture and short steps. Typically seen in cases of Parkinsonism.
- *Charlie Chaplin gait*: This is seen in cases of alkaptonuria, external rotation deformity of tibia, and flat feet with valgus deformity of ankle.
- *Drunkards or reeling gait*: The patient has wide base gait and he swings to each side with tendency to fall with every step. This is seen in cases of cerebellar lesions or alcohol poisoning.
- *Hysterical gait (helicopod gait)*: The patient walks in bizarre fashion with a tendency to fall on every step; often seen in females with a typical tendency to fold in themselves. Typically the patient does not fall or falls in safer position and places hence are never hurt. The pattern is present in front of others only.
- *Calcaneus gait*: The patient has broad heel due to malunion of the calcaneum fracture. The patient has no calcaneal pick up and push off due to weakness of triceps surae. The patient walks with tendency to rotating the foot outwards and genu recurvatum.
- *In-toeing gait*: Seen in clubfeet, metatarsus varus, medial tibial torsion, genu valgum, femoral intorsion, and acetabular dysplasia.
- *Peg-leg gait*: Congenital vertical talus.

11. What are the various crutch gaits and the gait patterns?

Ans. Depending upon the support assistance provided by the crutch and weight-bearing limb the gait patterns are divided on the total points of contact bearing the weight at a time.

Four-point gait:
- Partial weight bearing both feet

- Maximal support by crutches
- Constant shift of weight over points.

Gait-pattern:
- Advance right crutch
- Advance left foot
- Advance right crutch
- Advance right foot.

Three-point gait:
- Requires good balance and arm strength
- Nonweight-bearing one foot
- Faster gait
- Can be used with walker assistance.

Gait pattern (assuming right foot is affected):
- Advance left foot with both crutches
- Advance right foot
- Repeat sequence to move forward.

Two-point gait:
- Partial weight bearing both feet
- Minimal crutch support
- Faster than a four-point gait.

Gait pattern:
- Advance left foot and right crutch
- Advance right foot and left crutch
- Repeat sequence to move forward.

12. What do you understand by "swing-through" and "swing-to" gaits?

Ans. These are the manner in which the feet are brought forward in two-point gait.

Swing to gait:
- Weight-bearing both feet
- Requires stability and arm strength
- Faster gait
- Can be used with walker.

Gait pattern:
- Advance both crutches
- Lift feet → swing forward → land feet next to crutches
- Repeat the sequences again to move forward.

Miscellaneous Topics

Swing through gait:
- Weight-bearing both feet
- Requires stability and arm strength
- Most advanced gait.

Gait pattern:
- Advance both crutches
- Lift both feet → swing forward → land feet in front of the crutches
- Repeat the sequences again to move forward.

13. What is the advantage of walker and what are the various types of walker?

Ans. Walker provides more support and stability than a cane or a pair of crutches (*the obvious difference between a four-wheeler and a two-wheeler*).

Types of walker:
- *Pick-up walkers*: One that has to be picked up and moved forward with each step, it does not permit a natural walking pattern and is used for patients who have poor balance or limited cardiovascular reserve or who cannot use crutches.
- *Rolling walkers*: It allows automatic walking and is used by the patients who cannot lift or who inappropriately carry a pick-up walker.

14. What is the role of cane during walking?

Ans. Cane provides an additional point of contact that assists patient during gait by redistributing the weight and hence shifting the center of gravity and line of weight bearing.

Types of canes:
- Quad canes (four-footed canes) provide more stability
- Single foot cane one.

Placement of the cane:
- 15 cm lateral to the base of fifth toe
- Hold in the hands over less affected (or unaffected) side (line of weight bearing shifts to the side where cane is held; unloading the affected side)
- Hold the handle of cane at the level of greater trochanter.

PROSTHETICS AND ORTHOTICS

1. What is prosthesis?

Ans. Prosthesis is a device designed to replace as much as possible the function or appearance of a missing limb or body part.

2. How does it differ from an orthosis?

Ans. An orthosis [orthos (*Greek*)—straight] is a device designed to supplement or augment the function of an existing limb or body part. It controls the abnormal movement or allows restricted normal movements. The following can be devised as functions of splints:
- Static splints (immobilize or stabilize joints):
    - Protection
    - To put joints to rest
    - To decrease inflammation
    - To decrease pain
    - To prevent undesired motion
    - To resolve fixed joint contractures (e.g. serial casting)
    - To substitute for lost muscle function
    - To substitute for loss of a digit.
- Dynamic splints (mobilization or traction to joints):
    - To resolve tendon tightness
    - To resolve joint contracture
    - To increase activity range on motion to given joints
    - To increase muscle strength.

3. How do you classify prosthesis?

Ans. Prosthesis may be classified in three broad categories:
1. *Endoskeletal*: Most widely used for lower limbs throughout the world. This type of prosthesis consists of a central structural tube to which a joint and socket can be attached. The central tube is mostly made of carbon fiber or aluminum. This basic structure can then be covered by an outer cosmesis in form of shaped foam.
2. *Exoskeletal*: In these prostheses, the main structural component is the "outer visible skin". Nowadays, mostly *dural* (aluminum alloy) or plastic laminates are used. Majority of the upper limb prosthesis are of plastic exoskeletal structure.

Miscellaneous Topics

3. *Temporary "pylon" prosthesis*: This consists of two self-locking side struts resembling above knee calipers. They are rarely used in the current circumstances.

    The term *pylon* is also used to describe the central structural tube in the endoprostheses.

4. What components should you specify while prescribing prosthesis?

Ans. While prescribing prosthesis, following details have to be furnished:
- Type of prosthesis
- Level of amputation
- Type of socket
- Material of socket
- Hip, knee, and elbow mechanism
- Foot/ankle or hand/terminal appliance
- Suspension
- Cosmesis.

5. What are the various types of sockets?

Ans. From the viewpoint of patient, socket is the single most important factor in prosthesis.
- Sockets may be made of various materials, e.g. leather, polypropylene, fiberglass, etc.
- Sockets may be standard sockets, which are worn over a stump sock. Nowadays, suction sockets are available which remain in close contact to the skin and are worn without a sock.
- Recently, silicone impregnated sock or sock lined by a layer of polyurethane gel have been developed to increase comfort and reduce sweating.

6. What are the various types of suspension mechanisms?

Ans. The prosthesis may be:
- Suspended with the help of belt, cuff or sleeve.
- *Self-suspending*: These may again be divided into mechanical or suction.

7. What are the various knee mechanism options available?

Ans. The knee systems have met the most advancement, the simplest being single axis constant friction type. Other mechanisms are shown in **Table 1**.

Practical Orthopedic Examination Made Easy

Table 1: Various knee mechanism.			
Type	*Typical patient*	*Advantages*	*Disadvantages*
Single axis, constant friction	Sedentary, poor access to maintenance	<ul><li>Inexpensive</li><li>Durable</li><li>Easy to maintain</li><li>Light weight</li></ul>	<ul><li>No swing phase control</li><li>Gait optimal only at one speed</li><li>Little inherent stability</li></ul>
Weight activated stance phase control (safety knee)	<ul><li>Elderly</li><li>Neurologic compromise</li></ul>	<ul><li>Inexpensive</li><li>Durable</li><li>Provides stability during heel strike and stance phase</li></ul>	<ul><li>No swing phase control</li><li>Gait optimal at one speed only</li><li>Reduced flexibility</li></ul>
Polycentric four bar knee joint	<ul><li>Knee disarticulation</li><li>Amputation</li></ul>	<ul><li>Can be less expensive</li><li>Stable</li><li>Hydraulic swing phase control may be added</li><li>Inherent stability</li></ul>	<ul><li>Bulky</li><li>Poor cosmesis</li><li>Increased weight</li><li>Frequent maintenance</li></ul>
Hydraulic or pneumatic swing phase control	Active young patients with access to maintenance facility	<ul><li>Best swing phase control</li><li>Adapts to speed</li><li>Best gait pattern</li></ul>	<ul><li>Expensive</li><li>More frequent maintenance</li><li>Heavier</li><li>Bulky</li></ul>
Manual locking knee	<ul><li>Elderly/weak</li><li>Unstable</li></ul>	<ul><li>Maximum stability</li><li>Very light</li></ul>	<ul><li>Unnatural gait</li><li>Must be unlocked to sit</li></ul>

8. What are the various foot and ankle mechanisms available?

Ans. Main groups include:
- Articulated ankle joints
- Dynamic response and energy storing foot
- *Nondynamic response and/or energy storing foot*: The simplest mechanism is SACH which stands for "solid ankle, cushion heel". It consists of a nonarticulated

ankle and nondynamic response foot. It is least efficient. Articulated ankle has the following disadvantages:
- Heavier
- More frequent maintenance
- When combined with dynamic response foot, it prevents loading of toes to provide push off.

9. What is SCAH foot?

Ans. SACH stands for (solid ankle, cushion heel). No true ankle joint, contains a "simulated ankle joint" by compressed wedge-shaped rubber heel. Consists of a solid wooden keel, high density rubber for dorsum, low density rubber for toes and plantar aspect (ensures smooth transition from toe off to heel strike), and variable density rubber for heel. The advantages are as follows:
- Absorbs the impact of heel strike.
- ↓ vertical excursion of center of gravity.
- Allows some simulated movement of metatarsal head.

10. What is Jaipur foot?

Ans. It is developed by Professor PK Sethi. Contains two wooden keels (broken keel). There is provision of toe break. The fundamentals of these types of prosthetic foot and comparison between Jaipur foot and SACH foot are given in **Table 2**.

Table 2: Comparison between Jaipur foot and SACH foot.

Jaipur foot	SACH foot
Appearance similar to normal foot	Dissimilar to normal foot
Can be worn without shoe but if someone wishes to wear one he can use a flat heel shoe	Requires a closed shoe to protect and hide it
No restriction of movements at ankle as the metallic keel (carriage bolt) is confined to ankle only and all movements take place at natural site	Solid ankle consisting of long wooden keel restricts movements in nearly all directions

Contd...

Contd...

Jaipur foot	SACH foot
Squatting possible (dorsiflexion adequate)	Not possible
Cross-legged sitting is possible (adequate forefoot adduction and internal rotation possible)	Not possible
Walking on uneven ground possible (good inversion and eversion)	Suitable for walking only on level ground
Barefoot walking possible (cosmetic skin color, no heel and toe height difference)	Not possible

11. What are the various upper limb prostheses available?

Ans.

- *Passive/cosmetic*: They are useful in those individuals who want a customized own skin like cosmesis or those who have a high-level amputation and they want lightweight prosthesis for cosmetic reasons. These are nonfunctional.
- *Body powered*: This involves the use of gross body movements to move the components through a system of harnesses and straps.
    - *Advantages*:
        - Does not depend on battery power
        - Quicker reaction time
        - Less expensive
        - Durable
        - Maximum proprioception.
    - *Disadvantages*:
        - Repetitive injury to activating muscles and joints
        - Limited pinch force control of terminal device
        - Harnessing effect.
- *Externally powered (myoelectric and switch control)*: Myoelectric components are controlled by voluntary muscle action via an electronic signal. The signal is picked up and amplified by electrodes placed over muscle fibers and the downloaded over to a computer to

provide a specific function. Before prescribing this type of prosthesis, myoelectric testing has to be done.
- *Advantages*:
  - Better cosmesis
  - No need for harness
  - Prevents repetitive injury
  - Increased anatomic function
  - Voluntary wrist rotation.
- *Disadvantages*:
  - Heaviest
  - Slower response time
  - Expensive
  - Frequent maintenance
  - Battery dependent
  - Less durable and nonwaterproof
  - Longer training period.
- *Hybrid systems*: Hybrid system has a combination of body powered and myoelectric components. This combination reduces the weight as well as the cost of the prosthesis.

Various upper limb units:
- Terminal devices—passive or powered (myoelectric/body powered) hand or hook
- Wrist units—both body powered and myoelectric units are available
- Elbow units—passive, body powered, and myoelectric units
- Shoulder—only manual units are used.

12. What is immediate postoperative prosthesis?

Ans. Immediate postoperative prosthesis (IPOP)—this consists of a specialized dressing covered by a plaster cast molded to provide the patient with weight-bearing areas to enable them to ambulate as soon as possible.

The IPOP incorporates an adapter in the distal end that has a removable pylon with a prosthetic foot attached.

Disadvantages of IPOP are as follows:
- Pistoning action due to plaster loosening, leading to tissue breakdown
- Repeated changing of casts

- Heaviness of cast leading to reduced movement of contained joints and subsequent muscle atrophy
- Difficulty in regular monitoring of the wound
- Auxiliary suspension may be required.

13. What is postprosthetic care?
Ans.
- Balancing, stretching, and muscle strengthening exercises may be started as soon as possible. This helps in maintaining flexibility, prevent flexion contractures, and preserve muscle mass and strength.
- An aerobic conditioning program must be designed and incorporated in the rehabilitation process.
- Gait training should begin with first step. Initially walking stick or walker may be allowed, but its use should be terminated as soon as possible.
- In case of upper limb amputations, early fitting of prosthesis and promotion of two handed function leads to reduced rejection rate.

14. What is Milwaukee brace?
Ans. A brace designed by Blount, Schmidt, and Bedwell (1958) known by the city of origin of these men. This brace is used for controlling curve deterioration and to maintain the postoperative correction in patients with scoliosis. The brace has three parts:
1. The pelvic mold
2. Vertical bars
3. Mandibulo-occipital assembly.

The pelvic girdle uniformly fits over the iliac crests and is the most important part of brace. It helps in reducing lordosis, derotates the spine, and corrects frontal deformity. Uprights have localized pads to apply transverse force which is effective for smaller curves. The main corrective force is the thoracic pad which attaches to two posterior and one anterior upright. Discomfort from the same creates a righting response. Neck ring is another corrective force and is designed to give longitudinal traction. The throat mold allows the use of distraction force without producing jaw deformity.

Miscellaneous Topics

Complications:
- Pain
- Skin breakdown
- Jaw deformity
- Unsightly appearance
- Increased energy expenditure with ambulation, etc.

WOUND INFECTION, WOUND COVERAGE, AND DRESSINGS

This is typically a topic for DNB examination ward rounds and hardly if ever would be of any utility to MS Orth candidate. The practical utility is however immense and one may read it just out of interest.

Read times: 3–5 times for DNB candidate.

1. Describe the wound.

Ans. Wound or ulcer is basically described under following headings:
- *Inspection*:
  - Size and shape
  - Number
  - Position
  - Edge
  - Floor
  - Discharge
  - Surrounding area.
- *Palpation*:
  - Tenderness
  - Edge and margin
  - Base
  - Depth
  - Bleeding
  - Relations to deeper structure
  - Surrounding skin.
- *Inspection findings*: This is a single, oval shaped, roughly 3 cm in length, and ulcer (wound) situated over middle one-third of right leg on the medial aspect in healing stage. The edge of the ulcer is sloping and pale and smooth granulation tissue is visible at the floor.

Discharge is scanty. Surrounding skin is normal *(look for appendages and color)*.
- *Palpation findings*: The ulcer is slightly tender to palpation and it is 5 mm in depth. The base is indurated. It is mobile and not fixed to the deeper structures.

2. What else you would like to examine in this case?

Ans. I would like to examine the regional lymph nodes, peripheral pulses, vascular insufficiency, and sensory status *(for neurological status–neuropathic ulcer)*.

3. How do you classify an ulcer?

Ans. Ulcers can be classified either on the basis of clinical type or on the basis of pathological type.
- *Clinical types* are spreading ulcer, healing ulcer, chronic or callous ulcer.
- *Pathological ulcer*:
    - Nonspecific (traumatic, arterial, venous, and neurogenic)
    - Specific (tuberculous, syphilitic, and actinomycotic)
    - Malignant (epithelioma, Marjolin's ulcer, and rodent ulcer).

4. What are the characteristics of a healing ulcer?

Ans. The floor of a healing ulcer is covered with pinkish or red healthy granulation tissue. The edge is reddish with granulation, while the margin is bluish with growing epithelium. The discharge is slight and serous if at all present.

5. How can you say that an ulcer is a chronic ulcer?

Ans. These ulcers show no tendency towards healing. The floor is covered with pale granulation tissue. Discharge may be scanty or absent. The base is considerably indurated and so is the edge and surrounding skin.

6. When an ulcer or wound is called as infected?

Ans. Clinical indicators of infection seen on wound examination are:
- Poor quality granulation tissue
- Thinning of granulation tissue
- Increased volume of exudates
- Pain
- Formation of adherent fibrinous slough.

7. Classify a wound?
Ans. Classification of wound has been shown in **Table 3**.

Table 3: Classification of wound.		
According to the type	*According to the extent*	*According to local environment of wound*
Incisional wound	Deep wet wound	Necrotic wound
Partial thickness wound	Deep dry wound	Sloughing wound
Full thickness wound	Shallow wet wound	Granulating wound
	Shallow dry wound	Epithelializing wound

8. What is the principle of wound management and prerequisites for an ideal dressing material?
Ans. Wound management is based on stepwise approach consisting of:
- Assessment of both patient health and wound characteristics
- Planning the course of treatment
- Cleansing and debridement (establishment of open edge), application of dressing and adjunct therapy.

The ideal dressing should:
- Protect from external forces
- Allow appropriate gaseous exchange
- Provide moist environment
- Maintain high humidity
- Provide optimum pH (slightly acidic)
- Discourage infection
- Provide thermal insulation
- Reduce odor
- Absorb exudates
- Be easy to apply
- Be cost and resource effective.

9. What is the most accepted dressing method; wet dressing or dry dressing?
Ans. Wet dressing is most accepted method and conversion from wet to moist dressing is ideally suited in most cases.

Comparison between moist dressing and dry dressing has been shown in **Table 4**.

Table 4: Comparison between moist dressing and dry dressing.	
Moist	*Dry*
Reduced risk of infection	Encourages scab formation
Reduced healing time	Delays healing
Faster re-epithelization	Increases pain
Better cosmetic result	May produce scar tissue

10. Classify different dressing materials with examples.

Ans. Classified on the basis of construction and function.
- Absorptive
  - Gauze
    - Plain/impregnated
    - Foams and polymer dressing
    - Alginates
- Occlusive (moisture maintain) dressing
  - Film dressings
  - Hydrocolloids
  - Hydrogels
- Others
  - Oxidized regenerated cellulose and collagen
  - Silicone skin-substitute dressing
  - Amnion
  - Homograft/xenograft.

11. Where will you use paraffin gauze?

Ans. It is most commonly used in noninfective granulating wounds and on pink epithelializing wounds. Its major advantage is that it is nonsticky and can be left for several days.

12. Where will you use iodine or zinc impregnated gauge?

Ans. Skin graft donor site and graft.

13. What is foam dressing?

Ans. It consists of hydrophilic polyurethane open cell sheets and is highly absorptive. It provides moist environment and thermal insulation. It is useful in exudative wounds and needs to be changed in 3–4 days. No role in dry wound.

Miscellaneous Topics

14. What are alginates?
Ans. They are calcium and sodium salt of alginic acid. These are highly absorbent and hemostatic in nature and also provide moist environment. Commonly used in highly exudative wounds and infective wounds.

15. What are hydrocolloids?
Ans. They consists of two layers; an inner layer which consists of carboxymethylcellulose polymer absorbs exudates and forms gel. The outer layer which is of polyurethane seals the wound. It allows limited moisture and gas transmission and is impermeable to bacteria. It also has fibrinolytic property and is mainly useful in light to moderate level exudative wounds, e.g. Duoderm, nuderm, and comfeel. Mainly used in venous ulcers, pressure ulcers, diabetic ulcers, and first- and second-degree burns.

16. What is composition of betadine?
Ans. It is iodine combined with polyvinylpyrrolidone. It is broad spectrum—effective against gram-positive and gram-negative bacteria, fungi, viruses, and protozoa. Its preoperative application before surgical incision reduces colonization. It decreases fibroblast proliferation and neovascularization in chronic wound.

17. Tell something about hydrogen peroxide?
Ans. It is inexpensive and widely available. It uses free radical oxygen radical which scavenges the infective pathogens. Mainly used for cleaning and removing loose debris. It maintains aseptic environment but decreases neodermal regeneration and fibroblast proliferation.

18. What is EUSOL?
Ans. EUSOL stands for Edinburg University Solution. It is basically a chlorinated lime and boric acid solution 0.25% weight/volume of available chlorine. Better activity with freshly prepared solution.

19. What is oxoferin?
Ans. It is an aqueous solution which contains biocatalytically activated oxygen carrier. O_2 has good tissue penetration

capacity thus promotes phagocytosis. It provides good cleaning and good local defense against infection.

20. What are the properties of silver ointment used for dressing?

Ans. Silver ions destroy bacterial cell wall, enzymes, and DNA synthesis. Additional anti-inflammatory properties—reduces TNF-α which is responsible for rapid wound healing. It is useful in infective contaminated wound.

21. What are the constituents of neosporin ointment?

Ans. It is a combination of neomycin, bacitracin, and polymyxin B. It is effective against wide range of Gram-positive and gram-negative bacteria.

22. What is traditionally known as three-layer dressing?

Ans. The three-layer dressing consists of:
1. Contact layer (nonadherent material)
2. Absorptive layer
3. Binding layer (tape).

23. Enumerate the stages or grades of pressure sore?

Ans. Given by Shea, recommended by National Pressure Ulcer Advisory Panel.
- *Stage I*: Nonblanching erythema (after 30 seconds of pressure) of intact skin (partial thickness wound)
- *Stage II*: Partial thickness skin loss involving epidermis, dermis or both (partial thickness wound)
- *Stage III*: Full thickness skin involved and extending till fascia (full thickness wound)
- *Stage IV*: Full thickness skin involved and extending to supporting structures (bones and muscles) (full thickness wound).

PRINCIPLES OF FRACTURE FIXATION

The topic is added only in part to supplement the answers as the viva may be detailed to include the basics of plating and nailing principles. This makes it imperative to have the basic theoretical knowledge these principles. I fully understand that one has a good practical exposure of the same.

Read times: 2–4 times for MS and DNB candidates.

1. What are the various modes in which a plate can be applied?

Ans. The following are the various modes of plate fixation:

- *Neutralization*: Used to protect primary fixation from torsion, bending, and shear. The longer the plate the greater the neutralization capacity.
- *Buttressing*: Plate directly counters the bending, compressive and shear forces at fracture site to the applied axial compressive forces. Often used to stabilize periarticular and intra-articular fractures. Epiphyseal and metaphyseal fractures can displace to produce angular deformity.
- *Compression mode*: Reduces, stabilize, and compresses the fracture site (transverse and short oblique) when lag screw fixation is not possible.
- *Bridging mode*: To maintain length and alignment of a severely comminuted and segmental fracture. The plate goes over the main injury site as "bridge" without further disturbing the fracture region.
- *Tension band (adopted by Pauwels)*: Plates applied over the tensile surface prevent distraction of fracture fragment and by virtue of eccentric holding, also produces counteractive (compression) forces at the opposite side. Thus, the distraction forces are converted into compressive forces due to eccentric hold/fixation.
- *Antiglide*: The plate is applied in such a way as to hold the distal fragment indirectly and convert the displacing compression forces into reduction compressive forces, for example in Weber type B fractures the proximal spike of distal fragment is caught in the plate, with weight bearing the axial forces are transformed to compression forces at fracture site as the fragment is caught between fracture and plate.
- *Locked plates*: Where the internal fixation is actually a type of external fixation with the screws locked to both the plate and bone providing an extremely rigid

construct. This is beneficial for treatment of complex metaphyseal fractures and osteoporotic fractures but not simple diaphyseal fractures as the callus response may be suppressed and often compression at fracture site is not deliberately tried.

2. What are the principles of buttress plating?
Ans. This plating acts as a retaining wall if applied properly:
- Exactly contour the plate
- Screws should hold plate from moving with respect to bone
- Screw applied closest to the fracture through oval hole is said to be in buttress mode, minimizing axial movement at fracture
- Buttress plate applies force perpendicular to bone (compression plate applies force parallel to bone).

3. What is spring plate?
Ans. Plate is affixed to only one of the two fragments such that metallic properties of plate help reduce the fracture and hold it (buttress mode).

4. How do you achieve compression at fracture site?
Ans. By:
- Overbending the plate
- Compression device
- Using plates with dynamic holes that have two inclined and one horizontal cylinders merged together and lead to production of compression with screw tightening (DCP/LC-DCP).

5. What is a "wave plate" and what are its uses?
Ans. Similar to bridge plate but the plate is contoured away from fracture site. This gives space to insert bone graft in comminuted fractures and at pseudarthrosis site. In treating nonunions this plate allows for better in-growth of blood vessels, increases the area for bearing stress (decreasing stress at fracture site), can also act as a tension band by compressing the opposite side.

Miscellaneous Topics

6. What other modalities (aside from plate) can be used to utilize tension band principle and where all can it be used?

Ans. K-wires with metallic suture wires (encirclage wires), screws with encirclage wiring, and simple encirclage wiring can all be used at:
- Greater trochanter (femur)
- Patella
- Olecranon
- Greater tuberosity (humerus)
- Acromioclavicular joint
- Ulnar styloid
- Medial and lateral malleoli
- Tibial tuberosity fracture.

7. Where do you apply plate in a bone?

Ans. On the tensile surface:
- Humerus—anterior in extension and posterior in flexion (In elbow stiffness associated with nonunion the posterior surface is the tensile surface)
- Radius—lateral
- Ulna—posterior/posterolateral (actually in proximal third posteromedial is tensile but it is difficult to apply plate there)
- Femur—anterolateral
- Tibia—none specifically.

8. What is the principle of nailing?

Ans. The principle is—three-point fixation for snugly fitting and elastic nails. The solid unreamed interlocking nail acts as splints only. Nail is a load sharing device so that one does not see stress shielding and resulting osteoporosis. There is transmission of force also through the bone and hence fracture site which helps in bone formation and remodeling at fracture.

9. What is the principle of K-nail?

Ans. Kuntscher called the nailing as elastic nailing and described the mode of action of nailing to be elastic impingement or radial compliance to explain the mechanism of fixation. According to him the nail was released from the elastic constraint as soon as it is in the medullary canal and expands to grip the canal from inside. However, the mode of action is now considered to be three-point fixation only. K-nail provides angular (bending), translational (horizontal displacement) and to some extent torsional (rotatory) stability, and provides axial compression facilitating callus response.

10. What are the various generations of nailing?

Ans. Nailing has evolved over years and consecutive advancements can be grouped under three generations:

- *1st generation nailing* included K-nail, V-nail, clover-leaf nail, etc. that primarily acted as splints. The rotational stability was minimal and primarily relied on snug fit.
- *2nd generation nailing*: The major advantage was improved rotational stability due to locking screws at either ends. They also relied on snug fit. The proximal femoral entry was piriformis fossa in all. Here the nails were classified into centromedullary (Schneider self-broaching nail, Hansen-Street diamond nail, and Huckstep nail), cephalomedullary (G-K nail, SUN nail, MDN nail, etc.), caudocephalic nails (distal femoral nails), etc. depending on primary mode of action or technique of insertion. This was the most dynamic phase of nail evolution.
- *3rd generation nailing:* With the aid of CAD various design changes to make the nails as anatomical as possible and to aid the insertion and stability have led to development of multiple curve nails and multiple fixation systems, viz. greater trochanteric entry point for femoral nail with additional lateral curve, femoral nail with femoral neck fixation, tibial nail with malleolar fixation, etc.

11. What do you understand by nail length and working length?

Ans. The nail length is considered from the following viewpoints:
- Total nail length
- Length of nail bone contact
- Working length.

Total nail length is primarily an anatomical consideration. Nail-bone contact is difficult to calculate but practically determines the resistance to motion which is directly proportional to length of nail-bone contact.

Working length is the length of nail spanning the fracture site from its distal point of fixation in proximal fragment to the proximal point of fixation in distal fragment. This represents the part of nail not supported by bone and carries load across the fracture site.

12. What are the implications of working length?

Ans. Working length determines:
- Bending stiffness—inversely proportional to the square of working length
- Torsional stiffness—inversely proportional to the working length
- Strength of construct—the smaller is the working length the stronger is the construct.

[Interlocking screws reduce the working length in torsion by fixing the nail to specific part of bone. This also explains why you should impact the fracture before locking the nail. Similarly reaming the canal improves the working length by enhancing the nail-bone contact towards fracture].

13. What are the methods of reducing "hoop stresses" in nailing?

Ans. Hoop stresses (circumferential expanding forces on the bone walls) are generated when nail is inserted into medullary canal. These may rupture the bone and depend on the insertion force (axial forces converted into radial forces), which in turn depends on the resistance offered by medullary canal. The following can be done to reduce the hoop stresses:
- Using a flexible nail
- Over-reaming the canal
- Selecting proper entry point.

14. What is dynamization?

Ans. In general static locking is preferred in comminuted, segmental, long oblique, and spiral fractures. Dynamic locking is otherwise preferable if at least 50% cortical contact is established. Dynamic locking provides in situ dynamization with weight bearing (some 5–10 mm reserve is offered by most modern nails). Sometimes, however, in delayed union "proximal or distal" screw is removed to allow telescoping and compression at fracture site and aid healing. This allows axial compression but also takes away the rotational stability. Dynamization is preferably done between 6 weeks and 10 weeks.

ARTHROPLASTY OF HIP, ELBOW, AND SHOULDER

The basis of writing this chapter is to acquaint the students with the most popular arthroplasty procedures and not at all to detail them. Only those procedures have been dealt that have some significant mention in the book elsewhere—so deliberately quitting knee arthroplasty. It should be remembered however that the hip arthroplasty is so commonly performed nowadays that it is a favorite question once you cross the hurdles of examination points and diagnosis.

Read times: 3-5 times (MS Orth and DNB candidates).

HIP ARTHROPLASTY

1. **What is arthroplasty?**
Ans. Arthroplasty is a joint reconstructive procedure using natural or synthetic substitutes or reduction methods (excisional) that alter the structure and function of the joint.

2. **What is the principle of low friction arthroplasty as propounded by Sir John Charnley?**
Ans. Low friction arthroplasty principles of Sir John Charnley had the following components:
- *Thick plastic socket of high molecular weight polyethylene*: This is more suited than a metal bearing as it wears less and works best at high loads and slow speed. It is able to self-lubricate in dry state.
- *Small diameter femoral head of stainless steel*: The smaller the head the less the wear.
- *Greater trochanter transferred to more lateral position*: Increasing offset.
- *Fulcrum displaced medially*: Center of artificial joint is more medial than natural joint.

3. What are the various types of hip arthroplasty?

Ans.

- *Resection arthroplasty*: Girdle stone type
- *Interposition arthroplasty*: Various natural and synthetic materials interposed between two articulating surfaces. The materials used are muscle, fascia, fat, synthetic membranes (historically—wood. By Carnochan and gold foil by Sir Robert Jones), etc.
- *Cup arthroplasty:* Special interposition arthroplasty in which a cup was used to separate femoral and acetabular surfaces. Smith-Peterson used glass that was then changed to Vitallium cup.

Endoprostheses are of following two types:

1. *Hemiarthroplasty:*
   - Monoblock nonmodular prosthesis like Austin-Moore and Thompson prosthesis
   - Bipolar prosthesis (Bateman's prototype prosthesis, etc.)
   - Tripolar prosthesis (Jumbo head prosthesis)
2. *Total joint replacement arthroplasty:*
   - Cemented total hip replacement (THR)
   - Noncemented THR
   - Hybrid THR
   - Surface replacement arthroplasty (classically double cup arthroplasty)
   - Custom made THR with variable calcar/femoral replacing systems.

4. What is cemented THR?

Ans. A cemented THR is one in which both the femoral and acetabular components are fixed to bone with a cement interface.

5. What do you understand by hybrid THR?

Ans. In hybrid system only the femoral component is cemented whereas the acetabular component is used in a noncemented fashion.

6. Why was the need of this system felt?

Ans. Over the evolution of THR in the past 50 years it was seen that in a cemented system the acetabular component fails more frequently to the femoral component. There were more complications of cement-related bone degeneration like osteolysis on the acetabular side. So with the development of noncemented systems acetabulum was fixed to bone without cement interface. However, as regards the femoral component, sturdy fixation of the stem and early mobilization was possible with the use of cement interface. Also if at all revision would be required it often is limited to changing of acetabular component or liner so cementing of femoral component was retained as a "permanent" stem. The other major rationale emanates from different mechanisms of failure of cemented acetabular and femoral components (*see* below).

7. What are the various mechanisms of failure of cemented acetabular and femoral components? Can you correlate these to development of hybrid system?

Ans. Acetabular (cemented) component predominantly fails due to immunological-induced bone lysis destroying the fixation ultimately. This induction is done by wear particles.

Femoral (cemented) component whereas loosens predominantly for mechanical reasons. Early failure is related to thin cement mantle whereas long-term failure is due to loosening at cement metal interface at the tip and higher up seen more frequently with first-generation cementing techniques.

Cementless fixation of femoral stem developed with the hope of reducing above however fared poorly and on the contrary more frequent and progressive lysis was observed seen in anatomic modular locking (AML), Allopro prosthesis (APR), Harris-Galante prosthesis (HGP), and porous-coated anatomic (PCA) systems.

Considering the above results one would naturally be intended to use a cemented femoral and cementless acetabular component (hybrid system).

(*Philosophies and schools differ and may continue to do so endlessly—may be till total robotic age comes up! When there will be no "soft tissue" and only metal prevails*).

Miscellaneous Topics

8. What decides the use of a cemented or noncemented or a hybrid THR?

Ans. Primarily the decision is based upon the age of patient and bone stock [Dorr classification type A—complete finalization (ideal for cementless stem), type C—no funnel, type B—intermediate]. Requirement for mobility and disease condition for which replacement has been planned is also important while deciding type of prosthesis to use. Elderly patients with poor bone stalk are better dealt with cement augmentation of bone and hence cemented THR. Also, for patients requiring early mobilization and those with limited longevity (viz. tumor patients) cemented components are preferred. Noncemented prostheses are preferred for younger patients.

9. Can you name some cemented femoral and acetabular components that have evolved over time?

Ans. Cemented acetabular cups:
- Charnley's plastic cup
- Modified Charnley's cup
- Buchholtz cup
- Peg cups, etc.

Cemented femoral stems (these may be curved/straight, collared/collarless, textured/smooth, and bowed/straight):
- McKee-Farrar (metal-on-metal)
- Charnley femoral stem (metal-on-plastic) with 22.25 mm head
- Müller femoral stem with 32 mm head (medial ridge—"saber") and with a curve to ease insertion
- *Harris femoral component (HD-2)*: 32 mm head with moderate undercut and oval neck around 3 cm of proximal stem was precoated with PMMA for better fixation.
- *Amstutz femoral component (TR-28)*: Modified Charnley component to a head size of 28 mm and a thicker stem (but not wider).
- *Aufranc-Turner component*: Similar to Müller cup but the head is more undercut.
  (*A collarless, polished, and straight stem subsides well into the cement and converts load into hoop stresses*).

10. What are the various cementing techniques?

Ans. Over a time, refinements in the way cement was applied to the components have led to developments into generations in cementing:
- *First generation*: Finger packing and no distal plug.
- *Second generation*: Distal plug of canal, "preparation" of canal with pulsed lavage, distal centralizer, and use of cement gun to insert the cement in a retrograde fashion.
- *Third generation*: Precooling of cement, vacuum mixing and centrifugation, and pressurization of cement by use of proximal seal.
- *Fourth generation*: In addition, this uses a proximal centralizer to ensure symmetric cement mantle.

  During the same periods there were some "implant characteristics" that improved however they are not grouped into generations. In the first generation, the implants had "sharp" borders that used to split the mantle and were prone to "midstem pivot effect" whereby there was excessive medial pressure in the proximal portion and lateral pressure distally. In the second generation, the implants were made of superalloys and sharp corners were removed. During third generation, the surface characteristics were improved to increase bonding.

11. How much cement mantle is considered adequate?

Ans. It is about 2–5 mm. The place where cement is missing or very thin is called "mantle defect" and is often the site of failure.

12. What is cement disease?

Ans. "Cement disease" applies to the previously prevailing concept of ill effects on the body and local bone due to leakage of hot monomer, thermal injury during curing phase, degradation, and release of particles including contrast. Seemingly there is no strong biological backing for this mundane term.

13. What are the various types of cement available?

Ans. There is no standard classification, but the available types of cement evolved on the needs of different types of procedure:
- *High viscosity cements*: Standard arthroplasty procedures, now not preferred.

- *Low viscosity cements*: The most commonly used cement, surface replacement, and vertebroplasty (very low viscosity cement).
- *Antibiotic impregnated cements*: Revision and infection in arthroplasty, spacer, and cement beads for defect management in chronic osteomyelitis.
- Cold-curing cements (Mjoberg) using butyl methacrylate.
- Biodegradable aqueous gel phase cement.

14. What are the components of standard cement?

Ans. Cement is provided as biphasic module (two to three parts powder and one part monomer liquid). The solid phase comprises powder form microbeads (1–100 µm) of polymerized component (PMMA) with opacifier (barium sulfate or zirconium oxide) and initiator (benzoyl peroxide). The liquid phase consists of monomer methyl methacrylate and co-initiator [aka activator—dimethyl-p-toluidine (DMPT)] along with stabilizers to prevent autopolymerization (hydroquinone and/or ascorbic acid). The coloring agents like chlorophyllin can be added to any phase while antibiotics are added only to solid (powder) phase.

15. What are the various antibiotics that can be used?

Ans. Most commonly used are aminoglycosides and vancomycin. However, the β-lactams, cephalosporins, macrolides, quinolones, and doxycycline can all be used. Basically the antibiotic should be heat stable, water soluble, hypoallergic, bactericidal, and available as a powder.

16. What are the various phases of polymerization?

Ans.

1. *Mixing phase*: Wetting
2. *Waiting phase*: Swelling + polymerization, ↓ viscosity, and sticky dough
3. *Working phase*: Chain propagation, ↓ movability, and ↑ viscosity
4. *Setting phase*: Chain growth finished, no movability, and high temperature.
   There is shrinkage of the mix finally and the whole process is exothermic (heat of polymerization = 43–46°C).

17. What are the effects of precooling and warming of prosthesis?

Ans. Both are deleterious. Precooling leads to shrinkage of the material at cement-prosthesis interphase—early loosening. Prewarming leads to ↓ conductive capacity of prosthesis → heat necrosis → early loosening (*So warm prosthesis till body temperature*).

18. What are the effects of vacuum mixing and centrifugation?

Ans. Vacuum mixing results in ↑ in bending strength by 15–30%.

Centrifugation improves the fatigue strength by ≈ 9%. Precooling of monomer, polymer and mixing vessels decrease the number and volume of pores.

19. What are the various bearing surfaces?

Ans. The most popular one is metal (cobalt-chrome alloy) on UHMWPE (ultra-high molecular weight polyethylene). The others are:
- Metal-on-metal
- Ceramic-on-UHMWPE
- Ceramic-on-ceramic (alumina on alumina third-generation bearings)
- Failed bearing surfaces:
  - *Ceramic on metal*: High frictional torque and wear
  - *Titanium on polyethylene*: High wear typically third-body wear.

20. What are the various types of cementless stems?

Ans. There are three methods of cementless stem fixation:
1. *Press-fit*:
   - Moore and Thompson prototype stems
   - Lord and Sivash femoral stems.

   These rely on the development of bone "around" stem to give a tight fit.

2. *Macro-interlock*: Here the press-fit is supplemented by mechanically carving out ribs, threads, steps, etc. in the stem.

3. *Porous-coated stems (modern stems)*: The porous coating could be of hydroxyapatite (ceramic pore size ≈ 50 μm) or spongy metal porous coating in the form of small spherical beads (cobalt-chrome/titanium, pore size of

Miscellaneous Topics

50–400 μm) or mesh applied by sintering or diffusion bonding. Bone "ingrowth" is considered optimal if micromotion is <20 μm at bone-implant interface. Some examples are AML, HGP, and PCA stems. For porous-coated ceramic stems; the cells migrate into the pores (osteoconduction) and bone may form from the coating itself. The following characteristics are found:

- *Diaphyseal (distal) fit or metaphyseal (proximal) fit*: Latter is preferred. In the former one there is complete porosity over the surface that may stress shield the metaphysis due to early distal fit and lead to metaphyseal bone loss and are also prone to cause thigh pain. The metaphyseal fit stems to have only proximal porous coating.
- *Anatomical or straight stems*: The former have proximal posterior bow and a variable distal anterior bow (only for revision long stems). This mandates side determination for prosthesis as anteversion is also additionally built into the neck.
- *Circumferential or patchy porous coating*: Newer designs have circumferential coating earlier designs had patchy coating that served to circulate particulate debris around the stem—"effective joint space".
- *Collared or a collarless stem*: Collar in a cementless stem is useless! As if collar fits before stem fit—stability is compromised, if stem fits before collar is seated, it is ineffectual.

21. What is the rationale for using recently launched large head bearings?

Ans. Large head with limited endoprosthetic components that waste a very limited amount of patients bone have been popularized as surface replacement arthroplasty. Also there are various modular components which can fit large metal bearings on standard endoprosthetic components. The highly polished surfaces provide very limited wear and improved stability and range of motion as compared to the conventional arthroplasty.

22. What are various types of wear seen in THR?

Ans. Wear is the loss of rubbing surfaces due to repetitive motion and friction.

- *Abrasive*: Due to rubbing of two hard surfaces.
- *Adhesive*: Rubbing of a soft surface onto a hard one in which the former is transferred as a thin film over the latter.
- *Fatigue*: Due to repetitive loading.
- *Corrosive wear*: Due to different types of metals (galvanic), etc.
    - *Linear wear*: With linear wear the head penetrates into the acetabulum due to high contact pressure (linear distance traveled by head). This wear is more common with smaller heads (say 22 mm) (*The smaller heads may also penetrate the acetabulum due to "cold flow" of plastic—plastic deformation*).
    - *Volumetric wear*: This is due to frictional torque and is more with larger (say 32 mm) heads (*You see why we use 28 mm heads. The larger heads have again come in vogue due to improvement in plastic characteristics—the highly cross-linked polyethylene*).

23. What are the indications of total hip arthroplasty?

Ans. Primary and secondary osteoarthritis, osteonecrosis, inflammatory arthritis, dysplastic hip, PFFD, pathological fracture of proximal femur, conversion of arthrodesis into arthroplasty, etc.

24. What are the contraindications of hip arthroplasty?

Ans. *Absolute*: Active or latent infection at local/distant site, medically unfit patient with a high risk to benefit ratio.

Relative: Neuropathic arthropathy, rapid bone destruction, insufficiency of abductor mechanism, and rapidly progressive neurological disease.

25. What are the complications of THR?

Ans. Various complications are seen; all related to major surgical procedure and to prosthesis fixation itself: *Immediate*: Bleeding and vascular injury (external iliac, obturator, and superior gluteal), sciatic/femoral/obturator/peroneal nerve injury, fracture of femur/acetabulum, over-reaming and unstable implant, and bladder injury.

Early: Fat embolism, deep vein thrombosis, thromboembolism, dislocation, infection, and renal failure.

Late: Loosening and osteolysis, wear, thigh pain, lurch, protrusion, heterotopic ossification, and periprosthetic fractures.

ELBOW ARTHROPLASTY

1. **What are the indications of elbow arthroplasty?**
Ans. Age > 60 years, advanced arthritis or post-traumatic destruction of joint in a low demand patient.

2. **What are the various types of elbow prosthesis?**
Ans. Semiconstrained (linked prosthesis) like GBS III elbow and Coonrad-Morrey prosthesis and unconstrained or unlinked prosthesis like Kudo and iBP elbow.

3. **What are the prerequisites for unconstrained prosthesis?**
Ans. There should be good bone stock, little deformity, and stable capsuloligamentous support.

4. **What are the indications for unconstrained prosthesis?**
Ans. Elderly patients with rheumatoid arthritis, painless ankylosed elbow, e.g. juvenile rheumatoid arthritis.

5. **What is the prosthetic choice for post-traumatic elbow?**
Ans. Constrained (linked) prosthesis as the capsuloligamentous structures are damaged.

6. **What are the indications for constrained elbow prosthesis?**
Ans. Deficient bone stock, unstable capsuloligamentous support, and deformed joint.

7. **What is Bakshi's sloppy hinge prosthesis?**
Ans. It is a type of semiconstrained-linked prosthesis with a loose hinge (sloppy) to partially compensate for the rotational stress on the prosthesis hinge.

8. **What are the limitations after total elbow arthroplasty?**
Ans. The person cannot lift weight > 5 kg and should avoid contact sports for lifetime.

SHOULDER ARTHROPLASTY

1. What are the indications of shoulder arthroplasty?

Ans. In general, shoulder arthroplasty is recommended for patients with symptomatic glenohumeral arthritis (osteoarthritis and rheumatoid arthritis), traumatic arthritis, osteonecrosis, rotator cuff arthropathy, and four-part nonreconstructible proximal humerus fractures.

2. What are the various options available?

Ans.
- Hemiarthroplasty
- Total shoulder arthroplasty
- Reverse shoulder arthroplasty.

3. When do you decide between hemi and total shoulder replacements?

Ans. The demarcation is vague and controversial but the following guidelines are generally followed: Always first look at two crucial components to be restore—arthritis and instability.

Hemi-shoulder arthroplasty (HSA):
- Rough and destroyed humeral articular surface with intact glenoid cartilage with enough glenoid to stabilize the humeral prosthetic head
- There is insufficient bone to support glenoid component with irreparable cuff tears
- Fixed upward displacement of humeral head relative to glenoid
- History of remote joint infection
- Heavy demands anticipated for the joint
- Four-part nonreconstructible fracture of humeral head.

Total shoulder arthroplasty (TSA):
- Incongruent joint surfaces
- Normal or reparable cuff tears
- Loss of articular cartilage on both surfaces.

Reverse total shoulder arthroplasty (rTSA):
- Arthritis and/or instability from nonreconstructible soft tissue or osseous defects
- Posterior aspects of capsule and rotator cuff have been lost

Miscellaneous Topics

- "Anterior-superior escape" due to coracoacromial arch deficiency (wear, fracture, and acromioplasty)
- Slackened deltoid unable to lift the humerus for abduction "pseudoparalysis"
- Failed previous conventional arthroplasty.

4. What is reverse total shoulder prosthesis?
Ans. This prosthesis involves making glenoid 'ball' that articulates with concave humeral trumpet-shaped component, in effect it is reversal of the normal anatomical joint.

5. What are the prerequisites for hemiarthroplasty?
Ans. *This is the most popular procedure world over. Total shoulder needs expertise and overall the indications are not very clear. Reverse total shoulder is mentioned only for candidate to have an idea that this relatively new system exists. The experience is very limited and results not extensively quantified or qualified. So at the summit it becomes clear that if asked about shoulder arthroplasty then hemiarthroplasty will be the choice—unless furiously refrained to by an occasional examiner.*

- Concentric glenoid consisting of eburnated bone
- Nonconcentric glenoid that can be converted to a smooth concentric surface by reaming
- The humeral head can be centered in the glenoid by soft-tissue balancing and glenoid preparation
- The surgeon is proficient with soft tissue and osseous procedures.

6. What is the rationale for development of reverse total shoulder arthroplasty?
Ans. There are various limitations for conventional shoulder arthroplasty that could be addressed by reverse total shoulder arthroplasty as follows:

- *Limitation of TSA/HSA to manage glenohumeral translation*: For the exquisite ROM of a normal shoulder there is translation of humeral head, especially at the ends. This is limited in perfectly conforming joint surfaces of TSA/HSA.
- Limited fixation of glenoid component to bone in TSA.

- *Limited intrinsic stability of TSA/HSA (see above for indications of rTSA)*: The TSA/HSA can be done for the following conditions:
  - Arthritis/instability due to deficiency of humeral head (HSA)
  - Arthritis/instability due to deficient glenoid that can be reconstructed (TSA)
  - Arthritis + acute reparable rotator cuff tears (HSA/TSA)
  - Arthritis + excessive capsular laxity: Tightening + large head HSA/TSA with increased lateral offset and tissue balancing
  - Arthritis + upward displacement of humeral head (intact coracoacromial arch) (HSA/TSA).
- Limited ability for compensation of deltoid dysfunction (*These are the most preferred explanations for development and use of rTSA, results are beginning to come and have been satisfactory*).

7. What are the limitations of shoulder arthroplasty?

Ans.

- Skin, vascular, and osseous deficiency
- Infection
- Deltoid deficiency and limited scapular mobility
- Unfit patients (medical, emotional, and motivational issues).

8. What are the differences of shoulder arthroplasty as compared to hip arthroplasty?

Ans.

- Shoulder arthroplasty depends upon soft-tissue balancing primarily
- The humeral head is in retroversion (femoral head is anteverted)
- Glenoid is in minimal retroversion (acetabulum is anteverted)
- The approach to shoulder is anterior (hip is posterior/lateral)
- The glenoid surface (concave surface) is small and humeral surface (convex surface) is larger (in THR femoral head is smaller than acetabulum) (*This "issue" is also resolved by reverse shoulder*).

How to Read an X-ray and Some Common Radiographs as Examples?

Plain radiographs are the most commonly ordered initial investigation by an orthopedic surgeon to understand the pathology, make diagnosis or confirm clinical findings. The X-ray should be read in a systematic meticulous manner in order not to miss findings and pickup even subtle changes that will reveal some uncommon disorders. Also consistency of reading helps communication with colleagues. The listener should be able to visualize the findings as you are communicating (this essentiality has been nowadays lessened by picture or photo sharing apps or messaging services on smart phone!!).

1. **What are the steps of X-ray reading?**
Ans. Place the radiograph in anatomical position first.
- *Description*: Mention the anteroposterior (AP) view or views [AP/lateral (LAT)] followed by region observed (pelvis, cervical spine, thigh, etc.) on radiograph along with side (if not axial) followed by age and gender of the patient (if known, nowadays digital radiographs contain all these information). Lastly you should mention the date of examination (as follow-up radiographs would change for pathology; **Fig. 1**).
- The X-rays are read either from inside-out or outside-in approach (commonly we follow the former approach

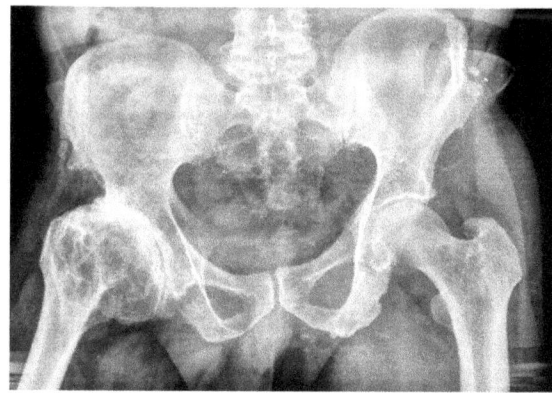

Fig. 1: *Radiograph 1:* The presented radiograph demonstrates anteroposterior (AP) view of pelvis with both hips in a 50-year-old male taken on April 15th, 2014. The radiograph shows whole bony pelvis, upper part of femora and lumbar fourth/fifth vertebra.

being in habit of jumping to diagnosis but the latter one is somehow considered better):

- *Soft tissues*: Note swelling, density of the tissues, and appearance of pathological signs like calcification, foreign bodies, and presence of air in the tissues.
- *Bones*: Note the outline, density (and contrast with soft tissues) as a whole (increased in fluorosis, reduced in osteoporosis).
  - *Periosteum*: Note the smoothness, periosteal reaction, new bone formation, lift-off of periosteum, thickness or bump (periostitis), break or absence of it.
  - *Cortex*: The cortex should be continuous and most thick in the diaphysis while thinning and virtually disappearing as a line in metaphysis. Note its continuity (especially break in it), its thickness, damage (lytic neoplasms), deformities (widening in Paget's, thinning in osteoporosis, bowing in

rickets, etc.). Finally note if any implant is present and reason for it. Note the nonunion or delayed union, changes of union, malunion, etc.
- *Endosteum*: Note as for periosteum. Loss of it is seen in lytic neoplasms, haziness in osteomyelitis, and disappearance due to bone forming neoplasms (like osteoid osteoma).
- *Medullary cavity*: Note the clear outline and differentiation from cortex (corticomedullary differentiation is lost in osteoporosis, Paget's and metabolic bone diseases). Identify the pathological structures like lytic/sclerotic lesions/cysts, presence of sequestrum (in osteomyelitis). Finally make a note of intramedullary implant if present and the reason for it.
- *Joints*: Identify the joint and note joint space, degenerative changes, pathology like deformity due to abnormal growth, angular deformity, and periarticular nonunion. Make a note of prosthetic replacement for the joint. Note the fitting (central placement, cementation, and articulation), deformity, loosening, and signs of infection.

2. How to read X-rays showing fracture?

Ans. Radiographs showing fracture should incorporate the following:
- *Level of fracture*: Divide the bone region into virtual thirds or halves and then dictate the site of fracture as upper/lower/middle-thirds or junction of upper/middle-thirds, etc.
- *Displacement*: Mention translation, angulation, rotation, and lengthening/shortening/overlap.
- *Geometry of fracture line*: Transverse, oblique, spiral, butterfly fragment, wedge, comminuted, segmental, bone-loss.
- Extension into joint.
- *Intra-articular fractures*: Impaction, comminution, condylar (or volar/dorsal involvement), displacement(s) of fragment and shift or tilt of joint.

3. **What are the prerequisites of taking X-rays?**

Ans.
- Two perpendicular views (oblique recommended for hand, foot, and spine).
- *Two joints*: The radiographs of limbs should incorporate joint above and below the target bone (especially in trauma series).
- *Two limbs*: Radiograph of contralateral limb is especially useful in children where fractures are often difficult to characterize.
- *Two occasions*: Some pathologies are better revealed after 2-3 weeks (like fracture of scaphoid). Nowadays litigation and peer pressure does not mandate waiting for so long as investigations like computed tomography (CT) scan can reveal it immediately.
- *Two injuries*: It is common place to find some group of injuries together so it is logical to order radiographs of expected other place injuries simultaneously.

RADIOGRAPH 1

1. **Describe the X-ray?**

Ans. This plain radiograph demonstrates AP and LAT projections of left forearm (which one is AP and which one lateral is difficult as position of elbow and forearm is different and expected in trauma patients!) taken for a skeletally mature patient. The radiograph shows whole forearm with elbow joint and wrist joint and metacarpals of hand **(Fig. 2)**.

The soft tissue shadow is unremarkable. There is a displaced transverse fracture at the junction of distal and middle-thirds of radius with dislocated ulnar head dorsally. The distal fragment is translated volarly with proximal

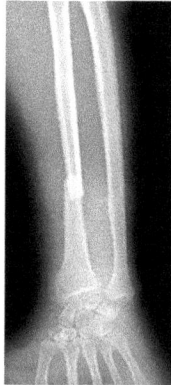

Fig. 2: Radiograph 1.

migration and there is dorsal angulation at fracture. The wrist and elbow joints are unremarkable.

2. What is your diagnosis?

Ans. This is a typical Galeazzi fracture dislocation.

3. Do you see something wrong in the radiograph and why?

Ans. There is a band or tie at wrist which should be immediately removed as it may cause strangulation effect producing compartment syndrome.

4. What is the importance of this injury?

Ans. The injury is classified as fracture of necessity and should be managed on emergency basis.

(Learn also other fractures of necessity and why are they called so? See fracture neck femur for description elsewhere in the book and read mechanism of injury and associations of the fracture from Essential Orthopedics: Principles and Practice, 2nd edition—annexure for trauma)

5. How will you proceed with the management?

Ans. I will immediately stabilize the fracture so that secondary complications like soft tissue injury do not occur and will counsel the patient and relatives for the grievous nature of injury. I will plan for open reduction/internal fixation (ORIF) of radius using AO principles and stabilize the distal radioulnar joint (DRUJ) with K-wire in supination.

RADIOGRAPH 2

1. Describe the X-ray?

Ans. The radiograph shows AP and LAT projections of left elbow joint in a skeletally mature patient. The elbow joint region with distal arm and proximal forearm is demonstrated in this roentgenogram **(Fig. 3)**.

The soft tissues show some wasting of forearm and disrupted elbow joint clearly visible on AP projection. The forearm is translated laterally at elbow with loss of elbow joint articulation. There is an intra-articular bony fragment with some calcification speck near radial head

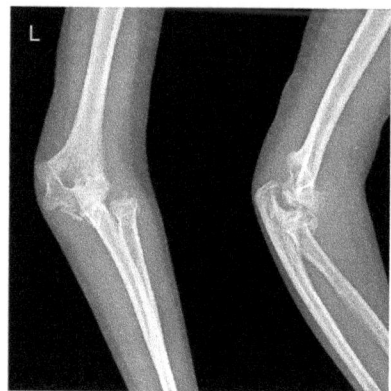

Fig. 3: Radiograph 2.

(indicative of old injury) on AP projection. Lateral projection demonstrates fracture of coronoid process of ulna and some anterior capsular calcification.

2. What is your diagnosis?

Ans. I will consider this dislocation of elbow keeping in mind the possibility of old unreduced injury (that will be ascertained on history taking).

(Learn about classification of elbow joint dislocation and associated injuries.)

3. What else you would keep in mind from this radiograph?

Ans. This is an unstable injury and if it is shown to be an old injury then I will have to keep in mind the difficulty in reduction due to capsular calcification and possibility of myositis.

4. How common is neglected elbow dislocation?

Ans. Uncommon injury and rare to see in practice.

5. Will you like to examine anything else clinically?

Ans. Definitely I will like to examine the distal neurovascular status as this could very well produce ulnar and/or radial nerve injury. I will also look for developing features of reflex sympathetic dystrophy (RSD).

6. How will you proceed?

Ans. After proper history taking and clinical evaluation, I would like to get magnetic resonance imaging (MRI) of the patient to see:
- Status of ligaments
- Myositis
- Status of articular cartilage, and
- Nerve entrapment in the joint (ulnar nerve may get entrapped in the joint).

I will discuss the options with family.

7. What options will you discuss?

Ans. Depending on the preservation of joint we can plan for open reduction of joint vs arthrodesis. Even after open reduction there is a high possibility of remaining stiffness as there is capsular calcification ± myositis and additional need for ligament reconstruction does not always produce highly functional joint in such neglected cases that have to be immobilized for a significant duration in postoperative period. The patient will also need 2–3 months of physiotherapy including multiple continuous passive motion (CPM) sessions. Also, the joint may remain painful after relocation.

(Learn about the arthrodesis of elbow joint additionally.)

RADIOGRAPH 3

1. Describe the radiograph?

Ans. The radiograph shows AP and LAT projections of left leg demonstrates whole tibia and fibula with barely visible knee articulation in a skeletally mature patient **(Fig. 4)**.

The soft tissue shadow demonstrates multiple irregularities, likely representative of puckered scars in the lower half, and hypertrophy in upper half of leg. The tibial bone overall demonstrates thickening well marked in the lower half with irregularity in cortex and irregular periosteal reaction. There is anterior and medial bowing of the bone in lower half with well-marginated lytic cortical lesions at lower and middle-thirds junction involving nearly one-third of the

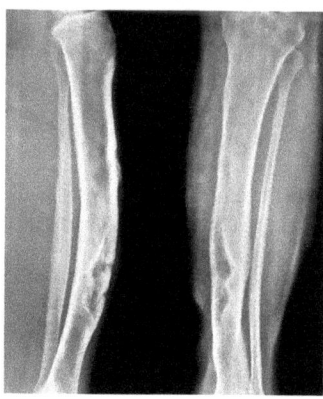

Fig. 4: Radiograph 3.

circumference of bone. The lesions are irregularly shaped, have a wide base and sclerotic margins. The endosteum is hazy in the middle-thirds with widening of medullary canal. There are multiple (three in number) poorly marginated lytic lesions in the medullary canal at proximal and middle-thirds junction without any definitive breach in cortex but a small solid periosteal reaction anteriorly.

Fibula also shows anterior and medial bowing with hypertrophy in middle-thirds prominent in lateral view.

2. What is your diagnosis?
Ans. I will give a differential diagnosis of:
- Multifocal osteomyelitis
- Operated case of osteomyelitis for distal lesions while active proximal lesions, and
- Operated case of fibrous dysplasia.

3. Why do you call this operated case?
Ans. The lower tibial lesions look like saucerization done for opening the medullary canal and drainage of pus as there is significant marginal sclerosis. Skin also shows scars.

4. How will you proceed if this is chronic osteomyelitis?
Ans. I will get sinogram done to look the culprit site of infection.

5. **Any other investigation you would do?**
Ans. I will get an MRI scan done with contrast to look for sites of active disease though it is commonly an overdiagnosis in such cases.

(Learn the classification and management aspect from elsewhere discussed case of chronic osteomyelitis).

RADIOGRAPH 4

1. **Describe the radiograph?**
Ans. The radiograph shows AP projection of pelvis with both hips in a skeletally mature male patient (look at the pubic angle and genitalia!) demonstrating whole of bony pelvis with both hip joints and lower lumbar spine **(Fig. 5)**.

The soft tissue shadows are unremarkable but there is overall increased density of the visualized bones. Shenton's line is broken at both the femoral neck region and there is external rotation deformity of the distal fragment. There is clear break of cortices in intracapsular femoral neck region and the trochanters are upridden. There is varus angulation at the fracture.

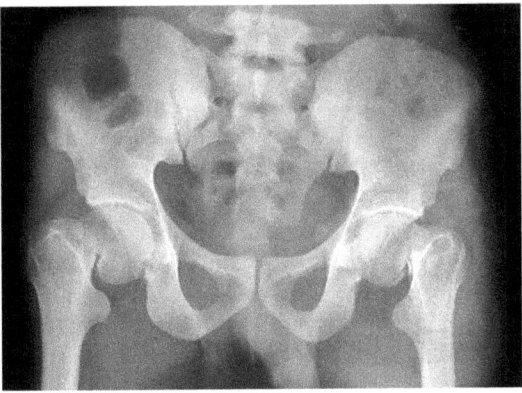

Fig. 5: Radiograph 4.

2. What is your diagnosis?

Ans. My diagnosis is displaced femoral neck fractures of both femurs with possibility of osteopetrosis or fluorosis.

(Learn about the classifications of fracture neck femur—kindly vide the case discussed for nonunion femoral neck fracture.)

3. Are you satisfied with the radiograph?

Ans. No, I would also like to obtain lateral views.

4. Why, the fractures and displacement is obvious here?

Ans. I would also like to look for posterior cortical comminution that has a bearing on treatment and stability of osteosynthesis if planned.

5. How common is bilateral femoral neck fracture and where do you see it?

Ans. It is quite uncommon but may be seen in:
- *Pathological fractures*: Osteoporosis, osteomalacia, osteopetrosis, Paget's, ankylosing spondylitis, renal osteodystrophy, hypocalcemia, etc.
- *Neoplasia*: Multiple myeloma, fibrous dysplasia
- Stress fractures of neck femur are also commonly bilateral.
- High-energy trauma and falls from height on both lower limbs standing straight landing on heels.

6. Will you order anything else if this is what you see in emergency department?

Ans. Definitely after resuscitation and a preliminary examination I would like to get screening of spine (lumbar, cervical, and thoracic), radiographs of both feet.

7. How will you proceed if this is the only injury?

Ans. I will thoroughly evaluate for any metabolic cause of bilateral femoral neck fracture in this patient as this may have a bearing on treatment plan. As the patient is young, I will discuss with the patient and relatives the pros and cons of hip preserving and sacrificing surgery thoroughly. I will be personally more tilted toward hip preservation.

RADIOGRAPH 5

1. Describe the radiograph?

Ans. This is a composite radiograph showing AP (standing) and LAT projections of both knee joints in a 74-year-old female depicting also the lower part of femur and upper tibia and fibula **(Fig. 6)**.

The soft-tissue shadows are unremarkable. There is degenerative change in both knees more marked in right knee joint with valgus deformity at knee, mild medial subluxation of femur, reduced lateral femorotibial space with tibial osteophytes and medial joint opening as visualized on AP view. On lateral radiographs there are prominent osteophyte formations quite obvious in the patellofemoral joint.

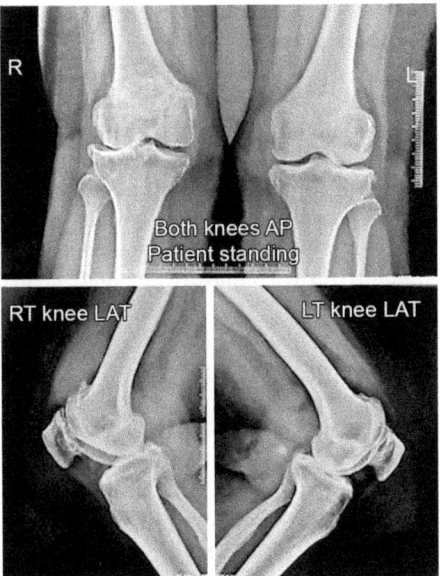

Fig. 6: Radiograph 5.

2. What is your diagnosis?

Ans. My radiological diagnosis is degenerative arthritis of right knee joint grade 4 and grade 2 for left knee joint (Kellgren-Lawrence radiographic grading).

3. Why do you say radiological diagnosis?

Ans. Valgus deformity in primary degenerative arthritis of knee joint is uncommon and is more commonly seen in patients with inflammatory arthritis so the diagnosis could change to rheumatoid arthritis clinically so I mentioned only the radiological diagnosis.

4. What will you do next?

Ans. I will evaluate the patient for inflammatory arthritis or crystal arthropathy and also evaluate the patient for disability due to disorder (western Ontario or a similar scoring system) then plan treatment.

5. What is the treatment for this case?

Ans. If the patient is sufficiently disabled so as not being able to do routine work and her functions are primarily limited due to knee pain and arthritis then I will suggest total knee joint arthroplasty if patient is also emotionally stable and understands the limitations of this treatment. Otherwise I will give a trial of conservative management with well-advised physiotherapy and strengthening exercises and functional rehabilitation of knee joint with adequate analgesia.

12

Long and Short Questions for Orthopedic Theory Examination

LONG QUESTIONS

Surgical Techniques and Approaches
1. Bone grafting, types, and technique. Describe bone graft substitutes.

Imaging in Orthopedics
1. Role of ultrasonics in orthopedics.
2. Role of magnetic resonance imaging (MRI) and computed tomography (CT) scanning in orthopedics.

The Hip
1. Describe the pathoanatomy of developmental dysplasia of the hip (DDH) with relevance to the treatment and the role of pelvic osteotomy.
2. What is the etiopathogenesis of slipped capital femoral epiphysis (SCFE) or slipped upper femoral epiphysis (SUFE)? Describe in detail the management of acute slip with a note of the advantages and disadvantages of various treatment methods for chronic slip.
3. Classify Perthes' disease with a note over the significance of changes in head and describe the management in various stages with a note on bracing and its role.

4. Give a note of the clinical and pathological aspects of septic arthritis. Describe the management of sequelae of septic arthritis.
5. Describe the etiopathogenesis of tuberculosis (TB) of hip and management of TB hip in stage III.
6. How will you manage ankylozed hip in a patient with ankylosis of both hip joints? Describe the principles of low-friction arthroplasty.
7. Describe the pathogenesis and management of coxa vara.
8. Describe the vascular supply of head. What is the role of steroids in production of osteonecrosis of femoral head and how do you manage stage III Ficat and Arlet hip in a 40-year-old male.
9. Describe the causes of loosening in total hip replacement (THR) and management of failed hip [also learn for total knee replacement (TKR)].
10. Describe the various dislocations around hip and management of a case of old neglected posterior dislocation of hip and its complications.
11. Classify fracture neck of femur in adults and what are the various complications. Outline the management of subcapital fracture neck of femur in a 35-year-old male.
12. How do you classify fracture of intertrochanteric region of femur? Describe the advances in management of intertrochanteric fractures.
13. Define femoral anteversion and clinical evaluation. What is the role of femoral anteversion in hip biomechanics, development, and clinical diagnosis?
14. Classify pelvic fractures and management of unstable patient with vertically unstable pelvis injury (basically also rule out abdominal injury).
15. Classify fracture acetabulum and management.
16. Briefly describe the valgus osteotomy of proximal femur and its role in orthopedics with merits and demerits.

The Knee Joint

1. Classify knee instability. How will you manage anterior cruciate ligament (ACL) deficient knee?

2. Classify patellar instability. How will you manage a case of habitual dislocation of patella in a 16-year-old female?
3. How will you manage a 60-year-old male with Kellgren grade III bilateral knee osteoarthritis? What is high tibial osteotomy and list the various methods to perform the same?
4. Describe the pathology of osteoarthritis and the biomechanics of malaligned knee. What is the role of surgery in correction of malalignment?
5. What are the various causes of anterior knee pain? Describe the pathoanatomy and management of patellofemoral overload syndrome.
6. Enumerate various methods of ACL reconstruction including types of grafts used and their relative merits and demerits.
7. How will you approach a patient with unstable knee? Briefly describe the treatment algorithm.

The Leg, Foot and Ankle

1. Describe the principles of distraction histogenesis. How will you manage a 21-year-old male with post-traumatic 8 cm limb shortening with anterior angulation of 30° of lower-thirds tibia?
2. Describe the pathoanatomy of clubfoot and the role of talo-calcaneo-navicular complex. How will you manage a 6-year-old child with neglected clubfoot?
3. Orthopedic management of leprosy foot.
4. Clinical features and management of old neglected Achilles tendon rupture?

The Shoulder Joint

1. Morbid anatomy of unstable shoulder and management.
2. Etiopathogenesis of rotator cuff tear and its management.

The Elbow and Arm

1. Management of neglected elbow dislocation.
2. Management of stiff elbow.
3. What are the various restraints for elbow and how will you manage an unstable elbow?
4. Describe in detail the pathoanatomy of ununited fracture of lateral condyle and detail its management.

5. What is nonunion? How will you manage a case of nonunion of humerus in a 30-year-old male?

The Hand and Forearm

1. Describe in detail the etiopathogenesis, clinical, and management perspectives of congenital radioulnar synostosis.
2. What is Madelung's disease? Describe in detail the management.
3. What do you understand by intercarpal instabilities? Describe in detail the morbid anatomy and management perspectives.
4. A 45-year-old female present with paresthesia and pain over radial 31/2 fingers, described in detail the morbid surgical anatomy, clinical features, and management of the patient.
5. Classify and describe Kienbock's disease with respect to etiology and surgical management of various stages.
6. Classify fracture scaphoid. What are the various complications, describe in detail the management of scaphoid nonunion?
7. What is tardy ulnar nerve palsy (ulnar neuritis), describe the surgical management?
8. How will you manage 6-month old case of posttraumatic radial nerve palsy associated with nonunion of fracture humerus?
9. Describe the components of extensor mechanism of fingers. Classify and describe the surgical management of boutonnière and swan neck deformities.
10. What are the various spaces in hand, describe with respect to deep hand infections and pathogenesis?
11. What are the various zones of flexor tendons? Describe the management of zone II injury?
12. Describe the etiopathogenesis, classification, anatomy and manipulative and surgical management of Volkmann ischemic contracture.
13. Describe the anatomy of peripheral nerve. How will you manage a case of high ulnar nerve palsy?
14. Outline the formation of brachial plexus and describe the course of ulnar nerve. What are the various sites of

compression of ulnar nerve and clinical and management perspectives?
15. Anatomy and pathology of brachial plexus injury. How will you differentiate preganglionic from postganglionic brachial plexus injury?

The Spine

1. Describe the structure of intervertebral disk (IVD). Describe in detail the clinical presentation of prolapsed IVD (PIVD) L4-L5 disk and current surgical management perspectives.
2. What is scoliosis and how do you classify the same. Describe the management of idiopathic scoliosis in a 17-year-old girl?
3. Describe the structure of spinal cord with respect to the location of spinal tracts. Describe in detail the rehabilitation of a traumatic paraplegic patient.
4. How do you define and classify spondylolisthesis? How will you manage grade III L5-S1 listhesis?
5. Classify traumatic injury to spine and describe the various spinal cord syndromes.
6. Describe the diagnostic and management perspectives of failed back syndrome.

Tumors

1. Describe in detail the etiopathogenesis, histopathology, and management of giant cell tumor of bone.
2. Classify and describe the osteosarcoma of long bones and its syndromic associations. Outline the management of a case of osteosarcoma of proximal tibia and the role of immunotherapy.
3. How will you approach a patient with metastasis and unknown primary?
4. Principles, evolution and practice of limb salvage surgery.
5. Describe in detail the radiologic and pathologic features of Ewing's sarcoma. Describe the surgical management of chemosensitive tumors.
6. Detail the work-up for a metastatic tumor to bone. Classify spinal metastasis and how will you manage a 55-year-old female with localized spinal metastasis with paraparesis?

General Orthopedics, Infections and Fractures

1. Describe the clinical anatomy of iliopsoas muscle and iliotibial tract.
2. What is osteoporosis; describe in detail the diagnostic and management perspectives?
3. What is the blood supply of talus? Classify and describe the management of fractures of talus.
4. Describe the etiopathological advances of cerebral palsy and classify the disease. When and how will you surgically manage a case of knee deformity due to cerebral palsy?
5. Biological therapy for osteoporosis.
6. Immunotherapy for rheumatoid arthritis.
7. Describe the management of post-polio residual paralysis and foot deformities in a 12-year-old child.
8. What is Pott's paraplegia? Classify and describe the causes and management of a case of late onset paraplegia.
9. Antitubercular chemotherapy.
10. What is gas gangrene and responsible pathogens? Describe the management of gas gangrene of lower limb (also learn for necrotizing fasciitis).
11. What are the various mechanisms for joint lubrication?
12. Describe in detail the clinical biomechanics of hip joint and correlate the use of rehabilitative devices.
13. Describe in detail the structure of physis. Classify physeal injuries. How will you manage a case of type three physeal injury (S-H) of distal femoral epiphysis?
14. Describe the management of disaster at state level [this was the long question in my Diplomatic National Board (DNB) exam!!].

SHORT QUESTIONS

1. Anterolateral decompression.
2. Spinal osteotomy.
3. Posterior fusion.
4. Pedicular screw.
5. Steps of diskectomy (fenestration).
6. Bankart repair.

7. Putti-Platt repair.
8. Anterior approach to shoulder for open reduction.
9. French and modified French osteotomy and difference.
10. Ulnar nerve transposition.
11. Max Page release.
12. Carpal tunnel release.
13. Darrach's reconstruction at wrist.
14. Wrist fusion, types and indications.
15. Drainage of various hand spaces.
16. Opponensplasty.
17. Southern approach, Harding's approach to hip.
18. Subtrochanteric valgus osteotomy.
19. McMurray's osteotomy.
20. Pauwels osteotomy.
21. Core decompression.
22. Girdlestone arthroplasty.
23. Shelf procedure.
24. High tibial osteotomy.
25. Approaches for total knee arthroplasty.
26. ACL repair.
27. Phemister grafting.
28. Sofield osteotomy.
29. Posteromedial soft tissue release.
30. Dwyer's osteotomy.
31. Lichtblau osteotomy.
32. Jone's transfer.
33. Lambrinudi, Grice-Green arthrodesis.
34. Hallux valgus.
35. Hallux rigidus.
36. Rigid flat foot.
37. Arches of foot.
38. Fungal infections of foot.
39. Calcaneal spur.
40. Trophic ulcer.
41. Diabetic foot.
42. Talocalcaneal bar.
43. Congenital pseudoarthrosis of tibia.

44. Varicose ulcer.
45. Congenital constriction band.
46. Fibular hemimelia.
47. Endobutton.
48. Patella alta, radiology and pathoanatomy.
49. Complications of TKA.
50. Bursae around knee, Clergyman's knee.
51. Arthroscopy of knee, optical principles and port designing.
52. Applied anatomy of quadriceps, quadriceps contracture.
53. Triple deformity of knee.
54. Osgood-Schlatter disease.
55. Osteochondritis dissecans.
56. Pivot-shift test.
57. Anterior drawer test.
58. Ober's test and iliotibial band (ITB) contracture.
59. Proximal focal femoral deficiency.
60. Bone cement.
61. Aseptic loosening.
62. Trendelenburg's gait.
63. Snapping hip.
64. Impingement syndrome.
65. Congenital pseudoarthrosis of clavicle.
66. Sprengel shoulder.
67. Cervical rib, thoracic outlet syndrome.
68. Milwaukee shoulder.
69. Subacromial bursitis.
70. Tennis elbow.
71. Congenital radial head dislocation.
72. Allen's test.
73. Mucous cyst and differentials with a note on giant cell tumor of tendon sheath.
74. Principles of tendon transfer.
75. Strength-duration curve.
76. Trigger finger.
77. Lobster hand.
78. Dupuytren's contracture.
79. Tenodesis.

Long and Short Questions for Orthopedic Theory Examination

80. Neurolysis.
81. Mallet finger.
82. Management of moderate Volkmann ischemic contracture (VIC).
83. Radial club hand.
84. Thumb aplasia.
85. Flexor pulley.
86. Glomus tumor.
87. Groin flap, skin grafting.
88. Myocutaneous flap.
89. Spina bifida.
90. Spinal shock.
91. Definition of global instability.
92. Klippel-Feil syndrome.
93. Fractures of spine and mechanism.
94. Lumbar canal stenosis.
95. Vertebra plana.
96. Microwave diathermy.
97. Transcutaneous electrical nerve stimulation (TENS).
98. Floor reaction orthosis.
99. Splints for radial and ulnar nerve palsy.
100. Milwaukee brace.
101. Jaipur foot and solid-ankle cushioned heel (SACH) foot.
102. Closed chain exercises.
103. Pavlik harness.
104. Hydrotherapy.
105. Lumbar and brachial plexus.
106. Structure of giant cell and giant cell lesions.
107. Structure of peripheral nerve and Wallerian degeneration.
108. Blood supply of scaphoid.
109. Vertebra plana.
110. Myositis ossificans progressiva.
111. Floating knee.
112. Stress fracture, pathological fracture, avulsion fracture.
113. Locking compression-dynamic compression plate (LC-DCP), DCP, LCP, interfragmentary compression (principles of lag screw).

114. Fracture disease.
115. AO principles of fracture management and evolution of ideology.
116. Biological fixation.
117. Reflex sympathetic dystrophy and complex regional pain syndrome.
118. Functional cast bracing.
119. Piezoelectric effect and bone healing.
120. Fracture healing and modulating factors, fracture healing enhancers.
121. Management of polytrauma patient and principles of triage.
122. Advanced trauma life support.
123. Management of pelvic injuries.
124. Crush syndrome.
125. Ankle fracture—classification and management.
126. Factors leading to nonunion lateral fracture of condyle and management.
127. Fat embolism.
128. Pulmonary embolism.
129. Low molecular weight heparins and prevention of deep vein thrombosis.
130. Septic shock.
131. Fluid and electrolyte imbalance.
132. Tension band principle.
133. Classification of compound fractures and management of compound tibial fractures.
134. Biodegradable implant.
135. Use of silicone in orthopedics.
136. Compartment syndrome—diagnosis and management.
137. Classification and management of calcaneal fractures.
138. Classification and management of talus fractures.
139. Plaster of Paris, resin based-fiber cast.
140. Soft tissue coverage of lower limb.
141. Acromioclavicular dislocations.
142. Sternoclavicular dislocations.
143. Trans-scapho-perilunate dislocation.
144. Carpometacarpal dislocation.

Long and Short Questions for Orthopedic Theory Examination

145. Lisfranc dislocation.
146. Divergent elbow dislocation.
147. Marble bone disease.
148. Osteogenesis imperfecta classification and management.
149. Pseudofractures, role and actions of vitamin D3.
150. Neo-osteogenesis.
151. Renal osteodystrophy.
152. Renal rickets.
153. Uses of LASER in orthopedics.
154. Uses of ultrasonics in orthopedics.
155. Charcot's arthropathy.
156. Gas gangrene.
157. Utility of MRI in differentiating infective from mitotic pathology.
158. Role of bone scans in diagnosing orthopedic infection and inflammation.
159. Role of fluoro-2-deoxyglucose positron emission tomography (FDG PET) in metastatic work-up.
160. Synovial disorders of joints.
161. Adamantinoma.
162. Diagnosis and management of solitary plasmacytoma.
163. Diagnosing and differentiating osteoid osteoma and osteoblastoma.
164. Methods and critical analysis of bone grafting and bone graft substitutes.
165. Café-au-lait spots.
166. Principle of limb salvage surgery.
167. Role of immunotherapy in bone tumors.
168. Compound palmar ganglion.
169. Regimen of ATT and drug interactions.
170. Histology of tubercular granuloma.
171. Fungal disease of bone.
172. Brodie's abscess.
173. Sequestrum.
174. Granulomatous osteomyelitis.
175. Role of reaming in femoral osteomyelitis.
176. Obstetrical palsy, its etiopathogenesis and management.

177. Stem cell therapy in orthopedics.
178. Posterior approach to hip joint.
179. Steps of fenestration for PIVD.
180. Steps of anterolateral decompression.
181. Use of tourniquet in orthopedics.
182. Radionuclide bone scan.
183. Bearing surfaces for THR.
184. Implant infections.
185. Trochanteric flip osteotomy for hip exposure.
186. Tribology.
187. Femoroacetabular impingement syndrome.
188. Autoimmune disorders in orthopedics.
189. Anticyclic citrullinated peptide (anti-CCP) test and significance in rheumatoid arthritis.
190. Pseudotumors and management (hemophilia and metal on metal hip arthroplasty).
191. Pigmented villonodular synovitis.
192. Single event multiple level resections (SEMLR).
193. Quadriga effect.
194. Giant cell tumor.
195. Paraffin wax and role in orthopedics.

Etc... etc..etc...etc.... virtually everything has been asked in DNB theory exams!!! And what you consider has not been asked will be asked in coming times?!?!?!

INDEX

Page numbers followed by *f* refer to figure and *t* refer to table.

A

Abdominal reflex, interpretations of superficial 504
Abduction 12, 13*f*, 57, 282, 363
    deformity 11, 30
    lurch gait 602
    shoulder splint 192
Abductor 126
    mechanism 37
    triangle 62
Above elbow amputation 566
Above knee amputation 566
Abscess 407
Acetabular procedure 122
Acetabulum, traveling 49
Achilles tendon 216, 267*f*, 268*f*
    rupture 274
        treatment of chronic 272
Acid-fast bacillus 399
Acquired clubfoot 223, 223*t*
    causes of 223
Active straight leg raise test 21
Adam's test 501*f*
    basis of 500
    interpretations of 501
Adamantinoma 575, 585
Adduction 12, 13*f*, 57, 282, 363
    deformity 30, 225
Adductor spasm 10
Adjacent joint, movements of 183
Adson's test 289
Allen test 369
Allis' sign 24
Allis' test 149
Allopro prosthesis 628
American Joint Committee Classification 576
Ames test 427
Amputation 564, 565, 567
    goals of 565
    level of 569, 569*t*, 609
    stump 564, 566
    surgery, complications of 568
Amstutz femoral component 629
Ancillary surgeries 406
Anconeus triangle 311, 311*f*
Andre-Thomas sign 390
Aneurysm 149
Ankle 30, 601
    dorsiflexion 458
    equinus 31
        deformity of 263
    joint
        arthrodesis 263
        articulated 610
Ankylosing spondylitis 7, 46
    diagnosis of 43
    pain of 7
Ankylosis
    bony 209, 465
    fibrous 465
Annular ligament, reconstruction of 356
Anterior cord syndrome 462
Anterior cruciate ligament 152, 195
    diagnosis of 196, 198
Anterior instrumentation, indications of 475
Antibiotic 631
    beads 532
    impregnated
        beads, disadvantages of 532
        cements 631
Antiglide 621

Anti-tubercular therapy 45
Anvil sign 11f
AO compression arthrodesis 293
Apley's compression test 150
Apley's distraction test 150
Apley's grinding test 290
Apley's test 150f
Aponeurectomy, segmental 412
Appendiceal spinal tuberculosis 465
Apprehension test 286f, 287
Arachnoiditis 497
Arch, medial longitudinal 217
Arm
    chair effect 69
    length 306
    swing 600
Arthrodesis 66, 314
    contraindications of 58
    indications of 55
    intra-articular 56f
    judge position of 293
    role of 131, 210
    triple 243, 255
Arthrogram, role of 122
Arthrogryposis multiplex congenita 179, 245
Arthrolysis, contraindications of 317
Arthropathy 7
Arthroplasty 66, 72, 314, 626
    distraction 317
    excisional 314
    fascial interposition 318
    interposition 318, 627
    role of 72, 140
    total joint replacement 627
Arthroscopic anterior cruciate ligament reconstruction 202
Arthroscopic procedures, role of 302
Arthrotomy 314
Articular cartilage, status of 645
Attitude 31
Aufranc-Turner component 629
Automatic bladder 460

B

Babcock's triangle 62
Babinski sign 454
Back pain, presentations of 486
Bacteriological index 398
Bado classification 354, 354f
Baker's cyst 146, 149
Bakshi's procedure 89
Bakshi's sloppy hinge prosthesis 635
Bankart's lesion 295
Barlow's maneuver 40
Barlow's tests 40
Barrel plate 137
    ideal angle of 136
Barton fracture 440
    reverse 440
Basal ganglia 600
Basilar neck osteotomy 104
Baumann's angle 337, 337f
Bead pouch technique 532, 533f
Beevor's sign 453
Beighton criteria 299f
Below elbow amputation 566
Below knee amputation 566
Bending films 506
Betadine, composition of 619
Bhattacharya procedure 317
Biceps
    femoris 194
    tendinitis, tests for 289
Bikini incision 122
Bilateral deformity 33
    causes of 167
Biodegradable beads 532
Biopsy, types of 581
Bisphosphonates 141, 320
Bitrochanteric compression test 41
Blackburne-Peel ratio 161
Bladder dysfunction 460
Blindness 600
Blood tests 50
Blount's disease 176
Blumensaat line 161
Bone 567
    age 511

Index

biopsy, principles of 580
cyst 7
    aneurysmal 463, 585
destructions, types of 579
disease 600
forearm 556
grafting 547
    intramedullary 563
    methods of 86
    substitutes 551
    types of 547
irregular thickened 521
loss 65
sarcoma, staging of 576t
scan 93, 580, 640
secondary malignancy of 585
transport, types of 555
true tumor of 183
tumor 580, 585
    benign 584
    common 584
    Enneking classification of 575, 576t
    excision, types of 582f
    malignant 575, 584
    secondary benign 584
Bony procedures 241t, 252
role of 240, 278
Bounce home test 150
Bouvier maneuver 389
Bower hemiresection interposition arthroplasty 440f
Boyd's approach 356
Boyd's dual onlay cortical bone grafting 563
Boyd's procedure 357
Boyes transfer 376
Brachial plexus, formation of 391
Bracing
    contraindications of 97
    end-point for 97
    prerequisites of 97
    role of 519
Bragard's test 455

Brittain's method 57, 58f
Broken Shenton's line 115
Broom test 310
Brown-Sequard syndrome 463
Brucellosis 464
Bruner incisions 417, 417f
Bryant's test 289
Bryant's triangle 19, 40, 41f, 62
    fallacies of 41
Buchholtz cup 629
Bulbar polio 191
Bulbospinal polio 191
Bunnel O sign 389, 389f
Bursitis 146
Buttress plating, principles of 622

C

Cabot's maneuver 150
Cabot's position 150
Café au lait spots 9, 499
Caffey's disease 522
Caffey's hypothesis 91
Caffey's sign 93
Caisson's disease 91
Calcaneal position 601
Calcaneocavus deformity 265
Calcaneous gait, transfer for 240
Calcaneum 248f
    posterior tuberosity of 218
Calcaneus deformity 255, 265
Calcar comminution 65
Calf atrophy 216
Callaway's test 289
Callus response, types of 558
Calve's disease 464
Camitz transfer 388
Campbell's posterior bone-block 263
Canes
    placement of 607
    types of 607
Card test 389, 390f
Caroll's two incision technique 237
Carpal canal stenosis 430
Carpal compression test 366
Carpal instability 367

Carpal tunnel syndrome 425, 428, 429, 431, 441
    nonsurgical treatment for 431
    risk factors for 429
    surgical approaches to 432
Carrying angle 329f
Cast immobilization 530
Cauda equina syndrome 490, 497
Cavus 226
Cech classification 541
Cell variant, small 585
Cellulitis 522
Cement
    available, types of 630
    disease 630
Cementing techniques 630
Cementless stems, types of 632
Central cord syndrome 462
Central disk 484
Cerebellum 600
Cerebral palsy 7, 600, 604
Cerebrospinal fluid leak 497
Cervical
    lesions 466
    spine 453, 473
        sniffing position of 448
Cervicodorsal scoliosis 304
Cervicothoracic region 473
Chaddock's sign 459
Chair test 309
Chandler's disease 79
Charcot's joint 39
Charcot-Marie-tooth disease 498
Charlie Chaplin gait 605
Charnley's cup 629
    modified 629
Charnley's femoral stem 629
Chauffeur fracture 440
Chemonucleolysis 493
Chemotherapy 401, 583
    adjuvant 583
    role of 51
    types of 583
Chest expansion 452
Chiari's osteotomy 98, 124
Chiene's test 20
Childress' test 150, 150f
Choi classification 107
Chondroblastic variant 585
Chondroblastoma 575
Chondrogenesis 546
Chondrosarcoma 575
Chordoma 585
Chronaxie 384, 385f
Chronic osteomyelitis 520, 521, 527, 530, 646
    complications of 535
    differential diagnosis for 522
Cierny-Mader classification 526
Circumduction test 287
Clasp test 394
Claw
    deformity 403
    foot 261
    hand 402-404, 586
    toe 258, 407
Clawing 259
    types of 258
Cleft
    lip 499
    palate 499
Clonus 461
Closed chain exercises 203
Closed fist
    sign 427
    test 366
Closed reduction
    maneuvers 72
    failure of 135
Clubfoot 224, 237, 240, 243
    clinical types of 228t
    congenital 223, 223t
    Kite's manipulative correction 229
    manipulative correction technique for 229
    Ponseti method of correction of 231
    types of 228
    untreated 240

Index

Cobb's angle 509
Cobb's method 507, 508*f*
   criticism of 509
Cobra-plate method 56*f*
Coccygodynia 10
Cock-up wrist splint 192
Codman angle 578
Cold abscess 466
Collared stem 633
Collarless stem 633
Collateral ligament, medial 152
Colles fracture 440, 441
   complications of 441
   reverse of 440
Column procedure 316
Comminution, posterior 65
Compactotomy 552
Compartment syndrome 586
Complete discectomy, signs of 494
Compression mode 621
Computed tomography 82, 429
   role of 428
Condylar blade plate 139
Congenital muscular torticollis,
      cause of 595
Congenital pseudoarthrosis of tibia,
      treatment for 562
Congenital vertical talus 212, 246,
      247, 248*f*
   complications of 251
Congruence angle 161*f*
Connective tissue disorder 8
Constant length phenomenon 588
Convex hemiepiphysiodesis 518
Copeland sphygmomanometer
      test 267
Cord
   branches of posterior 392
   involvement, level of 461, 461*t*
   like induration 586
   pathogenesis of 411
   poor recovery of 480
Core decompression 85
   methods of 86
   rationale of 85

Cortex 640
Corticosteroid 80
   injections, role of 431
   therapy 522
Corticotomy 552, 553
   complications of 554
   S-shaped 553
   types of 553
Cosmesis 609
Costotransversectomy,
      advantages of 481
Coxa breva 106
Coxa magna 98, 106
Coxa valga 600
Coxa vara 44, 600
   congenital 99, 100
   developmental 99
Cozen's test 309, 310*f*
Crackling egg-shell consistency 574
Craig's test 149
Cram test 456
Crank test 290, 290*f*
Crankshaft phenomenon 517
Crepitus 541
Critical median nerve
      compression 427
Crossed adductor's sign 459
Crutch gaits 605
Crystal arthropathies 600
Cubitus valgus 344, 348
   deformity
      causes of 344
      development of 348
Cubitus varus 328, 338, 350
   causes of 332
   correction of 342*f*
   deformity 330*f*, 338-340
      radiograph of 340*f*
Cuneiform 104
   osteotomy 105
Cup arthroplasty 627
Curly toe 258
Curve 506, 512
   determine flexibility of 503

D

De novo tumors, tumor differ from 187
De Quervain disease 369
Deep fibular nerve
    palsy 276
    supply 275
Deep mycotic infections 522
Deformity 31, 100, 143, 175, 213, 305, 358, 401, 446, 477, 521
    around hip 31
    correction 69, 232f
        techniques for 189
    magnitude of 171, 507
    Ponseti method of
        correction of 234
    progression 478, 478f, 479f, 479
    site 171
    worries orthopedician 100
Dejour's test 151
Deltoid contracture 302, 303
    causes of 303
Dennis-Browne
    bar with shoe 244f
    splint 244
Dental hygiene 9
Dentinogenesis 9
Deoxyribonucleic acid 584
Dermal nerves, integrity of 397
Dermatomyositis 600
Dermofasciectomy 412
Desault's sign 24
Diabetes mellitus 8
Diaphyseal fit 633
Diaphyseal lesions 575
Diaphyseal osteomyelitis, causes for 525
Dickson-Diveley procedure 260
Die-punch fracture 441
Digital Z-plasties 412
Digitorum longus, extensor 215, 458
Directly observed treatment in supervision 470
Disability 401
Discectomy
    complications of 497
    disk material removed in 495
Disease severity, classification of 591
Disk
    axillary presentation of 485
    herniations 482f
        sites of 483
        types of 482
    presentation of 489
    shoulder presentation of 485
    size of 489
    surgical removal of 494
Diskitis 497
Dislocated shoulder, tests for 288
Dislocation
    chronic 294
    complete 125
    incomplete 125
    old unreduced 127
    pathological 39
Displacement, degree of 73, 324
Distal amputation 569
Distal interphalangeal
    flexion 386
    joint 593
        hyperextension of 258
Distal neurovascular deficit 220
Distal phalanx 415
Distal radioulnar joint 437
    grinding test 367
    instability 367
Distal radius 436f
    fixation of 443
    fractures 442
    malunion of 435, 436
    parameters of 435
Distant metastasis 576
Distraction osteogenesis, physiological effect of 554
Divergent speculated pattern 579
Dome osteotomy 174f, 342f
Dorsal aspect 360, 362
Dorsal bunion 239, 262
Dorsal lesions 467

Index

Dorsal navicular subluxation 239
Dorsal spine tuberculosis 476
Dorsal tilt 437
    correction of 438*f*
Double bundle techniques 202
Double leg stance 602
Down's syndrome 121, 144, 497
Drawer test 287, 287*f*
    anterior 151, 152, 197, 197*f*, 198, 220
    causes of false negative 196, 204
    of Daniel, quadriceps active 153
Drop arm test 284, 285*f*
Drop-back phenomenon 153
Drunkards gait 605
Dry dressing 617
Duchenne's muscular dystrophy 600
Duchenne's sign 390
Duchenne's test 275*f*
    positive 275
Duck footed gait 146
Duck walk gait 603
Duga's test 289
Dunlop traction 338*f*
Dupuytren contracture 409
Dupuytren disease 409, 410, 412
Dupuytren nodules 410
Dural tear 497
Durkan median nerve compression test 366
Durkan test 367*f*, 427
Dwyer osteotomy 242
Dynamic compression screw 139
Dynamic hip screw
    failure of 140
    lag screw 138
Dynamization 557
Dysbarism 80
Dysplasia 9, 114, 145
    fibrous 522, 561, 575, 646

E

Ears
    lobe infiltration 395
    small 499
    tapering 499
Ectopic ossification 314, 318-320
    around elbow 321
Ehlers-Danlos syndrome 145
Eight-strand technique 419
Elbow 341, 609
    alignment of 329
    arthrodesis, optimal position of 314
    arthroplasty 317, 626, 635
        indications of 635
        total 635
    case, examination points for 305
    cubitus varus deformity of 330*f*
    dislocation 322, 331, 348, 644
        diagnosis of 322
        old unreduced 331*f*
    examination, prerequisites of 310
    flexed 586
    flexion
        deformity of 312
        resisted 310
        test 310
    injury, terrible triad of 328
    instability 324, 324*t*, 325
        causes of 325
    joint 305, 311, 315, 323
        tuberculosis of 313
    prosthesis 635
        types of 635
    recurrent dislocation of 328
    stability, Fortress concept for 324
    tuberculosis of 313
    unstable 322, 325
Elephant foot 540
Elizabethtown osteotomy 97
Ely's test 21, 22*f*
Encephalitis 191
Endoscopic release,
            contraindications for 432
Energy
    consumption 569
    storing foot 610
Enneking classification 575, 576*t*
Enzyme-linked immunosorbent assay 50
Eosinophilic granuloma 464, 522, 575, 585

Epidural injection
    indications of 492
    philosophy of 492
Epiphyseal lesions 575
Epiphyseal nonunions 556
Epiphysiodesis 105
Epithelioid sarcoma 412
Equinovalgus 265
Equinovarus 222
Equinus 225, 226
    deformity 263
Erichson's pelvis compression test 23
Erythema nodosum leprosum,
    types of 400
Erythrocyte sedimentation rate 526
Eusol 619
Ewing's sarcoma 522, 575, 583, 585
Excise exostosis 188
Exercises, types of 202
Exostosis 183, 186, 187
    complications of 186
Extension 13f, 65
    lurch gait 603
Extensor apparatus 146, 147
Extensor hallucis longus,
    tendon of 215
Extensor pollicis longus tendon,
    rupture of 441
Extensor tendon 416f
External bridging callus 558
External fixator 557
External rotation 282
    test 153
Extra-articular arthrodesis
    Brittain's method of 57
    role of 57
Extracapsular arterial ring 74
Extraperiosteal resection 188
Eyrebrook's delayed bone grafting 563

F

Facet dislocation 477
Failed back syndrome 497
Fairbank's and Hall classification 486
Fairbank's apprehension test 148f
Fairbank's triangle 62
False-negative test 38
False-positive test 37
Farmar's cross-legged vascularized
    pedicle bone grafting 563
Fascicle 381
Fasciectomy 412
Feagin maneuver 288
Femoral anteversion 19f, 146, 154
Femoral capital epiphysis, small 92
Femoral components 628
Femoral condyles 522
Femoral epiphyseal arrest 98
Femoral fracture 600
Femoral head
    blood supply of 74, 75f
    large malformed 98
    malformed 98
    osteonecrosis of 46, 77
Femoral length 153
Femoral neck 76
    fracture, bilateral 648
Femoral nerve stretch test 456
Femoral osteotomy, advantages of 122
Femoral torsion 600
Femoral triangle 27, 27f, 62
Femoral varus derotation
    osteotomy 97
Femorotibial alignment 165
Femur
    Babcock's triangle, head of 53
    fracture neck of 66, 72
    neck of 53
    non-union, fracture neck of 66
    old fracture neck of 62
    osteomyelitis of 106, 530
Fenestration 494
Ferguson's method 507, 508f
Fever 280
Fibrogenesis 546
Fibrosis 389
    epidural 497
Fibula 86
    vascularized 563

Index

Fibular nerve
    palsy 275
        causes of 276
        superficial 276
    supply, superficial 275
Ficat-Arlet classification 81, 81*t*
Figure of 4 sign 24
Finger 360-362
    flexion of 360*f*
    intrinsic function 387
    movements 363
Finkelstein test 369*f*
First metatarsal rise test 221
Fishtail deformity, causes of 341
Fite-Faraco stains 409
Five fingers quadriceps gait 603
Fix joint 57
Fixed abduction deformity 11, 30
Fixed adduction deformity 11, 30
Fixed flexion deformity 11, 16
Fixed rotational deformities 11
Fixed scar 520
Fixing osteotomy, methods of 342
Flaccid
    paralysis, acute 251
    paraplegia, causes of 470
Flail knee 195
    bilateral 195
Flaps
    configuring of 565
    vascularity of 566
Flat bones 575
Flexibility index 506
Flexible curves 498, 502*f*
Flexion 13*f*, 65, 306, 452
    anterior 282
    causes restriction of 333
    deformity 34, 35, 207, 312
    intertrochanteric osteotomy 88
    resisted 310
    rotation drawer test 152
Flexor digitorum
    profundus 415
        power 403
    superficialis 415, 588
        power 403
Flexor hallucis longus 588
Flexor tendon 416*f*
    injury 413
Focus, excision of 54
Foot 30
    after triple arthrodesis, appearance of 257
    and ankle 212, 610
        cases, examination points for 212
        common sarcoma of 585
        polio affection of 251
    deformity, correction of 231*f*
    drop 128, 274, 406
        causes of 276
        early 406
    flat 599
    inversion of 458
    position 601
    pronation of 226
    shape 601
    supination of 225, 226, 231
    surgery in polio, treatment in 253
    ulcers 407
Footwear 1
Forearm
    classification of 189*t*
    compartments in 594
    length 307
    supination, resisted 310
Forefoot 219
    adduction 225
    equinus of 261
Four-strand technique 418, 419
Fracture 64, 648
    affect treatment, status of 373
    comminution 64
    dislocation 127
    displaced 64
    fixation, principles of 620
    fresh intertrochanteric 134
    healing 141, 545
    intra-articular 641
    intramedullary fixation of 138
    irreducible 334

level of 641
line
    geometry of 641
    shape of 73
medial epicondyle 348
nonunion 67
old neglected 134
olecranon 348
pathological 648
posteromedial type 333
site 137
surfaces 66
type of 346
Fragments, telescopy of 541
Free-vascularized fibular grafting, principles of 86
French osteotomy 342
    modified 341, 341f, 342, 342t
Friedlander technique 549
Friedreich's ataxia 498, 600
Froment sign 389, 389f
Frozen hand 400
Fulcrum
    disruption of 38
    test 23
Fusion
    anterior 518
    indications of 495
    methods of 495
    posterior 518
F-wave 385

G

Gaenslen's test 23, 24f
Gage sign 94
Gait 177, 213, 451, 463, 499, 598, 600
    analysis 598
    antalgic 146, 602
    base of 602
    calcaneus 605
    circumduction 604f
    cycle 599, 599f
    evaluation 599
    festinating 605
    four-point 605
    hand to knee 603
    high stepping 603
    hysterical 605
    inspection of 146
    in-toeing 605
    pattern 498, 605-607
    short shuffling 605
    stamping 605
    stumbling 602
    three-point 606
    two-point 606
    types of 602
Galeazzi's lesion 355
Galeazzi's sign 18f, 149
    positive 113f
Ganglion, intraosseous 522
Garceau's cheilectomy 98
Garden's classification 73
Garden's index 73
Garre's osteomyelitis 536
Gaucher's disease 91, 522
Gauvain's sign 21
Gear-stick sign 24
Genu recurvatum
    causes of 192
    congenital 179
Genu valgum 145, 153, 163, 164f, 165, 207, 600
Genu varum 145, 153, 163, 164f, 165, 172f, 600
Gerdy's tubercle 16
Giant cell
    rich osteosarcoma 586
    tumor 463, 574, 575, 585
Gibbus 447f
Gill's sign 24
Girdlestone arthroplasty 39, 40, 59, 60
Girdlestone classification 468
Girdlestone-Taylor procedure 260
Glenoid
    rim, loss of 301
    sign, vacant 295
Glide test 148f

Index

Gluteal folds, asymmetry of 26
Gluteal inhibition 39
Gluteal tenderness 10
Gluteus maximus
    gait 603
    paralysis 127
    tendinitis 10
Gluteus medius 37
    gait 603
    paralysis 38, 127
Glycocalyx 533
Godfrey's sign 152
Gordon's sign 459
Gorlin's sign 299
Gout 600
Gracilis contracture 179
Grade muscle power 192
Graf's classification 117t
Grafting technique 68
Grafts
    enhance healing 548
    failure 476
    harvest nerve for 380
    heal 548
Graham and Hastings criteria 437t
Granular form 52
Grasp, reversal of 403
Great toe 219
    clawing 260
        mechanism of 260
    extension of 458
Greater trochanter 98, 626
    tip of 26
Greater tuberosity 300
Griffith's classification 468
Grind test 369
Grip strength 369
Growing rod
    complications of 519
    principle behind 518
    types of 518
Gunstock deformity 340, 340f
Gupta's method 130
Guyon canal 391f
    boundaries of 391

H

Haglund's deformity 216f
Hairy patch 499
    midline 449f
Hallucis longus, extensor 458
Hallux flexus 239
Hallux valgus 214f
Halsted's test 289
Hamilton ruler test 288
Hammer toe 258
Hand 361
    common sarcoma of 585
    elevation test 366, 427
    radial deviation of 359
    zones of 415, 415t
Hansen
    cardinal signs of 395
    disease 395, 408
    foot drop 406
Harmon's procedure, principles of 110
Harris femoral component 629
Harris-Galante prosthesis 628
Hart's classic signs 114
Hawkins impingement reinforcement test 284
Hawkins-Kennedy test 284f
Head
    blood supply of 91
    position of 448
Healed disease 480
Healing
    radiological signs of 50
    ulcer, characteristics of 616
Heel
    strike 599
    varus 225
Helicopod gait 605
Hemangioma 464, 585
Hematological disorder 8
Hematoma
    epidural 497
    formation, lack of 64
Hemiarthroplasty 627
    prerequisites for 637
Hemichondrodiastasis 175

Hemicircumduction gate 604
Hemiepiphyseal stapling,
    disadvantages of 174
Hemiepiphysiodesis,
    disadvantages of 174
Hemiparesis 604
Hemi-shoulder arthroplasty 636
Hemodynamic function, tests for 83
Hemophilia 9, 145, 522
Henri Dejour frog position 150
Herniation, level of 489
Heterotopic ossification 318
High median nerve palsy 400
High molecular weight
    polyethylene 626
High ulnar nerve palsy 400
    methods of 386
High viscosity cements 630
Hilgenreiner's epiphyseal angle 100
Hill-Sachs lesion 295, 301
    reverse 295, 301
Hilton law 394
Hindfoot
    score 235
    varus 241
Hinged abduction 98, 99
Hip 6, 16, 52, 609
    ankylosis of 106
    anterior dislocation of 63
    arthrodesis
        Brittain's method of 58f
        types of 56
    arthroplasty 626, 638
        contraindications of 634
        types of 627
    case, examination points for 6
    central fracture dislocation of 46
    chronic old unreduced posterior
        dislocation of 129
    contracture 126
    deformity, compensation for 30
    developmental dysplasia of 7, 25,
        39, 111, 113, 114, 117, 600
    dislocation
        complications of 129
        direction of 118
    dysplasia, Hart's classic signs of 114
    extended 13
    flexion
        deformity 34
        ipsilateral 458
    irritable 92
    joint 10, 25, 30, 32f, 39, 62, 72,
        105, 465
        causes out of 40
        osteoarthritis of 70
        pain of 42
        rest for 43
        tuberculosis of 45, 52
    osteonecrosis of 44, 79
    paralytic dislocation of 114
    pathology 43
    poliomyelitis affection of 125
    posterior dislocation of 25
    primary osteoarthritis of 78
    reduction of 115, 122
    rotation 15f
        measurement of 14f
    surgical dislocation of 105
    transient osteoporosis of 78
    tuberculosis of 40, 45, 78
Histoid leprosy 408
Hodgson's classification 469
Hoffa's disease 146
Hoffmann's reflex 459
Hoffmann's sign 459, 459f
Holstein Lewis fracture 377
Homan's sign 221f
Homan's test 221
Hompson-Simmonds test 269
Hong Kong procedure 474
Horse hoof 540
Hot foot syndrome 407
Howship's lacunae 50
H-reflex 385
Hughston's jerk test 152
Human immunodeficiency virus
    infection 80, 522
Humeral neck, profile of 295
Humerus fracture 378
    lateral condyle of 348
Hungerford technique 85

Index

Hunka classification 107, 108f
Hunter, circulus articuli vasculosus of 76
Hurler's syndrome 497
Hutchinson fracture 441
Hybrid system 613
　development of 628
Hydrocolloids 619
Hydrogen peroxide 619
Hyperabduction test 289
Hyperextension 258, 306
Hyperkeratosis 9
Hypermobility syndrome 9
Hypertension 8
Hyperuricemia 80
Hypervascular nonunion 547
Hypervitaminosis A 522
Hypotenuse, shortening of 41

I

Ilfeld phenomenon 118
Iliac crest 563
Iliac fossae 42
Iliac spine, anterior superior 498
Iliac tubercle 26
Iliopsoas transfer 127
Iliotibial band contracture produce 175
Ilizarov fixator, role of 243
Ilizarov method 549, 563
Ilizarov reconstruction osteotomy 111
Immobile joint 54
Implant, intramedullary 139
Inactive residual extremity syndrome 571
Indian Association of Leprologists 398
Infection 497
　cause of chronicity of 525
　chronic 7
　　cutaneous 522
　　subcutaneous 522
　foci of 291
　focus of 53
　throbbing of 7
Infraspinatus, test for 285
Infusion, intravenous 9

Injury 195, 203, 328, 643
　acute 162
　history of 414
Insall-Salvati ratio 161
　modified 161
Intercondylar distances 166f
Interepicondylar distance 311
Intermalleolar distances 166f
Intermittent compressive hydrostatic stress 546
Interpret finger flexion 414
Intertrochanteric fracture 135, 142
　malunion 132
　stable 135
　unstable 134, 138
Intervertebral disk disease 481
Intralesional excision 582
Intrinsic minus hand 382
Invasive test 427
Inversion stress test 220, 220f
Involucrum 524
Iodine 618
Ischial tuberosity 27
Ivory vertebra, isolated 464

J

Jacob's classification 346, 347f
Jaipur foot 611, 611t, 612
Jansen's sign 23
Japas osteotomy 262
Jaw, osteosarcoma of 585
Jeanne sign 389
Jerk test 287
Jobe's test 285
Jogerson Lewandoz law 397
Joints 255, 641
　arthritis 369
　basilar 361
　disease 600
　dislocated 106
　hypermobility of 404
　line 362
　multiple 7
　painless 54
　space, reduction of 48

stable 54
unstable 54
zygapophyseal 444
Jones procedure 260
modified 260
Joshi's external stabilization system 243
J-sign 159, 160f
Jug test 309
Jumper's knee 146

K

K-angle 477
Kapandji method 443
Keratin 585
Kernig's maneuver 455
Kiloh-Nevin sign 394
King and Moe classification 512f
Kite's error 233
Kite's manipulative correction 229
Kleinert regime 423
Klemm's triad 530
Klippel-Feil syndrome 281, 303
Klisic subgroups 117
K-nail, principle of 623
Knee 30, 143, 609
    amputation, advantages of 571
    angular deformity of 163
    ankle-foot orthosis 562
    case, examination points for 143
    congenital dislocation of 179
    flexion 226, 458
        test 268
    gait, flexed 146
    instabilities 199
    joint 211
        flexion contracture of 194
        lymphatic drainage of 208
        tuberculosis of 205, 207
    mechanism 609, 610t
    position 601
    Q-angle of 154f
    rehabilitation 202
    stiffness, causes of 530
    triple deformity of 207
Knock knee gait 603

Knuckle 447f
Kothari's parallelogram 19, 44
Kushtha 396
Kuwada's classification 272
Kyphosis 446f, 477
    partial reduction of 447
Kyphotic deformity 447, 463
    severe 480

L

Labral injuries 301
Labrum anterior to posterior, superior 289
Lachman test 151, 196, 196f
    advantages of 196
Lag screw 137
    ideal position of 135
Lambrinudi arthrodesis 263
Lamellar reaction, single 578
Laminectomy 494
    role of 475
Laminotomy 494
Larsen syndrome 144
Lasegue's test 455, 455f, 456
    modified 455, 455f
Lateral condyle fracture 339, 339t, 345, 346, 347f, 348
    components of 346
    displacements of 348
    Jacob's classification of 347f
Lateral cord, branches of 392
Lateral epicondylitis, tests for 309
Lateral ligament complex injury 146
Lateral limb
    decreased length of 311
    increased length of 311
Lateral translation sign 477
Lax nonunion 541
Laxity 144
Lazarine leprosy 408
Leg
    fracture of 555
    heel raise test, single 269
    hyperextension test, single 456
Legg-Calve-Perthes disease 90

Index

Lepra reaction 398
    types of 399, 399*t*
Lepromatous leprosy 399
Leprosy 396, 398, 400
    hand 394
        prerequisites for surgery in 404
        types of deformity in 401
Lesions, posterior 465
Lesser toes 219
Lesser tuberosity 300
Leukocyte imaging 528
Lhermitte's sign 454
Lichtblau procedure 242
Ligament
    status of 645
    tibionavicular 250
Ligamentous laxity 280, 299
    generalized 166
Ligamentum teres, artery of 76
Light-bulb procedure 86
Limb
    gait, short 602
    length
        discrepancy 8, 17
        inequality 600
        measurements 498
    malformations of 499
    motion 600
    neurological examination of 498
    two 642
Limp 7, 212
    painless 7
Lindequist and Tornkvist criteria 73
Linear measurements 306
Linear wear 634
Linton's classification 73
Liver
    dysfunction 80
    function test 526
Load-shift test 286
Long bones, nonunion of 537
Long finger extension test 309, 310
Lordotic deformities 451
Losee test 152
Low friction arthroplasty,
        principle of 626

Low median nerve palsy 400
Low ulnar nerve palsy 400
Low viscosity cements 631
Lowell's S-curves 73
Lower limb 192
    bones 556
Lower thoracic nerve roots 453
Lower trunk, anterior division of 393*f*
Ludloff sign 10
Ludloff test 24
Lumbar disk disease 481
Lumbar flatback 448
Lumbar interbody fusion
    anterior 496
    posterior 496
Lumbar lesions 467
Lumbar lift-off test 284
Lumbar lordosis 35
    increased 113*f*
Lumbar region 473
Lumbar spine 176
Lumbar triangle 467
Lumbrical plus finger 424
Lunotriquetral ballottement 368*f*
Lymphadenopathy 8, 149, 220
Lymphoma 464, 522, 575, 585

M

Magnetic resonance imaging 429, 468, 528, 645
Maisonneuve test 369
Malformations, congenital 499
Malignant transformation 187
Mallet toe 258
Malunion 537
    consequences of 435
    incidence of 435
    intra-articular 438
    type of 434
Malunited distal radius fracture 433
Malunited fracture 133
    acetabulum
        posterior wall 63
        superior wall 63

Malunited supracondylar fracture 333
Malunited tibial plateau fracture 146
Mandibular hypoplasia 499
Marfan's syndrome 121, 144, 497
Marginal excision 582
Martin-Gruber anastomosis 390
Mass 499
    maturity of 321
Masse sign 390
Matles knee flexion test 267, 268f
Maudsley's test 309
May's classification 536t, 540
McBab, bowstring sign of 455
McFarland type posterior bypass
        graft 563
McFarland's test 25
McMurray osteotomy 70
McMurray test 149, 150f
McMurray's osteotomy,
        principles of 70
Mechanical stimuli, low levels of 546
Medial cord, branches of 392, 393f
Medial limb
    decreased length of 311
    increased length of 311
Median nerve 369, 371, 384, 396, 590
    autonomous zones of 384
    compression 429
    tests for 393
Medullary canal 557
Medullary cavity 641
Melone classification 442
Meningomyelocele 121, 497
Meniscal cyst 146
Meniscal tear 146
    tests for 150f
Meniscus 290
    door stopper effect of 198
    tests for 149
Mesh cage bone graft technique 548
Metaphyseal
    cysts 94
    fit 633
    fragment 346
    lesions 574

Metastasis 575, 576, 585
Metatarsalgia 259
Metatarsophalangeal joint 213
    hyperextension of 258
Metatarsus adductus 241
Methylene blue test 397
Midfoot score 235
Midline defects 499
Midtarsal joint 601
Migrated disk 482f
Milch classification 346, 347f, 348
Milch-Batchelor osteotomy 61
Milgram's test 456
Mill's maneuver 310
Milwaukee brace 614
Mobile joint 54
Monoarticular rheumatoid 46, 78
    arthritis 7
Monteggia equivalents 355
Monteggia fracture dislocation 352-354
    old unreduced 351, 352
Monteggia lesion 354
    Bado classification of 354
Moore fracture 441
Morning stiffness 7
Morphological index 398
Morrey and Peterson's criteria 534
Morris bitrochanteric test 20
Morton's test 221
Moth-eaten destruction 579
Motion, range of 219
Movements
    functional range of 315
    limitation of 144, 280, 305
Müller femoral stem 629
Müller's test 153
Multidirectional instability 295, 301
Multifocal osteomyelitis 646
Multiple surgery 530
Muscle 319
    condition of 406
    contracture formation,
        causes of 177
    disease 600
    dysplasia, localized 179

Index

pedicle bone graft 68, 86
    advantages of 68
  pedicle periosteal graft 68
  power 283
  release of 126
  role of 300
  slide operation, disadvantages of 593
  stabilization 568
Musculoskeletal disorders 595
Mycobacterium leprae 395, 397
  characteristics of 408
  stains for 409
Myeloma 575
  multiple 585
Myeloproliferative disorders 80
Myerson's classification 272
Myodesis 568
Myopathy 145
Myoperiosteal graft 68
Myoplasty 568
Myositis 645
Myositis ossificans 106, 318, 319
  causes of 318
  circumscripta 318
  clinical features of 319
  differential diagnosis of 319
Myosteatosis 318

N

Naffziger's test 456
Nail 360, 557
  larger diameter 557
Nailing
  generations of 624
  intramedullary 563
  principle of 623
Narath sign 28
Nash and Moe method 510*f*
Natal cleft 10
National Leprosy Eradication Programme Classification 398
Navicular position 601

Neck femur
  fractured 64, 73
  stress fracture of 74, 648
Neck reconstruction 66, 68
Neck-shaft angle 101
Necrotic bone
  exposed 520
  removal, adequacy of 531
Needle test of O'Brien 268
Neer's impingement
  sign 283, 283*f*
  test 283*f*, 284
Neer's test, inferior drawer of 288
Neglected clubfoot 239
Nelaton's line 20, 20*f*
Neoadjuvant chemotherapy 583
Neoplasia 648
Neosporin ointment, constituents of 620
Nerve 395, 567
  anatomy of 372*f*
  entrapment 645
  gap 379
  grafting, types of 380
  injury 382
    type VI 382
  palsy 370
    causes of 388
  recovery, earliest sign of 383
  repair, types of 380
  root injury 497
  supply, variegated 42
  type of 377
Neuritis 402
Neurofibromatosis 146, 497
Neurofibromatosis, skin lesions of 561
Neurogenic claudication 487
Neurological disorders 8
Neurolysis
  internal 433
  types of 389
Neuromuscular curves, characteristics of 504
Neuromuscular defect 227
Neuromuscular disorder 7

Neuromuscular scoliosis 499
Neutral vertebra 507
Neutralization 621
Newspaper sign 389
Night cries 7, 463
  causes of 48
Nodule formation 410, 411*f*
Noncontained disk sequestration 482*f*
Non-Dupuytren disease 412
Noninfected nonunion 540
Nonoperative treatment,
  role of 273, 373
Nonparalytic aseptic meningitis 191
Nonsteroidal anti-inflammatory drugs
  320, 432
Nonunion 537-539, 555
  causes of 64, 539, 543
  develop 545
  fracture
    intertrochanteric 63
    neck of femur 46, 62, 66, 69, 72
  infected 543, 549
  lateral condyle fracture 345*f*
  occurrence of 543
  principles of treating 546
  small segment 552
  type of 64
Nonvascular graft 547
Normal hip 49

O

O'Brien's test 221, 267, 269, 289
Ober's test 21, 22*f*, 149, 149*f*, 166, 498
Oblique fracture, fixation of reverse
  138
Old femoral head fracture 78
Old Perthes disease 78
Onsall-Salvati ratio 162*f*
Open discectomy, failure of 496
Open reduction 356
  indications of 338
Open release, complications of 432
Opening-wedge osteotomy 172, 172*f*
Oppenheim's sign 459
Organ transplants 8

Organism reach vertebral column 464
Original Ficat's classification 81
Original French osteotomy 341, 342*t*
Orthopedic apparatus 191
Orthopedic procedures, aim of 192
Orthopedic residency program 1
Orthosis 608
Orthotics 608
Ortolani's tests 40
Osgood-Schlatter disease 146
Ossifying hematoma 318
Osteoarthritis 146, 600
Osteoblastic metastasis 464
Osteoblastoma 575, 585
Osteochondral grafting 86
Osteochondroma 181
Osteochondroses 464
Osteoconduction 548
Osteogenesis
  distraction 552
  imperfecta 498
Osteoid osteoma 522, 575, 585
Osteomalacia 133, 600
Osteomyelitis 521, 522, 524, 525,
  534*t*, 646
  acute 534
  affecting 534
  spread of 529*f*
Osteonecrosis 7, 65, 78, 79, 81, 522
  causes of 79, 80
Osteopenia 65, 65*f*
Osteophytes 214
Osteoporosis 65, 133, 141
Osteosarcoma 522
  multicentric 585
  secondary 585
  variants 585
Osteotomy 60, 66, 70, 71, 87, 88, 123,
  124, 173, 174, 342, 343, 356
  angulation 70
  barrel-vault 173
  closing-wedge 172*f*, 173
  complications of 344
  disadvantages of 124

Index

lineal 70
role of 69, 87
step-cut 343*f*
timing of 439
unstable 124
Oxoferin 619

P

Paget's disease 78, 464, 522, 600
Pain 7, 143, 212, 279, 305, 358, 444, 463
   causes of 481
      sudden onset of 187
   mediation of 482
Painless exostosis 187
Palate, arch of 9
Paley's classification 541, 541*f*
Palmar arch 386
Palmar aspect 362
Palmaris longus 405
Palms 361
Palpate pulses 283
Palpation 10, 362
   superficial 306
Pantalar arthrodesis 263
Papineau open bone grafting 549
Paradiskal involvement 464
Paraffin gauge 618
Parallel speculated reaction 578
Paralytic curve 503
Paralytic hip instability 125
Paralytic polio 190
   knee 195
Paralytic poliomyelitis 191
Paralytic talipes cavovarus 265
Paraplegia 480
   causes of 470
   grades of 469
   stage of 469
Paravertebral spasm 463
Parkinson's disease 600
Particle swarm optimization, types of 61
Passive extension test 150

Passive rotation test 285
Patella
   apparatus 146, 147
   chronic dislocation of 179
   faces 13
   habitual dislocation of 179, 181
   persistent dislocation of 155
   recurrent dislocation of 154
   restraints for 157
   subluxation of 156
Patellar aplasia 179
Patellar height 161
Patellar instability 160
Patellar position 601
Patellar rotation 601
Patellar shift 148*f*
Patellar tendinitis 146
Patellofemoral adhesions 530
Patellofemoral ligament, medial 148*f*
Path regimen, middle 470
Patrick's test 23, 23*f*
Pauwels' classification 71
Pauwels' osteotomy 71, 71*f*, 88
Pavlik harness
   contraindications of 121
   role of 121
Peg cups 629
Peg-leg gait 605
Pelvic support osteotomy, role of 61, 110
Pelvic tilt 600
Pelvis 30
   anteroposterior
      radiograph of 65*f*
      view of 640*f*
   bony 640*f*
   movements of 35
   unsquared 19
Pemberton's osteotomy 124
   indications of 123
Pen test 394
Percutaneous automated discectomy 496
Percutaneous fasciotomy 412
Percutaneous nucleotomy 496

Periarticular ossification 318
Periosteal reaction 525
    solid 578
    types of 577, 577f
Periosteum 640
Peripheral disk herniation 484
Peripheral nerve
    injuries 369
    structure of 381
Perkin's quadrants 115, 116f
Permeative destruction 579
Peroneal nerve 396
    palsy, complete 275
Peroneal tendon instability test 221
Persistent infection 106
Perthes disease 39, 40, 44, 89, 89f, 90, 92, 95, 98
    late-onset 46
Petit's triangle 467
Phalanx, middle 415
Phalen test 366, 366f
    reverse 366
Phantom limb
    pain 572
    sensation 572
Phelp's test 21
Phemister bone grafting 549
Phemister grafting
    modified 549
    philosophy of 550
Phemister triad 61
Piano key test 367
Pinning fracture 336
Pirani score card 236f
Piriformis test 23
Pitres-Testut sign 390
Pitres-Testut test 390
Pivot shift test 151, 152, 309
    reverse 153
Plane instability, single 199
Plantar fascia 218
Plantar fat pad 218
Plantar flexion 267f
Plantar reflex 454, 458
Plaster of Paris 314

Plate fixation 547
Polio 251, 497, 600
    foot 251, 253
        Peabody's classification of 254
    infection, types of 190, 191t
    knee 189, 192
    virus, types of 190
Poliomyelitis 7
Pollock sign 390
Polymerase chain reaction 50
Polymerization, phases of 631
Polymethylmethacrylate 532
Poncet's disease 53
Ponseti corrective casts 231f
Ponseti protocol 232
Poor bone quality 141
Popliteal region 467
Porous-coated anatomic systems 628, 632
Port-wine patch 499
Posterior cruciate ligament 152, 203
    tear 204
Posterior drawer test 153
Posterolateral laxity 146
Postinjection nerve palsy 388
Postpolio residual paralysis 179, 190
Postprosthetic care 614
Post-traumatic elbow 635
Post-traumatic malunited supracondylar fracture 330
Pott's disease 463, 464
Pott's paraplegia 468, 471
    causes of 469
Pott's paresis 471
Pott's spine 468
Pouteau fracture 440
Preprosthetic care 570
Prescapular abscess 281
Press test 368
Pressure
    intramedullary 83
    sore, grades of 620
Prominent humeral head, causes of 304
Prominent ulnar head 359

Index

Propulsion 601
Prosthesis 608
    immediate postoperative 613
    type of 609
    warming of 632
Prosthetic fitting, timing of 570
Protrusio acetabuli 49, 76
Protrusion acetabulum 77*f*
Provocative tests 285
Proximal femoral osteomyelitis 46
Proximal femur
    extracapsular fracture of 134
    intracapsular fracture of 134
Proximal interphalangeal joint 359
    hyperflexion of 258
Pseudarthrosis 541, 561
Pseudo valgum 175
Pseudo varum 175
Pseudoarthrosis 537, 538
Pseudocoxalgia 90
Pseudocubitus varus deformity 344
Pseudo-osteitis 522
Psoas abscess 9, 42, 467
Psoriatic arthropathy 9
Pubic tubercle 26
Pulsed lavage 531
Pylon prosthesis 570
Pyogenic arthritis 281
Pyogenic sinus 521

Q

Q-angle 154, 158, 159*f*
Quadriceps contracture 176, 178, 179, 530
Quadriceps gait 603
Quadriceps hypoplasia, congenital 179
Quadriceps paralysis 193
Quadriceps tethering 530
Quadriceps wasting 153
Quadriga effect 423
Quadruple deformity complex 207
Quorum sensing 533

R

Radial aspect 361, 363
Radial head 312
    dislocation
        congenital 352, 353*t*
        traumatic isolated 352, 353*t*
    fracture 348
    open reduction of 356
    recurrent dislocation of 328
Radial height, correction of 438*f*
Radial nerve 369-371, 378*f*, 384
    autonomous zones of 384
    injury, tendons transfers for 375
    palsy 372, 378
Radial osteotomy, contraindications of 439
Radial pulse disappears during plastering 336
Radial reflex, inverted 459, 460*f*
Radiation 80, 445
    therapy 320
Radical excision 582
Radiotherapy, role of 583
Reaction hand 400
Reconstruct annular ligament 356
Reconstruction surgeries, indications of 98
Reconstructive method 387
Rectus femoris 178
Rectus phenomenon 21
Recurrent clubfoot 239
Recurrent herniations 497
Recurrent patellar dislocation 157
Recurrent radial head instability 328
Recurrent shoulder instability, development of 295
Red flag signs 486, 491
Reeling gait 605
Reflex 459, 462
    sympathetic dystrophy 530, 644
Regional lymph nodes 576
Relapsed clubfoot 239
Relaxing gracilis 21
Relocation test 286, 286*f*
Renal function test 526

Resection arthroplasty 627
    Girdlestone type of 66
Resistant clubfoot 239
Rest and poultice method 530
Retrocalcaneal bursa 216
Retropulsion sign 477
Rheobase 384, 385*f*
Rheumatoid 145
    arthritis 7, 600
Rib vertebra angle
    difference 505*f*
    distance 511
Rice bodies 53
Rickets 464, 600
    signs of 168, 169
Rickettsial infection 91
Right femur, old fracture head of 63
Rigid clubfoot 229*f*
Rigid curve 498
Risser sign 511, 511*f*
Roll test 11
Rolling walkers 607
Rolling-pin test 310
Roos test 289
Rotation, hinge of 124
Rotational deformities 311
Rotational movements 12
Rotator cuff 300
    pathology 283
Rotatory tests 200
Russian march gait 603
Ryder method 149

S

Sacroilitis, bilateral 43
Salmonella typhi 464
Salter's innominate osteotomy 97
Salter's osteotomy 97, 124
    advantages of 98
    indications of 123
Salter's procedure 99
Salvage procedures 413
Saphena varix 8
Satellite lesions 583
Saucerization 531

Sauve-Kapandji procedure 439*f*
Scaphoid shift test of Watson 367
Scaphoid tuberosity 360*f*
Scapular protraction 282
Scapular retraction 282
Scarpa's triangle 10, 27, 42, 62, 467
    contents of 28
Scars 10, 146
Scheuermann's disease 447, 464
Schmidt technique 105
Schmorl's disease 464
Schober's test 25
    modified 452
Sciatic nerve injury 128
Sciatic stretch test 488
Sciatica 483
Scissors gait 603, 604*f*
Sclerosing nonsuppurative
                    osteomyelitis of Garre 536
Sclerotic margin 579
Scoliosis 446*f*, 450, 464, 497, 500
    congenital 499, 517, 519
    idiopathic 512, 513, 514*t*, 515
    infantile 513
    juvenile 513
    surgical treatment of 518
Sectoral sign 24
Seddon's classification 382, 469
Seddon's ellipsoid 589
Sensation testing 365
Sensory deficit 373
Sensory examinations 453
Sensory motor examination 456*t*
Sensory nerves 365*f*
Septic arthritis 114, 529*f*
    hip joint 106
    late sequelae of 105, 107
    sequel of 105
    subacute 45
Sequestra, types of 523
Sequestrum dense 523
Shanmugasundaram classification 49
Shanmugasundaram test, positive 303
Shell formation 577
Shilla 519
    procedure 519

Index

Shoe, examination of 214f
Shoemaker's lines 20, 21f
Shoulder 279
    anterior dislocation of 280
    arthrodesis 293
    arthroplasty 626, 636, 638
        indications of 636
        limitations of 638
        reverse total 636
        total 636, 637
    case, examination points for 279
    functional position of 293
    instability 294
        tests for 285
    joint, tuberculosis of 291
    Lachman test 287
    position 600
    posterior dislocation of 280
    prosthesis, total 637
    replacements, total 636
    restraints for 295, 296t
    unstable 294, 298
Silfverskiold test, reverse 269
Silliman and Hawkins
    augmentation test of 286
    release test of 286
Sinding-Larsen-Johansson
    syndrome 146
Single bundle techniques 202
Sinogram 529f
Sinus 10, 146, 520, 530
Six-strand techniques 419
Skew foot 239
Skin 146
    condition of 214
    dimples 499
    lesions 395
    tests 50
Skip lesions 465
Skull deformities 499
Slap lesion, tests for 289
Slew-footed gait 146
Sliding hip screw system 135
Slipped capital femoral
    epiphysis 7, 102
Slipped upper femoral epiphysis 102
Slocum's test 153
Slow union 538
Slump test 456
Smith fracture 440
Smith-Goyrand fracture 440
Smith-Petersen nail plate 140
Smooth shells 578
Socket
    material of 609
    type of 609
Sofield Miller's double
    distal osteotomy 563
    proximal osteotomy 563
Soft tissue 452, 520, 640
    nearby 521
    release 126, 237, 317
        posteromedial 237
    surgery 250
    tumor 584
        malignant 584
Solid-ankle cushioned heel foot 611,
    611t, 612
Solitary exostosis 182f
Solitary osteochondroma 185
Soltanpur method 344
Sonogram, role of 529
Speed test 289, 290f
Sphygmomanometer test 268
Spina bifida occulta 497
Spina ventosa 314
Spinal brace 192
Spinal cord injury 460
Spinal elements, posterior 585
Spinal fusion 494
Spinal level, localization of 456t
Spinal pathology 499
Spinal polio 191
Spinal tubercular infection 475
Spinal tuberculosis 463, 467
    adult 465
    apophyseal 465
    childhood 465
    prevent deformity in 480
    types of collapse in 466

Spinal tumor
  common anterior 585
  syndrome 465
Spine 30, 444, 477
  actinomycosis of 464
  deformity of 446f
  examination of 444
  lateral bending of 450f, 502f
  stiffness of 463
  types of 464
Splint, internal 377
Spondylolisthesis 449f
Spondylolysis 456
Spondylosis, ankylosing 11
Sprengel shoulder 281, 303
Spring plate 622
Spurious correction 235
Spurling's maneuver 454
Square pelvis 29, 34
  fallacies of 29
Squeezing calf 459
Squeezing heel cord 459
Stability, tests for 21, 150, 151t
Stainless steel, femoral head of 626
Standard cement, components of 631
Stasis ulcer 407
Steindler's fasciotomy 261
Stiff elbow 314, 315
  causes of 315
Stiff hip gait 603
Stiff knee gait 146, 603
Stiff nonunions, short 552
Stiffness 7
Stiles-Bunnel FF4T phasic transfer,
  modified 405
Stinchfield's test 21, 72
Stir-fry test 310
Straight leg raising test 455f
Strength duration curve 384
Streptococcus epidermidis 533
Stress fracture 522
Stress testing, significance of
  endpoint in 197
Stroking lateral malleolus 459
Structural scoliosis 503

Strut graft 474
Subligamentous extrusion 482f
Sublimis transfer 405
Subluxation test, posterior 288
Subscapularis 300
  Liftoff test 284
Subsynovial intra-articular arterial
  ring 76
Subtalar joint 219
Sugioka's anterior rotational
  osteotomy 87
Sulcus sign 288, 288f
Superficialis finger 421
Superficialis transfer 376
Supracondylar fracture 332-334,
  339, 339t
  acute 335
  complications of 334
  displacements of 333
  management of 337
  of elbow, types of 335f
Supracondylar ridges 306
Supraspinatus 300
Suprasternal notch 28
Sural cutaneous nerve 396
Sural insufficiency, triceps 240, 255
Surgery 180
  complications of 413, 596
  indications of 54, 320, 471
  prerequisites of 527
  role of 54
Surgical hardware 521
Suture techniques 418
Swelling 8, 143, 146, 183, 212, 217, 280,
  305, 358, 499, 574
  benign 573
  bony 575
  examination of 572
Swing phase 601
Swing through gait 606, 607
Swing to gait 606
Swollen hot foot 407
Symphysis pubis 28
Synergism 374
Synergistic muscles 382

Index

Synovial biopsy 209
Synovial sarcoma 585
Systemic lupus erythematosus 9

T

Tabes dorsalis 600
Talipes equinovarus 212, 264
    congenital 212
    idiopathic congenital 226
Talonavicular capsule 250
Talus, defective cartilage enlarge of 227
Tardy median palsy 425
Tardy ulnar nerve palsy
    causes of 349
    develop of 349
Tarsal joint, mid 248*f*
Tarsal tunnel syndrome, anterior 276
Tear, acute 273
Teardrop 115
    boundaries of 117
Telescoping hip, causes of 39
Telescopy 39
    prerequisites for 39
    test 72
Temporary pylon prosthesis 609
Tenderness over sacroiliac joint 10
Tenderness, bony 520
Tendo-Achilles 270
    discontinuity 268
    rupture 266, 266*f*
Tendon 218
    grafting and rationale,
        two-stage 420
    injury 414, 420
    repair of 273, 419*f*
        postoperative rehabilitation
            of 423
    rupture 272
    transfer 375, 385, 405
        prerequisites for 373, 406
        role of 240
Tennis leg 269
Tension 379
    band 621
Teratologic dislocation of hip 114
Teres minor 285, 300
Thick plastic socket 626
Thigh
    foot angle test 158*f*
    girth, measurement of 18*f*
    posterior aspect of 467
Thomas test 11, 12*f*, 16, 32, 32*f*
    causes of false positive 34
    principle behind 34
Thompson and Epstein
        classification 129
Thompson test 267*f*
    fallacies of 269
Thompson-Simmonds calf
        squeeze test 267
Thompson-Simmonds-Doherty
        test 268
Thomson's test 221
Thoracic disease, early 464
Thoracic outlet syndrome, tests for 289
Thoracic region 473
Three-layer dressing 620
Thrust tenderness 451
Thumb
    adduction 386, 387, 586
    and first MCP joint 361
    flexed 586
    function 405
    index finger 386
    movements 363
    opposition of 385, 387
Thyroid swelling 9
Tibia
    congenital pseudarthrosis of 559*f*,
        561, 562*t*
    fracture of 555, 600
        shaft of 543
    non-union, radiograph of 545*f*
    over femoral condyles, external
        rotation of 207
    posterolateral subluxation of 207
    pseudarthrosis of 559, 561
    rotations of 198
    vara 175

Tibial length 153
Tibial nerve, posterior 396
Tibial nonunion 541
Tibial position 601
Tibial rotation 601
Tibial tendon transfer, anterior 240
Tibial torsion 154, 600
    clinically 157
Tibialis transfer, split anterior 240
Tibiofemoral adhesions 530
Tinel sign 383
Tinel test 426
Tip pinch 386
Tip-apex distance 137f
Tissue injury, sequence of 325
Toe 214
    flexion 458
    position 601
    systolic blood pressure 566
Tom-Smith arthritis 105
Topographic sensitivity 382
Topple sign 477
Torticollis 594
    causes of 595
Total active elevation 282
Total hip
    arthroplasty, indications of 634
    replacement, complications of 634
Total knee
    arthroplasty, role of 211
    replacement, role of 195
Tourniquet test 366, 427
Toygar sign 271f
Traction, role of 53, 210, 337
Transcutaneous electrical nerve stimulation 492
Transferred tendon, amplitude of 374
Transforaminal lumbar interbody fusion 496
Transinterosseous membrane 406
Transverse defects 499
Trapdoor procedure 86
Trapeziometacarpal joint 369
Trauma 80, 446, 522

Trendelenburg test, positive 37, 38
Trendelenburg's gait 602
Trendelenburg's sign 39
Trendelenburg's test 36, 37f, 38
Trevor's disease 185
Triangular fibrocartilage complex test 368
Trillat modification 151
Tripod sign 21
Triradiate cartilage 512
Trochanter over Nelaton's line 112f
Trochanter shortening, upriding of 112f
Trochanteric arthroplasty
    limitation of 110
    principles of 110
Trochlear depth 161f
Tromner sign 459
Trophic ulcer 407
Trough sign 295
Trueta hypothesis 91
Tuber sulcus angle 154
Tubercular rheumatism 53
Tubercular sinus 521
Tubercular spondylitis, clinicoradiological classification of 468
Tuberculosis 7
    diagnosis of 291
    hip 47, 58, 208
        clinicoradiological types of 49f
        radiological signs of 50
    knee 208, 210
        joint 209
        pathological stages of 208
    shoulder 291
    spine, radiology of 467f
Tumor 146, 522
    primary 576
Two-strand techniques 418

U

Ulcer 616
    pathological 616

Index

Ulnar aspect 362
Ulnar bow 355
Ulnar claw hand 359
Ulnar deviation of hand 359
Ulnar nerve 369, 371, 384, 387, 390, 393, 396
    anomalous innervations for 390
    autonomous zones of 384
    palsy 349, 385, 387
        tests for 389
    protect 336
    transposition 351
    zones of 391f
Ulnar osteotomy, indications of 356
Ulnar paradox 386
Ultrasonogram 117t
Ultrasonography 93
    role of 117
Umbilicus 28
Unconstrained prosthesis 635
    prerequisites for 635
Unilateral deformity, causes of 167
University of Pennsylvania Classification 82t
Unstable fracture, stabilize 140
Upper dorsal spine, tuberculosis of 304
Upper extremity, bony landmarks for 307f
Upper limb 192, 372f
    prostheses available 612
    tension test 454
    units 613
Upper trunk, branches of 392

V

Vacuum mixing and centrifugation, effects of 632
Vacuum phenomenon 491
Valgus and varus
    laxity 150
    stress test 150
Valgus at knee 154
Valgus extension osteotomy 87
Valgus flexion osteotomy 88
Valgus overcorrection 239
Valgus stress test 153f, 309
Valgus thrust
    gait 146
    with circumduction 146
Valsalva maneuver 456
Varus angulation 65
Varus at knee 154
Varus derotation osteotomy, advantages of 98
Varus recurvatum
    test 153
    thrust 146
Varus stress 220
    test 153f, 309
Varus thrust gait 146
Vascular theory 227
Vastus intermedius 178
Vastus lateralis/intermedius, contracture of 178
Vaughan-Jackson lesion 359
Venus, dimple of 10
Vertebra
    apical 506
    measure rotation of 509
    posterior elements of 575
Vertebral body 575
Vibrio cholerae pyogenic diskitis 464
Volar aspect 361
Volar Barton fracture 440
Volar sensations 386
Volkmann's ischemic contracture 586, 587
Volkmann's sign 404, 587, 587f
    pathogenesis of 588
    positive 586
von Recklinghausen's disease 497

W

Waddling gait 602, 603
Walenkamp phenomenon 521
Walker
    advantages of 607
    types of 607

Wallerian degeneration 381
Wandering acetabulum 63
Ward's triangle 62
Wartenberg sign 389
Watson scaphoid shift test 368*f*
Wearing brace, schedule of 245
Weatherwax modification 197*f*
Weber and Cech classification 540*f*
    basis of 541
Weight-bearing caliper 192
Wet dressing 617
White blood cells 528
Whittle and Evans protractor
    method 508
Windswept deformity 145
Wound 615-617
    classification of 617*t*
    coverage 615
    excision 531
    infection 615
    management, principle of 617
Wright's maneuver 289
Wringing test 309

Wrist 361
    and hand 358
        case, examination points for
            358
    extension test 427
        resisted 309
    flexion 366, 386, 586
    motion 363

X

Xiphisternum 26, 28
Xiphoid process 26
X-ray reading, steps of 639

Y

Yeoman's test 21
    for sacroiliitis 23
Yergason test 289

Z

Ziehl-Neelsen stains 409
Zinc impregnated gauge 618

EU GSPR Authorised Reprsentative
Logos Europe, 9 rue Nicolas Poussin
1700, La Rochelle, France
Phone: +33 (0) 6 67 93 73 78
E-mail: contact@logoseurope.eu

www.ingramcontent.com/pod-product-compliance
Ingram Content Group UK Ltd.
Pitfield, Milton Keynes, MK11 3LW, UK
UKHW021257180426
11947UKWH00015B/884

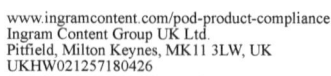